Neonatology Questions and Controversies

Neonatology Questions and Controversies

Series Editor

Richard A. Polin, MD
William T. Speck Professor of Pediatrics
College of Physicians and Surgeons
Columbia University;
Director Division of Neonatology
New York Presbyterian
Morgan Stanley Children's Hospital
New York, New York

Other Volumes in the Neonatology Questions and Controversies Series

GASTROENTEROLOGY AND NUTRITION

HEMATOLOGY, IMMUNOLOGY AND GENETICS

HEMODYNAMICS AND CARDIOLOGY

INFECTIOUS DISEASE AND PHARMACOLOGY

NEPHROLOGY AND FLUID/ELECTROLYTE PHYSIOLOGY

NEUROLOGY

Neonatology Questions and Controversies

Third Edition

Editor

Eduardo Bancalari, MD

Professor of Pediatrics, Obstetrics and Gynecology
Department of Pediatrics
University of Miami
Miller School of Medicine
Miami, Florida

Co-Editors

Martin Keszler, MD

Professor of Pediatrics
Warren Alpert Medical School of
  Brown University;
Director of Respiratory Services
Department of Pediatrics
Women and Infants Hospital
Providence, Rhode Island

Peter G. Davis, MBBS, MD, FRACP

Professor/Director
Newborn Research Centre
The Royal Women's Hospital;
Department of Obstetrics and Gynaecology
The University of Melbourne;
Department of Neonatology
The Royal Women's Hospital University of Melbourne
Melbourne, Victoria, Australia

Consulting Editor

Richard A. Polin, MD

William T. Speck Professor of Pediatrics
College of Physicians and Surgeons
Columbia University;
Director Division of Neonatology
New York Presbyterian
Morgan Stanley Children's Hospital
New York, New York

ELSEVIER

ELSEVIER

1600 John F. Kennedy Blvd.
Ste 1800
Philadelphia, PA 19103-2899

THE NEWBORN LUNG: NEONATOLOGY QUESTIONS AND
CONTROVERSIES, THIRD EDITION

ISBN: 978-0-323-54605-8

Notices

Knowledge and best practice in this field are constantly changing. As new research and experience broaden our understanding, changes in research methods, professional practices, or medical treatment may become necessary.

Practitioners and researchers must always rely on their own experience and knowledge in evaluating and using any information, methods, compounds, or experiments described herein. In using such information or methods they should be mindful of their own safety and the safety of others, including parties for whom they have a professional responsibility.

With respect to any drug or pharmaceutical products identified, readers are advised to check the most current information provided (i) on procedures featured or (ii) by the manufacturer of each product to be administered, to verify the recommended dose or formula, the method and duration of administration, and contraindications. It is the responsibility of practitioners, relying on their own experience and knowledge of their patients, to make diagnoses, to determine dosages and the best treatment for each individual patient, and to take all appropriate safety precautions.

To the fullest extent of the law, neither the Publisher nor the authors, contributors, or editors, assume any liability for any injury and/or damage to persons or property as a matter of products liability, negligence or otherwise, or from any use or operation of any methods, products, instructions, or ideas contained in the material herein.

Previous editions copyrighted 2012 and 2008.

Library of Congress Cataloging-in-Publication Data
Names: Bancalari, Eduardo, editor. | Polin, Richard A. (Richard Alan),
1945-editor.
Title: The newborn lung : neonatology questions and controversies / [edited
   by] Eduardo Bancalari ; consulting editor, Richard A. Polin.
Other titles: Neonatology questions and controversies.
Description: Third edition. | Philadelphia, PA: Elsevier, [2019] | Series:
   Neonatology questions and controversies | Includes bibliographical
   references and index.
Identifiers: LCCN 2018013382 | ISBN 9780323546058 (hardcover : alk. paper)
Subjects: | MESH: Infant, Newborn, Diseases | Lung Diseases | Infant, Newborn
   | Lung--growth & development | Respiration Disorders
Classification: LCC RJ312 | NLM WS 421 | DDC 618.92/2--dc23 LC record available at
https://lccn.loc.gov/2018013382

Content Strategist: Sarah Barth
Content Development Specialist: Lisa M. Barnes
Publishing Services Manager: Julie Eddy
Senior Project Manager: Rachel E. McMullen
Design Direction: Paula Catalano

Printed in China

Last digit is the print number: 9   8   7   6   5   4   3   2   1

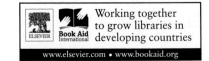

Working together
to grow libraries in
developing countries

www.elsevier.com • www.bookaid.org

Contributors

Steven H. Abman, MD
Professor
Department of Pediatrics
University of Colorado Health Sciences
    Center;
Director
Pediatric Heart Lung Center
The Children's Hospital
Aurora, Colorado
    *A Physiology-Based Approach to the
    Respiratory Care of Children With
    Severe Bronchopulmonary Dysplasia*

Namasivayam Ambalavanan, MD
Professor
Department of Pediatrics
University of Alabama at Birmingham
Birmingham, Alabama
    *The "-Omics" of the New
    Bronchopulmonary Dysplasia; Role of
    Microbiome in Lung Injury*

Lisa M. Askie, PhD
Director, Systematic Reviews & Health
    Technology Assessment
NHMRC Clinical Trials Centre
Sydney Medical School
University of Sydney
Camperdown, New South Wales,
    Australia
    *Optimal Oxygenation in Extremely
    Preterm Infants*

Eduardo Bancalari, MD
Professor of Pediatrics, Obstetrics and
    Gynecology
Department of Pediatrics
University of Miami
Miller School of Medicine
Miami, Florida
    *Definitions and Diagnostic Criteria of
    Bronchopulmonary Dysplasia: Clini-
    cal and Research Implications; Patent
    Ductus Arteriosus and the Lung: Acute
    Effects and Long-Term Consequences;
    Oxygenation Instability in the Premature
    Infant; Patient-Ventilator Interaction;
    Automation of Respiratory Support*

Vineet Bhandari, MBBS, MD, DM
Section Chief & Professor
Department of Neonatology (Pediatrics)
St. Christopher's Hospital for Children/
    Drexel University
Philadelphia, Pennsylvania
    *The "-Omics" of the New Bronchopul-
    monary Dysplasia*

Waldemar A. Carlo, MD
Edwin M. Dixon Professor of Pediatrics,
Director
Division of Neonatology
University of Alabama at Birmingham
Birmingham, Alabama
    *Optimal Oxygenation in Extremely
    Preterm Infants*

Jeanie L.Y. Cheong, MD
Consultant Neonatologist
Department of Neonatal Services
Royal Women's Hospital;
Associate Professor
Department of Obstetrics & Gynaecology
University of Melbourne;
Principal Research Fellow
Department of Clinical Sciences
Murdoch Childrens Research Institute
Melbourne, Victoria, Australia
Long-Term Pulmonary Outcome of Preterm Infants

Nelson Claure, MSc, PhD
Research Associate Professor of Pediatrics and Biomedical Engineering
Division of Neonatology
University of Miami
Miami, Florida
Definitions and Diagnostic Criteria of Bronchopulmonary Dysplasia: Clinical and Research Implications; Patent Ductus Arteriosus and the Lung: Acute Effects and Long-Term Consequences; Oxygenation Instability in the Premature Infant; Patient-Ventilator Interaction; Ventilator Strategies to Reduce Lung Injury and Duration of Mechanical Ventilation; Automation of Respiratory Support

Peter A. Dargaville, MBBS, FRACP, MD
Professorial Research Fellow in Neonatology
Menzies Institute for Medical Research
University of Tasmania;
Staff Specialist
Neonatal and Paediatric Intensive Care Unit
Royal Hobart Hospital
Hobart, Tasmania, Australia
Newer Strategies for Surfactant Delivery

Peter G. Davis, MBBS, MD, FRACP
Professor/Director
Newborn Research Centre
The Royal Women's Hospital;
Department of Obstetrics and Gynaecology
The University of Melbourne;
Department of Neonatology
The Royal Women's Hospital University of Melbourne
Melbourne, Victoria, Australia
Respiratory and Cardiovascular Support in the Delivery Room; Noninvasive Ventilation of Preterm Infants: An Alternative to Mechanical Ventilation

Juliann M. Di Fiore, BSEE
Research Engineer
Department of Pediatrics
Case Western Reserve University;
Division of Neonatology
Rainbow Babies & Children's Hospital
Cleveland, Ohio
Respiratory Control and Apnea in Premature Infants; Oxygenation Instability in the Premature Infant

Lex W. Doyle, MD, MSc
Associate Director of Research
Research Office
The Royal Women's Hospital;
Professor of Neonatal Paediatrics
Obstetrics and Gynaecology
The University of Melbourne;
Honorary Fellow
Critical Care and Neurosciences
Murdoch Children's Research Institute
Parkville, Victoria, Australia
Long-Term Pulmonary Outcome of Preterm Infants

Stuart B. Hooper, BSc (Hons), PhD
Professor
The Ritchie Centre
Hudson Institute for Medical Research, Monash University;
Professor
Department of Obstetrics and Gynaecology
Monash University
Melbourne, Victoria, Australia
Respiratory and Cardiovascular Support in the Delivery Room

Thomas A. Hooven, MD
Division of Neonatal-Perinatal Medicine
Vagelos College of Physicians and Surgeons
Columbia University
New York, NY
Ventilator-Associated Pneumonia

Alan H. Jobe, MD, PhD
Perinatal Institute
Division of Neonatology
Perinatal and Pulmonary Biology
Cincinnati Children's Hospital Medical Center
University of Cincinnati
Cincinnati, Ohio
Perinatal Events and Their Influence on Lung Development and Injury; Definitions and Diagnostic Criteria of Bronchopulmonary Dysplasia: Clinical and Research Implications; Prenatal and Postnatal Steroids and Pulmonary Outcomes

Suhas G. Kallapur, MD
Professor of Pediatrics
Department of Pediatrics
David Geffen School of Medicine
University of California Los Angeles
Los Angeles, California
    *Perinatal Events and Their Influence on
    Lung Development and Injury*

Martin Keszler, MD
Professor of Pediatrics
Warren Alpert Medical School of Brown
    University;
Director of Respiratory Services
Department of Pediatrics
Women and Infants Hospital
Providence, Rhode Island
    *Patient-Ventilator Interaction; Ventilator
    Strategies to Reduce Lung Injury and
    Duration of Mechanical Ventilation;
    Automation of Respiratory Support*

Martin Kluckow, MBBS, FRACP, PhD
Professor
Department of Neonatology
University of Sydney;
Senior Staff Specialist
Department of Neonatology
Royal North Shore Hospital
Sydney, Australia
    *Patent Ductus Arteriosus and the Lung:
    Acute Effects and Long-Term Conse-
    quences; Pulmonary-Cardiovascular
    Interaction*

Charitharth Vivek Lal, MD
Assistant Professor
Department of Pediatrics
University of Alabama at Birmingham
Birmingham, Alabama
    *The "-Omics" of the New
    Bronchopulmonary Dysplasia*

Matthew M. Laughon, MD, MPH
Neonatologist,
Professor
University of North Carolina at
    Chapel Hill
Chapel Hill, North Carolina
    *Definitions and Diagnostic Criteria of
    Bronchopulmonary Dysplasia: Clinical
    and Research Implications*

Brett J. Manley, MBBS, PhD
Consultant Neonatologist
Newborn Research Centre
The Royal Women's Hospital
Senior Lecturer
Department of Obstetrics and
    Gynaecology
The University of Melbourne
Melbourne, Victoria, Australia
    *Noninvasive Ventilation of Preterm
    Infants: An Alternative to Mechanical
    Ventilation*

Richard J. Martin, MD
Professor
Department of Pediatrics, Reproductive
    Biology, and Physiology & Biophysics
Case Western Reserve University School
    of Medicine
Cleveland, Ohio
    *Respiratory Control and Apnea in
    Premature Infants; Oxygenation Insta-
    bility in the Premature Infant*

Leif D. Nelin, MD
Director
Center for Perinatal Research
Research Institute at Nationwide
    Children's Hospital;
Professor
Department of Pediatrics
The Ohio State University
Columbus, Ohio
    *A Physiology-Based Approach to the
    Respiratory Care of Children With
    Severe Bronchopulmonary Dysplasia*

Shahab Noori, MD, MS CBTI, RDCS
Associate Professor of Pediatrics
Fetal and Neonatal Institute
Division of Neonatology
Department of Pediatrics
Children's Hospital Los Angeles
Keck School of Medicine, USC
Los Angeles California
    Pulmonary-Cardiovascular Interaction

Howard B. Panitch, MD
Director of Clinical Programs
Division of Pulmonary Medicine
The Children's Hospital of Philadelphia;
Professor of Pediatrics
Perelman School of Medicine
University of Pennsylvania
Philadelphia, Pennsylvania
    *A Physiology-Based Approach to the
    Respiratory Care of Children With
    Severe Bronchopulmonary Dysplasia*

Won Soon Park, MD
Department of Pediatrics
Sungkyunkwan University School of
    Medicine
Seoul, Korea
    *Cell-Based Therapy for Neonatal Lung
    Diseases*

Richard A. Polin, MD
Director Division of Neonatology
Department of Pediatrics
Morgan Stanley Children's Hospital
William T. Speck Professor of Pediatrics;
Department of Pediatrics
Vagelos College of Physicians and
    Surgeons
Columbia University
New York, New York
    Ventilator-Associated Pneumonia

Rashmin C. Savani, MBChB
Chief, Neonatal-Perinatal Medicine
Professor of Pediatrics
UT Southwestern Medical Center
Dallas, Texas
    *Molecular Bases for Lung Development,
    Injury, and Repair*

Vidhi P. Shah, MD
Department of Pediatrics
Rainbow Babies & Children's Hospital
Case Western Reserve University School
    of Medicine
Cleveland, Ohio
    *Respiratory Control and Apnea in Pre-
    mature Infants*

Ilene R.S. Sosenko, MD
Professor of Pediatrics
Department of Pediatrics
University of Miami
Miami, Florida
    *Patent Ductus Arteriosus and the
    Lung: Acute Effects and Long-Term
    Consequences*

Robin H. Steinhorn, MD
Senior Vice President
Children's National Health System;
Professor of Pediatrics
George Washington University
Washington, District of Columbia
    *Pulmonary Vascular Development and
    the Neonatal Circulation*

Bernard Thébaud, MD, PhD
Department of Pediatrics
University of Ottawa
Ottawa, Ontario, Canada
    *Cell-Based Therapy for Neonatal Lung
    Diseases*

Rose M. Viscardi, MD
Professor
Department of Pediatrics
University of Maryland School of
    Medicine
Baltimore, Maryland
    Role of Microbiome in Lung Injury

Gary M. Weiner, MD, FAAP
Associate Professor
Department of Pediatrics, Neonatal-
    Perinatal Medicine
University of Michigan
C.S. Mott Children's Hospital
Ann Arbor, Michigan
    *Respiratory and Cardiovascular
    Support in the Delivery Room*

Shu Wu, MD
Professor
Department of Pediatrics
University of Miami School of Medicine
Miami, Florida
    *Molecular Bases for Lung Development,
    Injury, and Repair*

Myra H. Wyckoff, MD
Professor
Department of Pediatrics, Neonatal-
    Perinatal Medicine
University of Texas Southwestern
    Medical Center
Dallas, Texas
    *Respiratory and Cardiovascular
    Support in the Delivery Room*

Bradley A. Yoder, MD
Professor
Department of Pediatrics
University of Utah School of Medicine
Salt Lake City, Utah
    *Noninvasive Ventilation of Preterm
    Infants: An Alternative to Mechanical
    Ventilation*

Karen C. Young, MD
Associate Professor
Department of Pediatrics
University of Miami
Miller School of Medicine
Miami, Florida
    *Cell-Based Therapy for Neonatal Lung
    Diseases*

Preface

We are very excited to introduce the Third Edition of *The Newborn Lung*.

Though gains in survival of extremely premature infants have slowed down in developing countries, there is an increasing awareness of the importance of reducing complications associated with intensive care and amelioration of the long-term consequences of preterm birth. Although we have witnessed important advances in the management of acute respiratory problems, some of the complications associated with neonatal respiratory support, such as pulmonary infections, bronchopulmonary dysplasia, and pulmonary hypertension, still occur at an unacceptably high rate.

The third edition of *The Newborn Lung* addresses many of the recent advances in the understanding of the mechanisms of normal and abnormal lung development and describes new strategies for the management of neonatal respiratory failure. The book emphasizes those areas where there have been major new developments in recent years. Several chapters deal with strategies that may reduce some of the chronic sequelae of neonatal respiratory failure.

Many of the leading clinicians and researchers in the specific areas have written these sections. We are certain that the reader will enjoy learning as much as we have from each of these chapters, and that the new knowledge will contribute to better neonatal outcomes in their units.

We are most grateful to all the authors who have contributed to this new edition of *The Newborn Lung*.

Peter G. Davis, MBBS, MD, FRACP
Martin Keszler, MD
Eduardo Bancalari, MD

Series Foreword

Richard A. Polin, MD

"To study the phenomena of disease without books is to sail an uncharted sea, while to study books without patients is not to go to sea at all."

—William Osler

Physicians in training generally rely on the spoken word and clinical experiences to bolster their medical knowledge. There is probably no better way to learn how to care for an infant than to receive teaching at the bedside. Of course, that assumes that the "clinician" doing the teaching is knowledgeable about the disease, wants to teach, and can teach effectively. For a student or intern, this style of learning is efficient because the clinical service demands preclude much time for other reading. Over the course of one's career, it becomes clear that this form of education has limitations because of the fairly limited number of disease conditions one encounters even in a lifetime of clinical rotations and the diminishing opportunities for teaching moments.

The next educational phase generally includes reading textbooks and qualitative review articles. Unfortunately, both of those sources are often outdated by the time they are published and represent one author's opinions about management. Systematic analyses (meta-analyses) can be more informative, but more often than not the conclusion of the systematic analysis is that "more studies are needed" to answer the clinical question. Furthermore, it has been estimated that if a subsequent large randomized clinical trial had not been performed, the meta-analysis would have reached an erroneous conclusion more than one-third of the time.

For practicing clinicians, clearly the best way to keep abreast of recent advances in a field is to read the medical literature on a regular basis. However, that approach is problematic given the multitude of journals, unless one reads only the two or three major pediatric journals published in the United States. That approach however, will miss many of the outstanding articles that appear in more general medical journals (e.g., *Journal of the American Medical Association, New England Journal of Medicine, Lancet,* and the *British Medical Journal*), subspecialty journals, and the many pediatric journals published in other countries.

Whereas there is no substitute to reading journal articles on a regular basis, the "Questions and Controversies" series of books provides an excellent alternative. This third edition of the series was developed to highlight the clinical problems of most concern to practitioners. The series has been increased from six to seven volumes and includes new sections on genetics and pharmacology. In total, there are 70 new chapters not included previously. The editors of each volume (Drs. Bancalari, Davis, Keszler, Oh, Baum, Seri, Kluckow, Ohls, Christensen, Maheshwari, Neu, Benitz, Smith, Poindexter, Cilio, and Perlman) have done an extraordinary job in selecting topics of clinical importance to everyday practice. Unlike traditional review articles, the chapters not only highlight the most significant controversies, but when possible, have incorporated basic science and physiological concepts with a rigorous analysis of the current literature.

As with the first edition, I am indebted to the exceptional group of editors who chose the content and edited each of the volumes. I also wish to thank Lisa Barnes (Content Development Specialist at Elsevier) and Judy Fletcher (VP, Content Development at Elsevier) who provided incredible assistance in bringing this project to fruition.

Contents

SECTION A

Lung Development and Injury

CHAPTER 1   Molecular Bases for Lung Development, Injury, and Repair   3
Shu Wu and Rashmin C. Savani

CHAPTER 2   Perinatal Events and Their Influence on Lung Development
and Injury   31
Suhas G. Kallapur and Alan H. Jobe

CHAPTER 3   Pulmonary Vascular Development and the Neonatal
Circulation   65
Robin H. Steinhorn

CHAPTER 4   The "-Omics" of the New Bronchopulmonary Dysplasia   87
Charitharth Vivek Lal, Namasivayam Ambalavanan, and
Vineet Bhandari

CHAPTER 5   Role of Microbiome in Lung Injury   97
Rose M. Viscardi and Namasivayam Ambalavanan

CHAPTER 6   Definitions and Diagnostic Criteria of Bronchopulmonary
Dysplasia: Clinical and Research Implications   115
Eduardo Bancalari, Nelson Claure, Alan H. Jobe, and Matthew M. Laughon

CHAPTER 7   Patent Ductus Arteriosus and the Lung: Acute Effects and
Long-Term Consequences   131
Martin Kluckow, Eduardo Bancalari, Ilene R.S. Sosenko, and
Nelson Claure

CHAPTER 8   Ventilator-Associated Pneumonia   147
Thomas A. Hooven and Richard A. Polin

CHAPTER 9   Long-Term Pulmonary Outcome of Preterm Infants   161
Jeanie L.Y. Cheong and Lex W. Doyle

SECTION B

Management of Respiratory Problems

CHAPTER 10   Respiratory and Cardiovascular Support in the Delivery Room   173
Gary M. Weiner, Stuart B. Hooper, Peter G. Davis, and Myra H. Wyckoff

CHAPTER 11   Noninvasive Ventilation of Preterm Infants: An Alternative to
Mechanical Ventilation   197
Brett J. Manley, Bradley A. Yoder, and Peter G. Davis

CHAPTER 12   Newer Strategies for Surfactant Delivery   221
Peter A. Dargaville

CHAPTER 13   Respiratory Control and Apnea in Premature Infants   239
Vidhi P. Shah, Juliann M. Di Fiore, and Richard J. Martin

CHAPTER 14   Oxygenation Instability in the Premature Infant   251
Nelson Claure, Richard J. Martin, Juliann M. Di Fiore, and
Eduardo Bancalari

CHAPTER 15   Optimal Oxygenation in Extremely Preterm Infants   261
Waldemar A. Carlo and Lisa M. Askie

CHAPTER 16   Patient-Ventilator Interaction   269
Nelson Claure, Martin Keszler, and Eduardo Bancalari

CHAPTER 17   Pulmonary-Cardiovascular Interaction   289
Shahab Noori and Martin Kluckow

CHAPTER 18   Ventilator Strategies to Reduce Lung Injury and Duration of
Mechanical Ventilation   307
Martin Keszler and Nelson Claure

CHAPTER 19   Automation of Respiratory Support   321
Nelson Claure, Martin Keszler, and Eduardo Bancalari

CHAPTER 20   Prenatal and Postnatal Steroids and Pulmonary Outcomes   335
Alan H. Jobe

CHAPTER 21   Cell-Based Therapy for Neonatal Lung Diseases   347
Karen C. Young, Bernard Thébaud, and Won Soon Park

CHAPTER 22   A Physiology-Based Approach to the Respiratory Care of Children
With Severe Bronchopulmonary Dysplasia   363
Leif D. Nelin, Steven H. Abman, and Howard B. Panitch

Corresponding color figures for select images are available on Expert Consult.

Lung Development and Injury

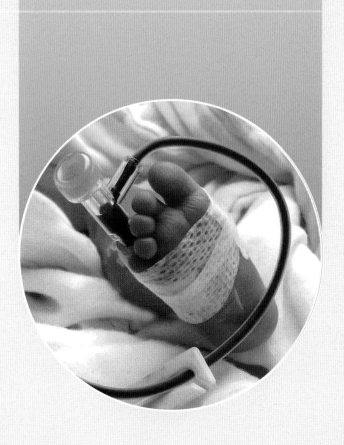

CHAPTER 1

Molecular Bases for Lung Development, Injury, and Repair

Shu Wu and Rashmin C. Savani

- Lung development involves lung bud initiation, branching morphogenesis, saccular formation, alveolar septation, and accompanying vascular development that begins in the embryonic period and continues through fetal and postnatal periods.

- These developmental processes are regulated by diverse crosstalk between the airway epithelium and surrounding mesenchyme, which are highly coordinated by localized expression of transcriptional factors, growth factors, and extracellular matrix.

- Temporospatially regulated specific cell differentiation, proliferation, and survival and extracellular matrix deposition give rise to the final complex lung structure.

- Bronchopulmonary dysplasia is a chronic lung disease of premature infants characterized by a developmental arrest of the immature lung caused by injurious stimuli such as mechanical ventilation, oxygen exposure, and intrauterine or postnatal infections.

- Animal studies suggest that dysregulation of key signaling pathways plays an important role in neonatal lung injury, repair and subsequent development of bronchopulmonary dysplasia.

The first breath taken by newborns after birth initiates the transition from fetal to neonatal life. Successful transition is dependent on the lung to transport oxygen from the atmosphere into the bloodstream and to release carbon dioxide from the bloodstream into the atmosphere. This exchange of gases takes place in the alveoli, the terminal units of the lung that consist of an epithelial layer surrounded by capillaries, and supported by extracellular matrix (ECM). The alveolocapillary barrier is thin and covers a large surface area to maximize gas exchange. The human lung achieves a final gas diffusion surface of 70 m^2 with 0.2 mm in thickness by young adulthood and is capable of supporting systemic oxygen consumption ranging between 250 mL/min at rest and 5500 mL/min during maximal exercise.[1-4] To facilitate the development of such a large, diffusible interface of the epithelial layer with the circulation, the embryonic lung undergoes branching morphogenesis to form a vast network of branched airways and subsequent formation and multiplication of alveoli by septation during the late stage of fetal lung development.[1] By the time the full-term infant is born there are about 50 million alveoli in the lungs that provide sufficient gas exchange to sustain extrauterine life.[4-6] Postnatally, alveoli continue to grow in size and number by septation to form approximately 300 million units in the adult lung.[4-6] A matching capillary network develops in close apposition to the alveolar surface beginning in the middle to late stage of fetal development and continuing through postnatal development, which in the adult can accommodate pulmonary blood flow rising from 4 L/min at rest to 40 L/min during maximal exercise.[1,3]

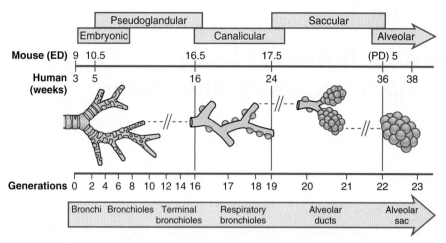

Fig. 1.1 **Phases of Human and Mouse Lung Development.** Human and mouse lung development follow the same phases—namely, embryonic, pseudoglandular, canalicular, saccular, and alveolar. Formation of the human lung bud occurs at 4 weeks of gestation, whereas mouse lung development begins at embryonic day *(ED)* 9. Trachea and major bronchi are formed by the end of the embryonic stage. The conducting airways are formed during the pseudoglandular stage up to the level of terminal bronchioles. Respiratory bronchioles are formed during the canalicular stage, whereas the alveolar ducts are formed during the saccular stage. Alveolarization in humans begins at around 34 weeks and continues at least through the first few years of childhood. Alveolarization in mouse begins in postnatal day *(PD)* 3 and continues for about 4 weeks.

Our understanding of basic lung developmental processes has been improved through extensive studies in mouse molecular genetics and genomics. It is well recognized that these developmental processes are regulated by diverse crosstalk between the airway epithelium and surrounding mesenchyme, which are highly coordinated by transcriptional factors, growth factors and ECM residing in the lung microenvironment. Specific temporospatial cell proliferation, differentiation, migration, and apoptosis orchestrated by this interplay give rise to the complex lung structure that prepares for the first breath. Genetic mutations, physical forces, intrauterine infection, and particularly premature birth, can disrupt these developmental processes, thus resulting in defective lung development that can lead to respiratory failure and death.

Bronchopulmonary dysplasia (BPD) is a chronic lung disease of premature infants characterized by a developmental arrest of the immature lung caused by injurious stimuli such as mechanical ventilation, oxygen exposure, and intrauterine or postnatal infections.[7] Data from animal studies suggest that dysregulation of key signaling pathways plays an important role in neonatal lung injury, repair, and subsequent development of BPD. Therefore basic knowledge about lung developmental processes and their cellular and molecular regulatory mechanisms is essential to understand lung injury and repair. This may lead to novel strategies to prevent and manage neonatal lung diseases, particularly BPD.

This chapter provides a brief overview of normal lung developmental processes, the key signaling pathways and proposed models of regulation of lung budding, branching morphogenesis, alveolarization, and vascular development. It also describes how injury from mechanical ventilation and oxygen exposure modulates key pathways, thus affecting neonatal lung development in the context of prematurity.

Overview of Lung Developmental Stages

Human lung development begins with the formation of airway primordia from the embryonic foregut that subsequently undergoes branching morphogenesis to form the conducting airways with expansion of the terminal airways, in combination with epithelial cell differentiation and vascular development to form the alveoli. Based on histologic appearance, lung development is classically divided into five overlapping stages: embryonic, pseudoglandular, canalicular, saccular, and alveolar (Fig. 1.1).[1,8] Distinctive histologic and structural changes at each stage of lung development have

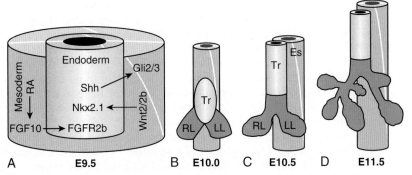

Fig. 1.2   Lung Bud Initiation and Tracheal-Esophageal Separation in Mice. Lung bud initiation on the foregut endoderm is controlled by a temporospatial expression of transcription factors and growth factors. A, At embryonic day (E) E9.5, *Nkx2.1* is expressed in the foregut endoderm which specifies the future trachea and lung. *Nkx2.1* expression is regulated by *Wnt2/2b*, expressed in the mesoderm. *Shh*, expressed in the endoderm and its signaling transducers, *Gli2/3*, expressed in the mesoderm, are required for lung budding. *Fgf10*, expressed in mesoderm and *Fgfr2b*, expressed in endoderm are also required for lung budding. Retinoic acid (RA) regulates *Fgf10* expression in the mesoderm. B, At E10, the primitive trachea (Tr), right lung (RL) bud, and left lung (LL) bud appear on the ventral face of the foregut. C, At E10.5, distinct tracheal and esophageal (Es) tubes emerge from the foregut tube. D, At E11.5, the trachea and esophagus are separated and connected only at the larynx. The RL bud gives rise to right main stem bronchus and subsequently four lobar bronchi, and the LL bud gives rise to single left lobar bronchus by branching into the ventrolateral mesenchyme derived from the splanchnic mesoderm. *FGF*, Fibroblast growth factor.

been well described, although the regulatory mechanisms responsible for these changes are not fully understood. There are striking similarities between human and mouse lung development. In fact, most of the current knowledge of lung developmental biology is acquired from mouse molecular genetics and genomic studies. This section reviews the key events during each of the lung developmental stages in mice and humans with a goal to better understand the regulatory mechanisms controlling this intricate process.

Embryonic Stage

The embryonic stage of human lung development occurs from 4 to 7 weeks of gestation. The lung bud originates as the laryngotracheal groove from the ventral surface of the primitive foregut. The proximal portion of the laryngotracheal groove separates dorsoventrally from the primitive esophagus to form the tracheal rudiment, which gives rise to the left and right main stem bronchi by branching into the ventrolateral mesenchyme derived from the splanchnic mesoderm. Subsequently, the right main bronchus branches to form three lobar bronchi, and the left main bronchus branches to form two lobar bronchi. The embryonic stage of mouse lung development occurs from embryonic day (E) 9 to E14, which begins as the formation of two endodermal buds from the ventral side of the primitive foregut. The single foregut tube then separates into the trachea containing the two primary lung buds and esophagus by inward movement of lateral mesodermal ridges, which proceed in a posterior to anterior direction. The two primary lung buds subsequently grow and branch into the splanchnic mesenchyme, with the right bud giving rise to four lobar bronchi and the left bud giving rise to a single lobar bronchus. During this stage, the trachea, primary bronchi, and major airways are lined with undifferentiated columnar epithelium.

Molecular Regulation of Lung Bud Initiation and Tracheoesophageal Separation

The processes and molecular regulators for lung bud initiation and tracheoesophageal separation are not fully established. However, mouse models have demonstrated that localized expression of key transcription factors and growth factors is essential during these processes (Fig. 1.2). Nkx2.1 (also known as thyroid transcription factor 1) is the earliest known transcriptional factor expressed in endodermal cells in the prospective lung/tracheal region of the anterior foregut.[9,10] Deletion of the *Nkx2.1* gene in mice results in abnormal lung formation with two main bronchi that give rise to cystic structures.[10] Additional studies have also demonstrated that *Nkx2.1* is essential for distal lung epithelial cell differentiation and expression of surfactant protein C (SP-C).[11] Expression of *Nkx2.1* in the foregut endoderm is regulated by wingless/int (Wnt)-β-catenin signaling. Combined loss of *Wnt2* and *Wnt2b*, which are expressed in the mesoderm surrounding the anterior foregut, or of β-catenin in the endoderm, leads to loss of *Nkx2.1* expression and failure of foregut separation.[12,13] *Nkx2.1* expression is inhibited by transforming growth factor β (TGF-β) signaling for lung epithelial progenitor cell fate determination.[14]

Sonic hedgehog (*Shh*) is expressed in the ventral foregut endoderm as early as E9.5 and appears to mediate early signaling between the endoderm and mesoderm.[15–17] *Shh* mediates its effects via GLI–Kruppel family member (*Gli*) 2/3 transcriptional factors present in the mesoderm. Mice with a targeted deletion of *Shh* gene have foregut defects with tracheoesophageal atresia/stenosis, tracheoesophageal fistula, and tracheal and lung anomalies.[18] *Gli2*[−/−] mice have unilobar left and right lungs[19] and *GLi3*[−/−] mice present with reductions in shape and size of pulmonary segmental branches.[20] Recent studies found that *Gli2*[−/−]*;GLi3*[−/−] double-knockout mice have a hypoplastic foregut that completely lacked Nkx2.1-positive respiratory progenitors.[21] In addition, *Wnt2/2b* transcripts were also lost or dramatically downregulated in these embryos.

Signaling mediated by fibroblast growth factor 10 (FGF10) and its receptor 2b (FGFR2b) is crucial for lung bud initiation. FGF10 belongs to an increasingly large and complex family of growth factors that signal through four cognate tyrosine kinases FGFRs.[1] FGF10 is a chemotactic and proliferation factor for lung endoderm that is expressed in the mesenchyme at the prospective sites of lung bud formation.[22] T-box transcription factors *Tbx2*, *Tbx3*, and *Tbx4* are coexpressed with *Fgf10* in the mesenchyme, which may positively regulate *Fgf10* expression.[23,24] The essential role of FGF10 in lung bud initiation is highlighted by the findings that deletion of *Fgf10* gene results in lung agenesis in mice.[25–27]

Retinoic acid (RA) also plays a role in lung bud formation. RA is produced in the mesoderm and can act on mesoderm and adjacent endoderm. RA, acting via the RA receptor β (RARβ) in the mesoderm, regulates *Fgf10* expression by integrating the Wnt and TGF-β pathways, to promote lung bud formation.[28,29] Dysregulation of bioactive RA synthesis through genetic mutation of retinaldehyde dehydrogenase 2 (*Raldh2*[−/−]), and pharmacologic inhibition of RA generation results in upregulation of TGF-β in the foregut and lung agenesis.[30] Thus RA–TGF-β–FGF10 interact with each other to control the initiation of the lung bud.

Our understanding of the critical signals required for initial lung budding and tracheoesophageal separation is incomplete and many other factors are likely to be involved. Knowledge gained from mouse studies will likely provide new insights into human congenital anomalies such as lung or tracheal agenesis, esophageal atresia, and tracheoesophageal fistula.

Pseudoglandular Stage

During the pseudoglandular stage (5–17 weeks in humans, E14–E16.5 in mice), the airway epithelial tubules undergo reproducible, bilaterally asymmetric, and stereotypical branching to form a treelike structure, which gives rise to 16 generations of conducting airways up to the level of terminal bronchioles.[1] There is also proximal airway epithelial differentiation with the appearance of basal cells, goblet cells, pulmonary neuroendocrine cells, ciliated cells, and nonciliated columnar (Clara) cells. The surrounding mesenchymal cells differentiate into fibroblasts, myofibroblasts, smooth muscle cells, and chondrocytes to form muscle and cartilage around the proximal airways. Vascular growth is in close proximity to airway branching during this stage. By the end of the pseudoglandular stage, the conducting airways and their accompanying pulmonary and bronchial arteries develop in a pattern corresponding to that found in the adult lung.

Airway branching morphogenesis in the pseudoglandular stage is controlled not only by intrinsic factors but also by physical space in the pleural cavity. Formation of

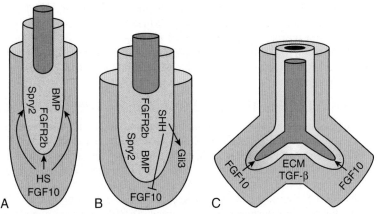

Fig. 1.3 Mechanisms of Branching Morphogenesis in Mice. A, Lung budding is induced by the localized expression of *Fgf10* in the distal mesenchyme, which acts on *Fgfr2b* expressed in epithelium. Heparan sulfate proteoglycan *(HS)* binds to FGF10 to provide location-specific patterning that drives branching. At the same time, FGF10 also induces expression of *Bmp4* and *Spry2* in epithelium. B, As the bud elongates, increased expression of *Spry2* in epithelium negatively regulates fibroblast growth factor *(FGF)* signaling and inhibits budding. Increased *Bmp* expression in epithelium may also inhibit budding. *Shh* expressed in the epithelium acting on *Gli3* expressed in the mesenchyme inhibits *Fgf* and *Fgfr2b* expression, thus inhibiting budding. C, *Fgf10* increases laterally to form new foci of lung buds that create a cleft. *Tgfβ1* expressed in the subepithelial mesenchyme increases extracellular matrix *(ECM)* deposition in the cleft areas that become the branching points. *BMP,* Bone morphogenetic protein; *TGF-β,* transforming growth factor β.

the diaphragm begins in the embryonic stage, continues through the pseudoglandular stage, and separates the pleural from the peritoneal cavities. Defects in the formation of the diaphragm, as in congenital diaphragmatic hernia, result in a decrease in the space within the pleural cavity, which in turn limits branching morphogenesis and vascularization, leading to variable degrees of pulmonary and vascular hypoplasia.[31]

Epithelial-Mesenchymal Interactions Control Branching Morphogenesis

Following the formation of primary lung buds, the airway epithelial tubules undergo branching morphogenesis to form the respiratory tree. Although the process of airway branching morphogenesis is still far from being fully understood, the interactions between epithelium and mesenchyme orchestrated by compartmental transcriptional factors, growth factors, as well as ECM play critical roles. These interactions involve FGF10, heparan sulfate proteoglycan, SHH, bone morphogenetic protein (BMP), TGF-β, Wnts, Hox, and RA.[29,32,33] These molecules are expressed in specific temporal, spatial, and cellular fashion, and together these signaling pathways coordinate reciprocal interactions between the epithelium and mesenchyme that control cell proliferation, differentiation, survival, and ultimately the number and size of airway branches (Fig. 1.3).

FGF10-FGFR2b Signaling: Driving Force for Branching Morphogenesis

At the early stages of branching morphogenesis, *Fgf10* is expressed in the mesenchyme surrounding the distal lung bud tip, whereas *Fgfr2b* is expressed at high levels along the entire proximal-distal axis of the airway endoderm.[34,35] Extensive in vitro studies have demonstrated the critical role of FGF10 in stimulating budding in mouse embryonic lung explants. In mesenchyme-free embryonic lung bud cultures, addition of recombinant FGF10 to culture medium induces budding.[22] Furthermore, placing an FGF10-soaked heparin bead, either in mesenchyme-free or whole lung bud cultures, induces bud elongation toward the FGF10 bead.[36] These in vitro data combined with in vivo data showing lung agenesis in *Fgf10* mutant mice indicate a critical role of FGF10 in driving branching morphogenesis. Interestingly, heparan sulfate side chains bind to growth factors, in particular, FGF10, to provide location-specific patterning that drives airway branching.[37,38] Thus spatiotemporal expression and the signaling activity of FGF10 need to be precisely regulated during branching morphogenesis to control the specific sites of budding, bud elongation, and branching. Further, recent studies of lung explant cultures have found that Rac1, a small Rho guanosine triphosphatase, regulates FGF10 expression and branching morphogenesis.[39]

Control of FGF10-FGFR2 Signaling by SHH and Sprouty

The exchange of signals between the growing bud and the surrounding mesenchyme establishes feedback responses that control the size and shape of the bud during branching. SHH, which is highly expressed in the distal lung epithelium, plays a role in controlling localized *Fgf10* expression in the mesenchyme surrounding the distal lung bud tip (see Fig. 1.3). In lung explant cultures, expression of *Fgf10* is inhibited by SHH.[40] Similarly, in *Shh* transgenic mice, *Fgf10* expression is downregulated in the lungs.[16] Furthermore, in *Shh*[−/−] mice, *Fgf10* expression is no longer restricted to the focal mesenchyme surrounding the distal bud, but becomes widespread through-out the distal mesenchyme.[41] Recent studies have identified the PEA3 group ETS domain transcription factors ETV4 and ETV5 as mediators of the FGF-SHH negative feedback loop during branching morphogenesis.[42]

Another antagonistic mechanism that interacts with FGF10 signaling is through Sprouty (Spry).[43] In the developing mouse lung, Spry2 is present at the tips of the growing epithelial buds. FGF10 induces Spry2 expression in lung epithelium.[44] Overexpression of *Spry2* in the distal lung epithelium of transgenic mice severely impairs branching.[44,45] However, *Spry2*-deficient mice have reduced branching and cystic formation and these structural anomalies are accompanied by reduced *Fgf10* expression and increased *Shh* and *Bmp4* expression.[46] Thus the interplay of FGF10-SHH-Spry2 regulates early lung branching morphogenesis.

BMP Signaling Regulates Branching Morphogenesis

The BMP family contains more than 20 members that regulate many developmental processes, including lung development, and BMP4 is the best studied in lung branching morphogenesis. *Bmp4*, *Alk3* (the type I receptor of *Bmp4*), and the BMP signaling transducer, *Smad1*, are present both in the epithelium and mesenchyme of the embryonic lung during early branching morphogenesis.[47–50] Transgenic overexpression of *Bmp4* in the distal epithelium causes abnormal lung morphogenesis with cystic terminal sacs.[49] Interestingly, blockade of endogenous *Bmp4* in embryonic mouse lung epithelium results in abnormal lung development with dilated terminal sacs, similar to those observed in *Bmp4* transgenic mice.[51] Conditional deletion of *Alk3* in embryonic lung epithelium causes retardation of branching morphogenesis.[52] Furthermore, abrogation of lung epithelial-specific *Smad1* also resulted in retardation of lung branching morphogenesis.[53] These findings suggest that balanced BMP4 signaling is important for in vivo lung branching morphogenesis, although the precise mechanisms remain unclear.

TGF-β Signaling Inhibits Branching

Members of the TGF-β family—TGF-β1, TGF-β2, and TGF-β3—have been implicated in lung airway branching.[54–56] During lung branching morphogenesis, *Tgfβ* messenger ribonucleic acid (mRNA) is expressed in the mesenchyme adjacent to the epithelium.[54] However, TGF-β1 protein accumulates in stalks and in regions between buds, where ECM components collagen I, collagen III, and fibronectin are also present. *Tgfβ1*[−/−] mice develop severe pulmonary inflammation postnatally,[57] whereas *Tgfβ2* gene deletion results in embryonic lethality at E14.5 with abnormal branching morphogenesis.[58] *Tgfβ3*[−/−] mice present with cleft palate, retarded lung development, and neonatal lethality.[55,56] In contrast, overexpression of *Tgfβ1* in embryonic lung epithelium decreases airway and vascular development as well as epithelial cell differentiation.[59,60] Many in vitro studies have demonstrated that exogenous TGF-β1 severely inhibits embryonic lung branching and epithelial differentiation, but stimulates mesenchymal differentiation by inducing ectopic expression of α-smooth muscle actin (α-SMA) and collagen.[61–63] TGF-β1 also markedly inhibits *Fgf10* expression in lung explant culture.[40] Abrogation of TGF-β signaling transducers *Smad2*, *Smad3*, and *Smad4* significantly affects branching.[64] Cumulatively, TGFβ signaling may be part of a mechanism that prevents FGF10 from being expressed in the mesenchyme of bud stalks or in more proximal regions of the lung. At these sites, TGF-β can also induce synthesis of ECM and prevent budding locally (see Fig. 1.3).

Wnt Signaling: Autocrine and Paracrine Effects on Branching Morphogenesis

The Wnt family constitutes a large family of secreted glycoproteins with highly conserved cysteine residues.[65] Wnt ligands bind to the membrane receptors, frizzled (Fzd) and low-density lipoprotein receptor-related protein (LRP) 5 or 6, thus activating a diverse array of intracellular signaling, targeted gene transcription, and cellular responses.[65] Canonical Wnt signaling, one of the best studied systems in lung development, involves nuclear translocation of β-catenin with subsequent interaction with members of T-cell–specific transcription factor (Tcf)/lymphoid enhancer-binding factor (Lef) family to induce target gene transcription.[65] Several Wnt ligands, receptors, and components of the canonical pathway, such as β-catenin and Tcf/Lef transcription factors, are expressed in a highly cell-specific fashion in the developing lung.[66–69] The role of Wnt/β-catenin signaling in branching morphogenesis has been examined by mouse mutagenesis as well as in embryonic lung explant culture. Epithelial-specific overexpression of *Wnt5a* results in decreased branching morphogenesis and increased enlargement of distal air spaces.[70] These lungs showed increased FGF signaling in the mesenchyme and decreased SHH signaling in the epithelium. Conversely, targeted deletion of *Wnt5a* leads to overexpansion of distal airways and expanded interstitium, accompanied by increased *Shh* expression.[71] Deletion of the *Wnt4* gene results in severe lung hypoplasia, tracheal abnormalities, and decreased expression of *Fgf10* and *Wnt2*.[72] Loss of *Fzd2* specifically in the developing lung epithelium results in defects in domain branch-point formation that alter the primary branching program of the lung.[73] Epithelial-specific deletion of β-catenin or overexpression of Wnt inhibitor, dickkopf1 (Dkk1) results in disruption of distal airway development and expansion of proximal airways.[74] Furthermore, inhibition of Wnt signaling by Dkk1 in vitro also results in disruption of branching morphogenesis and defective formation of pulmonary vascular network in embryonic lung explants.[75] Clearly, the mechanisms by which Wnt signaling regulates lung branching morphogenesis are very complex. These may be related to the fact that multiple Wnt ligands exist in the embryonic lung and Wnt signaling is known to regulate epithelial and mesenchymal cell biology in an autocrine and paracrine fashion. In addition, both canonical/β-catenin and noncanonical Wnt signaling pathways probably play a role in lung branching morphogenesis. Furthermore, how Wnt signaling interacts with other key signaling pathways such as FGF, SHH, and BMP remains unclear.

Hox5 Genes Control Lung Patterning by Regulating Wnt/BMP4 Signaling

Hox genes are a highly conserved group of transcription factors controlling complex developmental processes in various organs.[32,76] In human and mouse, 39 *Hox* genes are categorized into 13 paralog groups. Recent studies demonstrated that *Hoxa5;Hoxb5;Hoxc5* triple mutation results in severe embryonic lung hypoplasia with reduced branching and proximal-distal patterning defects.[32] Interestingly, loss of function of *Hox5* leads to loss of expression of *Wnt2/2b* in the distal lung mesenchyme and downregulation of downstream targets, including *Lef1*, *Axin2*, and *Bmp4*. Thus *Hox5* genes act as key upstream mesenchymal regulators of Wnt2/Wnt2b-BMP4 signaling that is critical for lung branching morphogenesis.

In summary, lung branching morphogenesis is controlled by epithelial-mesenchymal interactions that are orchestrated by a network of groups of transcriptional factors, growth factors, and ECM. Additionally, other molecules, such as integrins,[77–79] fibronectin,[80] and matrix metalloproteinases,[81,82] that are dynamically expressed during lung development also play a role in lung branching morphogenesis. Along with airway tubule budding, elongation, and branching, specific cell differentiation occurs in the endoderm and mesenchymal compartments. Furthermore, the regulatory mechanisms for proximal-distal patterning, establishing cell fate, and maintaining progenitor cells are likely even more complex. Physical forces such as intraluminal fluid pressure also play an important role in branching morphogenesis. Understanding the mechanisms of how the fluid is produced, and how fluid pressure is sensed and maintained has clinical implications in understanding congenital pulmonary hypoplasia. More importantly, defining these mechanisms may help developing fetal therapies to enhance lung growth in the face of lung hypoplasia.

Canalicular Stage

During the canalicular stage (16–26 weeks in humans, E16.5–E17.5 in mice), the terminal bronchioles continue to branch to form the final seven generations of the respiratory tree. The respiratory bronchioles branch out from the terminal bronchioles to form the prospective acini, which are accompanied by development of the capillary bed, the beginning of alveolar type II epithelial (ATII) cell differentiation to synthesize surfactant phospholipids and proteins, and the thinning of the surrounding mesenchymal tissues. The lung appears "canalized" as capillaries begin to arrange themselves around the air space and come into close apposition with the overlying epithelium. At sites of apposition, thinning of the epithelium occurs to form the first sites of the air-blood barrier. Thus if a fetus is born at around 24 weeks, the end of the canalicular stage, these primitive acini have the capacity to perform some gas exchange.

Saccular Stage

The saccular stage in humans occurs from 24 to 36 weeks. During this stage, primary septation results in clusters of thin-walled saccules in the distal lung to form the alveolar ducts, the last generation of airways before the development of alveoli. Small mesenchymal ridges develop on the saccular walls to initiate secondary septation. The capillaries form a "double capillary network" within the relatively broad and cellular intersaccular septae. The ATII cells are further differentiated and become functionally mature with the ability to produce surfactant. The alveolar type I epithelial (ATI) cells differentiate from the ATII cells in close apposition to the thinning capillaries to produce the final gas-exchange unit. The interstitium between the air spaces becomes thinner as the result of decreased collagen fiber deposition. Furthermore, elastic fibers are deposited in the interstitium, which lays the foundation for subsequent secondary septation and the formation of alveoli. The process of saccular formation in mice is quite similar to that in humans; however, the timing of the saccular stage in mice begins at E17.5 and continues up to postnatal day (P) 5.

Alveolar Stage

During the alveolar stage (36 weeks to childhood in humans, P5 to P30 in mice), the saccules are subdivided by the ingrowth of ridges or crests known as secondary septae. The ATII and ATI cells continue to differentiate. Postnatally, the alveoli continue to multiply by increasing secondary septation. Between birth and adulthood, the alveolar surface area expands nearly 20-fold.[83] In this stage, the double capillary network undergoes maturation, fusing into a single layer to allow for efficient gas exchange.[83] Thus capillary volume increases 35-fold from birth to adulthood.[83] In mouse lung development, alveolarization is completely a postnatal event. At birth, the mouse lung is in the saccular stage, equivalent to the human lung at 26 to 32 weeks' gestation. Mouse alveologenesis begins around P5 and continues up to P30. This postnatal pattern of mouse alveolar development provides an excellent model system for mechanistic studies to understand neonatal lung injury and repair in preterm infants.

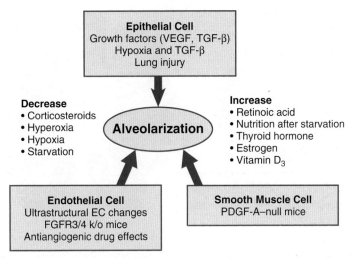

Fig. 1.4 Regulation of Alveolarization. Multiple cell types contribute to normal alveolarization, including epithelial cells that produce growth factors that both promote and inhibit the process, endothelial cells that are the primary cell that produce secondary septation, and myofibroblasts (smooth muscle cells) that define the sites of septal formation. Other factors influencing alveolarization include those that positively affect alveolarization vis-à-vis hormones such as vitamin D, retinoic acid, and thyroid hormone and that negatively affect alveolarization such as antiangiogenic drugs, corticosteroids, hyperoxia, hypoxia exposure, and nutrition deprivation. *EC,* Endothelial cell; *k/o,* knockout; *PDGF-A,* platelet-derived growth factor A; *TGF-β,* transforming growth factor β.

Regulatory Mechanisms of Alveologenesis

During the saccular stage, the primary septae are tightly associated with the vascular plexus, with ECM rich in elastin, and with still poorly defined mesenchymal cell types, including precursors of myofibroblasts. The endoderm begins to differentiate into two main specialized cell types of the future ATII and ATI cells. During alveolarization the sacs are subdivided by the ingrowth of secondary septae. Both myofibroblast progenitors and endothelial cells migrate into these crests, and a scaffold of matrix proteins is deposited, enriched in elastin at the tip. This development of secondary septae and formation of alveoli involves highly coordinated interactions of myofibroblasts, epithelial cells and microvascular endothelial cells, and proper deposition of ECM, particularly elastin (Fig. 1.4). In contrast to the extensive knowledge of the regulatory mechanisms of branching morphogenesis, it has been challenging to identify the molecular mechanisms that regulate cell proliferation, differentiation, migration, and ECM deposition in alveologenesis. This is in part because mouse mutagenesis often profoundly affects the earliest stages of lung development, thus resulting in cessation of lung development and/or death before the initiation of sacculation and alveolarization. Nevertheless, several signaling pathways have been proposed to play a role in regulating alveolar development.

Myofibroblast Differentiation and Elastin Deposition: Key Events for Alveolar Septation

The alveolar myofibroblasts have long been recognized to play an essential role in alveolar septation, and platelet-derived growth factor (PDGF) is probably one of the most important factors that regulates myofibroblast differentiation. It has been proposed that myofibroblasts are differentiated from alveolar interstitial lipofibroblasts, which "traffic" lipids and store retinoids.[84,85] Confocal microscopy revealed that lipofibroblasts with high lipid content are located at the base of alveolar septa and express low levels of PDGF receptor α (PDGFRα).[86] The same study showed that cells expressing high levels of PDGFRα have the characteristic of myofibroblasts located at the alveolar entry ring. These cells express α-SMA, contain contractile elements,[87,88] and also produce tropoelastin, the soluble precursor of elastin.[89] Elastin is assembled by cross-linking of tropoelastin under the action of lysyl oxidase in the ECM environment.[90]

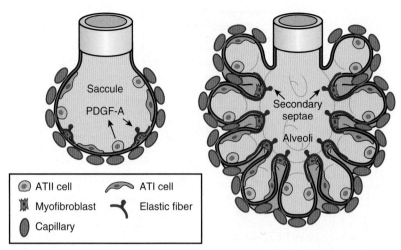

Fig. 1.5 Model of Alveolarization. A, During the later saccular stage, there is increased myofibroblast differentiation and elastin synthesis, stimulated by platelet-derived growth factor A *(PDGF-A)*, which is produced by alveolar type II epithelial *(ATII)* cells. B, During alveolar development, these myofibroblasts produce elastic fibers and migrate toward the alveolar airspaces. The ATII cells, type I epithelial *(ATI)* cells, and capillaries move together with the myofibroblasts into the alveolar air spaces that become the secondary septae.

PDGFα, a strong chemoattractant for fibroblasts, is produced by alveolar epithelial cells.[91] The importance of PDGFα, myofibroblasts, and elastin in alveolar septation was demonstrated by early studies in *Pdgfα*[−/−] mice that have a profound deficiency in alveolar myofibroblasts and associated bundles of elastin fibers, resulting in absence of secondary septa and definitive alveoli.[91,92] Inhibition of PDGF signaling by imatinib, a PDGF receptor antagonist, impaired alveolarization in the postnatal lung.[93] It has been suggested that in the absence of PDGFα, alveolar myofibroblasts or their precursors fail to migrate to the sites where elastin deposition and septation should occur. Furthermore, this migration to the sites of septal budding is not a random phenomenon, and a morphogen gradient is likely established to tightly regulate PDGFα production, myofibroblast differentiation and migration, and elastin deposition, thus providing instruction for the precise and specific localization of secondary septae (Fig. 1.5).

In addition, other molecules have been implicated in alveolarization by directly or indirectly affecting PDGF signaling, myofibroblast differentiation and migration, and elastin assembly. Members of the FGF family play an important role not only in branching morphogenesis but also in alveolarization. Multiple FGFs and FGFRs are expressed in the lung during late-stage development. The critical role for the FGF pathway in alveolar development was demonstrated by the phenotype of lungs of *Fgfr3/Fgfr4* double-mutant mice that failed to undergo secondary septation.[94] RA is known to be involved in not just early lung morphogenesis but also alveolar development. Synthesizing enzymes, receptors, and signaling transducers of RA are abundant during alveolar septation. Mice with deletions of RA receptors fail to form normal alveoli.[95] Precisely how RA signaling regulates alveolarization is not well understood. There is evidence for RA crosstalk with PDGF and FGF signaling.[96–98] There is also evidence that epithelial Notch signaling regulates alveolar formation through induction of PDGFα in ATII cells and activation of PDGFRα signaling in alveolar myofibroblast progenitors.[99]

External stressors also affect alveolarization (see Fig. 1.4). Thus exposure to starvation results in inhibition of alveolarization, which is reversed with refeeding.[100,101] Further, both hypoxia and hyperoxia during the neonatal period in mice are associated with increased TGF-β and disruption of alveolarization.[102,103] Interestingly, exposure to even low doses of corticosteroids completely inhibits alveolarization, which is irreversible and extends to adulthood.[104–106] These are relevant studies because preterm infants are often nutritionally deprived, exposed to repeated hyperoxemia and hypoxemia, and are given corticosteroids for blood pressure support and as antiinflammatory therapy to allow weaning from respiratory support.

Development of Airway Epithelial Lineages

Following branching morphogenesis, epithelial cell differentiation along distinct lineages into mature conducting airway and distal alveolar epithelial cells is necessary for appropriate lung function. Many transcription factors regulate proximal epithelial cell fate, including Sox2, FoxJ1, and Notch. Thus Sox2 regulates differentiation of proximal endotherm progenitors into mature lineages.[29,107] FoxJ1 is required for the formation of the multiciliated cells from Sox2-positive progenitors,[108] and Notch signaling is important in establishing and maintaining a proper balance of the various differentiated proximal airway cell types as well as directing the differentiation of basal cells in the adult lung.[109]

As lung development goes through canalicular, saccular, and alveolar stages, distal airway multipotent progenitors begin to generate differentiated distal alveolar epithelial cells, ATI and ATII. Although classical studies suggested that ATI cells arise from ATII cells, recent studies propose that distal tip progenitors contain bipotent progenitor cells that express both ATI and ATII markers late in gestation.[110] These data suggest that these pluripotent progenitors can differentiate into ATI and ATII cells as development prodeeds.[29]

The Surfactant System

Surfactant proteins (SPs) and lipids are synthesized primarily by ATII cells. There are four SPs—SP-A, SP-B, SP-C, and SP-D—that have been characterized to date. SP-A and SP-D are members of the collectin family and confer innate immunity as they have carbohydrate recognition domains that allow them to bind bacteria and viruses, promoting phagocytosis by macrophages.[111] SP-B and SP-C are highly hydrophobic, segregate into the lipid fraction of surfactant, and are assembled with surfactant phospholipids into lamellar bodies that are the storage organelles for surfactant before secretion.[111] Nkx2.1 regulates the surfactant-associated genes and is required for normal surfactant synthesis at birth.[111] Phospholipids, the principal component of pulmonary surfactant, consist primarily of phosphatidylcholine (PC) and phosphatidylglycerol. PC and phosphatidylglycerol are produced by ATII cells, dramatically increasing in late gestation. Adenosine triphosphate–binding cassette transporter 3 (ABCA3), located on the limiting membrane of the lamellar body, is required for PC to be transferred to the lamellar body.[111] In the lamellar body, SP-B and SP-C are assembled with PC into bilayer membranes. The surfactant contents in the lamellar body are secreted into the airway upon stimulation by catecholamines, purinoreceptor agonists, and cell stretch.[111] GPR116, an orphan G-protein–coupled receptor located on respiratory epithelial cells, regulates surfactant secretion because *Gpr116* mutation in mouse results in excess secretion of surfactant that accumulates in the air spaces after birth.[112,113]

Regulation of Pulmonary Vascular Development

The lung vasculature is constituted by the pulmonary and bronchial vascular systems. The pulmonary system consists of pulmonary arteries that carry blood to the alveolar capillary network to be oxygenated; oxygenated blood returns through pulmonary veins back to the heart. The bronchial system supplies oxygen and nutrients to the nonrespiratory portion of the lung, including the bronchial walls and perihilar region. The molecular basis of pulmonary vascular development is not well understood but is increasingly recognized as being controlled by epithelial-endothelial as well as endothelial-mesenchymal crosstalk.

Vascular Morphogenesis

It is generally believed that early pulmonary vascular development involves three processes to establish a circulatory network: angiogenesis, vasculogenesis, and fusion. Angiogenesis is defined as formation of new blood vessels from preexisting vasculature. New vessels sprout via a well-defined program: degradation of the basement membrane, endothelial cell differentiation and migration, formation of solid sprouts of endothelial cells, and restructuring of the sprout into a luminal line by endothelial cells that is finally integrated into the vascular network.[114] Vasculogenesis is defined as de novo formation of blood vessels from angioblasts or endothelial precursor cells arising in the mesodermal mesenchyme. Earlier studies by DeMello et al. indicated that the proximal vessels are generated by angiogenesis, whereas the distal vessels are formed by vasculogenesis during lung morphogenesis.[115] The proximal and distal vessels fuse to establish the luminal connection via a lytic process.[115] Using analysis of serial sections of human embryos, this group suggested that the same processes also occur during human lung formation.[116] However, this concept has been challenged in later studies. Work from Schachtner et al. suggested that vasculogenesis is primarily responsible for both proximal and distal vascular formation during lung development.[117] Studies by Hall et al. in human embryos have also indicated that intrapulmonary arteries originate from a continuous expansion and coalescence of a primary capillary plexus that would form by vasculogenesis during the pseudoglandular stage.[118] They have also indicated that the pulmonary veins are formed by the same mechanism. Parera et al. have proposed distal angiogenesis as a new concept for early pulmonary vascular morphogenesis.[119] Schwarz et al. have also proposed that initial pulmonary vessel formation within the mesenchyme is predominantly angiogenic.[120]

VEGF-Mediated Epithelial-Endothelial Interaction in Vascular and Alveolar Development

There is increasing evidence that epithelial-endothelial interactions play important roles in vascularization and alveolarization. Vascular endothelial growth factor (VEGF) is a key angiogenic factor known to play important roles in these processes.[121,122] VEGF stimulates proliferation, migration, differentiation, and tube formation in endothelial cells. These effects are largely elicited by VEGF binding to the high-affinity VEGF receptor 2 (VEGFR2) or Flk-1 on endothelial cells.[121] During normal mouse lung development, various VEGF isoforms (VEGF122, VEGF164, VEGF188) are present in epithelial cells, and their expression increases during later canalicular and saccular stages, when most of the vessel growth occurs in the lung.[123] In contrast, VEGFR2 and VEGFR1 (Flt-1) are expressed in the adjacent endothelial cells.[117,124] Individual knockouts for *Vegf*, *Vegfr2*, and *Vegfr1* result in embryonic lethality before the development of the lung capillary plexus.[125–128] Targeted deletion of the *Vegf* gene in respiratory epithelium results in an almost complete absence of pulmonary capillaries and this defective vascular formation is associated with a defect in primary septal formation.[129] Interestingly, these structural defects are coupled with suppression of epithelial proliferation and decreased hepatocyte growth factor (HGF) expression in endothelial cells. Furthermore, targeted deletion of the *Hgf* receptor gene in the epithelium results in a similar septation defect as seen in VEGF-deleted lungs. These data highlight the mechanisms by which VEGF and HGF signaling pathways orchestrate the reciprocal interactions between airway epithelium and the surrounding endothelium during septation. Recent studies showed that conditional inactivation of *Vegf* during alveologenesis not only decreased pulmonary capillary and alveolar development but also altered RA expression.[130] Treatment with RA partially improved vascular and alveolar development induced by VEGF inhibition. Thus VEGF and RA signaling interact to regulate vascularization and alveologenesis. VEGF signaling is also differentially regulated by FGF9 and SHH signaling during mouse lung development.[131] Mesenchymal expression of VEGF is regulated by gain and loss of function of *Fgf9* and *Vegf* is required for *Fgf9*-induced pulmonary blood vessel formation.[131] *Shh*, on the other hand, regulates the pattern of *Vegf* expression rather than the content because loss of *Shh* signaling did not affect *Vegf* expression in subepithelial mesenchyme, but decreased *Vegf* expression in the submesothelial mesenchyme. Nitric oxide (NO) is known to mediate VEGF angiogenic activity. In a neonatal rat model, treatment with SU5416, a VEGFR inhibitor, results in both disrupted angiogenesis and alveolarization and this is associated with a decreased content of endothelial NO synthase (eNOS) and NO production.[132] In contrast, inhaled NO improves alveolar development and pulmonary hypertension in VEGFR inhibitor-treated rats.[133] Further evidence of the importance of NO in alveolarization and vascularization was demonstrated by the combined disruption of alveolarization and paucity of distal arteries observed in *Nos*-deficient fetal and neonatal mice.[134,135]

Additional Angiogenic Factors in Vascular Development

Angiopoietins (Ang) and Tie signaling are also known to play important roles in vascular morphogenesis and homeostasis.[136–138] Ang/Tie signaling is known to play a primary role in the later stages of vascular development and in adult vasculature, where they control remodeling and stabilization of vessels.[138,139] Ang1 appears to work in complementary fashion with VEGF during early vascular development. VEGF appears to initiate vascular formation, and Ang1 promotes subsequent vascular remodeling, maturation, and stabilization, perhaps, in part, by supporting interactions between endothelial cells and surrounding support cells and ECM. The role of Ang/Tie in developmental angiogenesis is highlighted by the early embryonic lethality and significant abnormal vascular development observed in offspring of *Ang1*$^{-/-}$, *Tie1*$^{-/-}$, *Tie2*$^{--}$ as well as *Tie1*$^{-/-}$/*Tie2*$^{--}$ mice.[140–142] The specific role of Ang/Tie signaling in pulmonary vascular development is poorly understood. Studies have shown that *Ang1* is expressed in lungs of newborn mice and its expression is increased from P1 to P14, whereas *Ang2* is abundantly expressed at birth and decreases inversely with *Ang1*.[143] Transgenic overexpression of a potent form of *Ang1* protein, COMP-*Ang1* in lung epithelium resulted in abnormal alveolar and vascular structure and 50% lethality at birth owing to respiratory failure.[143] During postnatal lung development, Ang/Tie2 signaling is regulated by the Wnt ligand-receptor, LRP5.[144] Thus precise regulation of Tie2 signaling through an *Ang1* and *Ang2* expression switch is important to construct a mature lung vascular network required for normal lung development. Ang1 also plays a role in pulmonary hypertension because lung overexpression of *Ang1* causes severe pulmonary hypertension and Ang1 is increased in lungs from pulmonary hypertensive patients.[145,146] However, cell-based *Ang1* gene transfer protects against monocrotaline-induced experimental pulmonary hypertension.[147]

Other angiogenic signaling pathways, such as BMP, Notch, TGF-β, Wnts, and the Eph family of receptor tyrosine kinases and their membrane tethered ligands Ephrins, are likely involved in pulmonary vascular development.[83,148,149] More studies are needed to define the regulatory mechanisms of these important pathways and the interactions among these pathways during normal and abnormal lung vascular morphogenesis.

Lung Injury and Repair: Disruption of Normal Lung Development

With its vast airway and alveolar epithelium open to the atmosphere, the newborn lung is at great risk for harmful environmental insults, such as oxidative stress, physical forces, and infective agents. These environmental challenges place the lung under constant threat of injury, requiring coordinated defense repair and remodeling processes. The lungs of full-term neonates have a great ability to overcome various injuries, to generate needed repair and remodeling appropriately, and ultimately to maintain and/or restore normal lung architecture and function. When premature delivery occurs, particularly between 24 and 28 weeks, the lungs of these preterm infants are in the late canalicular to early saccular stage. Alveolarization has not yet begun and surfactant production is minimal. Lungs in the canalicular to early saccular stage are poorly compliant, whereas the chest wall is extremely compliant. A large proportion of infants born at these early gestational ages have significant respiratory failure and often require respiratory support including mechanical ventilation and oxygen therapy. These lungs are therefore at great risk for injury, altered development, and BPD.

Over the past four decades, with advances in neonatal intensive care—such as the introduction of antenatal corticosteroids, exogenous surfactant therapy, and gentler ventilator strategies—the survival of extremely premature infants has been significantly improved. However, during the same period, the incidence of BPD has

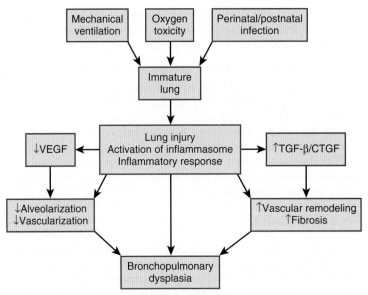

Fig. 1.6 Proposed Schematic for the Pathogenesis of Bronchopulmonary Dysplasia (BPD). The immature lung that is exposed to mechanical ventilation, oxygen, and perinatal and postnatal infection activates an inflammasome-mediated inflammatory response. The response to injury results in suppression of vascular endothelial growth factor *(VEGF)* expression, thereby decreasing alveolarization and vascularization, and an increase in TGF-β/CTGF expression, thereby causing vascular remodeling and fibrosis. These consequences of neonatal injury lead to abnormal alveolar and vascular growth, which are the hallmarks of BPD. *CTGF,* Connective tissue growth factor; *TGF-β,* transforming growth factor β.

not changed appreciably. This is likely due to the fact that infants of lower gestational ages are now surviving.[150] BPD is now recognized as a developmental arrest of lung development at the saccular stage caused by injurious stimuli, such as mechanical ventilation, oxygen exposure, and intrauterine or postnatal infections. Larger and simplified distal air spaces and decreased vascular growth are the key pathologic features observed in the lungs of infants dying of BPD.[7] The combination of decreased vascular growth and excessive pulmonary vascular remodeling leads to pulmonary hypertension, which significantly contributes to the morbidity and mortality of these infants.[83] The largely unchanged incidence of BPD has not only provided tremendous challenges in the management of these patients, but has also spurred the need for new knowledge of the molecular basis of neonatal lung injury and repair. Experimental models of BPD have used both larger animals such as preterm baboons and sheep, and smaller animals such as rats and mice. These studies attempt to create the BPD phenotype by exposing immature baboons and sheep, or neonatal rats and mice to noxious stimuli such as mechanical ventilation, hyperoxia, and/or infection. Extensive data generated from these studies indicate that the key signaling pathways regulating normal lung development can be disrupted by injurious stimuli in the immature lung, thereby playing important roles in the pathogenesis of BPD. Although many factors are involved in neonatal lung injury, this section emphasizes the role of inflammasomes, VEGF, TGF-β, and connective tissue growth factor (CTGF) (Fig. 1.6).

Innate Immunity, IL-1β, and the Development of BPD

It is clear that an inflammatory response and the elaboration of growth factors and cytokines are associated with the development of BPD.[151,152] The innate immune system is an early, nonspecific, yet robust system that senses endogenous danger signals and mobilizes inflammatory cells as a response. Microbes and other environmental challenges display unique structures called pathogen-associated molecular patterns, whereas tissue injury results in the production of endogenous ligands called danger-associated molecular patterns that are recognized by specific pattern recognition receptors. These include Toll-like receptors (TLRs), named after toll, a protein identified in

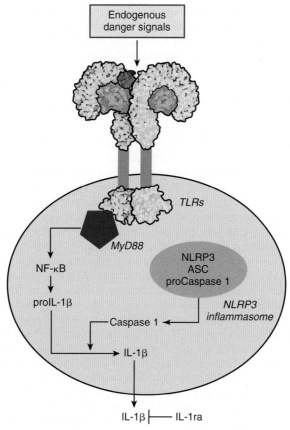

Fig. 1.7 **Mechanisms of NLRP3 Inflammasome Activation to Produce Mature Interleukin 1β** *(IL-1β)*. The innate immune system is largely activated by endogenous danger signals that signal via toll-like receptors *(TLRs)*, particularly TLR2 and TLR4. Signaling via the adaptor, myeloid differentiation primary response 88 *(MyD88)*, activates the transcription factor nuclear factor kappa B *(NF-κB)* and promotes transcription of pro-IL-1β. The TLR system, in conjunction with the extracellular adenosine triphosphate receptor P2X7 (not shown), promotes the formation of a complex of activating signal cointegrator *(ASC)*, NLRP3, and pro-caspase 1, the NLRP3 inflammasome, which then enzymatically processes and activates caspase 1. This enzyme, in turn, proteolytically processes pro-IL-1β to mature IL-1β, which is then secreted to promote an inflammatory response. Endogenous IL-1 receptor antagonist (IL-1ra) blocks the binding of IL-1β to its receptor and inhibits the inflammatory response. IL-1β and the NLRP3 inflammasome have been implicated in the pathogenesis of BPD.

Drosophilia that interacted with fungi and activated nuclear factor kappa B. There are at least 12 known mammalian TLRs with varying ligand specificities.[153] Interaction of bacterial and viral components with TLRs initiates a robust elaboration of cytokines and growth factors, as well as inducible NOS, leading to shock, surfactant deficiency, respiratory distress, and a systemic inflammatory response.[154] Lipopolysaccharide (LPS) of gram-negative organisms interacts with TLR4, whereas peptidoglycan of gram-positive organisms and zymosan of yeast cell walls interact with TLR2. Activation of each TLR results in intracellular signaling that activates growth factor and cytokine production, including interleukin 1β (IL-1β), TGF-β, and TNF-α. Further elucidation of innate immune pathways revealed the existence of a family of exclusively intracellular proteins called *nucleotide-binding oligomerization domain–like* (NOD-like) receptors (NLRs) that also bind to pathogen-associated molecular patterns or danger-associated molecular patterns.[155] One such NLR, NLRP3, forms a protein complex with the adaptor molecule *apoptosis-associated Speck-like protein containing a CARD* (ASC) and pro-caspase1 to form the *NLRP3 inflammasome*.[156,157] Inflammasome activation requires two signals (Fig. 1.7).[153,158,159] First, tissue injury results in the elaboration of endogenous danger signals that stimulate TLRs. Subsequent TLR signaling through the TLR/IL1R adaptor molecule, MyD88, activates a number of signaling pathways, including nuclear factor kappa B, and increases the expression of pro-IL-1β and pro-IL-18. The second signal is the activation of the purinergic receptor P2X7 by extracellular adenosine triphosphate that results in the formation of the NLRP3 inflammasome, consisting of NLRP3, ASC, and pro-caspase1, a response that has been demonstrated after hyperoxia exposure to adult mice[160] and in our studies of neonatal mice and rats exposed to hyperoxia.[161,162] Activation of this complex cleaves pro-caspase1 to caspase1 (p20), which in turn proteolytically cleaves pro-IL-1β and pro-IL-18 to produce mature IL-1β and IL-18. These cytokines are released and IL-1β interacts with its receptor, IL-1R, to signal inflammatory pathways. IL-1 receptor antagonist (IL-1ra) is an endogenous blocker of IL1R.

IL-1β, a key initiator of inflammation driven by the innate immune system, has a complex activation system and has been implicated in inflammatory disorders in humans. Neonatal-onset multisystem inflammatory diseases (NOMID) includes a collection of diseases (such as familial Mediterranean fever) characterized by relapsing fevers and recurrent bouts of inflammation that can affect the skin, joints, bones, eyes, gastrointestinal tract, and the nervous system.[163,164] The most common mutations in these diseases are either activating mutations of NLRP3 or inactivating mutations of IL-1ra that result in an imbalance in the ratio of IL-1β to IL-1ra.[165] NOMIDs are eminently treatable by a recombinant, non-glycosylated form of the human IL-1ra. Outcomes of patients with NOMIDs treated with rIL-1ra for 3 to 5 years show that the drug is well tolerated at doses of 1 to 5 mg/kg per day, suppresses inflammation systemically and in the central nervous system, and arrests any damage caused by inflammation.[166] With respect to the association of IL-1β with BPD, elevated concentrations of IL-1β in amniotic fluid[167,168] and in the lung postnatally[169] are associated with the development of BPD. Indeed, in preterm infants at risk of BPD, there is a balance of mature IL-1β to IL-1ra in the first few days of life, but the ratio of IL-1β to IL-1ra is increased in infants who subsequently develop BPD.[170] Further, transgenic lung overexpression of IL-1β in Clara cells, even in the absence of hyperoxia, results in inflammation, airway remodeling, and distal alveolar simplification, changes reminiscent of BPD.[171,172] Interestingly, in these studies, all other cytokines and growth factors, including TGF-β, were downstream of IL-1β, suggesting that IL-1β is a master regulator of innate immune response. Treatment with rIL-1ra of hyperoxia-exposed rats,[173] mice exposed in utero to LPS and subsequently to postnatal hyperoxia,[174] and in our own studies with neonatal hyperoxia in mice[161] is associated with less inflammation and improved alveolarization.

Increased TGF-β Signaling in Neonatal Lung Injury and BPD

Two decades ago, Kotecha et al. showed that higher concentrations of total and bioactive TGF-β were detected in bronchoalveolar lavage fluid from preterm infants who subsequently developed BPD.[175] Since then, cumulative data from both clinical and animal studies have indicated a critical role of dysregulated TGF-β signaling in neonatal lung injury, deranged repair, and the pathogenesis of BPD. One study has shown that increased TGF-β concentration in the amniotic fluid of preterm deliveries is correlated with histologic severity of chorioamnionitis, subsequent development of BPD, and duration of oxygen therapy in preterm infants.[176] In fetal sheep, chorioamnionitis-associated antenatal inflammation increases TGF-β concentrations and induces Smad2 phosphorylation in the lung, indicating activation of TGF-β signaling.[177] In preterm lambs, chronic mechanical ventilation increases TGF-β expression in the lung, which is associated with dysregulated pulmonary elastin synthesis and disrupted alveolar development.[178] In oxygen-exposed newborn mice, increased TGF-β signaling is responsible for aberrant lysyl oxidase expression, which may impede the matrix remodeling required for normal alveolarization.[179]

Studies in transgenic mouse models further support that increasing lung expression of *Tgfβ* disrupts alveolar development. For example, overexpression of *Tgfβ* in the respiratory epithelium, under the control of human SF-C gene promoter, results in arrested lung development at the pseudoglandular stage and perinatal death at E18.5.[59] Overexpression of *Tgfβ* in the developing fetal monkey lung also results in pulmonary hypoplasia.[180] To overcome the problem of prenatal death, one study used a triple-transgenic mouse to overexpress bioactive TGF-β under the doxycycline-induced control of the Clara cell secretory protein promoter.[181] Induction of *Tgfβ* expression from P7 to P14 resulted in larger alveoli with thick and hypercellular septae and abnormal capillary development. Overexpression of *Tgfβ* in the developing mouse lung also results in inflammation, apoptosis, and mortality via *Tgfβr2*.[182] However, a recent study found that genetic ablation of *Tgfβ*-induced matricellular proteins is associated with abnormal septal formation and BPD.[183]

Although increased TGF-β signaling is overwhelmingly linked to clinical and animal models of BPD, there have been very few studies examining the therapeutic potential of TGF-β antagonism in neonatal lung injury. Treatment with TGF-β–neutralizing antibody prenatally significantly attenuated hyperoxia-induced Smad2 activation and improved alveolar development, ECM assembly, and microvascular development in neonatal mice.[184] In addition, treatment with rosiglitazone, a peroxisome proliferator–activated receptor-gamma (PPARγ) agonist, blocked hyperoxia-induced TGF-β signaling activation and prevented alveolar damage.[185] Treatment with curcumin, a modulator of PPARγ and an antioxidant, also blocked TGF-β signaling and hyperoxia-induced lung injury.[186] Whether TGF-β inhibition will be beneficial in clinical BPD is yet to be determined. Given the exceptionally broad range of biologic activity ascribed to TGF-β and its fundamental physiologic roles, nonselective TGF-β blockade would likely have undesired consequences. Complete abrogation of TGF-β signaling could lead to loss of immune tolerance, spontaneous autoimmunity, and defective tissue repair.[187] Therefore identification of the upstream or downstream mediators and pathways of TGF-β may enhance our mechanistic understanding of neonatal lung injury and repair and provide more effective targets for treating BPD.

CTGF, a multimodular matrix-associated protein, is thought to be a downstream mediator and coactivator of TGF-β and plays an important role in tissue development and remodeling.[188,189] Historically, CTGF is best known for its fibroproliferative effect and is implicated in various forms of adult lung fibrosis.[188] Increasing evidence indicates that CTGF plays an important role in lung development and pathogenesis of BPD. CTGF is expressed in distal airway epithelium during embryonic lung development.[190] In mouse embryonic lung explant cultures, expression of CTGF is upregulated by TGF-β and CTGF inhibits branching morphogenesis.[63] *Ctgf*[-/-] mice die soon after birth with respiratory failure.[191] These mice display severe rib cage malformations and their lungs are hypoplastic with reduced cell proliferation and increased apoptosis, suggesting that CTGF deficiency may disrupt normal embryonic lung developmental processes.[191,192] In contrast, overexpression of *Ctgf* in respiratory epithelial cells under the control of the Clara cell secretory protein gene promoter resulted in thickened alveolar septae and decreased alveolarization and capillary density in neonatal mice.[193] Overexpression of *Ctgf* in ATII cells under the control of the SP-C gene promoter not only disrupted alveolarization and decreased vascular density, but also induced pulmonary vascular remodeling and pulmonary hypertension in neonatal mice.[194] Multiple studies have examined the role of CTGF in hyperoxia, mechanical ventilation, and LPS-induced neonatal lung injury. Chronic hyperoxia exposure increases CTGF expression in lungs of neonatal mice and rats.[195,196] Injurious mechanical ventilation with high tidal volume upregulates CTGF expression in newborn rat and lamb lungs.[197,198] Intraamniotic injection of LPS increases CTGF expression in ovine fetal lungs.[199] In addition, treatment with a CTGF-neutralizing antibody significantly improved alveolar and vascular development, and decreased pulmonary vascular remodeling and pulmonary hypertension in hyperoxia-induced lung injury in neonatal rats.[200] Furthermore, a recent study demonstrated that human mesenchymal stem cells attenuate both LPS-induced antenatal inflammation and postnatal hyperoxia-induced BPD in neonatal rats, and that these observations are associated with downregulation of CTGF expression.[201] The clinical relevance of CTGF with BPD is suggested by studies demonstrating increased CTGF in bronchoalveolar lavage fluid from premature infants with BPD[202] and in lungs of infants who died of BPD.[200] Together these data highlight an important role of CTGF in the pathogenesis of BPD.

Decreased VEGF Signaling in Neonatal Lung Injury and BPD

It is now established that lung VEGF expression is decreased in clinical as well as in experimental models of BPD. Preterm infants who subsequently developed BPD had lower VEGF concentration in their tracheal aspirates compared with those who did not develop BPD.[203] Expression of VEGF and VEGFR1 is decreased in lung autopsy specimens from preterm infants dying with BPD that is correlated with decreased expression of platelet endothelial cell adhesion molecule in alveolar capillary endothelial cells.[204] However, long-term ventilated preterm infants have increased total pulmonary microvascular endothelial volume and expression of platelet endothelial cell adhesion molecule, suggesting increased angiogenesis.[205] Subsequent studies have shown that although VEGF and its receptors were decreased in ventilated lungs from preterm infants, endoglin, a hypoxia-inducible TGF-β coreceptor and important regulator of angiogenesis, was increased.[206] This suggests that BPD is associated with a shift from traditional angiogenic growth factors to alternative regulators that may contribute to BPD-associated microvascular dysangiogenesis. In addition, a recent study in Japanese premature infants showed an association of the VEGF polymorphism, VEGF −634C>G with the development of BPD.[207]

Extensive studies in animal models of BPD have been conducted to explore how VEGF signaling is regulated and whether enhancing VEGF signaling could protect against alveolar and vascular damage. Exposure to hyperoxia decreases lung VEGF expression in neonatal rabbits and rodents and preterm baboons and lambs.[208–212] Hyperoxia also decreases VEGFR1 and VEGFR2 expression in neonatal rats and mice and preterm baboons.[178,209,212] Similarly, mechanical ventilation has been shown to decrease VEGF and VEGFRs expression in newborn mice and preterm baboons.[178, 211] However, exposure of pregnant rats to endotoxin on E20 and E21 significantly increased lung VEGF and VEGFR2 gene expression in their offspring at P2 to P14.[213] These changes were associated with alterations in gene expression of lysyl oxidase, fibulin, PDGFRα, and morphologic changes with fewer and larger alveoli, fewer secondary septae, and decreased peripheral vessel density. Studies have also shown that excess soluble VEGFR1 (sFlt1) in amniotic fluid impairs postnatal lung development.[214] Similarly, intraamniotic injection of sFlt1 also decreases VEGFR2 activation and increases apoptosis in endothelial cells and mesenchymal cells in these lungs. These data suggest that the timing, the length, and the type of lung injury variably modulate VEGF expression and signaling.

Given the importance of VEGF signaling in normal lung development and injury, the therapeutic potential of modulating VEGF signaling in experimental models of BPD has been examined. In a newborn rat model of BPD, treatment with recombinant VEGF during and after hyperoxia enhanced both vascular and alveolar development.[215,216] Adenovirus-mediated VEGF gene therapy increased survival, promoted lung angiogenesis, and prevented alveolar damage in hyperoxia-induced lung injury in newborn rats.[217] However, in these studies, increased VEGF also induced immature and leaky capillaries and lung edema. Using a transgenic mouse model, overexpression of VEGF in respiratory epithelial cells resulted in pulmonary hemorrhage, hemosiderosis, and air space enlargement in neonatal mice.[218] These adverse outcomes of capillary leakage and hemorrhage suggest the importance of tightly regulated VEGF expression in neonatal lung development and injury repair, and highlight the complexity of enhancing VEGF as a therapeutic approach to treat BPD. It was proposed that VEGF may work with other angiogenic factors, such as Angs, to form stabilized vessels during development. This hypothesis was supported by the data showing that combined VEGF and Ang1 gene therapy reduced capillary leakage and improved vascular and alveolar development in neonatal rats during hyperoxia.[217] Recent studies demonstrated that administration of mesenchymal stem cells improved alveolar and vascular development in antenatal LPS and postnatal hyperoxia-exposed newborn rats and this is associated with increased VEGF expression.[201]

MicroRNA in Lung Development and Injury Repair

MicroRNAs (miRNAs), small noncoding RNAs that regulate gene expression by inhibition of translation and mRNA stability of target genes, have recently been implicated in lung development. Thus deletion of Dicer, the enzyme responsible for the production of miRNAs, is associated with inhibition of branching.[219] Interestingly, the miR-17 family of miRNAs controls fibroblast growth factor 10-mediated lung branching morphogenesis.[220] Recent studies have also demonstrated potential roles of miRNAs in the pathogenesis of neonatal lung injury and BPD. Microarrays have identified multiple target miRNAs, including miR-206, miR-150, and miR-489, that are dysregulated in animal models of BPD and clinical BPD. All of these miRNAs are downregulated in both clinical and experimental mouse models of BPD, whereas their predicted target genes fibronectin (miR-206), glycoprotein nonmetastatic melanoma protein b (miR-150), and insulin-like growth factor 1, and tenascin (Tnc) (miR-469) are inversely upregulated.[221–225] Importantly, inhibition of miR-489 improved lung development in hyperoxia-induced BPD.[225] A recent study demonstrated that the miR-17-92 cluster is downregulated in autopsy specimens from patients with BPD, and low levels of miR-17 and miR-92 are detected in the plasma of patients who developed BPD.[226] Despite these studies, the functional role of miRNAs in the pathogenesis of BPD needs to be further elucidated.

Conclusions

Lung development involves lung bud initiation, branching morphogenesis, saccular formation, alveolar septation, and accompanying vascular development that begins in the embryonic period and continues through fetal and postnatal periods. These dynamic processes are tightly regulated by epithelial-mesenchymal crosstalk orchestrated by groups of body patterning genes, transcriptional factors, growth factors, and ECM components. Temporospatially regulated specific cell differentiation, proliferation, and survival and ECM deposition give rise to the final complex lung structure. To add to the complexity of these cell-cell as well as cell-ECM interactions, the need to form a coordinated air passage system and blood circulating system in the lung is paramount and unmatched by any other organ system. Furthermore, airway epithelium is exposed to the atmosphere and this puts the lung at great risk for environmental injury. Significant progress has been made in our understanding of basic lung developmental processes and identification of the regulatory pathways through mouse molecular genetics and genomic studies. Many of the same signaling pathways that control normal lung development are also key players in animal models of neonatal lung injury and BPD. However, there are still many unanswered questions as to how the disruption of these pathways affects human lung development, injury, and repair, particularly in the pathogenesis of BPD. It is also unknown whether aberrant pathways in the immature lung can be reversed or prevented, and if the structural defects observed in BPD can be regenerated through modulation of these pathways. Future studies are needed to clarify the interactions between these key regulatory pathways and to identify novel signaling in animal and human lung development. These may provide new insights into BPD pathogenesis, prevention, and therapy.

REFERENCES

1. Warburton D, Schwarz M, Tefft D, Flores-Delgado G, Anderson KD, Cardoso WV. The molecular basis of lung morphogenesis. *Mech Dev.* 2000;92:5–81.
2. Weibel ER. Design and development of the mammalian lung. *London Harvard.* 1984.
3. Comore JH. Physiology of respiration. In: *Year Book, Chicago.* 1965:11–16.
4. Jeffery PK, Hislop AA, Gibson GJ, et al. Embryology and growth. In: *Respiratory Medicine.* Saunders; 2003:50–63.
5. Angus GE, Thurlbeck WM. Number of alveoli in the human lung. *J Appl Phsiol.* 1972;32:483–485.
6. Thurlbeck WM. Postnatal growth and development of the lung. *Am Rev Respir Dis.* 1975;3:803–844.
7. Husain AN, Siddiqui NH, Stocker JT. Pathology of arrested acinar development in post surfactant bronchopulmonary dysplasia. *Hum Pathol.* 1998;29:710–717.
8. Burri PH. Lung development and pulmonary angiogenesis. In: Gaultier C, Bourbon JR, Post M, eds. *Lung Development.* Clinical Physiology Series. New York: Springer; 1999.

9. Kimura S, Hara Y, Pineau T, et al. The T/ebp null mouse: thyroid-specific enhancer-binding protein is essential for the organogenesis of the thyroid, lung, ventral forebrain, and pituitary. *Genes Dev.* 1996;10:60–69.

10. Minoo P, Su G, Drum H, Bringas P, Kimura S. Defects in tracheoesophageal and lung morphogenesis in Nkx2.1 ($-/-$) mouse embryos. *Dev Biol.* 1999;209:60–71.

11. Kelly SC, Bachurski CJ, Burhans MS, Glasser SW. Transcription of the lung-specific surfactant protein C gene is mediated by thyroid transcript factor 1. *J Biol Chem.* 1996;271:6881–6888.

12. Goss AM, Tian T, Tsukiyama T, et al. Wnt2/2b and beta-catenin signaling are necessary and sufficient to specify lung progenitors in the foregut. *Dev Cell.* 2009;17(2):290–298.

13. Harris-Johnson KS, Domyan ET, Vezina CM, Sun X. Beta-catenin promotes respiratory progenitor identity in mouse foregut. *Proc Natl Acad Sci U S A.* 2009;106:16287–16292.

14. Li C, Li A, Xing Y, et al. Apc deficiency alters pulmonary epithelial cell fate and inhibits Nkx2.1 via triggering TGF-beta signaling. *Dev Biol.* 2013;378:13–24.

15. Bitgood MJ, McMahon AP. Hedgehog and BMP genes are coexpressed at many diverse sites of cell-cell interaction in the mouse embryo. *Dev Biol.* 1995;172:126–138.

16. Bellusci S, Furuta Y, Rush MG, Henderson R, Winnier G, Hogan B. Involvement of Sonic hedgehog (Shh) in mouse embryonic lung growth and morphogenesis. *Development.* 1997;124:53–63.

17. Urase K, Mukasa T, Irigashi H, et al. Spatial expression of Sonic hedgehog in the lung epithelium during branching morphogenesis. *Biochem Biophys Res Commun.* 1996;225:161–166.

18. Chiang C, Litingtung Y, Lee E, et al. Cyclopia and defective axial patterning in mice lacking Sonic hedgehog gene function. *Nature.* 1996;383:407–413.

19. Motoyama J, Liu J, Mo R, Ding Q, Post M, Hui CC. Essential function of Gli2 and Gli3 in the formation of lung, trachea and esophagus. *Nat Genet.* 1998;20:54–57.

20. Grindley JC, Bellusci S, Perkins D, Hogan BL. Evidence for the involvement of the Gli gene family in embryonic mouse lung development. *Dev Biol.* 1997;188:337–348.

21. Rankin Scott A, Han L, McCracken Kyle W, et al. A retinoic acid-hedgehog cascade coordinates mesoderm-inducing signals and endoderm competence during lung specification. *Cell Rep.* 2016;16:66–78.

22. Bellusci S, Grindley J, Emoto H, Itoh N, Hogan BL. Fibroblast growth factor 10 (FGF10) and branching morphogenesis in the embryonic lung. *Development.* 1997;124:4867–4878.

23. Sakiyama J-i, Yamagishi A, Kuroiwa A. *Tbx4-Fgf10* system controls lung bud formation during chicken embryonic development. *Development.* 2003;130:1225–1234.

24. Lüdtke Timo H, Rudat C, Wojahn I, et al. Tbx2 and Tbx3 act downstream of Shh to maintain canonical Wnt signaling during branching morphogenesis of the murine lung. *Dev Cell.* 2016;39:239–253.

25. Min H, Danilenko DM, Scully SA, et al. Fgf-10 is required for both limb and lung development and exhibits striking functional similarity to Drosophila branchless. *Gene Dev.* 1998;12:3156–3161.

26. Sekine K, Ohuchi H, Fukiwara M, et al. Fgf10 is essential for limb and lung formation. *Nat Genet.* 1999;21:138–141.

27. Rawins EL, Hogan BL. Intercellular growth factor signaling and the development of mouse tracheal submucosal glands. *Dev Dyn.* 2005;233:1378–1385.

28. Chen F, Cao Y, Qian J, Shao F, Niederreither K, Cardoso WV. A retinoic acid–dependent network in the foregut controls formation of the mouse lung primordium. *J Clin Invest.* 120:2040–2048.

29. Swarr DT, Morrisey EE. Lung endoderm morphogenesis: gasping for form and function. *Annu Rev Cell Dev Biol.* 2015;31:553–573.

30. Chen F, Desai TJ, Qian J, Niederreither K, Lü J, Cardoso WV. Inhibition of Tgfβ signaling by endogenous retinoic acid is essential for primary lung bud induction. *Development.* 2007;134:2969–2979.

31. Gallot D, Marceau G, Coste K, et al. Congenital diaphragmatic hernia: a retinoid-signaling pathway disruption during lung development? *Birth Defects Res A: Clin Mol Teratol.* 2005;73:523–531.

32. Hrycaj Steven M, Dye Briana R, Baker Nicholas C, et al. Hox5 genes regulate the Wnt2/2b-Bmp4-signaling axis during lung development. *Cell Rep.* 2015;12:903–912.

33. Morrisey EE, Hogan BLM. Preparing for the first breath: genetic and cellular mechanisms in lung development. *Dev Cell.* 2010;18:8–23.

34. Peters KG, Chen WG, Williams LT. Two FGF receptors are differentially expressed in epithelial and mesenchymal tissue during limb formation and organogenesis. *Development.* 1992;114:233–243.

35. Cardoso WV, Itoh A, Nogawa H, Mason I, Brody JS. FGF-1 and FGF-7 induce distinct patterns of growth and differentiation in embryonic lung epithelium. *Dev Dyn.* 1997;208:398–405.

36. Weaver M, Dunn NR, Hogan BL. Bmp4 and Fgf10 play opposing roles during lung bud morphogenesis. *Development.* 2000;127:2695–2704.

37. Izvolsky KI, Zhong L, Wei L, Yu Q, Nugent MA, Cardoso WV. Heparan sulfates expressed in the distal lung are required for Fgf10 binding to the epithelium and for airway branching. *Am J Phys Lung Cell Mol Physiol.* 2003;285:L838–L846.

38. Izvolsky KI, Shoykhet D, Yang Y, Yu Q, Nugent MA, Cardoso WV. Heparan sulfate–FGF10 interactions during lung morphogenesis. *Dev Biol.* 2003;258:185–200.

39. Danopoulos S, Krainock M, Toubat O, Thornton M, Grubbs B, Al Alam D. Rac1 modulates mammalian lung branching morphogenesis in part through canonical Wnt signaling. *Am J Phys Lung Cell Mol Physiol.* 2016.

40. Lebeche D, Malpel S, Cardoso WV. Fibroblast growth factor interactions in the developing lung. *Mech Dev.* 1999;86:125–136.

41. Pepicelli CV, Lewis P, McMahon A. Sonic hedgehog regulates branching morphogenesis in the mammalian lung. *Cur Biol.* 1998;8:1083–1086.

42. Herriges John C, Verheyden Jamie M, Zhang Z, et al. Control FGF-SHH feedback loop in lung branching. FGF-regulated ETV transcription factors. *Dev Cell*. 2015;35:322–332.

43. Kim HJ, Bar-Sagi D. Modulation of signaling by sprout: a developing story. *Nat Rev Mol Cell Biol*. 2004;5:441–450.

44. Mailleux AA, Tefft D, Ndiaye D, et al. Evidence that Sprouty2 functions as an inhibitor of mouse embryonic lung growth and morphogenesis. *Mech Dev*. 2001:81–94.

45. Perl AK, Hokuto I, Impagnatiello MA, Christofori G, Whitsett JA. Temporal effects of Sprouty on lung morphogenesis. *Dev Biol*. 2003;258:154–168.

46. Zhao Y, O'Brien TP. Spry2 regulates signalling dynamics and terminal bud branching behaviour during lung development. *Genet Res*. 2015;97.

47. Weaver M, Yingling JM, Dunn NR, Bellusci S, Hogan BL. Bmp signaling regulates proximal-distal differentiation of endoderm in mouse lung development. *Development*. 1999;126:400–455.

48. Weaver M, Batts L, Hogan BL. Tissue interactions pattern the mesenchyme of the embryonic mouse lung. *Dev Biol*. 2003;258:169–184.

49. Bellusci S, Henderson R, Winnier G, Oikawa T, Hogan BL. Evidence from normal expression and targeted misexpression that bone morphogenetic protein (Bmp-4) plays a role in mouse embryonic lung morphogenesis. *Development*. 1996;122:1693–1702.

50. Chen C, Chen H, Sun J, et al. Smad1 expression and function during mouse embryonic lung branching morphogenesis. *Am J Physiol Lung Cell Mol Physiol*. 2005;288:L1033–L1039.

51. Eblaghie MC, Reedy M, Oliver T, Mishina Y, Hogan BL. Evidence that autocrine signaling through Bmpr1a regulates the proliferation, survival and morphogenetic behavior of distal lung epithelial cells. *Dev Biol*. 2006;672:291.

52. Sun J, Chen H, Chen C. Prenatal lung epithelial cell-specific abrogation of Alk3-bone morphogenetic protein signaling causes neonatal respiratory distress by disrupting distal airway formation. *Am J Pathol*. 2008;172:571–582.

53. Xu B, Chen C, Chen H, et al. Smad1 and its target gene Wif1 coordinate BMP and Wnt signaling activities to regulate fetal lung development. *Development*. 2011;138:925–935.

54. Pelton RW, Jonhson MD, Perkett EA, Gold LI, Moses HL. Expression of transforming growth factor-beta 1, -beta 2, and -beta 3 mRNA and protein in the murine lung. *Am J Respir Cell Mol Biol*. 1991;5:522–530.

55. Kaartinen V, Voncken JW, Shuler C. Abnormal lung development and cleft palate in mice lacking TGF-beta 3 indicates defects of epithelial-mesenchymal interaction. *Nat Genet*. 1995;11:41–51.

56. Shi W, Heisterkamp N, Groffen J, Zhao J, Warburton D, Kaartinen V. TGF-beta3-null mutation does not abrogate fetal lung maturation in vivo by glucocorticoids. *Am J Physiol*. 1999;277:L1205–L1213.

57. McLennan IS, Poussart Y, Koishi K, Bartram U, Molin DG, Wisse LJ. Development of skeletal muscles in transforming growth factor-beta 1 (TGF-beta1) null-mutant mice. *Dev Dyn*. 2001;217:250–256.

58. Bartram U, Molin DG, Wisse LJ. Double-outlet right ventricle and overriding tricuspid valve reflect disturbances of looping, myocardialization, endocardial cushion differentiation, and apoptosis in TGF-beta(2)-knockout mice. *Circulation*. 2001;103:2745–2752.

59. Zhou L, Dey CR, Wert SE, Whitsett JA. Arrested lung morphogenesis in transgenic mice bearing an SP-C-TGF-beta 1 chimeric gene. *Dev Biol*. 1996;175:227–238.

60. Zeng X, Gray M, Stahlman MT, Whitsett JA. TGF-beta1 perturbs vascular development and inhibits epithelial differentiation in fetal lung in vivo. *Dev Dyn*. 2001;221:289–301.

61. Serra R, Pelton RW, Moses HL. TGF beta 1 inhibits branching morphogenesis and N-myc expression in lung bud organ cultures. *Development*. 1994;120:2153–2161.

62. Serra R, Moses HL. pRb is necessary for inhibition of N-myc expression by TGF-beta 1 in embryonic lung organ cultures. *Development*. 1995;121:3057–3066.

63. Wu S, Peng J, Duncan MR, Kasisomayajula K, Grotendorst G, Bancalari E. ALK-5 mediates endogenous and TGF-beta1-induced expression of CTGF in embryonic lung. *Am J Respir Cell Mol Biol*. 2007;36:552–561.

64. Zhao J, Lee M, Smith S, Warburton D. Abrogation of Smad3 and Smad2 or of Smad4 gene expression positively regulates murine embryonic lung branching morphogenesis in culture. *Dev Biol*. 1998;194:182–195.

65. Konigshoff M, Eickelberg O. Wnt signaling in lung disease: a failure or a regeneration signaling? *Am J Cell Mol Biol*. 2010;42:21–31.

66. Lako M, Strachan T, Bullen P, Wilson DI, Robson SC, Lindsey S. Isolation, characterization and embryonic expression of WNT11, a gene which maps to 11q13.5 and has possible roles in the development of skeleton kidney and lung. *Gene*. 1998;219:101–110.

67. Tebar M, Destree D, de Vree WJ, Have-Opbroek AA. Expression of Tcf/Lef and sFrp and localization of beta-catenin in the developing mouse lung. *Mech Dev*. 2001;109:437–440.

68. Levay-Young BK, Navre M. Growth and developmental regulation of WNT-2 (IRP) gene in mesenchymal cells of fetal lung. *Am J Physiol*. 1992;262:L672–L683.

69. Shu W, Jiang YQ, Lu MM, Morrisey EE. WNT7b regulates mesenchymal proliferation and vascular development in the lung. *Development*. 2002;129:4831–4842.

70. Li C, Hu L, Xiao J, et al. WNT5a regulates SHH and FGF10 signaling during lung development. *Dev Biol*. 2005;287:86–97.

71. Li C, Xiao J, Hormi K, Borok Z, Minoo P. WNT5a participates in distal lung morphogenesis. *Dev Biol*. 2002:248.

72. Caprioli A, Villasenor A, Wylie LA, et al. Wnt4 is essential to normal mammalian lung development. *Dev Biol*. 2015;406:222–234.

73. Kadzik RS, Cohen ED, Morley MP, Stewart KM, Lu MM, Morrisey EE. Wnt ligand/Frizzled 2 receptor signaling regulates tube shape and branch-point formation in the lung through control of epithelial cell shape. *Proc Natl Acad of Sci*. 2014;111:12444–12449.

74. Shu W, Guttentag S, Wang Z, et al. WNT/beta-catenin signaling acts upstream of N-myc, BMP4, and FGF signaling to regulate proximal distal patterning in the lung. *Dev Biol*. 2005;283:226–239.

75. De Langhe SP, Sala FG, Moral PM, et al. Del Dickkopf-1 (DKK1) reveals that fibronectin is a marjor target of Wnt signaling in branching morphogenesis of the mouse embryonic lung. *Dev Biol*. 2005;277:316–331.

76. Boucherat O, Montaron S, Bérubé-Simard F-A, et al. Partial functional redundancy between *Hoxa5* and *Hoxb5* paralog genes during lung morphogenesis. *Am J Physiol Lung Cell Mol Physiol*. 2013;304:L817–L830.

77. Coraux C, Meneguzzi G, Rousselle P, Puchelle E, Gaillard D. Distribution of laminin 5, integrin receptors, and branching morphogenesis during human fetal lung development. *Dev Dyn*. 2002;225:176–185.

78. Benjamin JT, Gaston DC, Halloran BA, Schnapp LM, Zent R, Prince LS. The role of integrin alpha-8beta1 in fetal lung morphogenesis and injury. *Dev Biol*. 2009;335:407–417.

79. Chen J, Krasnow MA. Integrin beta 1 suppresses multilayering of a simple epithelium. *PLoS One*. 2012:7.

80. Sakai T, Larsen M, Yamada KM. Fibronectin requirement in branching morphogenesis. *Nature*. 2003;423:876–881.

81. Oblander SA, Zhou Z, Gálvez BG, et al. Distinctive functions of membrane type 1 matrix metalloprotease (MT1-MMP or MMP-14) in lung and submandibular gland development are independent of its role in pro-MMP-2 activation. *Dev Biol*. 2005;277:255–269.

82. Greenlee KJ, Werb Z, Kheradmand F. Matrix metalloproteinases in lung: multiple, multifarious, and multifaceted. *Physiol Rev*. 2007;87:69–98.

83. Abman SH, Baker C, Balasubramaniam V. Growth and development of the lung circulation: mechanisms and clinical implications. In: Bancalari E, Polin RA, eds. *The Newborn Lung*. Saunders: Elsevier; 2008:50–72.

84. Schultz CJ, Torres E, Londos C, Torday JS. Role of adipocyte differentiation-related protein in surfactant phospholipid synthesis by type II cells. *Am J Physiol Lung Cell Mol Physiol L288296*. 2002:283.

85. McGowan SE, McCoy DM. Regulation of fibroblast lipid storage and myofibroblast phenotypes during alveolar septation in mice. *Am J Physiol Lung Cell Mol Physiol*. 2014;307: L618–L631.

86. McGowan SE, Grossmann RE, Kimani PW, Holmes AJ. Platelet-derived growth factor receptor-alpha-expressing cells localize to the alveolar entry ring and have characteristics of myofibroblasts during pulmonary alveolar septal formation. *Anat Rec Hoboken*. 2008;291:1649–1661.

87. Adler KB, Low RB, Leslie KO, Mitchell J, Evans JN. Contractile cells in normal and fibrotic lung. *Lab Invest*. 1989;60:473–485.

88. Leslie KO, Mitchell JJ, Woodcock-Mitchell JL, Low RB. Alpha smooth muscle actin expression in developing and adult human lung. *Differentiation*. 1990;44:143–149.

89. Berk JL, Franzblau C, Goldstein RH. Recombinant interleukin-1 beta inhibits elastin formation by a neonatal rat lung fibroblast subtype. *J Biol Chem*. 1991;266:3192–3197.

90. Kagan HM, Li W. Lysyl oxidase: properties, specificity, and biological roles inside and outside of cell. *J Cell Biochem*. 2003;88:660–672.

91. Lindahl P, Karlsson L, Hellstrom M, et al. Alveogenesis failure in PDGF-A-deficient mice is coupled to lack of distal spreading of alveolar smooth muscle cell progenitors during lung development. *Development*. 1997;124:3943–3953.

92. Boström H, Willetts K, Pekny MPL, et al. PDGF-A signaling is a critical event in lung alveolar myofibroblast development and alveogenesis. *Cell*. 1996;85:863–873.

93. Lau M, Masood A, Yi M, Belcastro R, Li J, Tanswell AK. Long-term failure of alveologenesis after an early short-term exposure to a PDGF-receptor antagonist. *Am J Physiol Lung Cell Mol Physiol*. 2011;300:L534–L547.

94. Weinstein M, Xu X, Ohyama K, Deng CX. FGFR-3 and FGFR-4 function cooperatively to direct alveogenesis in the murine lung. *Development*. 1998;125:3615–3623.

95. McGowan S, Jackson SK, Jenkins-Moore M, Dai HH, Chambon P, Snyder JM. Mice bearing deletions of retinoic acid receptors demonstrate reduced lung elastin and alveolar numbers. *Am J Respir Cell Mol Biol*. 2000;23:162–167.

96. Chen H, Chang L, Liu H, et al. Effect of retinoic acid on platelet-derived growth factor and lung development in newborn rats. *Univ Sci Technolog Med Sci*. 2004;24:226–228.

97. Chailley-Heu B, Boucherat O, Barlier-Mur AM, Bourbon JR. J. FGF-18 is up-regulated in the postnatal rat lung and enhances elastogenesis in myofibroblasts. *Am J Physiol Lung Cell Mol Physiol. L4351*. 2005:288.

98. Perl AK, Gale E. FGF signaling is required for myofibroblast differentiation during alveolar regeneration. *Am J Physiol Lung Cell Mol Physiol*. 2009;297:L299–L308.

99. Tsao PN, Matsuoka C, Wei SC, et al. Epithelial Notch signaling regulates lung alveolar morphogenesis and airway epithelial integrity. *Proc Natl Acad Sci U S A*. 2016;113:8242–8247.

100. Massaro D, Alexander E, Reiland K, Hoffman EP, Massaro GD, Clerch LB. Rapid onset of gene expression in lung, supportive of formation of alveolar septa, induced by refeeding mice after calorie restriction. *Am J Physiol Lung Cell Mol Physiol*. 2007;292:L1313–L1326.

101. Londhe VA, Maisonet TM, Lopez B, Shin BC, Huynh J, Devaskar SU. Retinoic acid rescues alveolar hypoplasia in the calorie-restricted developing rat lung. *Am J Respir Cell Mol Biol*. 2013;48:179–187.

102. Ambalavanan N, Nicola T, Hagood J, et al. Transforming growth factor-β signaling mediates hypoxia-induced pulmonary arterial remodeling and inhibition of alveolar development in newborn mouse lung. *Am J Physiol Lung Cell Mol Physiol*. 2008;295:L86–L95.

103. Alejandre-Alcázar MA, Kwapiszewska G, Reiss I, et al. Hyperoxia modulates TGF-β/BMP signaling in a mouse model of bronchopulmonary dysplasia. *Am J Physiol Lung Cell Mol Physiol*. 2007;292:L537–L549.

104. Garber SJ, Zhang H, Foley JP, et al. Hormonal regulation of alveolarization: structure-function correlation. *Respir Res*. 2006;7:47.

105. Zhang H, Garber SJ, Cui Z, et al. The angiogenic factor midkine is regulated by dexamethasone and retinoic acid during alveolarization and in alveolar epithelial cells. *Respir Res*. 2009;10:77.

106. le Cras TD, Markham NE, Morris KG, Ahrens CR, McMurtry IF, Abman SH. Neonatal dexamethasone treatment increases the risk for pulmonary hypertension in adult rats. *Am J Physiol Lung Cell Mol Physiol*. 2000;278:L822–L829.

107. Que J, Luo X, Schwartz RJ, Hogan BLM. Multiple roles for Sox2 in the developing and adult mouse trachea. *Development*. 2009;136:1899–1907.

108. Rawlins EL, Ostrowski LE, Randell SH, Hogan BLM. Lung development and repair: contribution of the ciliated lineage. *Proc Natl Acad Sci*. 2007;104:410–417.

109. Guseh JS, Bores SA, Stanger BZ, et al. Notch signaling promotes airway mucous metaplasia and inhibits alveolar development. *Development*. 2009;136:1751–1759.

110. Treutlein B, Brownfield DG, Wu AR, et al. Reconstructing lineage hierarchies of the distal lung epithelium using single-cell RNA-seq. *Nature*. 2014;509:371–375.

111. Whitsett JA, Wert SE, Weaver TE. Diseases of pulmonary surfactant homeostasis. *Annu Rev Pathol*. 2015;10:371–393.

112. Bridges JP, Ludwig MG, Mueller M, et al. Orphan G protein-coupled receptor GPR116 regulates pulmonary surfactant pool size. *Am J Respir Cell Mol Biol*. 2013;49:348–357.

113. Yang Mi Y, Hilton Mary B, Seaman S, et al. Essential regulation of lung surfactant homeostasis by the orphan G protein-coupled receptor GPR116. *Cell Rep*. 2013;3:1457–1464.

114. Burri PH, Hlushchuk R, Djonov V. Intrussusceptive angiogenesis: its emergence, its characteristics, and its significance. *Dev Dynamics*. 2004;231:474–488.

115. DeMello DE, Sawyer D, Galvin N, Reid LM. Early fetal development of lung vasculature. *Am J Respir Cell Mol Biol*. 1997;16:568–581.

116. DeMello DE, Reid LM. Embryonic and early fetal development of human lung vasculature and its functional implications. *Pediatr Dev Pathol*. 2000;3:439–449.

117. Schachtner SK, Wang Y, Scott-Baldwin H. Qualitative and quantitative analysis of embryonic pulmonary vessel formation. *Am Cell Mol Biol*. 2000;22:157–165.

118. Hall SM, Hislop AA, Haworth SG. Origin, differentiation, and maturation of human pulmonary veins. *Am J Respir Cell Mol Biol*. 2002;26:333–340.

119. Parera MC, van Dooren M, van Kempan M, et al. Distal angiogenesis: a new concept for lung vascular morphogenesis. *Am J Physiol Lung Cell Mol Physiol*. 2005;288:L141–L149.

120. Schwarz MA, Caldwell L, Cafasso D, Zheng H. Emerging pulmonary vasculature lacks fate specification. *Am J Physiol Lung Cell Mol Physiol*. 2009;296:L71–L81.

121. Ferrara N, Hauck K, Jakeman L, Leung DW. Molecular and biological properties of the vascular endothelial growth factor families of protein. *Endocr Rev*. 1992;13:18–32.

122. Stenmark KR, Abman SH. Lung vascular development: implication for the pathogenesis of brochopulmoanry dysplasia. *Annu Rev Physiol*. 2005;67:623–661.

123. Ng YS, Rohan R, Sunday ME, Demello DE, D'Amore PA. Differential expression of VEGF isoforms in mouse during development and in the adult. *Dev Dyn*. 2001;220:112–121.

124. Millauer B, Wizigmann-Voos S, Schnurch S, et al. High affinity VEGF binding and developmental expression suggest Flk-1 as a major regulator of vasculogenesis and angiogenesis. *Cell*. 1993;72:835–846.

125. Carmeliet P, Ferreira V, Breier G, et al. Abnormal blood vessel development and lethality in embryos lacking a single VEGF allele. *Nature*. 1996;380:435–439.

126. Ferrara N, Gerber HP, LeCouter J. The biology of VEGF and its receptors. *Nat Med*. 2003;9:669–676.

127. Fong GH, Rossant J, Gertsenstein M, Breitman ML. Role of the Flt-1 receptor tyrosine kinase in regulating the assembly of vascular endothelium. *Nature*. 1995;376:66–70.

128. Shalaby F, Rossant J, Yamaguchi TP, et al. Failure of blood-island formation and vasculogenesis in Flk-1-deficient mice. *Nature*. 1995;376:62–66.

129. Yamamoto H, Jun Yun E, Gerber H-P, Ferrara N, Whitsett JA, Vu TH. Epithelial–vascular cross talk mediated by VEGF-A and HGF signaling directs primary septae formation during distal lung morphogenesis. *Dev Biol*. 2007;308:44–53.

130. Yun EJ, Lorizio W, Seedorf G, Abman SH, Vu TH. VEGF and endothelium-derived retinoic acid regulate lung vascular and alveolar development. *Am J Physiol Lung Cell Mol Physiol*. 2016;310:L287–L298.

131. White AC, Lavine KJ, Ornitz DM. FGF9 and SHH regulate mesenchymal Vegfa expression and development of the pulmonary capillary network. *Development*. 2007;134:3743–3752.

132. Le Cras TD, Markham NE, Tuder RM, Voelkel NF, Abman SH. Treatment of newborn rats with a VEGF receptor inhibitor causes pulmonary hypertension and abnormal lung structure. *Am J Lung Cell Mol Physiol*. 2002;283:L555–L562.

133. Tang JR, Markham NE, Lin YJ, et al. Inhaled nitric oxide attenuates pulmonary hypertension and improves lung growth in infant rats after neonatal treatment with a VEGF receptor inhibitor. *Am J Physiol Lung Cell Mol Physiol*. 2004;287:L344–L351.

134. Leuwerke SM, Kaza AK, Tribble CG, Kron IL, Laubach VE. Inhibition of compensatory lung growth in endothelial nitric oxide synthase-deficient mice. *Am J Physiol Lung Cell Mol Physiol*. 2002;282:L1272–L1278.

135. Han RN, Babaei S, Robb M, et al. Defective lung vascular development and fatal respiratory distress in endothelial NO synthase-deficient mice: a model of alveolar capillary dysplasia? *Circ Res*. 2004;94:1115–1123.

136. Sato TN, Qin Y, Kozak CA, Audus KL. Tie-1 and tie-2 define another class of putative receptor tyrosine kinase genes expressed in early embryonic vascular system. *Proc Natl Acad Sci U S A*. 1993;90:9355–9358.

137. Davis S, Aldrich TH, Jones PF, et al. Isolation of angiopoietin-1, a ligand for the TIE2 receptor, by secretion-trap expression cloning. *Cell*. 1996;87:1161–1169.

138. Augustin HG, Koh GY, Thurston G, Alitalo K. Control of vascular morphogenesis and homeostatsis through the angiopoietin-tie system. *Nat Rev Mol Cell Biol*. 2009;6:165–177.

139. Brindle NPJ, Saharinen P, Alitalo A. Signaling and functions of angiopoietin-1 in vascular protection. *Circ Res*. 2006;98:1014–1023.

140. Sato TN, Tozawa Y, Deutsch U, et al. Distinct roles of receptor tyrosin kinase Tie-1 and Tie-2 in blood vessel formation. *Nature*. 1995;376:70–74.

141. Suri C, Jones PF, Patan S, et al. Requisite role of angiopoietin-1, a ligand for tie2 receptor, during embryonic angiogenesis. *Cell*. 1996;87:1171–1180.

142. Dumont DJ, Gradwohl G, Fong GH, et al. Dominant-negative and targeted null mutations in the endothelial receptor tyrosin kinase, tek, reveal a critical role in vasculogenesis. *Genes Dev*. 1994;8:1897–1909.

143. Hato T, Kimura Y, Morisada T, et al. Angiopoietins contribute to lung development by regulating pulmonary vascular network formation. *Biochem Biophys Res Commun*. 2009;381:218–223.

144. Mammoto T, Chen J, Jiang E, et al. LRP5 regulates development of lung microvessels and alveoli through the angiopoietin-Tie2 pathway. *PLoS One*. 2012;7.

145. Rudge JS, Thurston G, Rancopoulos GD. Angiopoietin a and pulmonary hypertension: cause or cure? *Circ Res*. 2003;92:947–949.

146. Chu D, Sullivan CC, Du L, et al. A new animal model for pulmonary hypertension based on the overexpression of a single gene, angiopoietin-1. *Ann Thorac Surg*. 2004;77:449–456.

147. Zhao YD, Campbell AI, Robb M, Ng D, Stewart DJ. Protective role of angiopoietin-1 in experimental pulmonary hypertension. *Circ Res*. 2003;92:984–991.

148. Taichman DB, Loomes KM, Schachtner SK, et al. Notch1 and Jagged1 expression by the developing pulmonary vasculature. *Dev Dyn*. 2002;225:166–175.

149. Wilkinson GA, Schittny JC, Reinhardt DP, Klein R. Role for ephrinB2 in postnatal lung alveolar development and elastic matrix integrity. *Dev Dyn*. 2008;237:2220–2234.

150. Jobe AH. The new bronchopulmonary dysplasia. *Curr Opin Pediatr*. 2011;23:167–172.

151. Kallapur SG, Jobe AH. Contribution of inflammation to lung injury and development. *Arch Dis Child Fetal Neonatal Ed*. 2006;91:F132–F135.

152. Ryan RM, Ahmed Q, Lakshminrusimha S. Inflammatory mediators in the immunobiology of bronchopulmonary dysplasia. *Clin Rev Aller Immunol*. 2008;34:174–190.

153. Becker CE, O'Neill LAJ. Inflammasomes in inflammatory disorders: the role of TLRs and their interactions with NLRs. *Semin Immunopathol*. 2007;29:239–248.

154. Gao H, Leaver SK, Burke-Gaffney A, Finney SJ. Severe sepsis and Toll-like receptors. *Semin Immunopathol*. 2008;30:29–40.

155. Ye Z, Ting JP-Y. NLR, the nucleotide-binding domain leucine-rich repeat containing gene family. *Curr Opin Immunol*. 2008;20:3–9.

156. Mariathasan S, Monack DM. Inflammasome adaptors and sensors: intracellular regulators of infection and inflammation. *Nat Rev Immunol*. 2007;7:31–40.

157. Pétrilli V, Dostert C, Muruve DA, Tschopp J. The inflammasome: a danger sensing complex triggering innate immunity. *Cur Opin Immunol*. 2007;19:615–622.

158. Benko S, Philpott DJ, Girardin SE. The microbial and danger signals that activate Nod-like receptors. *Cytokine*. 2008;43:368–373.

159. Mariathasan S, Weiss DS, Newton K, et al. Cryopyrin activates the inflammasome in response to toxins and ATP. *Nature*. 2006;440:228–232.

160. Kolliputi N, Shaik RS, Waxman AB. The inflammasome mediates hyperoxia-induced alveolar cell permeability. *J Immunol*. 2010;184:5819–5826.

161. Liao J, Kapadia VS, Brown LS, et al. The NLRP3 inflammasome is critically involved in the development of bronchopulmonary dysplasia. *Nat Commun*. 2015;6.

162. Hummler JK, Dapaah-siakwan F, Vaidya R, et al. Inhibition of Rac1 signaling downregulates inflammasome activation and attenuates lung injury in neonatal rats exposed to hyperoxia. *Neonatology*. 2017;111:280–288.

163. Masters SL, Simon A, Aksentijevich I, Kastner DL. Horror autoinflammaticus: the molecular pathophysiology of autoinflammatory disease. *Annu Rev Immunol*. 2009;27:621–668.

164. Goldbach-Mansky R, Kastner DL. Autoinflammation: the prominent role of IL-1 in monogenic autoinflammatory diseases and implications for common illnesses. *J Allergy Clin Immunol*. 2009;124:1141–1151.

165. Goldfinger S. The inherited autoinflammatory syndrome: a decade of discovery. *Trans Am Clin Climatol Assoc.* 2009;120:413–418.

166. Sibley CH, Plass N, Snow J, et al. Sustained response and prevention of damage progression in patients with neonatal-onset multisystem inflammatory disease treated with anakinra: a cohort study to determine three- and five-year outcomes. *Arthritis Rheum.* 2012;64:2375–2386.

167. Yoon BH, Romero R, Jun JK, et al. Amniotic fluid cytokines (interleukin-6, tumor necrosis factor-α, interleukin-1β, and interleukin-8) and the risk for the development of bronchopulmonary dysplasia. *Am J Obstetr Gynecol.* 1997;177:825–830.

168. Kotecha S, Wilson L, Wangoo A, Silverman M, Shaw RJ. Increase in interleukin (IL)-1[beta] and IL-6 in bronchoalveolar lavage fluid obtained from infants with chronic lung disease of prematurity. *Pediatr Res.* 1996;40:250–256.

169. Rindfleisch MS, Hasday JD, Taciak V, Broderick K, Viscardi RM. Potential role of interleukin-1 in the development of bronchopulmonary dysplasia. *J Interferon Cytokine Res.* 1996;16:365–373.

170. Kakkera DK, Siddiq MM, Parton LA. Interleukin-1 balance in the lungs of preterm infants who develop bronchopulmonary dysplasia. *Neonatology.* 2005;87:82–90.

171. Bry K, Whitsett JA, Lappalainen U. IL-1β Disrupts postnatal lung morphogenesis in the mouse. *Am J Respir Cell Mol Biol.* 2007;36:32–42.

172. Lappalainen U, Whitsett JA, Wert SE, Tichelaar JW, Bry K. Interleukin-1β causes pulmonary inflammation, emphysema, and airway remodeling in the adult murine lung. *Am J Respir Cell and Mol Biol.* 2005;32:311–318.

173. Johnson B-H, Yi M, Masood A, et al. A critical role for the IL-1 receptor in lung injury induced in neonatal rats by 60% O_2. *Pediatr Res.* 2009;66:260–265.

174. Nold MF, Mangan NE, Rudloff I, et al. Interleukin-1 receptor antagonist prevents murine broncho-pulmonary dysplasia induced by perinatal inflammation and hyperoxia. *Proc Natl Acad Sci U S A.* 2013;110:14384–14389.

175. Kotecha S, Wangoo A, Silverman M, Shaw RJ. Increase in the concentration of transforming growth factor beta-1 in bronchoalveolar lavage fluid before development of chronic lung disease of prematurity. *J Pediatr.* 1996;128:464–469.

176. Ichiba H, Saito M, Yamano T. Amniotic fluid transforming growth factor-beta1 and the risk for the development of neonatal bronchopulmonary dysplasia. *Neonatology.* 2009;96:156–157.

177. Kunzmann S, Speer CP, Jobe AH, Kramer BW. Antenatal inflammation induced TGF-beta1 but suppressed CTGF in preterm lungs. *Am J Physiol Lung Cell Mol Physiol.* 2007;292:L223–L231.

178. Bland RD, Xu L, Ertsey R, et al. Dysregulation of pulmonary elastin synthesis and assembly in preterm lambs with chronic lung disease. *Am J Physiol Lung Cell Mol Physiol.* 2007;292:L1370–L1384.

179. Kumarasamy A, Schmitt I, Nave AH, et al. Lysyl oxidase activity is dysregulated during impaired alveolarization of mouse and human lungs. *Am Crit Care Med.* 2009;180:1239–1252.

180. Tarantal AF, Chen H, Shi TT, et al. Overexpression of transforming growth factor-β1 in fetal monkey lung results in prenatal pulmonary fibrosis. *Eur Respir J.* 2010;36:907–914.

181. Vicencio AG, Lee CG, Cho SJ, et al. Conditional overexpression of bioactive transforming factor-beta1 in neonatal mouse lung: a new model for bronchopulmonary dysplasia? *Am J Respir Cell Mol Biol.* 2004;31:650–656.

182. Sureshbabu A, Syed MA, Boddupalli CS, et al. Conditional overexpression of TGFβ1 promotes pulmonary inflammation, apoptosis and mortality via TGFβR2 in the developing mouse lung. *Respir Res.* 2015;16:4.

183. Ahlfeld SK, Wang J, Gao Y, Snider P, Conway SJ. Initial suppression of transforming growth factor-β signaling and loss of TGFBI causes early alveolar structural defects resulting in bronchopulmonary dysplasia. *Am J Pathol.* 2016;186:777–793.

184. Nakanishi H, Sugiura T, Streisand JB, Lonning SM, Roberts JD. TGF beta-neutralizing antibodies improve pulmonary alveologenesis and vasculogenesis in the injured newborn lung. *Am J Physiol Lung Cell Mol Physiol.* 2007;293:L151–161.

185. Dasgupta C, Sakurai R, Wang Y, et al. Hyperoxia-induced neonatal rat lung injury involves activation of TGF-{beta} and Wnt signaling and is protected by rosiglitazone. *Am J Physiol Lung Cell Mol Physiol.* 2009;296:L1031–L1041.

186. Sakurai R, Li Y, Torday JS, Rehan VK. Curcumin augments lung maturation, preventing neonatal lung injury by inhibiting TGF-β signaling. *Am J Physiol Lung Cell Mol Physiol.* 2011;301:L721–L730.

187. Varga J, Pasche B. Transforming growth factor beta as a therapeutic target in systemic sclerosis. *Nat Rev Rheumatol.* 2009;5:200–206.

188. Leask A, Abraham DJ. All in the CCN family: essential matricellular signaling modulators emerge from the bunker. *J Cell Sci.* 2006;119:4803–4810.

189. Grotendorst GR, Rahmanie H, Duncan MR. Combinatorial signaling pathways determine fibroblast proliferation and myofibroblast differentiation. *FASEB J.* 2004;18:469–479.

190. Kireeva ML, Latinkic BV, Kolesnikova TV, et al. Cyr61 and Fisp12 are both ECM-associated signaling molecules: activities, metabolism, and localization during development. *Exp Cell Res.* 1997;233:63–77.

191. Ivkovic S, Yoon BS, Popoff SN, et al. Connective tissue growth factor coordinates chondrogenesis and angiogenesis during skeletal development. *Development.* 2003;130:2779–2791.

192. Baguma-Nibasheka M, Kablar B. Pulmonary hypoplasia in the connective tissue growth factor (Ctgf) null mouse. *Dev Dyn.* 2008;237:485–493.

193. Wu S, Platteau A, Chen S, McNamara G, Whitsett J, Bancalari E. Conditional over-expression of connective tissue growth factor disrupts postnatal lung development. *Am J Respir Cell Mol Biol.* 2010;42:552–563.

194. Chen S, Rong M, Platteau A, et al. CTGF disrupts alveolarization and induces PH in neonatal mice: implication in the pathogenesis of severe bronchopulmonary dysplasia. *Am J Physiol Lung Cell Mol Physiol.* 2011;300:L330–L340.

195. Alejandre-Alcázar MA, Kwapiszewska G, Reiss I, et al. Hyperoxia modulates TGF-beta/BMP signaling in a mouse model of bronchopulmonary dysplasia. *Am J Physiol Lung Cell Mol Physiol.* 2007;292:L537–L549.

196. Chen CM, Wang LF, Chou HC, Lang YD, Lai YP. Up-regulation of connective tissue growth factor in hyperoxia-induced lung fibrosis. *Pediatr Res.* 2007;62:128–133.

197. Wu S, Capasso L, Lessa A, et al. High tidal volume ventilation up-regulates CTGF expression in the lung of newborn rats. *Pediatr Res.* 2008;63:245–250.

198. Wallace MJ, Probyn ME, Zahra VA, et al. Early biomarkers and potential mediators of ventilation-induced lung injury in very preterm lambs. *Respir Res.* 2009:10–19.

199. Collins JJP, Kunzmann S, Kuypers E, et al. Antenatal glucocorticoids counteract LPS changes in TGF-β pathway and caveolin-1 in ovine fetal lung. *Am J Physiol Lung Cell Mol Physiol.* 2013;304:L438–L444.

200. Alapati D, Rong M, Chen S, et al. CTGF antibody therapy attenuates hyperoxiainduced lung injury in neonatal rats. *Am J Respir Cell Mol Biol.* 2011;45:1169–1177.

201. Chou HC, Li YT, Chen CM. Human mesenchymal stem cells attenuate experimental bronchopulmonary dysplasia induced by perinatal inflammation and hyperoxia. *Am J Transl Res.* 2016;8:342–353.

202. Kambas K, Chrysanthopoulou A, Kourtzelis I, et al. Endothelin-1 signaling promotes fibrosis in vitro in a bronchopulmonary dysplasia model by activating the extrinsic coagulation cascade. *J Immunol.* 2011;186:6568–6575.

203. Lassus P, Ristimäki A, Ylikorkala O, Viinikka L, Andersson S. Vascular endothelial growth factor in human preterm lung. *Am J Crit Care Med.* 1999;159:1429–1433.

204. Bhatt AJ, Pryhuber GS, Huyck H, Watkins RH, Metlay LA, Maniscalco WM. Disrupted pulmonary vasculature and decreased vascular endothelial growth factor, Flt-1, and TIE-2 in human infants dying with bronchopulmonary dysplasia. *Am J Respir Crit Care Med.* 2001;164:1971–1980.

205. De Paepe ME, Mao Q, Powell J, et al. Growth of pulmonary microvasculature in ventilated preterm infants. *Am J Respir Crit Care Med.* 2006;173:204–211.

206. De Paepe ME, Patel C, Tsai A, Gundavarapu S, Mao Q. Endoglin (CD105) up-regulation in pulmonary microvasculature of ventilated preterm infants. *Am J Respir Crit Care Med.* 2008;178:180–187.

207. Fujioka K, Shibata A, Yokota T, et al. Association of a vascular endothelial growth factor polymorphism with the development of bronchopulmonary dysplasia in Japanese premature newborns. *Sci Rep.* 2014:4.

208. Maniscalco WM, Watkins RH, D'Angio CT, Ryan RM. Hyperoxic injury decreases alveolar epithelial cell expression of vascular endothelial growth factor (VEGF) in neonatal rabbit lung. *Am J Respir Cell Mol Biol.* 1997;16:557–567.

209. Hosford GE, Olson DM. Effects of hyperoxia on VEGF, its receptors, and HIF-2alpha in the newborn rat lung. *Am J Physiol Lung Cell Mol Physiol.* 2003;285:L161–L168.

210. Mokres LM, Parai K, Hilgendorff A, et al. Prolonged mechanical ventilation with air induces apoptosis and causes failure of alveolar septation and angiogenesis in lungs of newborn mice. *Am J Physiol Lung Cell Mol Physiol.* 2010;298:L23–L35.

211. Maniscalco WM, Watkins RH, Pryhuber GS, Bhatt A, Shea C, Huyck H. Angiogenic factors and alveolar vasculature: development and alterations by injury in very premature baboons. *Am J Respir Lung Cell Mol Physiol.* 2002;282:L811–L823.

212. Tambunting F, Beharry KD, Waltzman J, Modanlou HD. Impaired lung vascular endothelial growth factor in extremely premature baboons developing bronchopulmonary dysplasia/chronic lung disease. *J Investig Med.* 2005;53:253–262.

213. Cao L, Wang J, Tseu I, Luo D, Post M. Maternal exposure to endotoxin delays alveolarization during postnatal rat lung development. *Am J Physiol Lung Cell Mol Physiol.* 2009;296:L726–L737.

214. Tang JR, Karumanchi SA, Seedorf G, Markham N, Abman SH. Excess soluble vascular endothelial growth factor receptor-1 in amniotic fluid impairs lung growth in rats: linking preeclampsia with bronchopulmonary dysplasia. *Am J Physiol Lung Cell Mol Physiol.* 2012;302:L36–L46.

215. Kunig AM, Balasubramaniam V, Markham NE, Seedorf G, Gien J, Abman SH. Recombinant human VEGF treatment transiently increases lung edema but enhances lung structure after neonatal hyperoxia. *Am J Physiol Lung Cell Mol Physiol.* 2006;291:L1068–L1078.

216. Kunig AM, Balasubramaniam V, Markham NE, et al. Recombinant human VEGF treatment enhances alveolarization after hyperoxic lung injury in neonatal rats. *Am J Physiol Lung Cell Mol Physiol.* 2005;289:L529–L535.

217. Thébaud B, Ladha F, Michelakis ED, et al. Vascular endothelial growth factor gene therapy increases survival, promotes lung angiogenesis, and prevents alveolar damage in hyperoxia-induced lung injury: evidence that angiogenesis participates in alveolarization. *Circulation.* 2005;112(16):2477–2486.

218. Le Cras TD, Spitzmiller RE, Albertine KH, Greenberg JM, Whitsett JA, Akeson AL. VEGF causes pulmonary hemorrhage, hemosiderosis, and air space enlargement in neonatal mice. *Am J Physiol Lung Cell Mol Physiol.* 2004;287:L134–L142.

219. Harris KS, Zhang Z, McManus MT, Harfe BD, Sun X. Dicer function is essential for lung epithelium morphogenesis. *Proc Natl Acad Sci U S A.* 2006;103:2208–2213.

220. Carraro G, El-Hashash A, Guidolin D, et al. miR-17 family of microRNAs controls FGF10-mediated embryonic lung epithelial branching morphogenesis through MAPK14 and STAT3 regulation of E-Cadherin distribution. *Dev Biol*. 2009;333:238–250.
221. Bhaskaran M, Xi D, Wang Y, et al. Identification of microRNAs changed in the neonatal lungs in response to hyperoxia exposure. *Physiol Genomics*. 2012;44:970–980.
222. Nardiello C, Morty RE. MicroRNA in late lung development and bronchopulmonary dysplasia: the need to demonstrate causality. *Mol Cell Pediatr*. 2016:3.
223. Zhang X, Xu J, Wang J, et al. Reduction of micro-RNA contributes to the development of broncho-pulmonary dysplasia through up-regulation of fibronectin 1. *PLoS One*. 2013:8.
224. Narasaraju T, Shukla D, More S, et al. Role of microRNA-150 and glycoprotein nonmetastatic melanoma protein B in angiogenesis during hyperoxia-induced neonatal lung injury. *Am J Respir Cell Mol Biol*. 2015;52:253–261.
225. Olave N, Lal CV, Halloran B, et al. Regulation of alveolar septation by microRNA-489. *Am J Physiol Lung Cell Mol Physiol*. 2016;310:L476–L487.
226. Rogers LK, Robbins M, Dakhlallah D, et al. Attenuation of miR-17~92 cluster in bronchopulmonary dysplasia. *Ann Am Thorac Soc*. 2015;12:1506–1513.

1

CHAPTER 2

Perinatal Events and Their Influence on Lung Development and Injury

Suhas G. Kallapur and Alan H. Jobe

- Multiple antenatal exposures have effects on the fetal lung—some adverse and other beneficial for postnatal survival.
- Antenatal exposures can alter lung development and interact with postnatal exposures.
- Early gestational lung maturation is common and promoted by both antenatal steroids and fetal exposure to inflammation.
- Trials indicate that antenatal steroid use may expand to late preterm infants and elective cesarean section.
- Antenatal steroid is a common exposure that may interact with postnatal care practices in presently unknown ways.
- Sepsis with chorioamnionitis is an infrequent event in term and near-term infants.
- Fetal exposure to inflammation/chorioamnionitis results in complex immunomodulation that may alter postnatal exposure.
- Growth restriction and maternal tobacco and alcohol use alter fetal lung development with effects on post-delivery outcomes.

Overview of Lung Development and Perinatal Events

Lung growth and development are the substrate on which all lung outcomes ultimately depend. This chapter emphasizes four categories of events that can modulate fetal and subsequent postnatal lung development and thus alter lung outcomes for a lifetime (Fig. 2.1). McElrath and colleagues[1] propose that there are two pathologic pathways that result in deliveries at very early gestational age (GA): intrauterine inflammation that is often chronic and aberrations of placentation/vascular development. Other examples of clinically relevant modulators of lung development are small for gestational age/intrauterine growth restriction (SGA/IUGR) and environmental exposures such as maternal tobacco and alcohol use. Lung maturation is a late phase of lung development that can be accelerated by antenatal corticosteroids and by fetal exposure to inflammation. Although infection can induce lung maturation, fetal exposures to acute or chronic chorioamnionitis also can injure the lung. There are two "elephants in the room" for this discussion of events that influence lung development. The first is the concept of what is considered normal. Any discussion of premature lungs is complicated by the lack of a normal comparison group with which to evaluate the impact of the perinatal event of interest. Although the words *all* or *never* should be sparingly used in biology and medicine, all very low-birth-weight (VLBW) deliveries must be regarded as adverse pregnancy outcomes. The 24-week GA newborn who does not have respiratory distress syndrome (RDS) is a true wonder of nature.

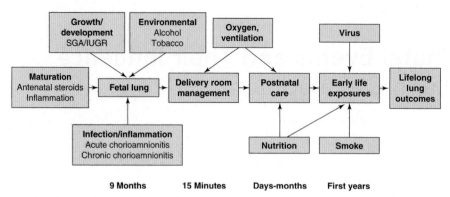

Fig. 2.1 Sketch of factors that modulate the fetal lung development and function. Some effectors that alter lung development after delivery also are indicated. *IUGR*, Intrauterine growth retardation; *SGA*, small for gestational age.

The second "elephant" is the complexity of the entangled pathways that regulate lung development, injury, and repair for any perinatal event that affects the lung. These three cellular and molecular response programs share signaling pathways superimposed simultaneously or sequentially on the immature lung. This complexity confounds simple interpretations about what mediator is causing which outcome. Finally, outcomes such as bronchopulmonary dysplasia (BPD) and asthma/airway disease in childhood and later life may be initiated by fetal events that then are modulated by postnatal responses of the lungs. An example is early life exposures to viral infections.[2] This biologic complexity generates inconsistencies in clinical data and controversies. In this chapter, we provide our current understanding of how prenatal exposure to various conditions can change postnatal lung function based on both clinical information and animal models.

Lung Development: The Substrate for Adverse Events

Lung development is programmed by the fetus to be sufficiently mature to adapt rapidly to air breathing at birth. The timing of the structural development of the lung in Fig. 2.2 is given as weeks from the last menstrual period and from conception to emphasize the 2-week difference. Infants born by elective cesarean section as early term infants (38 weeks postmenstrual age) have more problems with pulmonary adaptation than infants born at 40 weeks postmenstrual age.[3,4] Late preterm infants have more lung adaptation problems and more RDS for each week of birth prior to 37 weeks.[5] Finally, lung adaptation abnormalities, RDS, and subsequently BPD become increasingly frequent as GA decreases into the early GA and very early GA categories of preterm infants.[6]

Lung development includes development of the structural elements as well as functional maturation of fluid clearance pathways and the surfactant system. The major structural events are the completion of airway branching by about 18 weeks of gestation, followed by three generations of airway divisions to form respiratory bronchioles, and three more divisions to form alveolar ducts to about 32 to 36 weeks.[7] Subsequently, secondary septation or alveolarization occurs to term and for several years after birth. Septation events are dynamic with about 0.06×10^6 distal structures at 18 to 20 weeks that increase to about 100×10^6 alveoli at term—a 1700-fold increase. Alveolar numbers increase only about fivefold from the term birth lung to the adult lung.[8] There is essentially no information about the variability of the timing of normal septation in the human lung. It is also not known whether very early lung maturation changes the timing of the later gestational septation events that generate respiratory bronchioles and alveolar ducts. Some forms of pulmonary hypoplasia may result from altered septation and airway development. The injury and repair associated with BPD do inhibit and delay alveolarization of the developing lung.[9]

Recent human anatomic and experimental data demonstrate that the healthy lung probably grows new alveoli and loses old alveoli continuously at a very slow rate.[10,11] Empirically, very preterm infants with a BPD-associated "arrest" in alveolar septation must be able to grow alveoli or they could not grow and survive. These

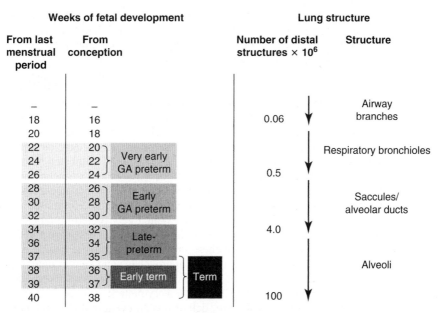

Weeks of fetal development		Lung structure	
From last menstrual period	**From conception**	**Number of distal structures × 10⁶**	**Structure**
–	–		
18	16	0.06	Airway branches
20	18		
22	20 ⎫ Very early GA preterm		Respiratory bronchioles
24	22		
26	24 ⎭	0.5	
28	26 ⎫ Early GA preterm		Saccules/ alveolar ducts
30	28		
32	30 ⎭		
34	32 ⎫ Late-preterm	4.0	
36	34		
37	35 ⎭		Alveoli
38	36 ⎫ Early term		
39	37 ⎭ Term		
40	38	100	

Fig. 2.2 Timing of fetal lung development, emphasizing the 2-week difference in weeks between postmenstrual age and conceptional age. The lung progressively branches from airways to alveoli with a large increase in distal structures. The adult lung contains about 500 × 10⁶ alveoli. *GA*, Gestational age.[13]

lungs may "catch up" to have lung volumes or alveolar numbers equivalent to normal lungs.[12] The questions for the future include how alveoli grow after very preterm birth and how lung injury can be prevented.

Lung Maturation

From the clinical perspective, questions about lung maturation have focused on RDS and the surfactant system since the seminal report from Avery and Mead[13] in 1959 that the lungs of infants who died of RDS had less surfactant. Lung maturation also includes epithelial development of ion/water regulation, thinning of the alveolar capillary barrier, and microvascular development. The first challenge is to define the timing of normal lung maturation, which is not an easy task if one assumes that most preterm infants are abnormal. In the 1970s, amniotic fluid was sampled from women with relatively normal gestations to test for lung maturation using surfactant components.[14] The lecithin/sphingomyelin (L/S) ratio was less than 2 until after 34 to 35 weeks of gestation, and phosphatidylglycerol was seldom detected prior to 34 weeks of gestation in normal pregnancies.[15] The true time course and the variability for the timing for normal lung maturation are not known with any precision for the human. However, lung maturity testing and inadvertent experiences with non-indicated cesarean sections prior to 37 weeks demonstrate that lung maturation, defined as absence of RDS, normally occurs after about 34 to 36 weeks in normal pregnancies.

The diagnosis of RDS for very early GA preterm infants has been confounded in clinical series and epidemiologic studies by intubation and ventilation with or without surfactant treatment shortly after birth. These intubated and ventilated infants likely carry the diagnosis of RDS even if they are not receiving supplemental oxygen.[16] Furthermore, if these infants have infection, transient tachypnea of the newborn, a degree of pulmonary hypoplasia, or apnea requiring ventilatory support, they likely will be said to have RDS. The successful use of continuous positive airway pressure (CPAP) to minimize lung injury in very early GA infants demonstrates that many very preterm infants do not have enough RDS to need surfactant or mechanical ventilation.[17–19] Infants born at 24 to 25 weeks' GA without RDS are surprisingly common.[20] Because lung maturation (and RDS) is a continuum from severe immaturity to sufficient maturation to avoid RDS, we think that most very preterm infants have some degree of induced lung maturation.[21] The infant born at 24 to 26 weeks of gestation with severe respiratory failure and a poor response to surfactant and who dies soon after birth is an infant with "normal" 25-week lungs or an infant with RDS-plus (RDS plus infection or pulmonary hypoplasia, for example). Very few infants die of RDS in the United States unless they are of extremely low GA.

At the margin of lung maturity in preterm sheep, a surfactant pool size of about 4 mg/kg is sufficient to support normal gas exchange with CPAP,[22] demonstrating that a small amount of surfactant is sufficient to protect the preterm lung from RDS. No good tests are available to quantify the lung maturation status prior to or soon after delivery. The L/S ratio or phosphatidylglycerol measurements in amniotic fluid are no longer commonly available, and other tests such as lamellar body number in amniotic fluid are imprecise. Samples of fetal lung fluid (intubated infants) or gastric aspirates soon after birth could provide information about surfactant and inflammation, but they are not used routinely. An evaluation of the messenger ribonucleic acid (mRNA) in amniotic fluid may provide a maturation profile for multiple fetal organs in the future.[23] A clinical controversy is: Which very preterm infant should receive surfactant/ventilation or CPAP after birth? The controversy is based on the perceived risk for RDS and the ability of these infants to transition if treated by CPAP. The clinical trials demonstrate that the two approaches yield similar outcomes that marginally favor an initial trial of CPAP.[24] However, individualized treatments could be given if the functional potential of the very preterm lung could be assessed prior to delivery. Clearly, very preterm delivery is an event that profoundly changes the developing lung. However, there is no good information about how preterm delivery and breathing, independent of oxygen exposure and injury, change the trajectory of subsequent lung development. Lung stretch from breathing and the striking changes in hormone milieu alter lung development in experimental models.[25,26] The implication is that independent of injury, lung structure at 40 weeks will be different for infants born at 25 weeks or 35 weeks from those for infants born at 40 weeks.[27]

Antenatal Corticosteroids

The antenatal administration of corticosteroids for women at risk for preterm delivery at 24 to 34 weeks of gestation is the standard of care. This therapy was developed to reduce the risk of RDS, but it also decreased the incidences of intraventricular hemorrhage and death. The therapy is supported by two National Institutes of Health Consensus Conferences,[28] and an extensive meta-analysis.[29] Nevertheless, there are controversies about repeated treatments,[30] the drug and dose to be used,[31] and the responses of selected populations of patients.[5,32] We briefly review the effects of antenatal corticosteroids on fetal lungs and identify some of the remaining questions.

Maternal corticosteroid treatments have pleiotropic effects on the lung and other fetal organ systems. Corticosteroids upregulate families of genes and downregulate other genes.[33] The net responses in an organ such as the lung are changes in anatomy, physiology, and clinical outcomes (Table 2.1). The fetal primate lung responds to a 3-day maternal corticosteroid treatment, beginning at 63 days of gestation with a thinning of the mesenchyme and enlargement of air spaces (Fig. 2.3).[34] The functional effect is to increase lung gas volume. This increase in lung gas volume reflects two events: mesenchymal thinning and an interruption in alveolar septation such that saccular/alveolar numbers decrease and the sizes increase.[35] These anatomic changes in the lung to increase lung gas volumes occur within 15 hours and prior to an increase in alveolar surfactant in fetal sheep.[36] Antenatal steroids increase the risk for pneumothorax for about 24 hours after treatment in preterm sheep and rabbits by reducing the rupture pressures of the lung, presumably by thinning the mesenchyme without increasing support structures.[37,38]

The physiologic changes that accompany the changes in lung structure and increased surfactant are increased lung compliance, improved gas exchange, and decreased permeability of the air space epithelium. Antenatal corticosteroid treatments improve surfactant treatment responses in animal models and in infants.[39,40] The fetal corticosteroid exposure decreases the amount of surfactant to achieve better responses[41,42] because surfactant composition is altered.[43] Endogenous surfactant is

Table 2.1 EFFECTS OF ANTENATAL CORTICOSTEROIDS ON FETAL LUNGS

Anatomy/biochemistry	Thin mesenchyme of alveolar-capillary structures
	Increased saccular/alveolar gas volumes
	Decreased alveolar septation
	Increased antioxidant enzymes
	Increased surfactant
Physiology	Increased compliance
	Improved gas exchange
	Decreased epithelial permeability
	Protection of preterm lung from injury during resuscitation
Interactions with exogenous surfactant	Improvement in surfactant treatment responses
	Improvement in surfactant dose-response curve
	Decreased inactivation of surfactant
Clinical	Decreased incidence of respiratory distress syndrome
	No effect on incidence of bronchopulmonary dysplasia
	Decreased mortality

less susceptible to inactivation by proteinaceous pulmonary edema. The decreased epithelial permeability also protects surfactant from inactivation. Lung injury during resuscitation with high tidal volumes was decreased by fetal exposure to corticosteroids in preterm surfactant-deficient sheep.[44] The surfactant lipids and proteins do not increase in fetal sheep until 4 to 7 days after corticosteroid treatment.[45] Therefore the early physiologic effects of antenatal corticosteroids result primarily from anatomic and other associated effects. The clinical correlates are a decrease in RDS and improved surfactant treatment responses. There was no consistent decrease in BPD in the placebo-controlled trials of antenatal corticosteroids conducted before 1990 or in clinical series since that era (Fig. 2.4).[29] Antenatal corticosteroids decrease mortality and salvage a population of infants who are at high risk for BPD, and the great majority of infants at the highest risk for BPD are exposed to maternal corticosteroids. Any difference in a BPD outcome will depend on the comparison group, and currently 80% to 90% of the at-risk population of extremely low-birth-weight (ELBW) infants have been exposed to antenatal steroids.[46] Those not exposed will have different antenatal histories, perinatal management, and outcomes (Table 2.2).

A number of questions remain about the appropriate use and benefits of antenatal corticosteroids. Current practice is to treat with either 12 mg of betamethasone acetate plus betamethasone phosphate given as a 2-dose treatment separated by 24 hours or a 4-dose 12-hour interval treatment with dexamethasone phosphate.[31] These drugs are not equivalent, having different and complex pharmacokinetics in the mother and the fetus. In animal models, fetal lung maturation is induced with low and prolonged fetal exposures to betamethasone, but not with single high-dose exposures to betamethasone.[47] The presently recommended drug doses probably cause peak fetal exposures to betamethasone phosphate or dexamethasone phosphate that are higher than necessary, and treatment intervals may not be optimal.[48] Research is needed to optimize the benefits of antenatal corticosteroid treatments while minimizing risks.

Trials with antenatal corticosteroids were completed by about 1990, and only about 100 randomly assigned infants were delivered prior to 28 weeks' GA. However, in clinical practice, the use of corticosteroids is routine for infants who are to be offered intensive care of GAs as low as 22 to 23 weeks.[49] Because most of these extremely preterm infants have a diagnosis of RDS (appropriate or not), a decrease in RDS may not be a good indicator of benefit. For example, Garite and coworkers[50] found no decrease in RDS but did document decreased severity of RDS in early GA infants. As demonstrated in Fig. 2.3, the primate lung can respond to antenatal corticosteroids at very early (previable human equivalent) GAs, as do explants of human fetal lung at less than 20 weeks of gestation. Antenatal corticosteroids should be used if a very preterm delivery is likely to occur within the next 7 days if the goal is for the infant to survive.[51]

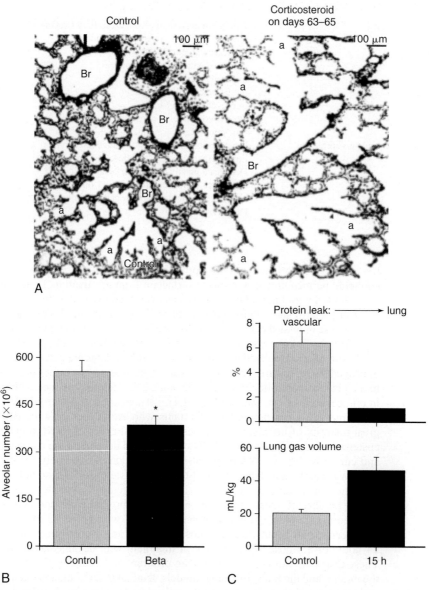

Fig. 2.3 Examples of fetal corticosteroid responses. A, Corticosteroid responses of the very immature fetal mon-key lung. Maternal triamcinolone (10 mg) treatment on days 63 to 65 of pregnancy cause mesenchymal loss and air space enlargement at 90 days of gestation. B, Alveolar numbers in fetal sheep lung were decreased 7 days follow-ing maternal treatments with 0.5 mg/kg betamethasone. C, An interval between fetal betamethasone treatment and delivery of 15 hours was sufficient to decrease vascular to alveolar leaks and increase lung gas volumes in beta-methasone-exposed preterm and ventilated lambs. *a,* Distal saccule; *Br,* bronchiole. (A, From Bunton TE, Plopper CG. Triamcinolone-induced structural alterations in the development of the lung of the fetal rhesus macaque. *Am J Obstet Gynecol.* 1984;148:203–215. B, Reprinted with permission of the American Thoracic Society. Copyright © 2018 American Thoracic Society. Willet KE, Jobe AH, Ikegami M, et al/2001/American Journal of Respiratory and Critical Care Medicine/Lung Morphometry after Repetitive Antenatal Glucocorticoid Treatment in Preterm Sheep/163/1437–1443. The American Journal of Respiratory and Critical Care Medicine is an official journal of the American Thoracic Society. C, From Ikegami M, Polk D, Jobe A. Minimum interval from fetal betamethasone treatment to postnatal lung responses in preterm lambs. *Am J Obstet Gynecol.* 1996;174:1408–1413.)

Although the neonatal community is primarily concerned about the lung out-comes of very preterm infants, large populations of term infants delivered by elective cesarean section and late preterm infants delivered for multiple indications require respiratory care after birth. Sinclair[52] pointed out in 1995 that the early clinical tri-als demonstrated lung benefits for infants exposed to antenatal corticosteroids who were delivered after 32 to 34 weeks of gestation. The respiratory morbidities RDS and transient tachypnea of the newborn increase greatly for deliveries at less than 38

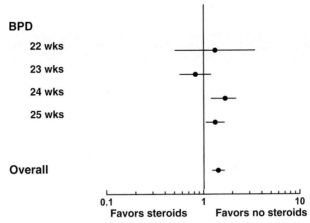

BPD

22 wks

23 wks

24 wks

25 wks

Overall

0.1   1   10
Favors steroids   Favors no steroids

Fig. 2.4 Antenatal corticosteroids and bronchopulmonary dysplasia *(BPD)* for 10,541 infants from 1993 to 2009 in the National Institutes of Child Health and Human Development (NICHD) Neonatal Network. While mortality decreased with antenatal steroids, BPD did not decrease for the large populations of very preterm infants cared for in NICHD Neonatal Network Centers. (Data from Carlo WA, McDonald SA, Fanaroff AA, et al. Association of antenatal corticosteroids with mortality and neurodevelopmental outcomes among infants born at 22 to 25 weeks' gestation. *JAMA.* 2011;306:2348–2358.)

Table 2.2 CHARACTERISTICS OF ANTENATAL VARIABLES FOR 22 TO 28 WEEKS GESTATIONAL AGE INFANTS CARED FOR IN NICHD NEONATAL RESEARCH NETWORK CENTERS[a]

Characteristic	Percentage of Population Affected from 1993 to 2012	% Change from 1993 to 2012
Antenatal corticosteroids	80	62% Increase
Antenatal antibiotics	66	33% Increase
Cesarean delivery	56	19% Increase
Small for gestational age	7	No change
Multiple births	24	8% Increase

[a]A total of 34,636 infants received care at National Institutes of Child Health and Human Development (NICHD) centers from 2003 to 2012.
Data from Stoll BJ, Hansen NI, Bell EF, et al. Trends in care practices, morbidity, and mortality of extremely preterm neonates, 1993–2012. *JAMA.* 2015;314:1039–1051.

weeks' GA for even modest prematurity.[5] The recently completed randomized controlled trial of corticosteroid use for deliveries between 34[0] and 34[6] weeks enrolled 2831 patients and demonstrated that steroids improved the combined primary outcome of need for respiratory support, stillbirth, or death (Table 2.3).[53] The benefit was for respiratory morbidity, but an unanticipated complication was hypoglycemia. There presently is no follow-up for this trial. The benefits are modest and the risks are poorly defined.[54,55]

A provocative randomized trial of antenatal corticosteroids using betamethasone (Celestone) for 998 women scheduled for elective cesarean delivery demonstrated that respiratory distress after use of corticosteroids decreased from 11.4% to 5.4% for deliveries at 37 weeks and from 1.5% to 0.6% for deliveries at 39 weeks.[56] A second trial used an untested treatment schedule of 3 doses of 8-mg dexamethasone given 12 hours apart prior to elective cesarean section at 38 weeks. The steroid treatment decreased admission to the neonatal intensive care unit from 3.9% to 1.6% in 1290 randomly assigned women with a number needed to treat of 43.[3] These trials identify much larger populations of women for treatment with antenatal corticosteroids beyond prematurity. There are minimal long-term outcome data to assure safety for such widespread use.

Repeated courses of antenatal corticosteroids are conceptually attractive because many early GA fetuses are not delivered within 7 days of maternal treatment and the benefits of therapy seem to decrease with time after treatment.[29] In one report, about 60% of women who received an initial treatment with corticosteroids

Table 2.3 ANTENATAL STEROIDS FOR INFANTS BORN AT 34^0 THROUGH 36^0 WEEKS OF GESTATIONAL AGE

	Placebo (N = 1400)	Antenatal Steroid (N = 1427)	P Value
Gestational age at delivery (weeks)	36.1	36.1	—
Primary outcome (%)	14.4	11.6	.023
Severe respiratory morbidity (%)	12.1	8.1	<.001
Surfactant treatment (%)	3.1	1.8	.031
Hypoglycemia (%)	15	24	<.001

From Gyamfi-Bannerman C, Thom EA. Antenatal betamethasone for women at risk for late preterm delivery. *N Engl J Med.* 2016;375(5):486–487.

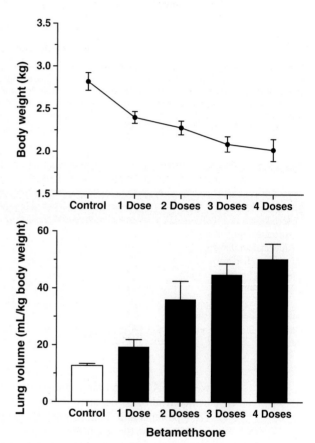

Fig. 2.5 Birth weight and lung functional effects of repeated weekly antenatal corticosteroid treatments of fetal sheep. All animals were delivered at 125 days of gestational age following a maternal steroid treatment at 104, 111, 118, and 124 days' gestation for 4 doses or 1, 2, or 3 doses only. Birth weight decreased linearly with doses. Lung gas volume is measured at 40 cm H_2O after a period of ventilation increased with dose. (Data from Ikegami M, Jobe AH, Newnham J, et al. Repetitive prenatal glucocorticoids improve lung function and decrease growth in preterm lambs. *Am J Respir Crit Care Med.* 1997;156:178–184.)

delivered more than 7 days later.[57] In animal models, second courses of corticosteroids progressively increase the indicators of fetal lung maturation.[58] The risks are adverse effects of repeated fetal exposures on fetal somatic and brain growth, effects that occur in animal models (Fig. 2.5).[58] A meta-analysis of 4733 randomized pregnancies in trials reported a modest benefit for RDS and severe lung disease with modest growth effects for repeated courses of treatment.[59] A subsequent trial of 1858 women randomly assigned to a 14-day retreatment interval versus no retreatment found no benefit for RDS, mortality, or other outcomes, but a decrease in birth weights and head circumferences.[60] Reports of 2-year neurodevelopment outcomes are reassuring for infants exposed to fewer than four courses of antenatal corticosteroids.[61,62] Another option is a rescue treatment when a woman has received an initial treatment and again has a high risk of delivery prior to 34 weeks. There are no recommendations from learned societies about the use of repeated corticosteroid treatments.

Antenatal Infection/Inflammation

Overview of Fetal Inflammation

The human fetus is normally considered to be in an environment protected from infection. However, the human fetus can be exposed to a variety of pathogens, which may initiate an inflammatory process in the placenta, chorioamnion, or fetus. For example, human fetuses are exposed to viral pathogens as a consequence of maternal viremia. The patterns of fetal injury after exposure to agents such as varicella and cytomegalovirus depend on the period of gestation during which the infection occurs. Similarly, the fetus can acquire a spirochete infection with syphilis or a parasitic infection with toxoplasmosis secondary to maternal infection, and each causes characteristic syndromes depending on the gestational timing of exposure. These infections are not generally viewed as predominantly inflammatory, although the fetal injury and immune responses have inflammatory characteristics. Asphyxia with injury to fetal tissue also causes inflammation as part of the injury and the repair process. Similarly, normal labor is associated with an increase in proinflammatory mediators.[63] Both innate and acquired inflammatory responses of the fetus are generally considered less robust than those in the child or adult because the response systems in the fetus are immature and pregnancy is an immune-suppressive environment.[64] For example, fetal inflammatory responses to pathogens such as group B streptococcus and *Listeria monocytogenes* are blunted, resulting in severe infection and often death of the fetus or newborn. The most common fetal infectious exposure is to chorioamnionitis, which is associated with preterm labor and delivery.[65] In this section, we identify the questions and controversies about the associations of chorioamnionitis with a range of effects on the fetal and newborn lung.

Diagnosis of Chorioamnionitis

Chorioamnionitis can be either a clinical syndrome or a silent, indolent process. The clinical diagnosis of chorioamnionitis is made when a pregnant woman has a constellation of findings that include fever, a tender uterus, an elevated blood granulocyte count, and bacteria and/or inflammatory cells in amniotic fluid and often preterm or prolonged rupture of membranes.[66] Clinical chorioamnionitis is an imprecise diagnosis that has little prognostic or treatment value.[67] The diagnosis of clinical chorioamnionitis is frequently made for near-term or term labors, and occasionally infection can be caused by highly virulent organisms. Before 30 weeks of gestation, *clinical chorioamnionitis* is most often diagnosed after attempts to delay preterm delivery or with preterm prolonged rupture of membranes. Another method to diagnose chorioamnionitis is by histopathology of the chorioamnion with inflammation, indicating *histologic chorioamnionitis*. The amount of infiltration of the chorioamnion by inflammatory cells and the intensity of secondary changes are used to grade the severity of the fetal exposure to inflammation.[68] Inflammation of the cord, called *funisitis*, is generally considered to indicate a more advanced inflammatory process that involves the fetus.[69] Another diagnostic approach is to culture amniotic fluid or fetal membranes for organisms or to assay amniotic fluid for proinflammatory inflammatory mediators such as tumor necrosis factor α (TNF-α) and interleukin-1 (IL-1) and IL-6.[70] With the recognition that only a minority of organisms in the human biome can be cultured, polymerase chain reaction (PCR) and DNA sequencing techniques are being used to demonstrate that chorioamnionitis is often polymicrobial with organisms that cannot be cultured.[71] Technologies to identify multiple proteins in biologic fluids also are being adapted to develop proteomic biomarkers for chorioamnionitis in amniotic fluid.[72] These technologies have the potential to rapidly diagnose inflammation and to identify specific organisms. Such approaches will change the understanding of fetal exposures to inflammation and pathology related to specific organisms.

The chorioamnion is fetal tissue, and the amniotic fluid surrounding the fetus is in direct contact with the fetal gut, skin, and lung.[69] Therefore the fetus will be exposed to inflammation if there is histologic chorioamnionitis or if the amniotic fluid contains mediators of inflammation. The Venn diagram in Fig. 2.6 illustrates the diagnostic conundrum. Clinical chorioamnionitis does not correlate well with the subsequent diagnosis of histologic chorioamnionitis, and an amniotic fluid diagnosis of infection may or may not predict chorioamnionitis associated with preterm delivery. PCR-based analyses of amniotic fluid call into question the assumption that fetal colonization with organisms is abnormal and will cause preterm delivery. Gerber and associates[73] demonstrated that 11% of 254 presumably normal amniotic fluid samples collected at 15 to 19 weeks of gestation for genetic analysis were PCR-positive for *Ureaplasma urealyticum*. Although 17 of the 29 *Ureaplasma*-positive pregnancies had preterm labor, only 2 fetuses were delivered before 34 weeks of gestation. Perni and colleagues[74] analyzed 179 amniotic fluid samples and found that 13% were positive for *Ureaplasma* and 6% were positive for *Mycoplasma hominis*, and in 28 of the 33 pregnancies with positive amniotic fluid samples infants were not delivered preterm. Deep sequencing of the microbial genome reveals "colonization" of the amniotic fluid in some women without apparent adverse effects, suggesting the presence of an amniotic biome.[75,76] Attempts to extensively culture the placenta/chorioamnion have recovered multiple organisms of low virulence that include vaginal flora.[77] The severity of the chorioamnionitis does not correlate well with the organisms but tends to be more severe with *Ureaplasma* and *Mycoplasma* species.[78–80] Furthermore, in many preterm deliveries, polymicrobial organisms are recovered by culture or PCR from the amniotic fluid. The unknowns are the association of organisms with pregnancies that are not delivered preterm and the variety of organisms that can be identified by PCR. For example, Steel and coworkers[81] used a fluorescent probe for a common 16S ribosomal RNA bacterial sequence and identified organisms deep within the membranes of all preterm deliveries and many term deliveries. These results suggest that the human pregnancy can tolerate colonization/infection with low-pathogenicity organisms. The provocative question is: Does the fetus need exposure to a biome for normal development?

There is no clear answer to the question "What is chorioamnionitis?" The multiple ways to make the diagnosis are not necessarily congruent. Furthermore, if one accepts that chorioamnionitis results from colonization/infection, then the diagnosis is imprecise in the extreme in relation to how infectious diseases are generally diagnosed. The diagnosis of an infection includes the identity of the organism, an estimate of the duration of infection, its intensity, and specific sites of involvement. The diagnosis of chorioamnionitis contains none of these elements. Research is now linking genetically determined inflammatory response characteristics of the mother and fetus with prematurity.[82] The chronic indolent chorioamnionitis associated with

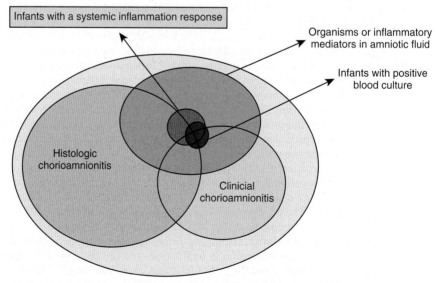

Fig. 2.6 Venn diagram illustrating the overlapping relationships among different ways to diagnose chorioamnionitis and the outcomes of sepsis and systemic inflammatory syndromes. The *outer circle* represents preterm deliveries prior to 30 weeks of gestation.

prematurity may result from the interaction of the environment and the genetically determined immunomodulatory characteristics of the mother and fetus. Challenges for the future are how to better diagnose and to understand what makes patients susceptible to chorioamnionitis, and how to quantify the severity potential for fetal injury from the chorioamnionitis.[67]

Clinical Pulmonary Outcomes of Fetal Exposure to Inflammation/Infection

An important perspective is how infrequent severe sepsis and pneumonia are in large delivery populations where the diagnosis of clinical chorioamnionitis will apply to 5% to 10% of the population. A clinical experience from Dallas is representative: of 23,321 deliveries; 7% (1660) of cases were diagnosed as clinical chorioamnionitis and 1571 infants were asymptomatic.[83] Only 61 (0.26%) infant were ultimately thought to be sick and in need of the neonatal intensive care unit, primarily for respiratory and sepsis symptoms. The occurrence of culture-proven sepsis is very infrequent and of 396,586 infants, 389 (0.1%) had early-onset sepsis; 60% of these had clinical chorioamnionitis. Most of the septic infants were born preterm and had symptoms (Fig. 2.7).[84] Another concern is a sepsis/pneumonia risk for infants born before term after prolonged rupture of membranes (PROM). Should women with PROM have immediate delivery on presentation or expectant management with maternal treatment with antibiotics? A recent trial demonstrated that expectant management was associated with fewer cesarean sections, less RDS, and no difference in neonatal sepsis.[85] While a risk of infection is associated with chorioamnionitis, the risk is very low for asymptomatic infants and overtreatment with antibiotics is prevalent.

The fetal effects of chorioamnionitis are much more frequent in preterm populations. A decreased incidence of RDS was associated with preterm PROM, a surrogate marker for chorioamnionitis, as early as 1974.[86] Watterberg and associates[87] reported in 1996 that ventilated preterm infants exposed to histologic chorioamnionitis had a lower incidence of RDS but a higher incidence of BPD than infants not exposed to chorioamnionitis. Furthermore, the initial tracheal aspirates from infants exposed to chorioamnionitis contained proinflammatory mediators such as IL-1, IL-6, and IL-8, indicating that the lung inflammation was of antenatal origin. Other reports support that association.[88,89] Clinical chorioamnionitis was associated with decreased death in all infants born at or before 26 weeks of gestation in the United Kingdom and Ireland in 1995.[90] Hannaford and colleagues[91] identified *U. urealyticum* as an organism of fetal origin that was associated with a decreased

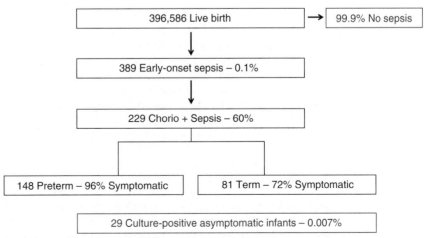

Fig. 2.7 Culture-proven sepsis is infrequent and usually symptomatic. The flow diagram is for almost 400,000 deliveries with assessments for early-onset sepsis by blood culture. The overall occurrence of sepsis was only 0.1% and the majority of the septic infants were premature and symptomatic. (Data from Wortham JM, Hansen NI, Schrag SJ, et al. Chorioamnionitis and culture-confirmed, early-onset neonatal infections. *Pediatrics.* 2016;137(1).)

risk of RDS. Lahra and coworkers[92] noted, in a population of 724 preterm infants, that RDS was decreased for infants exposed to histologic chorioamnionitis (odds ratio [OR] 0.49, 95% confidence interval [95% CI] 0.31–0.78) or chorioamnionitis plus funisitis (OR 0.23, 95% CI 0.15–0.35) relative to no chorioamnionitis. This group also reported its 13-year experience that histologic chorioamnionitis (with or without funisitis) was associated with a decreased risk of BPD (OR 0.58, 95% CI 0.51–0.67).[93] A recent systematic meta-analysis showed that histologic chorioamnionitis was associated with BPD, but there was low confidence in the findings because of evidence of publication bias.[94]

In contrast, other reports associate chorioamnionitis with poor pulmonary and other outcomes. Hitti and associates,[95] for example, reported that high levels of TNF-α in amniotic fluid predicted prolonged postnatal ventilation, suggesting early and persistent lung injury from chorioamnionitis. Ramsey and colleagues[96] also demonstrated that chorioamnionitis increased neonatal morbidities. Laughon and coworkers,[97] after extensively evaluating and culturing the placentas of 1340 infants born before 28 weeks of gestation, found no association between histologic chorioamnionitis, funisitis, or specific organisms and the initial oxygen requirements of the infants or subsequent development of BPD. The Canadian Neonatal Network also reported that clinical chorioamnionitis was not predictive of RDS or BPD.[98]

These discrepant reports need to be understood within the complexities of the diagnosis of chorioamnionitis as well as the factors contributing to the diagnosis of RDS or BPD. Van Marter and associates[99] evaluated the outcomes of ventilated and VLBW infants and found that chorioamnionitis was associated with a decreased incidence of BPD (OR 0.2). However, BPD was increased if the infant had been exposed to chorioamnionitis and either was mechanical ventilated for more than 7 days (OR 3.2) or had postnatal sepsis (OR 2.9). Lahra and coworkers[93] noted the same associations in an unselected population of 761 infants with gestations less than 30 weeks. BPD was lower in infants exposed to histologic chorioamnionitis than in infants without chorioamnionitis, as noted previously. However, the combination of histologic chorioamnionitis and postnatal sepsis increased the risk for BPD (OR 1.98, 95% CI 1.15–3.39). These reports demonstrate that antenatal and postnatal exposures interact to change outcomes such as BPD. Been and colleagues[100,101] reported that newborns exposed to chorioamnionitis with fetal involvement had more severe RDS and impaired surfactant treatment responses. In contrast, infants exposed to chorioamnionitis without fetal involvement had minimal lung disease. The severity of the chorioamnionitis and postnatal interventions confound simple correlations between chorioamnionitis and outcomes such as RDS and BPD.

Other studies have explored the associations of antenatal inflammation with postnatal lung outcomes with measurements of proinflammatory cytokines in cord plasma and tracheal aspirates collected shortly after birth. In general, cord plasma from early gestational deliveries had higher proinflammatory cytokine levels than cord plasma from term deliveries, but the median values were not greatly different,[102] suggesting little useful resolution between the preterm and term populations. Although Ambalavanan and coworkers[103] could detect differences in blood cytokines collected within 4 hours of birth for infants in whom BPD developed from those without BPD, the resolution between the populations was not clinically useful for the prediction of risk of BPD. Similarly, Paananen and associates[104] found higher selected cord plasma cytokine levels in infants exposed to severe chorioamnionitis. The cord cytokine levels decreased with age for infants at lower risk for BPD, but cord cytokine levels were not reliable predictors of BPD. De Dooy and colleagues[88] could predict chorioamnionitis from IL-8 levels in tracheal aspirates collected soon after birth, but the clinical utility of that information also is unclear. Been and colleagues[105] did find that vascular endothelial growth factor levels in initial tracheal aspirates were predictive of BPD. However, there is no compelling evidence that measurements of proinflammatory mediators in cord plasma or tracheal aspirates will identify high-resolution biomarkers for either chorioamnionitis or the pulmonary outcomes RDS and BPD.

Table 2.4 PULMONARY AND SYSTEMIC OUTCOMES FOR CONSECUTIVELY DELIVERED INFANTS BORN BEFORE 30 WEEKS OF GESTATION AND EXPOSED TO INFECTION[a]

	Percentage of Population		
	Yes	No	P Value
Histologically Diagnosed Chorioamnionitis			
Respiratory distress syndrome	61	73	.008
Bronchopulmonary dysplasia	17	17	NS
Fetal inflammatory response syndrome	44	18	.001
Positive Result of Cord Blood Culture			
Respiratory distress syndrome	66	65	NS
Bronchopulmonary dysplasia	27	10	.001
Fetal inflammatory response syndrome	41	26	.007

[a]A comparison of fetal exposures diagnosed by histologic chorioamnionitis or positive results of cord blood cultures for *Ureaplasma* or *Mycoplasma*.
NS, Not significant.
Data from Andrews WW, Goldenberg RL, Faye-Petersen O, et al. The Alabama Preterm Birth Study: polymorphonuclear and mononuclear cell placental infiltrations, other markers of inflammation, and outcomes in 23- to 32-week preterm newborn infants. *Am J Obstet Gynecol.* 2006;195:803–808; and Goldenberg RL, Andrews WW, Goepfert AR, et al. The Alabama Preterm Birth Study: umbilical cord blood *Ureaplasma urealyticum* and *Mycoplasma hominis* cultures in very preterm newborn infants. *Am J Obstet Gynecol.* 2008;198:43.e41–43.e45.

Fig. 2.8 Overview of outcomes of acute clinical or chronic subclinical chorioamnionitis. Acute chorioamnionitis with virulent organisms is likely to cause severe lung disease or death. In contrast, chronic chorioamnionitis may improve lung outcomes by inducing lung maturation. However, bronchopulmonary dysplasia *(BPD)* may occur if the inflammation in the fetal lung is increased by postnatal exposures to oxygen, ventilation or postnatal sepsis. *RDS*, Respiratory distress syndrome.

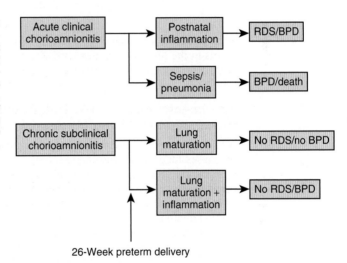

26-Week preterm delivery

The inconsistent clinical correlates most likely result from the imprecise nature of the diagnosis of chorioamnionitis and its association with different populations of infants. An example of the inconsistency is the diagnosis of fetal exposures by histologic chorioamnionitis or by blood culture for *Ureaplasma* collected from the cord at delivery and the outcomes of RDS and BPD for the same cohort of consecutive patients (Table 2.4).[106,107] The associations with histologic chorioamnionitis and culture positivity for *Ureaplasma* for BPD are the *opposite* of those for RDS in the same cohort of patients. The diagram in Fig. 2.8 may help frame the question about the variable outcome. A progressive chorioamnionitis caused by virulent organisms may cause severe postnatal lung and systemic inflammation with the outcomes of more severe RDS, BPD, or sepsis/death. Such outcomes are relatively infrequent in VLBW infants who are not stillborn. Fewer than 2% of VLBW infants have positive blood culture results at birth.[108] Chronic, indolent chorioamnionitis caused by organisms such as *Ureaplasma* can induce lung maturation (less RDS), but that early maturation may be associated with more BPD.[87] These associations may depend on how the diagnosis of chorioamnionitis is made (clinical, histopathologic, other), and the population of infants studied (ventilated only, all VLBW infants, other selected populations). In an attempt to better establish a cause-and-effect relationship, Viscardi

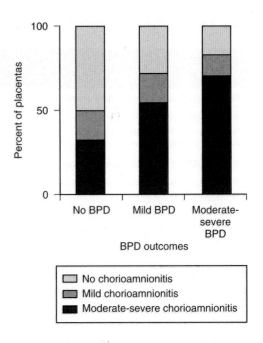

Fig. 2.9 Relationship of severity of chorioamnionitis by histologic grading with the severity of bronchopulmonary dysplasia *(BPD)*. Infants with moderate to severe BPD were more likely to have been exposed to more severe histologic chorioamnionitis. (Data from Viscardi RM, Muhumuza CK, Rodriguez A, et al. Inflammatory markers in intrauterine and fetal blood and cerebrospinal fluid compartments are associated with adverse pulmonary and neurologic outcomes in preterm infants. *Pediatr Res.* 2004;55:1009–1017.)

and associates[109] correlated the intensity of the inflammatory response to chorioamnionitis in the fetal membranes with the clinical outcome of BPD (Fig. 2.9). More severe chorioamnionitis at delivery predicted a higher incidence and greater severity of BPD.

Experimental Results: The Link Between Fetal Exposure to Inflammation and Lung Maturation and Lung Remodeling

Animal models have consistently demonstrated that fetal exposure to inflammation causes lung injury and induces lung maturation. In a strict sense, lung maturation should probably be called "dysmaturation" because the beneficial effects of improved lung mechanics are also accompanied by altered lung development. Bry and colleagues[110] first demonstrated in 1997 that inflammation induced lung maturation by intraamniotic injection of IL-1α. Our group found that intraamniotic injection of the proinflammatory mediator endotoxin from *Escherichia coli* in sheep caused chorioamnionitis (inflammatory cells and increased IL-1β and IL-6 mRNA expression in the chorioamnion), inflammatory cells in amniotic fluid, and increased IL-8 protein levels in amniotic fluid.[111,112] The chorioamnionitis was accompanied by inflammation of the fetal lung, as demonstrated by recruitment of granulocytes to the fetal lung tissue and air spaces within 24 hours and expression of multiple proinflammatory mediators (Fig. 2.10).[113,114] Apoptosis of lung cells increased at 24 hours, and proliferation increased at 3 days. This lung inflammation/injury sequence included multiple indicators of lung microvascular injury—epithelial nitric oxide synthase and vascular endothelial growth factor decreased, and medial smooth muscle hypertrophied.[113] Thus intraamniotic endotoxin caused lung inflammation and an injury sequence that resulted in lung remodeling.

There are very few studies of respiratory muscle function in preterms. Recently Song et al. reported that intraamniotic endotoxin exposure in preterm fetal lambs resulted in transient inflammation in fetal diaphragm followed by atrophic gene expression resulting in impaired diaphragm contractility.[115]

Inflammation was associated with the induction of the mRNAs for the surfactant proteins within 12 to 24 hours, persistent elevation of those mRNAs for weeks, and an increase in alveolar surfactant proteins and lipids with improved lung function within 5 to 7 days.[111,116] The improvement in lung function was accompanied by a decrease in mesenchymal tissue and an increase in potential gas volume in the fetal lung. The residual effects of the injury at 7 days were greater thickness of the

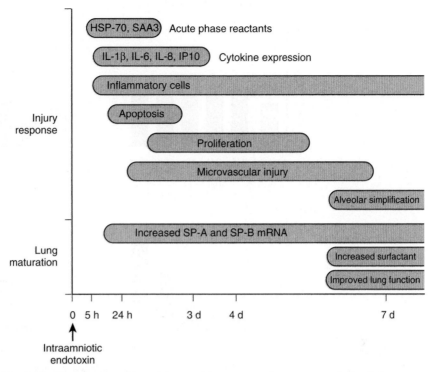

Fig. 2.10 Time course of lung injury and lung maturation responses in fetal sheep to an intraamniotic injection of endotoxin. The lung initially has an inflammation and injury response, which are followed by lung maturation. *d,* Day(s); *h,* hour(s); *HSP-70,* heat shock protein 70; *IL,* interleukin; *IP10,* interferon gamma–inducing protein 10; *mRNA,* messenger ribonucleic acid; *SP,* surfactant protein.

pulmonary microvessels and a reduction in secondary septation of the alveoli.[38,113] However, the net effect was a lung that was easier to ventilate because of improved compliance and that had better gas exchange (Fig. 2.11). Of note, the lung injury followed by maturation sequence did not result from "fetal stress," because fetal blood cortisol levels did not increase. Intraamniotic endotoxin also increased surfactant protein mRNA in the primate.[117] Lung inflammation results in accelerated lung maturation.

To understand whether the signal for lung inflammation/maturation during chorioamnionitis is systemic versus local, Moss and colleagues[118] isolated the lung from the amniotic fluid surgically with collection of the fetal lung fluid in a bag placed in the amniotic cavity. Intraamniotic endotoxin without exposure to fetal lung induced chorioamnionitis but not lung inflammation or lung maturation. In contrast, a 24-hour tracheal infusion of endotoxin induced both lung inflammation and lung maturation. This same result also was achieved with a fetal tracheal infusion of IL-1 as the proinflammatory agonist.[119] Therefore the sequence from fetal lung inflammation to maturation did not result from a lung response to a systemic fetal inflammatory response. Also, new mediators resulting from the chorioamnionitis were not required for the response. Rather, direct contact of the fetal lung—presumably the airway epithelium—with endotoxin or IL-1 given by intraamniotic injection or tracheal infusion induced the lung maturation. The initial inflammation is thought to result from responses to the mediators by the airway epithelium, because the airways express the acute-phase reactants heat shock protein 70 (Hsp70) and serum amyloid A3 (SAA3), and there are very few monocytes/macrophages present in the fetal lung to initiate an inflammatory response. However, in chronic chorioamnionitis, the inflammatory products of the chorioamnionitis or organisms in the amniotic fluid probably are mediating the responses of the fetal lungs.

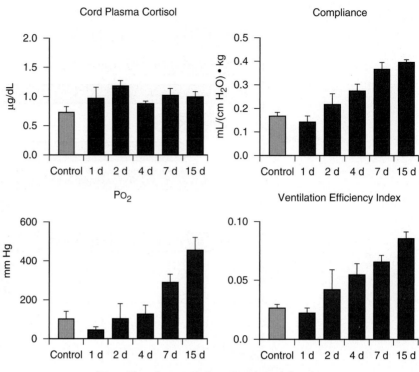

Mediators That Induce Fetal Lung Inflammatory Responses

Innate immune responses are signaled by a family of pattern recognition molecules called the toll-like receptors (TLRs). TLR4 recognizes endotoxin from gram-negative organisms, TLR2 signals gram-positive organisms, and TLR3 recognizes double-stranded RNA from viral pathogens, for example. The chorioamnion has TLRs, but there is very little information about the pattern of responses or the expression of the TLRs in the human fetus.[120] The inflammatory cells in the chorioamnion are likely of maternal origin when organisms localized between the endometrium and chorioamnion initiate the inflammation.[121] The fetal rabbit lung expresses low levels of TLR2 and TLR4, and mRNA levels remain unchanged for the last third of gestation in the fetal mice and sheep.[122,123] Empirically, *E. coli* endotoxin induces a rapid inflammatory response in the fetal sheep lung, as does IL-1, a cytokine that signals inflammation through a receptor that shares receptor elements and the signaling pathways with endotoxin. A high dose of a TLR2 agonist given by intraamniotic injection in sheep induced less inflammation than did endotoxin and had inconsistent effects on lung maturation. Blood monocytes from preterm sheep also do not respond as well as monocytes from adult sheep to challenge with TLR agonists.[124] The fetus may not respond uniformly to different TLR agonists.

Ureaplasma given by intraamniotic injection in sheep can colonize the amniotic fluid and fetal lung as early as 50 days of gestation (term is 150 days) and cause low-grade chronic lung inflammation and lung maturation (Table 2.5).[125] In fetal sheep, the innate inflammatory response to *Ureaplasma* is modest, with an increase in neutrophils by 3 days and persistent increase in lymphocyte populations in the lung.[126] The organism is not cleared from the fetal lungs. Colonization with

Table 2.5 MEASUREMENTS AFTER INTRAAMNIOTIC INJECTION OF *UREAPLASMA PARVUM* IN SHEEP FETUSES[A]

	Controls	*Ureaplasma* Group
Culture for *Ureaplasma*	Negative	Positive
Plasma cortisol (mg/dL)	1.04 ± 0.20	0.89 ± 0.09
Measurements in Bronchoalveolar Lavage Fluid[b]		
Inflammatory cells ($\times 10^6$/kg)	0.01 ± 0.01	3.5 ± 1.4
Protein (mg/kg)	16.1 ± 2.4	32.3 ± 4.7
Saturated phosphatidylcholine (µmol/kg)	0.07 ± 0.02	0.81 ± 0.19
Lung gas volume (mL/kg)	7.1 ± 0.8	19.7 ± 3.3

[a]Intraamniotic injection of 2×10^7 colony-forming units of *Ureaplasma parvum* at 67 days gestational age (GA) for sheep fetuses; measurements made at 124 days GA.
[b]Values per kilogram are expressed per kilogram of body weight; all values for the *Ureaplasma* animals are different from those in controls except plasma cortisol.
Data from Moss TJ, Nitsos I, Ikegami M, Jobe AH, Newnham JP. Experimental intrauterine *Ureaplasma* infection in sheep. *Am J Obstet Gynecol*. 2005;192(4):1179–1186.

Ureaplasma also does not cause fetal death or injury, a result similar to the outcomes of human pregnancies in which amniotic fluid samples were PCR-positive for *Ureaplasma* at 15 to 19 weeks of gestation.[73,74] However, the fetal lungs have increased surfactant and persistent elevations in mRNAs for surfactant proteins. This model of chronic colonization/infection of the fetal lung with *Ureaplasma* may closely resemble the clinical effects of *Ureaplasma* associated with preterm deliveries in humans.

These experiments demonstrate that fetal sheep can respond to a variety of proinflammatory agonists and can be colonized with *Ureaplasma*, the organisms most frequently associated with preterm delivery in the human. However, fetal responses do not simply replicate responses in the adult. For example, fetal sheep do not respond to intraamniotic or intravascular injections of sheep recombinant TNF-α,[127] and as noted previously, responses to TLR2 agonist were insufficient to consistently induce lung maturation. The spectrum of the response potential of the fetus and the fetal lung to the multiple mediators of innate immune responses remains to be studied. Clinical responses also may reflect the polymicrobial nature of the chorioamnionitis. Questions that remain relate to receptor expression, the cell localization of that expression, the response potential of the signaling pathways, and the maturity of the integration of innate and acquired immune responses.

Early Gestational Fetal Lung Responses to Inflammation

The interval from fetal exposure to chorioamnionitis and lung inflammation or lung maturation to delivery is not known in the human, primarily because of the lack of precision about the diagnosis of chorioamnionitis. In fetal sheep, significant lung maturation is not detected until 4 to 7 days after an intraamniotic injection of endotoxin.[116] Lung maturation is striking if the interval between intraamniotic endotoxin injection and preterm delivery is 15 days. Intraamniotic *Ureaplasma* did not induce lung maturation within 7 days but did induce lung maturation when given 14 to 45 days before preterm delivery.[125] Intraamniotic endotoxin given at 60 days of gestation (40% of gestation) to fetal sheep resulted in a doubling of lung-saturated phosphatidylcholine; increased surfactant protein A (SP-A), SP-B, and SP-C mRNA; and improved in lung function 65 days later.[128] The fetal sheep lung can respond to intraamniotic endotoxin/chorioamnionitis across a wide range of GAs. The question of how early in gestation an inflammatory stimulus can modulate fetal lung development remains unanswered in the clinical context. However, the frequent occurrence of early lung maturation and chorioamnionitis suggests that inflammation is the major mediator of lung maturation in the very preterm infant.

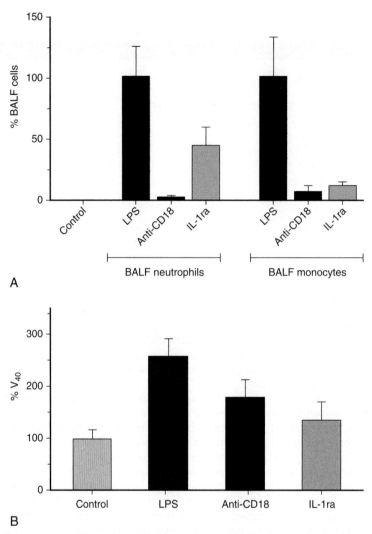

Fig. 2.12 Anti–CD18 antibody and IL-1 receptor antagonist *(IL-1ra)* block lung inflammation and maturation in fetal sheep. A, Fetal sheep were given an anti-CD18 antibody by intramuscular injection or IL-1ra into the amniotic fluid 3 hours before intraamniotic lipopolysaccharide *(LPS)*. Both treatments decreased the numbers of neutrophils and monocytes in bronchoalveolar lavage fluid *(BALF)*, indicating almost complete blockade of the endotoxin-induced lung inflammation at 2 days. B, The treatments also decreased lung gas volumes, measured at 40 cm H_2O pressure *(V_{40})* relative to LPS, indicating decreased lung maturation. (Data from Kallapur SG, Moss TJ, Ikegami M, et al. Recruited inflammatory cells mediate endotoxin-induced lung maturation in preterm fetal lambs. *Am J Respir Crit Care Med*. 2005;172:1315–1321; and Kallapur SG, Nitsos I, Moss TJ, et al. IL-1 mediates pulmonary and systemic inflammatory responses to chorioamnionitis induced by lipopolysaccharide. *Am J Respir Crit Care Med*. 2009;179:955–961.)

Mechanisms of Inflammation-Mediated Lung Maturation

The mechanisms responsible for inflammation-induced lung maturation are not well understood. The minimal amount of *E. coli* endotoxin given by intraamniotic injection that will induce lung maturation in the fetal sheep is 1 to 4 mg, and doses as high as 100 mg induce lung maturation without increasing the amount of lung inflammation or causing fetal injury or preterm delivery.[112,116] In general, the amount of lung inflammation induced by chorioamnionitis correlated with the amount of lung maturation. Our group used a monoclonal antibody to the integrin CD18 to block endotoxin-induced lung inflammation, which also prevented lung maturation (Fig. 2.12).[129] In contrast, inflammation and lung maturation induced by IL-I was not blocked by this anti-CD18 antibody. This experiment directly links inflammation to lung maturation and further demonstrates that different proinflammatory agonists can recruit inflammatory cells to the fetal lungs by different mechanisms.

This inflammation-maturation relationship was further examined with an IL-1 receptor blocker.[130] IL-1α and IL-1β are potent inducers of chorioamnionitis, lung inflammation, and lung maturation. When the IL-1 receptor antagonist IL-1ra was given into the amniotic fluid, about 80% of the lung inflammatory response to intraamniotic endotoxin was blocked, and lung maturation decreased. Since IL-1β is a potent cytokine, its secretion is exquisitely controlled in the cytoplasm by inflammasomes—a collection of interacting proteins that ultimately activate caspase 1, which cleaves pro-IL-1β to active IL-1β. When inflammasome NLRP3 was knocked out in mice, there was a significant reduction of lung IL-1β in neonatal mice in response to a hyperoxia challenge with a corresponding protection against BPD-like changes in response to hyperoxia.[131] These experiments demonstrate that lung inflammation in response to multiple stimuli is mediated, at least in part, by IL-1 signaling and that lung inflammation can drive lung maturation responses. There currently is no information about which products of lung inflammation signal lung maturation. Presumably, mediators produced locally in the distal lung parenchyma, possibly by granulocytes and/or monocytes, induce a signaling cascade resulting in the mesenchymal and type II cell changes that result in lung maturation. Insight into this signaling sequence may provide clues for the development of clinically practical strategies to induce lung maturation.

Experimental Chronic Chorioamnionitis

Although the majority of VLBW infants may be exposed to chronic chorioamnionitis, the duration and the intensity of the inflammatory exposure to the fetus remain undefined. A single proinflammatory fetal exposure from intraamniotic injections of mediators caused acute lung inflammation, mild microvascular injury, and an arrest in alveolar septation by 7 days.[38,113] Low-grade inflammation (increased inflammatory cells) persisted for weeks. Live *Ureaplasma* caused mild inflammation despite prolonged persistence in the fetal lung.[125] The clinically relevant question is how the fetal lung copes with prolonged exposures to inflammatory agonists such as endotoxin. Surprisingly, few VLBW infants seem to have severe pneumonia after preterm birth despite exposure to infection/inflammation. Although a single intrauterine exposure to endotoxin caused histologic changes consistent with a mild BPD phenotype in experimental animals, infants are not born with BPD. A possible exception is the rapid development of the BPD variant described by radiologic changes as the Wilson-Mikity syndrome, which has been associated with chorioamnionitis.[132] However, in general, severe lung injury and pneumonia are infrequent after the histologic chorioamnionitis associated with preterm birth.

Our group has modeled chronic endotoxin-induced chorioamnionitis with repeated weekly intraamniotic injections of endotoxin and with osmotic pumps that deliver endotoxin continuously over 28 days to the amniotic fluid. A prolonged fetal exposure resulting from a 28-day intraamniotic infusion of endotoxin from 53% to 72% of gestation caused striking lung maturation and increases in surfactant with decreased alveolar septation at 125 days (83% of gestation).[128] When the lungs of the fetal sheep were examined at 138 days of gestation, low-grade inflammation persisted 30 days after the end of endotoxin administration and surfactant was increased as a residual effect of the induced lung maturation (Fig. 2.13).[133] Remarkably, all anatomic indicators of the arrest of alveolar septation seen at 125 days of gestation had disappeared. There also were no biochemical or histologic indicators of microvascular injury.

Weekly intraamniotic injections with 10 mg endotoxin given at 100 days, 107 days, 114 days, and 121 days of gestation resulted in the persistence of inflammatory cells in the bronchoalveolar lavage just prior to term.[133] The mRNA for the proinflammatory cytokine IL-1β in lung tissue was higher than in controls, as was the amount of surfactant, but there were no changes in the lung architecture or microvasculature. These results demonstrate that the fetal lung can adapt to chronic inflammation and that despite a brief interference with alveolar septation and microvascular development, the fetal lung corrects the deficits and can continue to develop. *Ureaplasma* also causes subtle alterations in lung structure after a 14-day exposure, but the changes do not persist with more chronic exposures.[126,134]

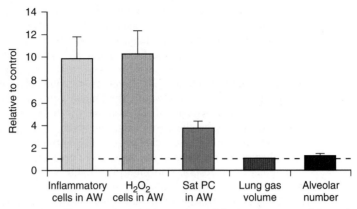

Fig. 2.13 Residual effects at 138 days of gestation of the intraamniotic infusion of 1 mg/day of endotoxin for 28 days of gestation, from day 80 to day 108 days, in fetal sheep. All measurements are expressed relative to the control group, which was normalized to 1.0 *(dashed line)*. Residual indicators of inflammation were the number of inflammatory cells in bronchoalveolar lavage and their ability to produce hydrogen peroxide *(H₂O₂)*. Although the amount of saturated phosphatidylcholine *(Sat PC)* in alveolar wash *(AW)* was increased, lung structure was not altered. (Data from Kallapur SG, Nitsos I, Moss TJ, et al. Chronic endotoxin exposure does not cause sustained structural abnormalities in the fetal sheep lungs. *Am J Physiol Lung Cell Mol Physiol.* 2005;288:L966–L974.)

Immune Response and Modulation from Fetal Exposures to Inflammation

A central question is how the naive immune system of the fetus responds to an intrauterine inflammatory challenge. In a rhesus macaque model of chorioamnionitis induced by intraamniotic injection of endotoxin, the frequency of the proinflammatory cytokines IL-17+ and IL-22+ CD4+–expressing T cells increased in the spleen of endotoxin-exposed fetuses, and the normally antiinflammatory regulatory T cell (Treg) frequency decreased.[135] Compounding the decrease in Tregs, larger proportions of the normally antiinflammatory Tregs expressed the proinflammatory cytokine 1L-17 (IL-17+ Forkhead box protein 3 [FoxP3+]–designated inflammatory Tregs). The emergence of inflammatory Tregs was largely dependent on IL-1 signaling. These results demonstrate that a prenatal inflammatory environment can lead to inadequate Treg generation in the thymus with a switch of splenic Tregs toward an inflammatory phenotype.

The sentinel immune cell of the lung is the alveolar macrophage. In adult humans and animals, macrophages are located in the air spaces directly in contact with the alveolar hypophase. Fetuses do not normally have alveolar macrophages. In mice, macrophages can be detected in the lung interstitium from early gestation, whereas in other species including nonhuman primates and sheep, very few mature macrophages are found in the fetal lung. In all species, mature alveolar macrophages begin populating the lung in large numbers postnatally with the onset of air breathing. Immature lung monocytes from preterm sheep have a minimal IL-6 secretory response to an in vitro challenge to endotoxin and do not respond to TNF-α.[136] However, intraamniotic endotoxin matures the lung monocytes by stimulating granulocyte-macrophage colony-stimulating factor (GM-CSF) and transcription factor PU.1 expression in the fetal lung (Fig. 2.14). These monocytes migrate into the fetal alveolar spaces and respond vigorously to both endotoxin and TNF-α in vitro.[136] Thus exposure to a proinflammatory agonist in the amniotic fluid is a potent stimulus for maturation and responsiveness of monocytes in the lung.

Intraamniotic endotoxin also can cause an innate immune tolerance in the fetus. In adult animals and humans, endotoxin tolerance is the suppression of endotoxin signaling caused by a complex reprogramming of inflammatory responses. As part of endotoxin tolerance, proinflammatory cytokine expression is downregulated, while there is no change or an increase in the expression of antiinflammatory

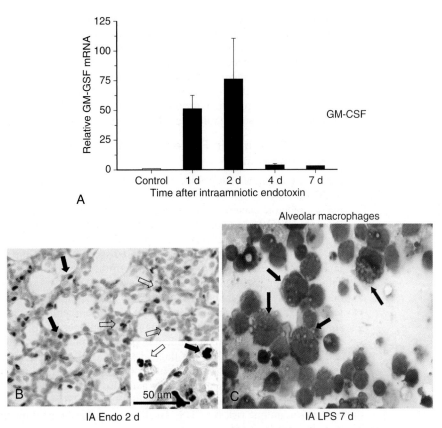

Fig. 2.14 Intraamniotic administration of lipopolysaccharide *(LPS)* matures alveolar macrophages in the fetal lungs. A, Following the intraamniotic injection *(IA)* of 10 mg LPS, granulocyte-monocyte colony-stimulating factor *(GM-CSF)* is induced in the fetal lung and, B, PU.1-positive cells appear in the lung at 2 days, indicating maturation from monocytes to macrophages. Expression is localized to nuclei of monocyte cells *(solid black arrows)* and neutrophils *(outlined arrows)*. Insert is similarly labeled with a scale bar = 50 μm. C, By 7 days, mature-appearing alveolar macrophages *(arrows)* are in high numbers in alveolar washes. *Endo,* Endotoxin; *mRNA,* messenger ribonucleic acid. (Data from Kramer BW, Joshi SN, Moss TJ, et al. Endotoxin-induced maturation of monocytes in preterm fetal sheep lung. *Am J Physiol Lung Cell Mol Physiol.* 2007;293:L345–L353.)

genes, antimicrobial genes, and genes mediating phagocytosis. In the preterm fetal sheep, exposure to intraamniotic endotoxin 2 days before delivery induces a robust expression to cytokines in the fetal lung. However, if the fetus is exposed to two intraamniotic endotoxin injections of the same dose 7 days and 2 days before delivery, the fetal lung is refractory to the second endotoxin injection.[137] Interestingly, both lung and blood monocytes are refractory to an in vitro challenge with endotoxin.

The phenomenon of innate immune tolerance is not restricted solely to exposure to endotoxin. Exposure to intraamniotic *Ureaplasma parvum* almost completely abolished responsiveness of the fetal lung to endotoxin, implying a profound immune paralysis in the fetal lung induced by *Ureaplasma* exposure.[138] The lung and blood monocytes from fetal sheep exposed to two injections of intraamniotic endotoxin were also refractory to stimulation by other TLR agonists, indicating a cross-tolerance.[139] Other interactive phenomena between antenatal endotoxin and postnatal inflammatory insults have also been reported. Intraamniotic endotoxin alone induced aberrant lung development and pulmonary hypertension in rats similar to that in sheep. When fetal mice exposed to endotoxin were exposed as newborns to moderate hyperoxia, the lung abnormalities were no longer evident. However, exposure to severe hyperoxia as newborns further enhanced the pulmonary abnormalities induced by antenatal endotoxin.[140] Thus the interactive phenomena between different inflammatory insults can be complex and either increase or reduce lung injury responses. The innate immune tolerance is time-dependent; thus it is not clear how these immune phenomena will translate into clinical scenarios when the timing of exposure to different inflammatory insults is not known. Although the precise mechanisms of innate immune tolerance are not known, the expression of the negative regulator of toll/IL-1 signaling, IRAK-M (IL-1 receptor–associated kinase-M), was increased in both the lung and blood monocytes,[137] suggesting a possible mechanism for innate immune tolerance in the fetus.

Immune Changes in Preterm Infants Exposed to Chorioamnionitis

Studies on immune changes in response to chorioamnionitis in humans are limited. In 2010, the National Institutes of Health initiated a collaborative network of five major academic centers in the United States (Prematurity and Respiratory Outcomes Program [PROP]) to understand the epidemiology and pathogenesis of BPD and to facilitate biomarker discovery.[141] As part of PROP, studies were conducted to identify immunologic alterations that might predispose to BPD. In a study of 35 ELBW infants, adverse ratios of the antiinflammatory Treg to the proinflammatory Th17 cells in the peripheral blood were detected in ELBW infants exposed to funisitis but not to BPD.[142] The infants with severe BPD had increased expression of IL-4 mRNA in peripheral blood mononuclear cells in response to stimulation. However, another study suggested involvement of Tregs in the pathogenesis of BPD.[143] A proinflammatory CD4[+] T-cell status was noted in preterm infants exposed to chorioamnionitis and those developing BPD, but those developing BPD also had decreased numbers of the antiinflammatory Tregs.[143] In another study from the PROP cohort, CD8[+] T cells from the more immature infants had a loss of regulatory coreceptor CD31 and greater effector differentiation than the more mature infants. This may place preterm neonates at unique risk for CD8[+] T-cell–mediated inflammation and impaired T-cell memory formation.[144]

Inflammatory Mediators and BPD

To understand the pathogenesis of BPD, the National Institutes of Child Health and Human Development (NICHD) enrolled a cohort of 1067 VLBW infants at multiple Neonatal Research Network sites in the United States.[103] Dried blood spots were collected from these infants serially over the first 21 days of life. Plasma cytokines in infants surviving without BPD were compared with those developing BPD or who died. In early samples from the BPD group (0–3 days) IL-8 and IL-10 were increased and RANTES and IL-17 were decreased. In the late samples (14–21 days) IL6 and interferon gamma were increased in infants who later had BPD. D'Angio et al.[145] recently reanalyzed these data for the surviving infants with BPD using the different respiratory patterns identified by Laughon et al.[97] The premise of this analysis was that because BPD is a heterogeneous disease, better insights might be gained by comparing cytokines in infants who developed BPD and had persistently high oxygen needs for the first 14 days (classic BPD) with those needing very low oxygen for the first 14 days of life (new BPD). IL-6, IL-8, IL-10, IL-18, C-reactive protein, macrophage inflammatory protein 1 alpha (MIP-1α), and matrix metalloproteinase 9 (MMP9) were increased in new versus classic BPD. In another report[146] increased IL-8, intracellular adhesion molecule 1 (ICAM-1) and decreased RANTES, vascular endothelial growth factor (VEGF), and MMP1 were demonstrated in plasma from infants developing BPD/death versus those surviving without BPD. Thus these different studies, while suggesting that inflammatory pathways underlie BPD, do not identify a particular inflammatory pathway. A limitation of these studies is that the inflammatory mediators associated with BPD may be missed because the expression and effect may be restricted to the lungs and not be present in the blood. Tissue cannot be sampled clinically. Because multiple different etiologies contribute to BPD (e.g., oxygen, mechanical ventilation, antenatal inflammation, postnatal infections), the complexity of inflammatory pathways induced may preclude identification of common pathways leading to BPD.

Table 2.6 META-ANALYSIS OF OBSERVATIONAL STUDIES OF ANTENATAL CORTICOSTEROID TREATMENTS FOR WOMEN WITH CHORIOAMNIONITIS

	Odds Ratio	95% Confidence Interval
Histologic Diagnosis of Chorioamnionitis (Five Studies)		
Mortality of newborn	0.45	0.30–0.68
Respiratory distress syndrome	0.53	0.40–0.71
Bronchopulmonary dysplasia	0.79	0.35–1.83
Severe intraventricular hemorrhage	0.39	0.19–0.82
Clinical Diagnosis of Chorioamnionitis (Four Studies)		
Mortality of newborn	0.77	0.36–1.65
Respiratory distress syndrome	0.73	0.48–1.12
Bronchopulmonary dysplasia	0.80	0.37–1.74
Severe intraventricular hemorrhage	0.29	0.10–0.89

Data from Been JV, Degraeuwe PL, Kramer BW, et al. Antenatal steroids and neonatal outcome after chorioamnionitis: a meta-analysis. *BJOG.* 2011;118:113–122.

Antenatal Corticosteroid Treatments and Chorioamnionitis

Corticosteroids are given antenatally to more than 80% of the women at risk for preterm delivery before 30 weeks of gestation, and the majority of these women have undiagnosed (histologic) chorioamnionitis.[66,97] The majority of women with preterm rupture of membranes have histologic chorioamnionitis. Thus preterm rupture of membranes is a surrogate marker for chorioamnionitis. The current recommendation is to give antenatal corticosteroids to women with preterm rupture of membranes because the treatment reduces the incidences of RDS, intraventricular hemorrhage, and death.[147] In clinical series, antenatal corticosteroids are of benefit for preterm deliveries that in retrospect had associated histologic chorioamnionitis.[148] A 2011 meta-analysis of observational studies identified benefit of corticosteroid treatment in infants from women with chorioamnionitis (Table 2.6).[149] Antenatal corticosteroids also decrease the fetal inflammatory response syndrome in preterm infants exposed to histologic chorioamnionitis.[148]

Although there is no specific clinical information available about how corticosteroids influence chorioamnionitis, the corticosteroids might suppress inflammation—a potential benefit—or increase the risk of progressive inflammation—a potential risk. Both outcomes seem possible on the basis of the small amount of information available from experimental studies. Maternal treatment with betamethasone suppressed the inflammation caused by intraamniotic endotoxin in the chorioamnion and lungs of fetal sheep (Fig. 2.15).[150,151] Inflammatory cells and proinflammatory cytokine expression were suppressed for about 2 days after the betamethasone treatment, but subsequently inflammation was *increased* in the lungs of lambs exposed to both maternal betamethasone and intraamniotic endotoxin compared with lambs exposed to endotoxin alone 5 and 15 days after the exposures. Lung maturation was greater in lambs exposed to both betamethasone and endotoxin at the same time than to either treatment alone (Fig. 2.16).[152] A surprising result was that growth restriction induced by betamethasone did not occur with concurrent endotoxin exposure. These results in fetal sheep support the clinical observations that betamethasone can further decrease RDS in the presence of histologic chorioamnionitis.[148] In fetal sheep the lung maturational response to endotoxin was larger and more uniform than the response to betamethasone. A distinct difference in the responses is the improvement in lung function within 15 hours after administration of betamethasone and the delay for an improvement in lung function of at least 4 days following intraamniotic endotoxin.[36,116] Betamethasone also can augment the lung maturation induced by chronic fetal *Ureaplasma* colonization.[153]

The increased inflammation in the fetal sheep lungs that occurs 5 to 15 days after combined betamethasone and endotoxin exposures is a potential concern. A potential mechanism to explain the increased inflammation is that both

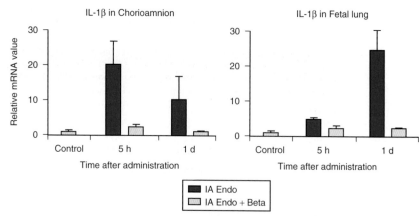

Fig. 2.15 Maternal betamethasone suppressed the inflammation induced by intraamniotic *(IA)* administration of endotoxin *(Endo)* in the chorioamnion and fetal lung. The expression of interleukin-1β (IL-1β) messenger RNA *(mRNA)* was decreased to control values by maternal betamethasone given to sheep 3 hours *(h)* before IA endotoxin. (Data from Newnham JP, Kallapur SG, Kramer BW, et al. Betamethasone effects on chorioamnionitis induced by intra-amniotic endotoxin in sheep. *Am J Obstet Gynecol.* 2003;189:1458–1466; and Kallapur SG, Kramer BW, Moss TJ, et al. Maternal glucocorticoids increase endotoxin-induced lung inflammation in preterm lambs. *Am J Physiol Lung Cell Mol Physiol.* 2003;284:L633–L642.)

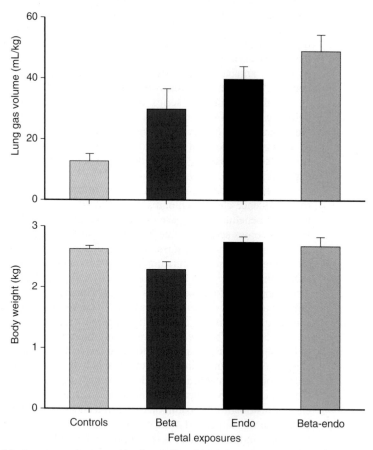

Fig. 2.16 Lung gas volumes and body weights of fetal sheep 7 days after exposure to maternal betamethasone *(Beta)*, intraamniotic endotoxin *(Endo)*, or both *(Beta-endo)*. Maximal lung gas volume, measured at an airway pressure of 40 cm H_2O, increased with either treatment but was largest with both treatments. Only maternal betamethasone decreased fetal weight, and this effect was prevented by concurrent endotoxin exposure. (Redrawn from Newnham JP, Moss TJ, Padbury JF, et al. The interactive effects of endotoxin with prenatal glucocorticoids on short-term lung function in sheep. *Am J Obstet Gynecol.* 2001;185:190–197.)

betamethasone and the endotoxin "mature" an immature innate immune system. Blood monocytes from fetal sheep have decreased responses in vitro to endotoxin stimulation compared with monocytes from adult sheep.[154] However, 7 days after the fetal exposures, the monocytes respond to endotoxin in vitro similarly to monocytes from adult sheep. Maternal betamethasone also initially suppresses the fetal monocyte, but function is increased 7 days after the maternal treatment.[155] These results illustrate just how clinically complex interactions between these two clinically relevant exposures may be.

These experiments in fetal sheep describe simultaneous exposures to betamethasone and chorioamnionitis. The more likely clinical scenarios are the superposition of maternal betamethasone treatments on chronic, subclinical chorioamnionitis, or maternal betamethasone treatments followed by the acute onset of chorioamnionitis. In fetal sheep exposure to endotoxin 14 days followed by betamethasone 7 days before preterm delivery qualitatively induced the largest lung maturation response.[156] There is no information about how the timing of exposures may alter clinical outcomes. Repetitive courses of betamethasone treatments may be a concern, particularly when chorioamnionitis is present. The clinical dilemma is that histologic chorioamnionitis is a retrospective diagnosis of a process that is frequently clinically silent.

Intrauterine Growth Restriction/Small for GA

Fetuses identified as having IUGR on the basis of estimates of fetal size and Doppler flow patterns of the fetal circulation and infants born SGA according to standardized growth charts are overlapping populations with varied causes for the inadequate growth. For the preterm segment of this population, the majority of infants are from pregnancies with associated hypertension or preeclampsia,[157] excluding genetic and chromosomal abnormalities. Lung disease after term or near-term delivery has not been well studied but is not appreciated as a clinical problem. In contrast, preterm growth-restricted infants and infants of preeclamptic pregnancies have an increased risk for RDS, despite the severe chronic stress experienced by the fetuses.[158,159] Jelin and associates[160] also reported that preeclampsia with onset early in pregnancy increased the risk for SGA infants (OR 3.9, 59% CI 2.5–6.2) and for RDS (OR 1.5, 95% CI 1.1–2.2). The concept has been that fetal stress will increase fetal cortisol levels and induce lung maturation, but the stresses causing fetal growth restriction and preeclampsia do not decrease RDS relative to the comparison populations of preterm infants. We suspect that the comparison group simply illustrates one "elephant in the room" in that the comparison population may be enriched for infants exposed to chorioamnionitis, which is less frequent in IUGR/SGA infants. This interpretation suggests decreased RDS in both populations relative to a theoretical population of normal preterm infants. A reasonable conclusion is that preeclamptic/IUGR/SGA preterm infants are not protected from respiratory problems soon after birth, as captured by the diagnosis of RDS.

These small infants are at increased risk for mortality and BPD. In one study, IUGR or SGA status at birth raised mortality for infants at all gestations and increased the need for respiratory support at 28 days of age primarily for infants born at 26 to 29 weeks GA.[161] Reiss and colleagues[162] reported an increased risk in BPD for infants with birth weights below the 10th percentile (OR 3.8, 95% CI 2.1–6.8). This relationship of increased BPD with low birth weight for GA is a continuum that includes less BPD at high birth weights for GA (Fig. 2.17).[157] Bose and coworkers[163] also demonstrated an increased risk of BPD with logistic regression models for 1241 infants who were born prior to 28 weeks of gestation and survived to 36 weeks GA. The predictors of BPD were GA and birth weights for GA with a z score below −1 (OR 3.2, 95% CI 2.1–5.0), or z scores of −2 (OR 4.4, 95% CI 2.2–8.2). There are several possible explanations for the increased risk of BPD in infants born SGA. The somewhat trivial explanation is that the respiratory and nutritional care of smaller infants are more difficult technically than that for larger infants. For example, the 600-g 27-week infant may be ventilated longer because of perceived fragility than

Fig. 2.17 Odds ratios *(circles)* and 95% confidence intervals *(lines)* for bronchopulmonary dysplasia *(BPD, solid circles)* and mortality *(open circles)* for infants grouped by birth weight percentiles adjusted for gestational ages. The risks for BPD and mortality increase as birth weight percentiles decrease from the reference group for the 50th to 74th percentiles. The risks of BPD and death are lower for the larger infants. (Data from Zeitlin J, El Ayoubi M, Jarreau PH, et al. Impact of fetal growth restriction on mortality and morbidity in a very preterm birth cohort. *J Pediatr.* 2001;157:733.e1–739.e1.)

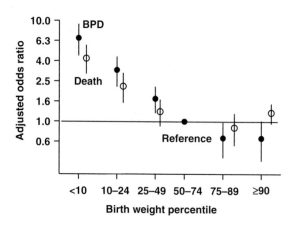

the 1000-g 27-week infant, with the consequence being increased BPD. However, biologic explanations likely contribute to this association. McElrath and associates[1] hypothesize that most severe prematurity results from either inflammation/infection or vascular developmental abnormalities that may progress from implantation. These vascular abnormalities (preeclampsia) are highly associated with fetal growth failure and an increased risk for BPD.[164] Therefore the clinical data are consistent with the likelihood that small infants may have abnormal lung vascular development.

IUGR may interact with hypoxemia to cause adverse outcomes in preterm infants. In a secondary analysis of the SUPPORT trial designed to evaluate optimal oxygen targeting, and less invasive respiratory support to decrease BPD, Walsh et al. report that the unexpected finding of increased mortality in infants randomized to the low oxygen targeting group was almost exclusively in the IUGR population.[165] Collectively, these studies highlight the importance of intrauterine growth as a potent modulator for the risk of BPD or death in preterm infants.

Antenatal corticosteroids decrease fetal growth in animal models and can decrease fetal growth with repetitive treatments in humans.[60] Thus the combined effects of antenatal corticosteroid treatments in growth-restricted fetuses could be adverse. There are no targeted randomized trials of antenatal corticosteroids for these at-risk pregnancies, although antenatal corticosteroids are routinely used for pregnancies with preeclampsia and at risk for preterm delivery.[161] Data from the early randomized trials show no adverse effects of corticosteroid use with maternal hypertension or for SGA infants.[29] The available data from clinical series do not suggest that antenatal corticosteroids are of benefit for growth-restricted fetuses.[166] Thus questions remain about the benefit of antenatal corticosteroids for the growth-restricted fetus.

Experimental models demonstrate clear effects of decreased fetal growth on lung development. Fetal sheep become growth restricted if placental implantation sites are decreased prior to pregnancy. Lipsett and colleagues[167] reported that fetal growth restriction caused a reduction in the gas exchange surface density of the fetal lung with smaller alveoli. Growth-restricted preterm fetal sheep had reduced surfactant protein levels, indicating delayed lung maturation despite high fetal cortisol levels.[168] Similarly, fetal growth restriction caused by a hypoxic environment in mice decreased mRNA expression of the surfactant proteins.[169] Exposure of growth-restricted fetal sheep to corticosteroids altered cardiovascular responses and increased indicators of brain injury relative to comparison groups with normal growth.[170,171] Although the causes of fetal growth restriction in humans differ from those in the animal models, the lungs may have abnormal structure and maturation. Multiple questions remain about the mechanisms by which growth restriction increases BPD.

Environmental Factors and Lung Disease

Multiple environmental factors could modulate lung development in the fetus and have consequences after birth. Fetal and early neonatal exposures that may increase risks for asthma in children and chronic lung diseases in adults are included in the research on early origins of adult diseases and the hygiene hypothesis. Studies have focused primarily on term infant populations, and these subjects are beyond the scope of this chapter. However, we briefly explore two fetal exposures that may be underappreciated modulators of fetal lung development and that have not been adequately explored in relation to lung diseases in preterms. In a perspective written in 2001, Pierce and Nguyen[172] itemized the multiple effects of maternal cigarette smoking on fetal and newborn lung growth and function in animal models. These effects include decreased lung size and volume, changes in lung collagen and elastin, greater alveolar size, and increased type II cell numbers. Maternal smoking induced airway remodeling in fetal mice,[173] the presumed substrate for the airway disease reported in infants exposed to environmental smoke.[174] Maternal smoking was associated with increases in tests of lung maturation and cortisol in amniotic fluid in humans,[175] and nicotine altered developmental programs in the fetal lungs of rats.[176] In fetal monkeys, prenatal exposure to nicotine also caused lung hypoplasia and increased collagen deposition around large airways and vessels.[177] Infants who were exposed to maternal smoking and who died of sudden infant death syndrome had fewer alveolar attachment points on airways.[178] A striking example of prevention of adverse lung function in infants born to mothers smoking cigarettes is maternal treatment with vitamin C. In a randomized, double-blind trial enrolling 159 newborns of pregnant smokers, supplemental vitamin C improved newborn pulmonary function tests and decreased wheezing through 1 year.[179] These observations are consistent with the hypothesis that maternal smoking may alter lung structural and maturational development in both term and preterm infants, an effect that should be reflected in disease incidences of RDS, BPD, and more frequent airway reactivity in childhood. Populations of very preterm infants have not been evaluated for such effects.

A less studied exposure with possible effects on the preterm lung is maternal alcohol use. The fetal alcohol syndrome that includes fetal growth restriction and impaired neurodevelopment is well described. Exposure of fetal sheep to alcohol for the last third of gestation decreased surfactant protein mRNA expression but increased extracellular matrix deposition.[180] Changes in cytokine levels in the fetal lungs could result in altered immune status. Alcohol abuse alters the redox state of the adult lung, in which adult respiratory distress syndrome is more likely to develop with an injury.[181] The effects of maternal alcohol abuse on lung function and injury in preterm infants remain unexplored.

Summary: The Complexities

Premature delivery is an abnormal event, and the preterm infant must have sufficiently developed lungs to survive, often with the help of multiple interventions such as antenatal corticosteroids, surfactant, and mechanical ventilation. The experimental literature relating to lung development and maturity is vast and informative, but the story becomes quite muddled when clinical experiences are considered. There are just too many variables that influence the status of the preterm lung at delivery. GA and birth weight are the overriding predictors of outcomes. Maternal/fetal diseases such as preeclampsia and chorioamnionitis have potent effects on the fetal lung, but both have a spectrum of effects ranging from decreased risks to increased risks of RDS or BPD. Antenatal corticosteroids clearly benefit preterm infants overall, but how they further modulate the pregnancy abnormalities resulting in preterm delivery probably differ for each abnormality and with the timing of the fetal exposures. Environmental exposures such as smoke and alcohol are seldom considered relative to lung disease in the preterm. Other factors, such as genetic background, race, and fetal sex, are not discussed in this chapter. Finally, the diagnoses of RDS and BPD are imprecise and also represent spectrums of severity. The pathophysiology that accompanies RDS or BPD results in large part from clinical management of the preterm infants. As clinicians, we can understand populations of infants, but we are poor at predicting the outcomes for individual very preterm infants. Our failures result from a lack of a basic understanding of how lung developmental programs interact with injury programs and repair programs that are superimposed during the fetal period on the abnormalities that result in preterm delivery. The fetus then is assaulted by postnatal events—oxygen, mechanical ventilation, infection. It is a wonder of nature that VLBW infants can survive and that most of the survivors have relatively normal lung function in childhood.

REFERENCES

1. McElrath TF, Hecht JL, Dammann O, et al. Pregnancy disorders that lead to delivery before the 28th week of gestation: an epidemiologic approach to classification. *Am J Epidemiol.* 2008;168(9):980–989.
2. Berry CE, Billheimer D, Jenkins IC, et al. A distinct low lung function trajectory from childhood to the fourth decade of life. *Am J Respir Crit Care Med.* 2016;194(5):607–612.
3. Nada AM, Shafeek MM, El Maraghy MA, Nageeb AH, Salah El Din AS, Awad MH. Antenatal corticosteroid administration before elective caesarean section at term to prevent neonatal respiratory morbidity: a randomized controlled trial. *Eur J Obstet Gynecol Reprod Biol.* 2016;199:88–91.
4. Tita AT, Landon MB, Spong CY, et al. Timing of elective repeat cesarean delivery at term and neonatal outcomes. *N Engl J Med.* 2009;360(2):111–120.
5. Consortium on Safe Labor, Hibbard JU, Wilkins I, et al. Respiratory morbidity in late preterm births. *JAMA.* 2010;304(4):419–425.
6. Stoll BJ, Hansen NI, Bell EF, et al. Trends in care practices, morbidity, and mortality of extremely preterm neonates, 1993–2012. *JAMA.* 2015;314(10):1039–1051.
7. Burri PH. Structural aspects of prenatal and postnatal development and growth of the lung. In: McDonald JA, ed. *Lung Growth and Development.* New York: Marcel Dekker, Inc; 1997:1–35.
8. Ochs M, Nyengaard JR, Jung A, et al. The number of alveoli in the human lung. *Am J Respir Crit Care Med.* 2004;169(1):120–124.
9. Coalson JJ, Winter V, deLemos RA. Decreased alveolarization in baboon survivors with bronchopulmonary dysplasia. *Am J Respir Crit Care Med.* 1995;152(2):640–646.
10. Burri PH. Structural aspects of postnatal lung development—alveolar formation and growth. *Biol Neonate.* 2006;89(4):313–322.
11. Schittny JC, Mund SI, Stampanoni M. Evidence and structural mechanism for late lung alveolarization. *Am J Physiol Lung Cell Mol Physiol.* 2008;294(2):L246–L254.
12. Narayanan M, Beardsmore CS, Owers-Bradley J, et al. Catch-up alveolarization in ex-preterm children: evidence from (3)He magnetic resonance. *Am J Respir Crit Care Med.* 2013;187(10):1104–1109.
13. Avery ME, Mead J. Surface properties in relation to atelectasis and hyaline membrane disease. *AMA J Dis Child.* 1959;97(5, Part 1):517–523.
14. Gluck L, Kulovich MV, Borer RC Jr, Brenner PH, Anderson GG, Spellacy WN. Diagnosis of the respiratory distress syndrome by amniocentesis. *Am J Obstet Gynecol.* 1971;109(3):440–445.
15. Hallman M, Kulovich M, Kirkpatrick E, Sugarman RG, Gluck L. Phosphatidylinositol and phosphatidylglycerol in amniotic fluid: indices of lung maturity. *Am J Obstet Gynecol.* 1976;125(5):613–617.
16. Bancalari EH, Jobe AH. The respiratory course of extremely preterm infants: a dilemma for diagnosis and terminology. *J Pediatr.* 2012;161(4):585–588.
17. Morley CJ, Davis PG, Doyle LW, et al. Nasal CPAP or intubation at birth for very preterm infants. *N Engl J Med.* 2008;358(7):700–708.
18. SUPPORT Study Group of the Eunice Kennedy Shriver NICHD Neonatal Research Network, Finer NN, Carlo WA, et al. Early CPAP versus surfactant in extremely preterm infants. *N Engl J Med.* 2010;362(21):1970–1979.
19. Verder H, Albertsen P, Ebbesen F, et al. Nasal continuous positive airway pressure and early surfactant therapy for respiratory distress syndrome in newborns of less than 30 weeks' gestation. *Pediatrics.* 1999;103(2):E24.
20. Ammari A, Suri M, Milisavljevic V, et al. Variables associated with the early failure of nasal CPAP in very low birth weight infants. *J Pediatr.* 2005;147(3):341–347.
21. Jobe AH. "Miracle" extremely low birth weight neonates: examples of developmental plasticity. *Obstet Gynecol.* 2010;116(5):1184–1190.
22. Mulrooney N, Champion Z, Moss TJ, Nitsos I, Ikegami M, Jobe AH. Surfactant and physiologic responses of preterm lambs to continuous positive airway pressure. *Am J Respir Crit Care Med.* 2005;171(5):488–493.
23. Kamath-Rayne BD, Du Y, Hughes M, et al. Systems biology evaluation of cell-free amniotic fluid transcriptome of term and preterm infants to detect fetal maturity. *BMC Med Genomics.* 2015;8:67.
24. Schmolzer GM, Kumar M, Pichler G, Aziz K, O'Reilly M, Cheung PY. Non-invasive versus invasive respiratory support in preterm infants at birth: systematic review and meta-analysis. *BMJ.* 2013;347:f5980.
25. Bland RD, Ertsey R, Mokres LM, et al. Mechanical ventilation uncouples synthesis and assembly of elastin and increases apoptosis in lungs of newborn mice. Prelude to defective alveolar septation during lung development? *Am J Physiol Lung Cell Mol Physiol.* 2008;294(1):L3–L14.
26. Mokres LM, Parai K, Hilgendorff A, et al. Prolonged mechanical ventilation with air induces apoptosis and causes failure of alveolar septation and angiogenesis in lungs of newborn mice. *Am J Physiol Lung Cell Mol Physiol.* 2010;298(1):L23–L35.
27. Hjalmarson O, Sandberg K. Abnormal lung function in healthy preterm infants. *Am J Respir Crit Care Med.* 2002;165(1):83–87.
28. Effect of corticosteroids for fetal maturation on perinatal outcomes. NIH consensus development panel on the effect of corticosteroids for fetal maturation on perinatal outcomes. *JAMA.* 1995;273(5):413–418.

29. Roberts D, Dalziel S. Antenatal corticosteroids for accelerating fetal lung maturation for women at risk of preterm birth. *Cochrane Database Syst Rev*. 2006;(3):CD004454.
30. Antenatal corticosteroids revisited: repeat courses. *NIH Consens Statement*. 2000;17(2):1–18.
31. Brownfoot FC, Crowther CA, Middleton P. Different corticosteroids and regimens for accelerating fetal lung maturation for women at risk of preterm birth. *Cochrane Database Syst Rev*. 2008;(4): CD006764.
32. Hayes EJ, Paul DA, Stahl GE, et al. Effect of antenatal corticosteroids on survival for neonates born at 23 weeks of gestation. *Obstet Gynecol*. 2008;111(4):921–926.
33. Borowski KS, Clark EA, Lai Y, et al. Neonatal genetic variation in steroid metabolism and key respiratory function genes and perinatal outcomes in single and multiple courses of corticosteroids. *Am J Perinatol*. 2015;32(12):1126–1132.
34. Bunton TE, Plopper CG. Triamcinolone-induced structural alterations in the development of the lung of the fetal rhesus macaque. *Am J Obstet Gynecol*. 1984;148(2):203–215.
35. Willet KE, Jobe AH, Ikegami M, Kovar J, Sly PD. Lung morphometry after repetitive antenatal glucocorticoid treatment in preterm sheep. *Am J Respir Crit Care Med*. 2001;163(6):1437–1443.
36. Ikegami M, Polk D, Jobe A. Minimum interval from fetal betamethasone treatment to postnatal lung responses in preterm lambs. *Am J Obstet Gynecol*. 1996;174(5):1408–1413.
37. ElKady T, Jobe A. Corticosteroids and surfactant increase lung volumes and decrease rupture pressures of preterm rabbit lungs. *J Appl Physiol (1985)*. 1987;63(4):1616–1621.
38. Willet KE, Jobe AH, Ikegami M, Newnham J, Sly PD. Pulmonary interstitial emphysema 24 hours after antenatal betamethasone treatment in preterm sheep. *Am J Respir Crit Care Med*. 2000;162(3 Pt 1):1087–1094.
39. Ikegami M, Polk D, Tabor B, Lewis J, Yamada T, Jobe A. Corticosteroid and thyrotropin-releasing hormone effects on preterm sheep lung function. *J Appl Physiol (1985)*. 1991;70(5):2268–2278.
40. Jobe AH, Mitchell BR, Gunkel JH. Beneficial effects of the combined use of prenatal corticosteroids and postnatal surfactant on preterm infants. *Am J Obstet Gynecol*. 1993;168(2):508–513.
41. Ikegami M, Jobe AH, Yamada T, Seidner S. Relationship between alveolar saturated phosphatidylcholine pool sizes and compliance of preterm rabbit lungs. The effect of maternal corticosteroid treatment. *Am Rev Respir Dis*. 1989;139(2):367–369.
42. Seidner S, Pettenazzo A, Ikegami M, Jobe A. Corticosteroid potentiation of surfactant dose response in preterm rabbits. *J Appl Physiol (1985)*. 1988;64(6):2366–2371.
43. Ueda T, Ikegami M, Jobe AH. Developmental changes of sheep surfactant: in vivo function and in vitro subtype conversion. *J Appl Physiol (1985)*. 1994;76(6):2701–2706.
44. Hillman NH, Pillow JJ, Ball MK, Polglase GR, Kallapur SG, Jobe AH. Antenatal and postnatal corticosteroid and resuscitation induced lung injury in preterm sheep. *Respir Res*. 2009;10:124.
45. Bachurski CJ, Ross GF, Ikegami M, Kramer BW, Jobe AH. Intra-amniotic endotoxin increases pulmonary surfactant proteins and induces SP-B processing in fetal sheep. *Am J Physiol Lung Cell Mol Physiol*. 2001;280(2):L279–L285.
46. Carlo WA, McDonald SA, Fanaroff AA, et al. Association of antenatal corticosteroids with mortality and neurodevelopmental outcomes among infants born at 22 to 25 weeks' gestation. *JAMA*. 2011;306(21):2348–2358.
47. Jobe AH, Nitsos I, Pillow JJ, Polglase GR, Kallapur SG, Newnham JP. Betamethasone dose and formulation for induced lung maturation in fetal sheep. *Am J Obstet Gynecol*. 2009;201(6):611. e611–e617.
48. Kemp MW, Saito M, Usuda H, et al. Maternofetal pharmacokinetics and fetal lung responses in chronically catheterized sheep receiving constant, low-dose infusions of betamethasone phosphate. *Am J Obstet Gynecol*. 2016;215(6):775.e771–e712.
49. Onland W, de Laat MW, Mol BW, Offringa M. Effects of antenatal corticosteroids given prior to 26 weeks' gestation: a systematic review of randomized controlled trials. *Am J Perinatol*. 2011;28(1):33–44.
50. Garite TJ, Rumney PJ, Briggs GG, et al. A randomized, placebo-controlled trial of betamethasone for the prevention of respiratory distress syndrome at 24 to 28 weeks' gestation. *Am J Obstet Gynecol*. 1992;166(2):646–651.
51. Tucker Edmonds B, McKenzie F, Robinson BK. Maternal-fetal medicine physicians' practice patterns for 22-week delivery management. *J Matern Fetal Neonatal Med*. 2016;29(11):1829–1833.
52. Sinclair JC. Meta-analysis of randomized controlled trials of antenatal corticosteroid for the prevention of respiratory distress syndrome: discussion. *Am J Obstet Gynecol*. 1995;173(1):335–344.
53. Gyamfi-Bannerman C, Thom EA. Antenatal betamethasone for women at risk for late preterm delivery. *N Engl J Med*. 2016;375(5):486–487.
54. Kamath-Rayne BD, Rozance PJ, Goldenberg RL, Jobe AH. Antenatal corticosteroids beyond 34 weeks gestation: what do we do now? *Am J Obstet Gynecol*. 2016;215(4):423–430.
55. Society for Maternal-Fetal Medicine (SMFM) Publications Committee. Implementation of the use of antenatal corticosteroids in the late preterm birth period in women at risk for preterm delivery. *Am J Obstet Gynecol*. 2016;215(2):B13–B15.
56. Stutchfield P, Whitaker R, Russell I. Antenatal Steroids for Term Elective Caesarean Section (ASTECS) Research Team. Antenatal betamethasone and incidence of neonatal respiratory distress after elective caesarean section: pragmatic randomised trial. *BMJ*. 2005;331(7518):662.
57. Makhija NK, Tronnes AA, Dunlap BS, Schulkin J, Lannon SM. Antenatal corticosteroid timing: accuracy after the introduction of a rescue course protocol. *Am J Obstet Gynecol*. 2016;214(1):120. e121–e126.

58. Ikegami M, Jobe AH, Newnham J, Polk DH, Willet KE, Sly P. Repetitive prenatal glucocorticoids improve lung function and decrease growth in preterm lambs. *Am J Respir Crit Care Med.* 1997;156(1):178–184.

59. Crowther CA, McKinlay CJ, Middleton P, Harding JE. Repeat doses of prenatal corticosteroids for women at risk of preterm birth for improving neonatal health outcomes. *Cochrane Database Syst Rev.* 2015;(7):CD003935.

60. Murphy KE, Hannah ME, Willan AR, et al. Multiple courses of antenatal corticosteroids for preterm birth (MACS): a randomised controlled trial. *Lancet.* 2008;372(9656):2143–2151.

61. Crowther CA, Doyle LW, Haslam RR, et al. Outcomes at 2 years of age after repeat doses of antenatal corticosteroids. *N Engl J Med.* 2007;357(12):1179–1189.

62. Wapner RJ, Sorokin Y, Mele L, et al. Long-term outcomes after repeat doses of antenatal corticosteroids. *N Engl J Med.* 2007;357(12):1190–1198.

63. Stjernholm-Vladic Y, Stygar D, Mansson C, et al. Factors involved in the inflammatory events of cervical ripening in humans. *Reprod Biol Endocrinol.* 2004;2:74.

64. Marshall-Clarke S, Reen D, Tasker L, Hassan J. Neonatal immunity: how well has it grown up? *Immunol Today.* 2000;21(1):35–41.

65. Goldenberg RL, Culhane JF, Iams JD, Romero R. Epidemiology and causes of preterm birth. *Lancet.* 2008;371(9606):75–84.

66. Goldenberg RL, Hauth JC, Andrews WW. Intrauterine infection and preterm delivery. *N Engl J Med.* 2000;342(20):1500–1507.

67. Higgins RD, Saade G, Polin RA, et al. Evaluation and management of women and newborns with a maternal diagnosis of chorioamnionitis: summary of a workshop. *Obstet Gynecol.* 2016;127(3):426–436.

68. Redline RW, Wilson-Costello D, Borawski E, Fanaroff AA, Hack M. Placental lesions associated with neurologic impairment and cerebral palsy in very low-birth-weight infants. *Arch Pathol Lab Med.* 1998;122(12):1091–1098.

69. Romero R, Espinoza J, Chaiworapongsa T, Kalache K. Infection and prematurity and the role of preventive strategies. *Semin Neonatol.* 2002;7(4):259–274.

70. Yoon BH, Romero R, Jun JK, et al. Amniotic fluid cytokines (interleukin-6, tumor necrosis factor-alpha, interleukin-1 beta, and interleukin-8) and the risk for the development of bronchopulmonary dysplasia. *Am J Obstet Gynecol.* 1997;177(4):825–830.

71. DiGiulio DB, Romero R, Amogan HP, et al. Microbial prevalence, diversity and abundance in amniotic fluid during preterm labor: a molecular and culture-based investigation. *PLoS One.* 2008;3(8):e3056.

72. Buhimschi IA, Christner R, Buhimschi CS. Proteomic biomarker analysis of amniotic fluid for identification of intra-amniotic inflammation. *BJOG.* 2005;112(2):173–181.

73. Gerber S, Vial Y, Hohlfeld P, Witkin SS. Detection of *Ureaplasma urealyticum* in second-trimester amniotic fluid by polymerase chain reaction correlates with subsequent preterm labor and delivery. *J Infect Dis.* 2003;187(3):518–521.

74. Perni SC, Vardhana S, Korneeva I, et al. Mycoplasma hominis and *Ureaplasma urealyticum* in midtrimester amniotic fluid: association with amniotic fluid cytokine levels and pregnancy outcome. *Am J Obstet Gynecol.* 2004;191(4):1382–1386.

75. Combs CA, Gravett M, Garite TJ, et al. Amniotic fluid infection, inflammation, and colonization in preterm labor with intact membranes. *Am J Obstet Gynecol.* 2014;210(2):125.e121–e115.

76. DiGiulio DB. Diversity of microbes in amniotic fluid. *Semin Fetal Neonatal Med.* 2012;17(1):2–11.

77. Onderdonk AB, Delaney ML, DuBois AM, Allred EN, Leviton A. Extremely low gestational age newborns study I. detection of bacteria in placental tissues obtained from extremely low gestational age neonates. *Am J Obstet Gynecol.* 2008;198(1):110.e111–e117.

78. Hecht JL, Onderdonk A, Delaney M, et al. Characterization of chorioamnionitis in 2nd-trimester C-section placentas and correlation with microorganism recovery from subamniotic tissues. *Pediatr Dev Pathol.* 2008;11(1):15–22.

79. Oh KJ, Lee KA, Sohn YK, et al. Intraamniotic infection with genital mycoplasmas exhibits a more intense inflammatory response than intraamniotic infection with other microorganisms in patients with preterm premature rupture of membranes. *Am J Obstet Gynecol.* 2010;203(3):211.e211–e218.

80. Sweeney EL, Kallapur SG, Gisslen T, et al. Placental infection with *Ureaplasma* species is associated with histologic chorioamnionitis and adverse outcomes in moderately preterm and late-preterm infants. *J Infect Dis.* 2016;213(8):1340–1347.

81. Steel JH, Malatos S, Kennea N, et al. Bacteria and inflammatory cells in fetal membranes do not always cause preterm labor. *Pediatr Res.* 2005;57(3):404–411.

82. Reiman M, Kujari H, Ekholm E, et al. Interleukin-6 polymorphism is associated with chorioamnionitis and neonatal infections in preterm infants. *J Pediatr.* 2008;153(1):19–24.

83. Shalak LF, Laptook AR, Jafri HS, Ramilo O, Perlman JM. Clinical chorioamnionitis, elevated cytokines, and brain injury in term infants. *Pediatrics.* 2002;110(4):673–680.

84. Wortham JM, Hansen NI, Schrag SJ, et al. Chorioamnionitis and culture-confirmed, early-onset neonatal infections. *Pediatrics.* 2016;137(1).

85. Morris A, Meaney S, Spillane N, O'Donoghue K. The postnatal morbidity associated with second-trimester miscarriage. *J Matern Fetal Neonatal Med.* 2016;29(17):2786–2790.

86. Richardson CJ, Pomerance JJ, Cunningham MD, Gluck L. Acceleration of fetal lung maturation following prolonged rupture of the membranes. *Am J Obstet Gynecol.* 1974;118(8):1115–1118.

87. Watterberg KL, Demers LM, Scott SM, Murphy S. Chorioamnionitis and early lung inflammation in infants in whom bronchopulmonary dysplasia develops. *Pediatrics.* 1996;97(2):210–215.

88. De Dooy J, Colpaert C, Schuerwegh A, et al. Relationship between histologic chorioamnionitis and early inflammatory variables in blood, tracheal aspirates, and endotracheal colonization in preterm infants. *Pediatr Res*. 2003;54(1):113–119.

89. Groneck P, Goetze-Speer B, Speer CP. Inflammatory bronchopulmonary response of preterm infants with microbial colonisation of the airways at birth. *Arch Dis Child Fetal Neonatal Ed*. 1996;74(1):F51–F55.

90. Costeloe K, Hennessy E, Gibson AT, Marlow N, Wilkinson AR. The EPICure study: outcomes to discharge from hospital for infants born at the threshold of viability. *Pediatrics*. 2000;106(4):659–671.

91. Hannaford K, Todd DA, Jeffery H, John E, Blyth K, Gilbert GL. Role of *Ureaplasma urealyticum* in lung disease of prematurity. *Arch Dis Child Fetal Neonatal Ed*. 1999;81(3):F162–F167.

92. Lahra MM, Beeby PJ, Jeffery HE. Maternal versus fetal inflammation and respiratory distress syndrome: a 10-year hospital cohort study. *Arch Dis Child Fetal Neonatal Ed*. 2009;94(1):F13–F16.

93. Lahra MM, Beeby PJ, Jeffery HE. Intrauterine inflammation, neonatal sepsis, and chronic lung disease: a 13-year hospital cohort study. *Pediatrics*. 2009;123(5):1314–1319.

94. Hartling L, Liang Y, Lacaze-Masmonteil T. Chorioamnionitis as a risk factor for bronchopulmonary dysplasia: a systematic review and meta-analysis. *Arch Dis Child Fetal Neonatal Ed*. 2012;97(1):F8–F17.

95. Hitti J, Krohn MA, Patton DL, et al. Amniotic fluid tumor necrosis factor-alpha and the risk of respiratory distress syndrome among preterm infants. *Am J Obstet Gynecol*. 1997;177(1):50–56.

96. Ramsey PS, Lieman JM, Brumfield CG, Carlo W. Chorioamnionitis increases neonatal morbidity in pregnancies complicated by preterm premature rupture of membranes. *Am J Obstet Gynecol*. 2005;192(4):1162–1166.

97. Laughon M, Allred EN, Bose C, et al. Patterns of respiratory disease during the first 2 postnatal weeks in extremely premature infants. *Pediatrics*. 2009;123(4):1124–1131.

98. Soraisham AS, Singhal N, McMillan DD, Sauve RS, Lee SK, Canadian Neonatal Network. A multicenter study on the clinical outcome of chorioamnionitis in preterm infants. *Am J Obstet Gynecol*. 2009;200(4):372.e371–e376.

99. Van Marter LJ, Dammann O, Allred EN, et al. Chorioamnionitis, mechanical ventilation, and postnatal sepsis as modulators of chronic lung disease in preterm infants. *J Pediatr*. 2002;140(2):171–176.

100. Been JV, Rours IG, Kornelisse RF, Jonkers F, de Krijger RR, Zimmermann LJ. Chorioamnionitis alters the response to surfactant in preterm infants. *J Pediatr*. 2010;156(1):10–15.e11.

101. Been JV, Rours IG, Kornelisse RF, et al. Histologic chorioamnionitis, fetal involvement, and antenatal steroids: effects on neonatal outcome in preterm infants. *Am J Obstet Gynecol*. 2009;201(6):587.e581–e588.

102. Matoba N, Yu Y, Mestan K, et al. Differential patterns of 27 cord blood immune biomarkers across gestational age. *Pediatrics*. 2009;123(5):1320–1328.

103. Ambalavanan N, Carlo WA, D'Angio CT, et al. Cytokines associated with bronchopulmonary dysplasia or death in extremely low birth weight infants. *Pediatrics*. 2009;123(4):1132–1141.

104. Paananen R, Husa AK, Vuolteenaho R, Herva R, Kaukola T, Hallman M. Blood cytokines during the perinatal period in very preterm infants: relationship of inflammatory response and bronchopulmonary dysplasia. *J Pediatr*. 2009;154(1):39–43.e33.

105. Been JV, Debeer A, van Iwaarden JF, et al. Early alterations of growth factor patterns in bronchoalveolar lavage fluid from preterm infants developing bronchopulmonary dysplasia. *Pediatr Res*. 2010;67(1):83–89.

106. Andrews WW, Goldenberg RL, Faye-Petersen O, Cliver S, Goepfert AR, Hauth JC. The Alabama Preterm Birth Study: polymorphonuclear and mononuclear cell placental infiltrations, other markers of inflammation, and outcomes in 23- to 32-week preterm newborn infants. *Am J Obstet Gynecol*. 2006;195(3):803–808.

107. Goldenberg RL, Andrews WW, Goepfert AR, et al. The Alabama Preterm Birth Study: umbilical cord blood *Ureaplasma urealyticum* and *Mycoplasma hominis* cultures in very preterm newborn infants. *Am J Obstet Gynecol*. 2008;198(1):43.e41–e45.

108. Stoll BJ, Hansen N, Fanaroff AA, et al. Changes in pathogens causing early-onset sepsis in very-low-birth-weight infants. *N Engl J Med*. 2002;347(4):240–247.

109. Viscardi RM, Muhumuza CK, Rodriguez A, et al. Inflammatory markers in intrauterine and fetal blood and cerebrospinal fluid compartments are associated with adverse pulmonary and neurologic outcomes in preterm infants. *Pediatr Res*. 2004;55(6):1009–1017.

110. Bry K, Lappalainen U, Hallman M. Intraamniotic interleukin-1 accelerates surfactant protein synthesis in fetal rabbits and improves lung stability after premature birth. *J Clin Invest*. 1997;99(12):2992–2999.

111. Kallapur SG, Willet KE, Jobe AH, Ikegami M, Bachurski CJ. Intra-amniotic endotoxin: chorioamnionitis precedes lung maturation in preterm lambs. *Am J Physiol Lung Cell Mol Physiol*. 2001;280(3):L527–L536.

112. Kramer BW, Moss TJ, Willet KE, et al. Dose and time response after intraamniotic endotoxin in preterm lambs. *Am J Respir Crit Care Med*. 2001;164(6):982–988.

113. Kallapur SG, Bachurski CJ, Le Cras TD, Joshi SN, Ikegami M, Jobe AH. Vascular changes after intra-amniotic endotoxin in preterm lamb lungs. *Am J Physiol Lung Cell Mol Physiol*. 2004;287(6):L1178–L1185.

114. Kramer BW, Kramer S, Ikegami M, Jobe AH. Injury, inflammation, and remodeling in fetal sheep lung after intra-amniotic endotoxin. *Am J Physiol Lung Cell Mol Physiol*. 2002;283(2):L452–L459.

115. Song Y, Karisnan K, Noble PB, et al. In utero LPS exposure impairs preterm diaphragm contractility. *Am J Respir Cell Mol Biol*. 2013;49(5):866–874.

116. Jobe AH, Newnham JP, Willet KE, et al. Endotoxin-induced lung maturation in preterm lambs is not mediated by cortisol. *Am J Respir Crit Care Med*. 2000;162(5):1656–1661.

117. Kallapur SG, Presicce P, Rueda CM, Jobe AH, Chougnet CA. Fetal immune response to chorioamnionitis. *Semin Reprod Med*. 2014;32(1):56–67.

118. Moss TJ, Nitsos I, Kramer BW, Ikegami M, Newnham JP, Jobe AH. Intra-amniotic endotoxin induces lung maturation by direct effects on the developing respiratory tract in preterm sheep. *Am J Obstet Gynecol*. 2002;187(4):1059–1065.

119. Sosenko IR, Jobe AH. Intraamniotic endotoxin increases lung antioxidant enzyme activity in preterm lambs. *Pediatr Res*. 2003;53(4):679–683.

120. Kim YM, Romero R, Chaiworapongsa T, et al. Toll-like receptor-2 and -4 in the chorioamniotic membranes in spontaneous labor at term and in preterm parturition that are associated with chorioamnionitis. *Am J Obstet Gynecol*. 2004;191(4):1346–1355.

121. Steel JH, O'Donoghue K, Kennea NL, Sullivan MH, Edwards AD. Maternal origin of inflammatory leukocytes in preterm fetal membranes, shown by fluorescence in situ hybridisation. *Placenta*. 2005;26(8–9):672–677.

122. Harju K, Glumoff V, Hallman M. Ontogeny of Toll-like receptors Tlr2 and Tlr4 in mice. *Pediatr Res*. 2001;49(1):81–83.

123. Hillman NH, Moss TJ, Nitsos I, et al. Toll-like receptors and agonist responses in the developing fetal sheep lung. *Pediatr Res*. 2008;63(4):388–393.

124. Kramer BW, Jobe AH. The clever fetus: responding to inflammation to minimize lung injury. *Biol Neonate*. 2005;88(3):202–207.

125. Moss TJ, Nitsos I, Ikegami M, Jobe AH, Newnham JP. Experimental intrauterine *Ureaplasma* infection in sheep. *Am J Obstet Gynecol*. 2005;192(4):1179–1186.

126. Collins JJ, Kallapur SG, Knox CL, et al. Inflammation in fetal sheep from intra-amniotic injection of *Ureaplasma parvum*. *Am J Physiol Lung Cell Mol Physiol*. 2010;299(6):L852–L860.

127. Ikegami M, Moss TJ, Kallapur SG, et al. Minimal lung and systemic responses to TNF-alpha in preterm sheep. *Am J Physiol Lung Cell Mol Physiol*. 2003;285(1):L121–L129.

128. Moss TJ, Newnham JP, Willett KE, Kramer BW, Jobe AH, Ikegami M. Early gestational intra-amniotic endotoxin: lung function, surfactant, and morphometry. *Am J Respir Crit Care Med*. 2002;165(6):805–811.

129. Kallapur SG, Moss TJ, Ikegami M, Jasman RL, Newnham JP, Jobe AH. Recruited inflammatory cells mediate endotoxin-induced lung maturation in preterm fetal lambs. *Am J Respir Crit Care Med*. 2005;172(10):1315–1321.

130. Kallapur SG, Nitsos I, Moss TJ, et al. IL-1 mediates pulmonary and systemic inflammatory responses to chorioamnionitis induced by lipopolysaccharide. *Am J Respir Crit Care Med*. 2009;179(10):955–961.

131. Liao J, Kapadia VS, Brown LS, et al. The NLRP3 inflammasome is critically involved in the development of bronchopulmonary dysplasia. *Nat Commun*. 2015;6:8977.

132. Hodgman JE. Relationship between Wilson-Mikity syndrome and the new bronchopulmonary dysplasia. *Pediatrics*. 2003;112(6 Pt 1):1414–1415.

133. Kallapur SG, Nitsos I, Moss TJ, et al. Chronic endotoxin exposure does not cause sustained structural abnormalities in the fetal sheep lungs. *Am J Physiol Lung Cell Mol Physiol*. 2005;288(5):L966–L974.

134. Polglase GR, Hillman NH, Pillow JJ, et al. Ventilation-mediated injury after preterm delivery of *Ureaplasma parvum* colonized fetal lambs. *Pediatr Res*. 2010;67(6):630–635.

135. Rueda CM, Presicce P, Jackson CM, et al. Lipopolysaccharide-induced chorioamnionitis promotes IL-1-dependent inflammatory FOXP3+ CD4+ T cells in the fetal rhesus macaque. *J Immunol*. 2016;196(9):3706–3715.

136. Kramer BW, Joshi SN, Moss TJ, et al. Endotoxin-induced maturation of monocytes in preterm fetal sheep lung. *Am J Physiol Lung Cell Mol Physiol*. 2007;293(2):L345–L353.

137. Kallapur SG, Jobe AH, Ball MK, et al. Pulmonary and systemic endotoxin tolerance in preterm fetal sheep exposed to chorioamnionitis. *J Immunol*. 2007;179(12):8491–8499.

138. Kallapur SG, Kramer BW, Knox CL, et al. Chronic fetal exposure to *Ureaplasma parvum* suppresses innate immune responses in sheep. *J Immunol*. 2011;187(5):2688–2695.

139. Kramer BW, Kallapur SG, Moss TJ, Nitsos I, Newnham JP, Jobe AH. Intra-amniotic LPS modulation of TLR signaling in lung and blood monocytes of fetal sheep. *Innate Immun*. 2009;15(2):101–107.

140. Tang JR, Seedorf GJ, Muehlethaler V, et al. Moderate postnatal hyperoxia accelerates lung growth and attenuates pulmonary hypertension in infant rats after exposure to intra-amniotic endotoxin. *Am J Physiol Lung Cell Mol Physiol*. 2010;299(6):L735–L748.

141. Pryhuber GS, Maitre NL, Ballard RA, et al. Prematurity and respiratory outcomes program (PROP): study protocol of a prospective multicenter study of respiratory outcomes of preterm infants in the united states. *BMC Pediatr*. 2015;15:37.

142. Jackson CM, Wells CB, Tabangin ME, Meinzen-Derr J, Jobe AH, Chougnet CA. Pro-inflammatory immune responses in leukocytes of premature infants exposed to maternal chorioamnionitis or funisitis. *Pediatr Res*. 2016.

143. Misra RS, Shah S, Fowell DJ, et al. Preterm cord blood CD4(+) T cells exhibit increased IL-6 production in chorioamnionitis and decreased CD4(+) T cells in bronchopulmonary dysplasia. *Hum Immunol*. 2015;76(5):329–338.

144. Scheible KM, Emo J, Yang H, et al. Developmentally determined reduction in CD31 during gestation is associated with CD8+ T cell effector differentiation in preterm infants. *Clin Immunol*. 2015;161(2):65–74.

145. D'Angio CT, Ambalavanan N, Carlo WA, et al. Blood cytokine profiles associated with distinct patterns of bronchopulmonary dysplasia among extremely low birth weight infants. *J Pediatr*. 2016;174:45–51.e45.

146. Bose C, Laughon M, Allred EN, et al. Blood protein concentrations in the first two postnatal weeks that predict bronchopulmonary dysplasia among infants born before the 28th week of gestation. *Pediatr Res*. 2011;69(4):347–353.

147. Harding JE, Pang J, Knight DB, Liggins GC. Do antenatal corticosteroids help in the setting of preterm rupture of membranes? *Am J Obstet Gynecol*. 2001;184(2):131–139.

148. Goldenberg RL, Andrews WW, Faye-Petersen OM, Cliver SP, Goepfert AR, Hauth JC. The Alabama Preterm Birth Study: corticosteroids and neonatal outcomes in 23- to 32-week newborns with various markers of intrauterine infection. *Am J Obstet Gynecol*. 2006;195(4):1020–1024.

149. Been JV, Degraeuwe PL, Kramer BW, Zimmermann LJ. Antenatal steroids and neonatal outcome after chorioamnionitis: a meta-analysis. *BJOG*. 2011;118(2):113–122.

150. Kallapur SG, Kramer BW, Moss TJ, et al. Maternal glucocorticoids increase endotoxin-induced lung inflammation in preterm lambs. *Am J Physiol Lung Cell Mol Physiol*. 2003;284(4):L633–L642.

151. Newnham JP, Kallapur SG, Kramer BW, et al. Betamethasone effects on chorioamnionitis induced by intra-amniotic endotoxin in sheep. *Am J Obstet Gynecol*. 2003;189(5):1458–1466.

152. Newnham JP, Moss TJ, Padbury JF, et al. The interactive effects of endotoxin with prenatal glucocorticoids on short-term lung function in sheep. *Am J Obstet Gynecol*. 2001;185(1):190–197.

153. Moss TJ, Nitsos I, Knox CL, et al. *Ureaplasma* colonization of amniotic fluid and efficacy of antenatal corticosteroids for preterm lung maturation in sheep. *Am J Obstet Gynecol*. 2009;200(1):96.e91–e96.

154. Kramer BW, Ikegami M, Moss TJ, Nitsos I, Newnham JP, Jobe AH. Endotoxin-induced chorioamnionitis modulates innate immunity of monocytes in preterm sheep. *Am J Respir Crit Care Med*. 2005;171(1):73–77.

155. Kramer BW, Ikegami M, Moss TJ, Nitsos I, Newnham JP, Jobe AH. Antenatal betamethasone changes cord blood monocyte responses to endotoxin in preterm lambs. *Pediatr Res*. 2004;55(5):764–768.

156. Kuypers E, Collins JJ, Kramer BW, et al. Intra-amniotic LPS and antenatal betamethasone: inflammation and maturation in preterm lamb lungs. *Am J Physiol Lung Cell Mol Physiol*. 2012;302(4):L380–L389.

157. Zeitlin J, El Ayoubi M, Jarreau PH, et al. Impact of fetal growth restriction on mortality and morbidity in a very preterm birth cohort. *J Pediatr*. 2010;157(5):733–739.e731.

158. Chang EY, Menard MK, Vermillion ST, Hulsey T, Ebeling M. The association between hyaline membrane disease and preeclampsia. *Am J Obstet Gynecol*. 2004;191(4):1414–1417.

159. Tyson JE, Kennedy K, Broyles S, Rosenfeld CR. The small for gestational age infant: accelerated or delayed pulmonary maturation? Increased or decreased survival? *Pediatrics*. 1995;95(4):534–538.

160. Jelin AC, Cheng YW, Shaffer BL, Kaimal AJ, Little SE, Caughey AB. Early-onset preeclampsia and neonatal outcomes. *J Matern Fetal Neonatal Med*. 2010;23(5):389–392.

161. Garite TJ, Clark R, Thorp JA. Intrauterine growth restriction increases morbidity and mortality among premature neonates. *Am J Obstet Gynecol*. 2004;191(2):481–487.

162. Reiss I, Landmann E, Heckmann M, Misselwitz B, Gortner L. Increased risk of bronchopulmonary dysplasia and increased mortality in very preterm infants being small for gestational age. *Arch Gynecol Obstet*. 2003;269(1):40–44.

163. Bose C, Van Marter LJ, Laughon M, et al. Fetal growth restriction and chronic lung disease among infants born before the 28th week of gestation. *Pediatrics*. 2009;124(3):e450–e458.

164. Hansen AR, Barnes CM, Folkman J, McElrath TF. Maternal preeclampsia predicts the development of bronchopulmonary dysplasia. *J Pediatr*. 2010;156(4):532–536.

165. Walsh MC, Di Fiore JM, Martin RJ, Gantz M, Carlo WA, Finer N. Association of oxygen target and growth status with increased mortality in small for gestational age infants: further analysis of the surfactant, positive pressure and pulse oximetry randomized trial. *JAMA Pediatr*. 2016;170(3):292–294.

166. Torrance HL, Derks JB, Scherjon SA, Wijnberger LD, Visser GH. Is antenatal steroid treatment effective in preterm IUGR fetuses? *Acta Obstet Gynecol Scand*. 2009;88(10):1068–1073.

167. Lipsett J, Tamblyn M, Madigan K, et al. Restricted fetal growth and lung development: a morphometric analysis of pulmonary structure. *Pediatr Pulmonol*. 2006;41(12):1138–1145.

168. Orgeig S, Crittenden TA, Marchant C, McMillen IC, Morrison JL. Intrauterine growth restriction delays surfactant protein maturation in the sheep fetus. *Am J Physiol Lung Cell Mol Physiol*. 2010;298(4):L575–L583.

169. Gortner L, Hilgendorff A, Bahner T, Ebsen M, Reiss I, Rudloff S. Hypoxia-induced intrauterine growth retardation: effects on pulmonary development and surfactant protein transcription. *Biol Neonate*. 2005;88(2):129–135.

170. Miller SL, Chai M, Loose J, et al. The effects of maternal betamethasone administration on the intrauterine growth-restricted fetus. *Endocrinology*. 2007;148(3):1288–1295.

171. Miller SL, Supramaniam VG, Jenkin G, Walker DW, Wallace EM. Cardiovascular responses to maternal betamethasone administration in the intrauterine growth-restricted ovine fetus. *Am J Obstet Gynecol*. 2009;201(6):613.e611–e618.

172. Pierce RA, Nguyen NM. Prenatal nicotine exposure and abnormal lung function. *Am J Respir Cell Mol Biol*. 2002;26(1):10–13.

173. Blacquiere MJ, Timens W, Melgert BN, Geerlings M, Postma DS, Hylkema MN. Maternal smoking during pregnancy induces airway remodelling in mice offspring. *Eur Respir J*. 2009;33(5):1133–1140.

174. Hylkema MN, Blacquiere MJ. Intrauterine effects of maternal smoking on sensitization, asthma, and chronic obstructive pulmonary disease. *Proc Am Thorac Soc*. 2009;6(8):660–662.

2

175. Lieberman E, Torday J, Barbieri R, Cohen A, Van Vunakis H, Weiss ST. Association of intrauterine cigarette smoke exposure with indices of fetal lung maturation. *Obstet Gynecol*. 1992;79(4):564–570.

176. Rehan VK, Wang Y, Sugano S, et al. In utero nicotine exposure alters fetal rat lung alveolar type II cell proliferation, differentiation, and metabolism. *Am J Physiol Lung Cell Mol Physiol*. 2007;292(1):L323–L333.

177. Sekhon HS, Jia Y, Raab R, et al. Prenatal nicotine increases pulmonary alpha7 nicotinic receptor expression and alters fetal lung development in monkeys. *J Clin Invest*. 1999;103(5):637–647.

178. Elliot JG, Carroll NG, James AL, Robinson PJ. Airway alveolar attachment points and exposure to cigarette smoke in utero. *Am J Respir Crit Care Med*. 2003;167(1):45–49.

179. McEvoy CT, Schilling D, Clay N, et al. Vitamin C supplementation for pregnant smoking women and pulmonary function in their newborn infants: a randomized clinical trial. *JAMA*. 2014;311(20):2074–2082.

180. Sozo F, O'Day L, Maritz G, et al. Repeated ethanol exposure during late gestation alters the maturation and innate immune status of the ovine fetal lung. *Am J Physiol Lung Cell Mol Physiol*. 2009;296(3):L510–L518.

181. Joshi PC, Guidot DM. The alcoholic lung: epidemiology, pathophysiology, and potential therapies. *Am J Physiol Lung Cell Mol Physiol*. 2007;292(4):L813–L823.

CHAPTER 3

Pulmonary Vascular Development and the Neonatal Circulation

Robin H. Steinhorn

- Lung vascular development occurs as highly choreographed sequence, regulated by hypoxia inducible factors, vascular endothelial growth factor, nitric oxide, and other transcription factors and mediators.
- In addition to arterial vessels, pulmonary veins are now understood to be highly reactive vessels that contribute to the overall regulation of pulmonary vascular resistance in the fetus and newborn.
- Antenatal pulmonary vascular development can be disrupted by events such as placental insufficiency, genetic abnormalities such as Down syndrome, prolonged oligohydramnios, and congenital diaphragmatic hernia.
- Postnatal development of the lung circulation can be disrupted by numerous stressors such as preterm birth, asphyxia, and hypoxia or hyperoxia.
- Numerous questions and controversies remain, including the role of cardiac dysfunction in congenital diaphragmatic hernia and the causes of acute and chronic pulmonary hypertension in the premature infant.

Development of the Fetal Pulmonary Circulation

The development of the pulmonary vasculature during fetal and neonatal life is highly coordinated with airway growth and plays a key role in normal lung development. Compared with adult pulmonary vascular disease, disruption of lung vascular development plays a central role in the pathobiology of pulmonary vascular disease and airway development in the neonate and young infant.[1]

Lung development is classically divided into five overlapping stages in humans and rodents on the basis of gross histologic features. They are termed the embryonic (weeks 4–7 of gestation), pseudoglandular (weeks 5–17), canalicular (weeks 16–26), saccular (weeks 24–38), and alveolar stages (week 36 to infancy).[2] The development of the pulmonary vasculature is closely correlated with and interacts with airway growth. Lung vascularization initially originates in the mesenchyme, distal to the epithelium. In response to epithelial-derived vascular endothelial growth factor (VEGF), the endothelial cells move toward the epithelium, where they form the epithelium-capillary interface needed for gas exchange.[3] Growth of the lung vasculature continues after birth and into adulthood.

Physiology of the Fetal Pulmonary Circulation

Pulmonary hypertension (PH) is a normal physiologic state during fetal life and permits survival on placental support. Fetal pulmonary vascular resistance (PVR) is high in part because of hypoxic pulmonary vasoconstriction (Fig. 3.1). In the fetal

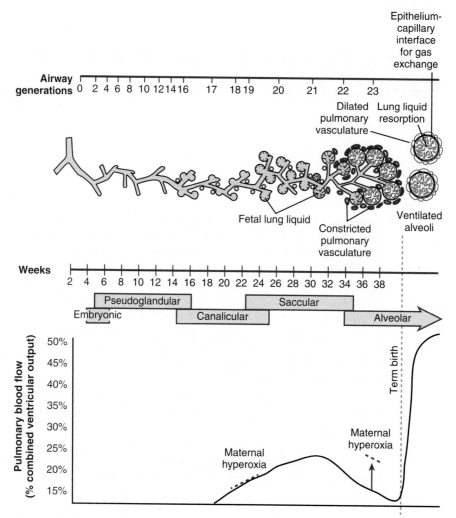

Fig. 3.1 **Stages of Lung Development.** Changes in airway morphology and pulmonary vasculature during various stages of lung development and at birth. The cross-sectional area of pulmonary vasculature increases with gestation. However, the pulmonary vasculature develops sensitivity to oxygen during later gestation, leading to hypoxic pulmonary vasoconstriction (*thick red vessels*). Pulmonary vasodilation secondary to ventilation and oxygenation at birth increase pulmonary blood flow. Changes in pulmonary blood flow (as a percentage of combined ventricular output) during the last half of human pregnancy and immediate postnatal life are shown in the bottom graph. During the early second trimester, the pulmonary vasculature does not respond to changes in oxygen tension induced by maternal hyperoxia (*dashed red line*). During the third trimester, pulmonary blood flow increases with changes in oxygen tension (*dashed red line* and *red arrow*). After birth, after normal transition, the entire right ventricular output and left-to-right ductal shunt perfuse the lung, establishing this organ as the site of gas exchange during postnatal period. (Copyright Satyan Lakshminrusimha and Robin H. Steinhorn.)

lamb, pulmonary arterial blood has a partial pressure of oxygen (Po_2) of approximately 18 mm Hg and oxygen saturation of 50%.[4] Because of high PVR, only about 16% of the combined ventricular output is directed to the lungs; the remainder passes through the ductus arteriosus to the descending aorta. The blood is then oxygenated in the placenta and returns to the body through the umbilical vein, with a Po_2 of ~32 to 35 mm Hg in lambs.[4] The difference in oxygen saturation between the umbilical vein (85%) and umbilical artery (52%) during fetal life is similar to the difference between the pulmonary vein/aorta (95%–100%) and pulmonary artery (60%–70%) in an adult. The fetus thus achieves normal oxygen delivery at the low Po_2 levels needed for normal lung development.

In human fetuses, Doppler studies demonstrate that the pulmonary blood flow is only 13% of combined ventricular output at 20 weeks' gestation (canalicular stage), representing a nadir during lung development (see Fig. 3.1).[5] This finding is largely secondary to the lower cross-sectional area of the very immature pulmonary vascular bed. Furthermore, in fetal lambs at an equivalent point in gestation (~65% gestation), pulmonary blood flow does not increase in response to hyperoxia and PVR does not increase in response to hypoxia.[6,7] Similarly, in human pregnancies, maternal hyper-oxygenation with face mask oxygen at 20 to 26 weeks' gestation does not result in pulmonary vasodilation.[8] Birth at this gestational age (23–26 weeks) is associated with a 2% risk of clinical PH[9,10] and perhaps explains the high rates of inhaled nitric oxide (NO) therapy (6%–8%) in extremely premature infants.[11–13]

As the lung develops through the early saccular stage, rapid proliferation of pulmonary vessels and a marked increase in cross-sectional area of the pulmonary vascular bed occurs, which decreases fetal PVR. At the same time, pulmonary vessels become more reactive to vasoconstrictors such as hypoxia and endothelin and vasodilators such as oxygen. The net result is higher PVR and increased reactivity of the pulmonary vasculature. The maternal hyperoxygenation test (administered with 60% oxygen by face mask) has been proposed to measure the ability of fetal pulmonary arteries to vasodilate in response to oxygen in late gestation and predict pulmonary vascular reactivity and survival in congenital diaphragmatic hernia (CDH).[14] Later in fetal life, PVR becomes very sensitive to small changes in Po_2. In nonhuman primate fetuses, Arraut et al. evaluated the effect of maternal hypoxemia (by administration of 12% oxygen) and hyperoxemia (by administration of 100% oxygen) on the pulsatility index (PI) of the right pulmonary artery.[15] Maternal hypoxemia increased fetal right pulmonary arterial PI by fivefold, suggesting fetal pulmonary vasoconstriction, and maternal hyperoxemia decreased right pulmonary arterial PI by fourfold and increased ductus arteriosus PI. Maternal oxygenation status did not affect the umbilical arterial PI or ductus venosus PI, suggesting that umbilical flow is not influenced by and does not regulate fetal oxygenation.[15] Similarly, Konduri et al. showed that an increase in pulmonary arterial Po_2 of 7 mm Hg resulted in a threefold increase in pulmonary blood flow in fetal lambs.[16] These changes in PVR will determine the distribution of fetal cardiac output and oxygen delivery to the brain and heart. In pathologic conditions such as CDH, reduced pulmonary venous return and left ventricular filling may contribute to left ventricular hypoplasia, emphasizing the important role of pulmonary blood flow during fetal life.[17,18]

Pulmonary veins have been traditionally regarded as passive conduit vessels, but they are now recognized as reactive vessels that contribute to the overall regulation of PVR.[19] In the fetus, pulmonary veins contribute a significant fraction to total PVR, and they may play a more important role in regulating the fetal and newborn pulmonary circulation than in adults (Fig. 3.2). In perinatal sheep, NO stimulated endogenously by acetylcholine or given exogenously causes greater relaxation and accumulation of cyclic guanosine monophosphate (cGMP) in pulmonary veins than in arteries.[20] At birth, the veins, as well as the arteries, relax in response to NO and dilator prostaglandins, thereby assisting in the fall in PVR (Fig. 3.3). These effects are oxygen dependent and modulated by protein kinase G.[21] In a number of species, including the human, pulmonary veins are also the primary sites of action of certain vasoconstrictors, such as endothelin and thromboxane (see Figs. 3.2 and 3.3).

Mediators of Early Pulmonary Vascular Development

The hypoxic conditions of fetal life support the tremendous lung vascular growth that occurs before birth. Hypoxia-inducible factors (HIFs) are regarded as the "master regulators" of the transcriptional response to hypoxia and are involved in angiogenesis, survival, and metabolic pathways (Fig. 3.4). HIFs are heterodimers consisting of oxygen-sensitive α-subunits (HIF-1α, HIF-2α) and constitutively expressed β-subunits. Hypoxia stabilizes the α-subunit, leading to nuclear accumulation and activation of multiple target genes. HIF-1 regulates genes involved in angiogenesis (e.g., VEGF), oxygen transport (e.g., erythropoietin), and energy metabolism (e.g., glycolytic enzymes), among others.[22] HIFs are constitutively expressed in multiple fetal pulmonary cell types, including endothelial, smooth muscle, and epithelial cells.[23] The importance of HIFs in fetal lung development has been demonstrated by studies revealing that deletion of HIF-1 causes embryonic lethality, and deletion of

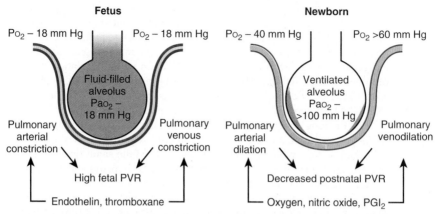

Fig. 3.2   Changes in Pulmonary Arterial and Venous Resistance at Birth. Relative hypoxia with Po_2 in the 15- to 20-mm Hg range in the fluid-filled alveoli, pulmonary arterial, and venous blood contributes to high fetal pulmonary vascular resistance *(PVR)*. The pulmonary veins are highly responsive to vasoconstrictors such as endothelin and thromboxane. At birth with ventilation of the lungs, Pao_2 increases, resulting in marked elevation of pulmonary venous Po_2. Pulmonary arterial Po_2 increases to a lesser extent. These changes contribute to a precipitous decrease in PVR at birth. Pulmonary veins are exquisitely sensitive to vasodilators such as oxygen, nitric oxide, and prostacyclin *(PGI₂)*. *Pao₂*, Arterial partial pressure of oxygen; *Po₂*, partial pressure of oxygen; *PVR*, pulmonary vascular resistance. (Copyright Satyan Lakshminrusimha and Robin H. Steinhorn.)

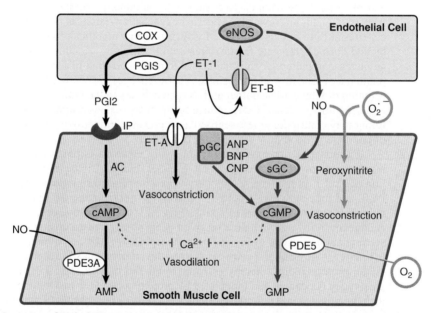

Fig. 3.3   Overview of Endothelium-Derived Vasodilator (Prostacyclin and Nitric Oxide *[NO]*) and Vasoconstrictor (Endothelin, *ET-1*) Pathways. *AC,* Adenylate cyclase; *AMP,* adenosine monophosphate; *ANP,* atrial natriuretic peptide; *BNP,* brain natriuretic peptide; *Ca²⁺,* calcium ion; *cAMP,* cyclic adenosine monophosphate; *CNP,* C-type natriuretic peptide; *COX,* cyclooxygenase; *eNOS,* endothelial nitric oxide synthase; *ET-A,* endothelin A; *ET-B,* endothelin B; *GMP,* guanosine monophosphate; *IP,* PGI2 receptor; *PDE,* phosphodiesterase; *ET,* endothelin; *pGC,* particulate guanylate cyclase; *PGIS,* prostacyclin synthase; *PG12,* prostaglandin 12; *sGC,* soluble guanylate cyclase. (Copyright Satyan Lakshminrusimha and Robin H. Steinhorn.)

HIF-2 reduces VEGF levels and leads to early death owing to respiratory failure.[24] In the adult lung, hypoxia induces abnormal vascular remodeling, potentially by inducing HIF activity. In contrast, hypoxia is the normal fetal condition and is a required environmental stimulus to sustain normal fetal lung and vascular development.

Although NO is best known for its vasoactive properties, it also plays an important role in the structural development of the pulmonary vasculature. Lung endothelial NOS (eNOS) mRNA and protein are present in early fetal life in rats and sheep and increase with advancing gestation in utero.[25,26] The expression and activity of

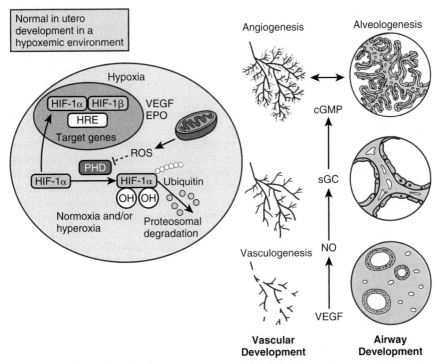

Fig. 3.4 Lung Development Occurs In Utero in a Relatively Hypoxic Environment. Under hypoxic conditions, the hypoxia-inducible factor *(HIF)*-1α is stabilized, and it dimerizes with HIF-1β and translocates to the nucleus and binds to target genes that stimulate vascular endothelial growth factor *(VEGF)* production and angiogenesis. Under hyperoxic conditions, HIF is hydroxylated by prolyl hydroxylases *(PHD)* and ubiquinated for proteosomal degradation. Vascular and alveolar growth is mediated by VEGF through nitric oxide *(NO)* and soluble guanylate synthase *(sGC)* pathways. Fetal or neonatal disruption of these pathways in animal models is associated with respiratory and vascular abnormalities. *cGMP,* Cyclic guanosine monophosphate; *EPO,* erythropoietin; *HRE,* hypoxia-responsive elements; *OH,* hydroxyl anion; *ROS,* reactive oxygen species. (Copyright Satyan Lakshminrusimha and Robin H. Steinhorn.)

eNOS are regulated by multiple factors, including hemodynamic forces, hormonal stimuli (e.g., estradiol), paracrine factors (including VEGF), substrate and cofactor availability, oxygen tension, and others.[25,26] Numerous studies suggest the importance of NO-cGMP signaling in lung development. Lungs of fetal and neonatal mice deficient in eNOS have reduced alveolarization and vascularization and are more susceptible to the effects of hypoxia on vascular and alveolar growth.[27,28] Furthermore, mice deficient in soluble guanylate cyclase (sGC), the main target enzyme for NO, have decreased lung volumes and small airways.

VEGF is a key regulator of lung vascular growth and development during fetal and postnatal life. VEGF transcription is regulated by HIF, and its signaling is transduced via two transmembrane tyrosine kinase receptors: VEGFR-2 and VEGFR-1. VEGF ribonucleic acid (RNA) and protein are localized to distal airway epithelial cells, whereas VEGFR-1 and VEGFR-2 messenger RNA (mRNA) expression is localized to the pulmonary endothelial cells closely approximated to the developing epithelium.[29]

The fundamental importance of VEGF for vascular development has been demonstrated by several studies that inactivate or knock out VEGF or its receptors. Each of these produces a lethal phenotype that is characterized by deficient organization of endothelial cells. Furthermore, VEGFR-1 and VEGFR-2 inhibitors (e.g., SU5416) impair alveolar development in fetal and newborn rodent models, producing pathologic findings similar to those seen in clinical bronchopulmonary dysplasia (BPD). Even in adult rats, long-term treatment with SU5416 causes PH and enlarges the air spaces, suggesting that normal VEGF function is required not only for the formation but also for the maintenance of the pulmonary vasculature and alveolar structures well after lung development is completed.[30]

Recent studies suggest that VEGF-induced lung angiogenesis is in part mediated by NO. VEGF inhibition is associated with decreased lung eNOS protein expression and NO production; treatment with inhaled NO improves vascular and alveolar growth after VEGF inhibition. However, in neonatal mice that are eNOS deficient, recombinant human VEGF protein treatment restores lung structure after exposure to mild hyperoxia, suggesting that VEGF operates in part through mechanisms independent of eNOS.

Numerous transcription factors important to lung vascular development have been identified.[31] The forkhead box (Fox) family of transcription factors regulates expression of genes involved in cellular proliferation and differentiation. Newborn mice with low Foxf1 levels die with defects in lung vascularization and alveolarization,[32] and endothelial-specific deletion of Foxf1 produces embryonic lethality, growth restriction, and vascular abnormalities in the lung, placenta, and retina.[33] These findings are directly relevant to human lung development, as Foxf1 haploinsufficiency is found in 40% of infants with alveolar capillary dysplasia (ACD), a lethal disorder of lung vascular development.[34]

Nuclear factor kappa B (NF-κB) is a transcription factor traditionally associated with inflammation, but recent data suggest it may play a very different, protective role in the neonatal lung. Constitutive NF-κB expression is higher in the neonatal lung than in the adult lung and inhibiting it impairs in vitro pulmonary endothelial cell proliferation and angiogenesis. Blocking NF-κB activity during the alveolar stage of lung development in neonatal mice induced alveolar simplification and reduced pulmonary capillary density similar to that observed in BPD, effects that appear to be regulated by VEGFR-2.[35]

Lung endothelial progenitor cells (EPCs) have been recently identified as mediators of lung development, although their mechanistic role is not yet well understood. In rats, microvascular pulmonary endothelial cells proliferate twice as fast as endothelial cells isolated from large pulmonary arteries.[36] These cells, called resident microvascular endothelial progenitor cells (RMEPCs), are highly proliferative and express endothelial cell markers (CD31, CD144, eNOS, and von Willebrand factor) and progenitor cell antigens (CD34 and CD309). Thus the pulmonary microcirculation seems to be enriched with EPCs that support vasculogenesis while maintaining endothelial microvascular functionality.[37]

Resident microvascular EPCs also share features of human cord blood–derived endothelial colony-forming cells (ECFCs). Developing human fetal and neonatal rat lungs contain ECFCs with robust proliferative and vasculogenic potential. The functionality of these cells can be disrupted during or after birth: for instance, human fetal lung ECFCs exposed to hyperoxia in vitro proliferate less and form fewer capillary-like networks. These findings suggest a role for ECFCs in lung repair and if their function is impaired, it could contribute to the arrested alveolar growth after extremely preterm birth. Consequently, in rodents, exogenous administration of human cord blood–derived ECFCs restored alveolar and lung vascular growth in hyperoxic rodents. However, lung engraftment was low, suggesting that the ECFCs support lung growth and repair through paracrine effects.

Mediators of Early Pulmonary Vascular Function

As gestation progresses, NO and cGMP become central to the emergence of pulmonary vascular reactivity. VEGF acutely releases NO and causes rapid pulmonary vasodilation in vivo; conversely, chronic inhibition of VEGF receptors downregulates eNOS and induces PH in the late-gestation fetus.[38] Both findings point to its importance in the development and function of the developing pulmonary vasculature. Inhibition of eNOS increases basal PVR as early as 75% gestation (112 days) in the fetal lamb, indicating that endogenous NOS activity contributes to vasoregulation during late gestation. Pulmonary vasodilation in response to NO (an endothelium-independent mediator) precedes the response to endothelium-dependent mediators such as acetylcholine and oxygen. The response to NO is dependent on activity of soluble guanylate cyclase in the smooth muscle cell (see Fig. 3.3). In the ovine fetus, sGC mRNA levels are low during early preterm (126-day) gestation and markedly increase toward the end of third trimester.[39] Low levels of pulmonary arterial sGC activity during late canalicular and early saccular stages of lung development could partly explain the variable response to inhaled NO (iNO) observed in some extremely preterm infants.[9] Intracellular cGMP levels are also tightly regulated by cGMP-specific phosphodiesterase type 5 (PDE5) activity. PDE5 expression and activity increase during late gestation, and it plays a critical role in pulmonary vasoregulation during the perinatal period.

Pulmonary endothelial cells produce the prostaglandin (PG) molecules PGI_2 and PGE_2, which are both potent vasodilators. Prostacyclin (PGI_2) acts on its receptor in the smooth muscle cell to produce cyclic adenosine monophosphate (cAMP), which also mediates smooth muscle cell vasodilation (similar to cGMP, see Fig. 3.3). cAMP is inactivated by cAMP-specific phosphodiesterase 3A (PDE3A). In isolated pulmonary resistance vessels of term fetal lambs, the cyclooxygenase inhibitor indomethacin constricts arteries under higher oxygen tensions but has no effect under lower concentrations, suggesting that oxygen may regulate the synthesis or downstream signaling of the dilator prostanoids.[40] Although stimuli such as shear stress induce release of PgI_2, overall, prostaglandin release appears to play a less important role than NO in regulating fetal and transitional pulmonary vascular tone.[41]

Constrictors also play a role in regulating the pulmonary vascular tone of the fetus. Lipid mediators, such as thromboxane A_2, leukotrienes C_4 and D_4, and platelet-activating factor are potent pulmonary vasoconstrictors. Although thromboxane A_2 has been implicated in animal models of group B streptococcal sepsis, it does not appear to influence PVR in the normal fetus. Some data suggest that leukotrienes and platelet-activating factor may influence PVR during fetal life and transition but remain inconclusive. Endothelin-1 (ET-1) is produced by vascular endothelium and acts on the ET-A receptors in the smooth muscle cell to induce vasoconstriction by increasing ionic calcium concentrations. A second endothelial receptor, ET-B, on the endothelial cell stimulates NO release and vasodilation (see Fig. 3.3). Prepro-ET-1 mRNA (the precursor to ET-1) has been identified in fetal rat lung early in gestation, and high circulating ET-1 levels are present in umbilical cord blood. Although capable of both vasodilator and constrictor responses, ET-1 appears to primarily act as a pulmonary vasoconstrictor in the fetal pulmonary circulation.

Endogenous serotonin (5-HT) production is another contributor to the high PVR of the fetus. Infusions of 5-HT increase PVR[42,43] and infusions of ketanserin, a 5-HT 2A receptor antagonist, decrease fetal PVR in a dose-related fashion. Conversely, brief infusions of selective serotonin reuptake inhibitors (SSRIs), such as sertraline and fluoxetine, cause potent and sustained elevations of PVR. Together, these findings suggest that 5-HT causes pulmonary vasoconstriction and contributes to maintenance of high PVR in the normal fetus through stimulation of 5-HT 2A receptors and Rho kinase activation. These findings have important implications for SSRI treatment for maternal depression, as described in later text.

Transitional Circulation and Postnatal Pulmonary Vascular Development

A rapid and dramatic series of circulatory events occur at birth as the fetus transitions to extrauterine life. After birth and initiation of air breathing, a number of mechanisms operate simultaneously to rapidly reduce pulmonary arterial pressure and increase pulmonary blood flow. Of these, the most important stimuli appear to be ventilation of the lungs and an increase in oxygen tension (see Figs. 3.1 and 3.2).[44] Pulmonary blood flow increases by eightfold, resolving fetal PH.[45] Clamping of the umbilical cord removes the low-resistance placental circulation, increasing systemic arterial pressure as pulmonary arterial pressure falls. In some infants with in utero adverse events or with abnormalities of pulmonary transition at birth, PH persists into the newborn period, resulting in the syndrome of persistent pulmonary hypertension of the newborn (PPHN).

The vascular endothelium releases vasoactive products that play a critical role in achieving rapid pulmonary vasodilation. Pulmonary endothelial NO production increases markedly at the time of birth. Inhibitors of NOS activity (e.g., nitro-L-arginine) attenuate the decline in PVR after delivery of fetal lambs,[46,47] suggesting that the release of NO may be responsible for 50% of the rise in pulmonary blood flow at birth. Oxygen is an important catalyst for this increased NO production. In near-term fetal lambs, maternal hyperoxia induced by hyperbaric oxygenation increased pulmonary arterial Po_2 from 19 ± 1.5 to 48 ± 9 mm Hg, and pulmonary blood flow from 34 ± 3.3 to 298 ± 35 mL/kg per minute, a rise that nearly replicates the normal transition and is blocked by pretreatment with NOS inhibitors.[48] However, mice deficient in eNOS can successfully make the transition at birth without evidence of PPHN, suggesting the presence of alternate or compensatory vasodilator mechanisms, such as upregulation of other NOS isoforms or dilator prostaglandins.[49] Interestingly, eNOS-deficient mouse pups develop PH after relatively mild decreases in arterial partial pressure of oxygen (Pao_2) and have higher neonatal mortality when exposed to hypoxia after birth.[50] It is possible that eNOS deficiency alone may not be sufficient for the failure of postnatal adaptation, but that a decreased ability to produce NO in the setting of a perinatal stress such as hypoxia or inflammation may contribute to the development of postnatal PH. Expression of sGC also peaks in late gestation in rats and sheep,[51] which may explain why the immediate response to NO is greater in neonates than in any other reported age group. Pulmonary expression of PDE5 also peaks in the immediate newborn period in sheep and rats (see Fig. 3.4).[52,53] Together, these events appear to create the ability to finely regulate vascular cGMP concentrations in the transitional and early neonatal period.

The arachidonic acid–prostacyclin pathway also plays an important role in the transition at birth. Rhythmic lung distention and shear stress stimulate both PGI_2 and NO production in the late-gestation fetus, although the effect of oxygen tension is predominantly on NO activity. Phosphodiesterase 3A catalyzes the breakdown of cAMP (see Fig. 3.3) and appears to create important crosstalk with the cGMP pathway.

Less is known about the pulmonary vascular transition after preterm birth, although similar mechanisms appear to be in effect.[54] In premature lambs at ~70% of gestation (112–115 days), the pulmonary vasodilator responses to rhythmic distention of the lung or increased Pao_2 are partly due to stimulation of NO release.[54] In human preterm infants, the decrease in pulmonary arterial pressure after birth is significantly slower compared with term infants, particularly if respiratory distress syndrome also exists.[55] Pulmonary arterial pressure elevations may persist for a number of days in extremely preterm infants.[56,57] Skimming et al. have questioned whether a "natural" increase in PVR benefits the preterm infant by reducing the ductal steal and stabilizing systemic circulation.[58] However, recent prospective studies clearly indicate that early PH in extremely preterm infants is associated with BPD and late PH,[59] so it is more likely that this indicates abnormal vascular development or function.

After birth, structural development of the lung and its vasculature continues. More than 90% of lung alveolarization occurs postnatally, with a prominent surge between birth and 6 months of age. Similarly, there is marked growth and development of the microvascular network during the alveolarization phase. A double capillary network is characteristic of the fetal and neonatal lung, but as alveolarization progresses, the interalveolar septae thin and the double capillary layer fuses into the single layer characteristic of the mature vasculature. The capillary network continues to expand its surface area through childhood by nearly 20-fold.[31]

Features of Abnormal Pulmonary Vascular Development

The histologic features of early neonatal PPHN have been described in animal models and in fatal cases of PPHN in term infants.[60,61] In two autopsy series of infants with PPHN, vascular remodeling resulted in muscularization of the smallest arteries (<30 µM external diameter) at the level of the alveolar duct and wall[61,62] and a doubling of the medial wall thickness of the intraacinar arteries (Fig. 3.5). These findings suggest that structural maldevelopment of the peripheral pulmonary arterial bed begins in utero and does not merely represent a failure of the fetal pattern to regress. Very similar patterns of remodeling are observed in animal models of PPHN, including the lamb model of antenatal ductal ligation.[63]

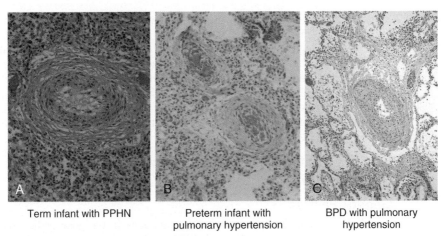

| Term infant with PPHN | Preterm infant with pulmonary hypertension | BPD with pulmonary hypertension |

Fig. 3.5   Vascular Remodeling in Neonatal Pulmonary Hypertension. Histology of pulmonary arteries in the lung sections from three patients with pulmonary hypertension. A, A 14-day-old, 37-week gestation infant with trisomy 21 (note the significant thickening of the medial and adventitial layers). B, A 5-day-old, 25-week gestation preterm infant with pulmonary hypertension and severe hypoxemic respiratory failure. C, A 4-month-old, former 23-week gestation infant with bronchopulmonary dysplasia and pulmonary hypertension. *BPD,* Bronchopulmonary dysplasia; *PPHN,* persistent pulmonary hypertension of the newborn.

Thickening of the adventitia is observed in remodeled pulmonary vessels (see Fig. 3.5)[63] and likely contributes to pulmonary artery stiffness.[64] The adventitial cells (including fibroblasts, pericytes, progenitor cells, and so on) also appear to be regulators of vascular wall function from the "outside in."[65,66] For example, NO is less potent when administered to the adventitial side of vessels. This may be partly due to the presence of constitutively active NADPH oxidase in adventitial cells, which generate superoxide anions that actively scavenge NO.

In contrast to PPHN, after very preterm birth, the developing lung is exposed to an extrauterine environment that disrupts the normal fetal vascular developmental patterns. On histology, the lungs of very preterm infants with BPD display evidence of arrested development, with reduced numbers of both alveoli and intraacinar arteries. The pulmonary circulation in animal models and infants with BPD is characterized by vascular pruning, decreased vascular branching, and altered patterns of vascular distribution within the lung interstitium. Similar to early PPHN, smooth muscle proliferation also extends abnormally into the smaller peripheral arteries. In addition, intrapulmonary bronchopulmonary anastomoses have recently been identified that act as arteriovenous shunts that contribute to hypoxemia.[67] These anastomotic vessels may represent a compensatory mechanism to overcome the reduction in vascular surface area or act as a protective "pop-off" mechanism to reduce the severity of PH and protect the right ventricle.[68]

Signaling abnormalities in the remodeled vasculature include decreased expression of endothelial NOS and reduced urinary levels of NO metabolites.[69,70] sGC expression and activity is also diminished in animal models of neonatal PH and CDH,[71,72] which is partly secondary to oxidation of sGC that renders it NO-insensitive.[73,74] Because NO and cGMP also inhibit vascular smooth muscle growth, it is likely that a combination of diminished eNOS expression, inactivation of sGC, and reduced cGMP levels also contribute to excessive muscularization of pulmonary vessels in PPHN and BPD. Ventilation with high concentrations of inspired oxygen and exposure to reactive oxygen species also decreases cGMP levels through increasing PDE5 activity, effects that appear to be mediated by reactive oxygen species produced from the mitochondria (see Fig. 3.3).[75] In fetal lambs with PPHN, pulmonary prostacyclin synthase and PGI_2 receptor (IP) protein levels in the lung are decreased, but levels of adenylate cyclase and PDE3A are not altered.[76]

Circulating levels of endothelin (ET-1), a potent vasoconstrictor and smooth muscle mitogen, are increased in human infants with PPHN,[77] and lung and vascular ET-1 levels are increased in fetal lambs with PPHN.[78,79] ET-1 also appears to be a marker for chronic PH, in that infants with CDH and poor outcomes have higher plasma ET-1 levels at 2 weeks of age and severity of PH than infants discharged breathing room air.[80] The constrictor effects of endothelin are mediated in part through activation of the RhoA-Rho-kinase (ROCK) pathway.[79] Increased Rho-kinase activity leads to phosphorylation of myosin light-chain kinase, which in turn increases intracellular calcium and causes vascular contraction. The ROCK pathway plays an important role in hypoxic pulmonary vasoconstriction[81] and as a mediator of the impaired angiogenesis and increased contractility associated with chronic fetal PH (see Fig. 3.3).[82]

Factors That Disrupt Fetal Pulmonary Vascular Development

Genetic Factors

A number of gene mutations, including mutations in the gene coding bone morphogenic protein receptor type 2 (BMPR2) and other genes (e.g., CAV1, KCNK3, EIF2AK4), have been identified in adults with PH. In contrast, few genetic mutations have been identified in neonates with PH. Although eNOS mRNA expression was found to be reduced or absent in umbilical venous endothelial cells of infants with PPHN,[69] candidate gene analysis did not identify any polymorphisms of the eNOS gene in infants with PPHN.[83] In that same study, no variants for BMPR2, VEGF, cGMP-specific phosphodiesterase, or other plausible causes of fetal vascular remodeling were found in infants with PPHN.[83] Interestingly, higher rates of genetic variants for cortisol signaling (corticotropin-releasing hormone receptor-1 [CRHR1] and CRH-binding protein) were observed in neonates with PPHN, as well as evidence for functional adrenal insufficiency.[83] The CRH-binding protein decreases bioavailability of CRH and may diminish the activity of the hypothalamic-pituitary-adrenal axis and affect fetal lung functional development or the capacity to adequately transition to ex utero life. Additionally, CRHR1 single-nucleotide polymorphisms are located close to the transcription factor binding site for peroxisome proliferator-activated receptor-gamma (PPARγ), which is an essential regulator of pulmonary arterial smooth muscle cell proliferation and vascular tone.

Other genetic abnormalities of the NO pathway have been associated with PPHN. Endothelial cells generate NO from the precursor L-arginine, an amino acid supplied by the urea cycle. Carbamoyl-phosphatase synthetase catalyzes the first, rate-determining step of the urea cycle.[70] In term neonates with respiratory failure, with and without PPHN, a polymorphism in the rate-limiting enzyme of the urea cycle, carbamoyl-phosphate synthetase-1, was associated with PH, low plasma arginine concentrations, and low plasma NO metabolites.[70]

Children with Down syndrome (trisomy 21) commonly develop PH in association with structural heart defects, but they also have a 10-fold increased risk for idiopathic PPHN. In a Dutch cohort, PPHN was documented in 5.2% of infants with Down syndrome without cardiac disease.[84] In addition, infants with Down syndrome have worse pulmonary artery hypertension in conjunction with anatomic cardiac disease than genetically normal infants with similar lesions and they are more likely to require extracorporeal membrane oxygenation (ECMO) support for PPHN.[85] One recent study showed that 85% of autopsy specimens from children with Down syndrome displayed pulmonary vascular remodeling, suggesting that PH may occur even more commonly than clinically recognized.[86]

Chromosome 21 includes at least three genes with potent antiangiogenic properties that could affect fetal vascular development. One of these genes, endostatin, is a known antiangiogenic factor that downregulates signaling of VEGF, so it is plausible that endostatin upregulation could impair angiogenesis and adversely affect lung structure. A threefold increase of endostatin mRNA expression has been reported in prenatal Down syndrome lungs, along with reduced microvascular density, thickened large and small pulmonary artery walls, and a persistent double capillary network.[87] These results strongly suggest a role for genetically driven antiangiogenic signals in the pathogenesis of impaired lung vascular development and PH in Down syndrome.

Antenatal Ductal Closure

A patent ductus arteriosus is critical for the normal fetal circulation. It directs right ventricular output to the aorta, but it also protects the pulmonary circulation from volume overload and the right ventricle from pressure overload. Either partial or complete ductal ligation in the fetal lamb increases pulmonary arterial pressure without sustained elevation in pulmonary blood flow or in utero hypoxemia.[63,88,89] Endothelial dysfunction rapidly emerges and results in poor response to endothelium-dependent vasodilators such as oxygen and acetylcholine, along with decreased expression and activity of pulmonary eNOS.[90] There is also a strong constrictor "myogenic response" that may exist to protect the pulmonary capillary bed from high pulmonary blood flow, and may by mediated by activation of the ROCK pathway.[91] Downstream signaling abnormalities emerge within days of ductal closure, including decreased activity and expression of soluble guanylate cyclase and increased activity of PDE5.[92] After birth the newborns develop severe PH, a model that has been extensively used for preclinical studies to evaluate inhaled NO and other pulmonary vasodilators in PPHN.[93]

Placental Insufficiency

Recent epidemiology studies have reported an association between fetal growth restriction and the later development of PH in premature infants with BPD.[94] This association suggests that intrauterine stress could initiate the cascade that results in abnormal pulmonary vascular development and PH in preterm infants. In fetuses with severe fetal growth restriction and absent end-diastolic flow in the umbilical artery, PH with right-to-left shunting across the patent foramen ovale and patent ductus arteriosus was commonly observed.[95]

Animal models have suggested that pulmonary vascular maldevelopment and PH associated with chronic lung disease begin before birth in response to chronic fetal hypoxia.[96] Recent studies examining the placental and cord blood findings in preterm infants in whom PH later developed showed a striking association with placental pathologic changes of maternal vascular underperfusion and decreased villous vascularity.[97,98] Moreover, cord blood angiogenic factors such as placental growth factor and VEGF-A were decreased in premature infants exposed to placental underperfusion, and these fetal blood markers predicted the subsequent development of PH.[99] It is possible that disruption of placentation and placental vascular perfusion represents failed angiogenesis, as reflected by these biomarkers, and that this abnormal developmental angiogenesis may reflect global abnormalities of vascular signaling that contribute to postnatal vascular disease.[100] Additional preclinical studies suggest that disruption of angiogenesis because of adverse antenatal factors such as chorioamnionitis, preeclampsia, or maternal smoking, can cause pulmonary vascular disease that not only leads to PH but also impairs lung growth and alveolarization.[68]

Oligohydramnios/PH in Preterm Infants

Some preterm infants develop severe early PH after prolonged rupture of membranes with oligohydramnios and some degree of pulmonary hypoplasia.[101,102] Preterm infants with prolonged rupture of membranes and PH were found to have low tracheal aspirate levels of nitrates/nitrites, suggesting a specific deficiency of NO; these infants responded promptly and dramatically to iNO.[10] In animal studies, the pulmonary circulation of lambs with hypoplastic lungs created by a tracheoamniotic shunt had significantly increased PVR with high pulmonary artery pressure and reduced pulmonary blood flow.[103] Furthermore, changes in indices of lung ventilation were proportional to the changes in lung size, but accompanied by disproportionate changes in the pulmonary circulation associated with reduced density of pulmonary arterioles.[103] These findings suggest that oligohydramnios-induced pulmonary hypoplasia exerts a selective effect on lung vascular development, and raises important questions about the role of the amniotic fluid in maintaining levels of lung vascular growth factors. Histologic changes of the pulmonary vasculature include reduced volume density of pulmonary arteries and increased acinar arterial wall muscle thickness.[104]

Maternal Drug Exposures

Two classes of medications, nonsteroidal antiinflammatory agents (NSAIDs) and SSRIs, have the most evidence to suggest a direct effect on pulmonary vascular development. An association between PPHN and prostaglandin synthase inhibitor use during late gestation was first reported 40 years ago.[105] Experimental closure or constriction of the ductus arteriosus in fetal lambs produces rapid development of pulmonary vascular remodeling and severe PPHN.[63] Prostaglandins maintain ductal patency in utero and are important mediators of pulmonary vasodilation in response to ventilation at birth. Analysis of meconium from newborn infants with PPHN revealed the presence of NSAIDs in approximately half of the samples,[106] linking antenatal NSAID exposure to PPHN. However, a recent epidemiologic study suggests these relationships are more complex than initially appreciated: an association was found only for aspirin use during the third trimester and PPHN, with no effect of ibuprofen at any point in gestation.[107]

Exposure of pregnant rats to fluoxetine, an SSRI, produces PH, hypoxia, and increased mortality in the pups.[108,109] In human epidemiology studies, the use of SSRIs during the last half of pregnancy has been associated with an increase in the incidence of PPHN, although recent reports indicate the risk is modest when controlling for maternal depression.[110–114] In addition, the severity of PPHN has not been well described, and one recent report found that neonatal mortality rates were not higher in SSRI-exposed versus nonexposed neonates with PPHN (3.4% vs. 8.3%, P not significant).[115] The mechanism by which SSRIs induce PPHN remains poorly understood, although a recent study shows that SSRIs induce concentration-dependent constriction of the ductus arteriosus and reduce sensitivity to prostaglandin-induced dilation, and that SSRI-exposed mice exhibit inappropriate ductus arteriosus constriction in utero.[116] These findings are in agreement with a recent report from a large Swedish registry, which suggested that SSRI-exposed infants are more likely to have idiopathic PPHN without lung disease.[115]

Maternal medications also have the potential to reverse pathologic fetal vascular development. In fetal lambs with PPHN induced by ductal ligation, maternal betamethasone reduced oxidative stress and improved the relaxation response to NO donors.[117] Although not specifically examined, lower rates of PPHN could partially explain the benefit of antenatal steroids in late preterm infants.[118] In fetal rats with nitrofen-induced CDH, antenatal administration of sildenafil to the dam improved lung morphology, and reduced pulmonary vascular remodeling and right ventricular hypertrophy.[119] Maternal administration of sildenafil is under investigation for severe fetal growth restriction.[120]

Congenital Diaphragmatic Hernia

CDH occurs in approximately 1 in 2500 to 3000 pregnancies and represents ~8% of all major congenital anomalies. CDH includes abnormal diaphragm development, herniation of abdominal viscera into the chest, and a variable degree of lung hypoplasia. Herniation occurs most often in the posterolateral segments of the diaphragm, and 80% of the defects occur on the left side. Of the various causes of PH in term and late-preterm infants, CDH is associated with the most intractable PH and has become the leading neonatal respiratory indication for ECMO.

Severe CDH develops early in the course of lung development. An incomplete closure of the diaphragm results in a diaphragm defect, herniation of the abdominal contents into the chest, and compression of the intrathoracic structures (Fig. 3.6). An arrest in the normal pattern of airway branching occurs in both lungs, resulting in reduced lung volume and impaired alveolarization. A similar developmental arrest occurs in pulmonary arterial branching, resulting in reduced cross-sectional area of the pulmonary vascular bed, thickened media and adventitia of small arterioles, and abnormal medial muscular hypertrophy extending distally to the level of the acinar arterioles.

In utero lung compression by herniated viscera was assumed to be the primary mechanism causing the lung abnormalities of CDH. However, comparisons with fetuses with lung compression caused by other space-occupying lesions such as congenital pulmonary adenomatoid malformations suggest that lung compression alone

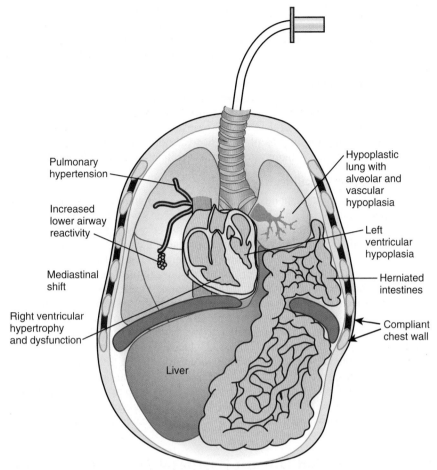

Fig. 3.6 Congenital Diaphragmatic Hernia (CDH). A defect in the diaphragm (usually on the left side) results in herniation of abdominal contents (intestines and liver) to the thorax, leading to compression and abnormal development of the ipsilateral and contralateral lung. Paucity of air space and vascular bed leads to hypoxic respiratory failure and pulmonary hypertension. Right ventricular hypertrophy and dysfunction along with left ventricular hypoplasia and dysfunction are associated with pulmonary arterial and venous hypertension, respectively, in infants with CDH. (Copyright Satyan Lakshminrusimha and Robin H. Steinhorn.)

is not sufficient to explain the pulmonary vascular pruning, vascular remodeling, and refractory PH seen in CDH.[121] Additional evidence suggests that decreased pulmonary blood flow alone is sufficient to cause lung hypoplasia.[122] Newer investigations into the pathophysiologic processes responsible for CDH suggest that environmental and/or genetic factors exert an effect before the development of the diaphragm, leading to arrested development of the parenchyma and vasculature of both lungs.[123]

Histologic findings of CDH show pulmonary vascular remodeling superimposed on pulmonary vascular bed hypoplasia[124]; such findings are clinically associated with increased vascular tone and altered vasoreactivity after birth. High or suprasystemic PVR is commonly observed in the newborn with CDH, and extrapulmonary right-to-left shunting across the foramen ovale and ductus arteriosus produce profound hypoxemia. High PVR is caused by multiple factors, including the small cross-sectional area of pulmonary arteries, structural vascular remodeling, vasoconstriction with altered reactivity, as well as left ventricular hypoplasia/dysfunction causing pulmonary venous hypertension. The mediators of altered pulmonary vascular reactivity in CDH are not well understood, although substantial evidence points to disruptions in NO-cGMP and endothelin signaling.[80] Chronic PH is seen in infants with severe disease and is associated with persistently high endothelin levels.[80]

Abnormalities of cardiac development and function are increasingly recognized as key determinants of CDH pathophysiology.[123] The left ventricle, left atrium, and intraventricular septum are hypoplastic in infants who die of CDH relative to age-matched controls, perhaps because of low fetal and postnatal pulmonary blood flow and/or compression by the hypertensive right ventricle. Left ventricular hypoplasia and dysfunction increase left atrial and pulmonary venous pressures, and the resulting pulmonary venous hypertension diminishes the clinical response to iNO during the first few days of life. This may explain why in the early clinical trials of iNO, infants with CDH did not experience a reduction in ECMO use or mortality. Some infants may have exceptionally severe left ventricular dysfunction that leads to dependence on the right ventricle for systemic perfusion[125]; this subset may depend on patency of the ductus arteriosus for survival in the early postnatal period. Determining the origins of these heart abnormalities will be key to understanding and treating the pathophysiology of severely affected infants with CDH.

Alveolar Capillary Dysplasia

ACD, with or without misalignment of the pulmonary veins, is a rare form of vascular and parenchymal lung disease that presents as severe PH and refractory hypoxemia early in life.[34] The etiology of ACD is believed to be a genetic defect or early antenatal insult that prevents normal development of the pulmonary capillary bed. Findings include remodeling of the pulmonary arterioles, simplification of the alveolar architecture, and development of congested "misaligned pulmonary veins" residing in the same adventitial sheath. These so-called veins have recently been recognized as bronchopulmonary anastomoses that link the systemic and pulmonary circulations and bypass the alveolar capillary bed.[126] Although ACD classically presents in the neonatal period, presentation occasionally occurs later at several months of life.[127] No long-term survivors of ACD have been reported despite treatment with all known modalities, including extracorporeal support, although limited survival after lung transplantation was recently reported.[127] Mutations or deletions in the Foxf1 transcription factor gene have been identified in up to 40% of infants with ACD.[128] Other anomalies of the genitourinary, cardiovascular, and gastrointestinal systems are seen in up to half of infants with ACD and could also be explained by abnormal Foxf1 signaling.

Factors That Disrupt Postnatal Pulmonary Vascular Development

Asphyxia

Perinatal asphyxia interferes with the adaptation of the perinatal pulmonary vasculature by impeding the fall in PVR and increasing the risk for PH.[129] Multiple antenatal and postnatal mechanisms combine to cause respiratory failure and affect pulmonary circulation in asphyxia—for instance, fetal hypoxemia, ischemia, meconium aspiration, left ventricular dysfunction, and acidosis can all increase PVR.[129] Moreover, animal studies demonstrate exaggerated hypoxic pulmonary vasoconstriction with pH < 7.25.[130] Acute asphyxia is associated with reversible pulmonary vasoconstriction,[131] but chronic in utero asphyxia with or without meconium aspiration may be associated with vasoconstriction and vascular remodeling.[62] Thus it is not surprising that PH complicates the course of 25% of infants with perinatal asphyxia. Severe hypothermia (temperature decreased to 30°C) increased mean pulmonary arterial pressure by 30% in neonatal lambs.[132] However, the effect of moderate hypothermia (33.5°C) on PVR appears to be modest, and analysis of randomized trials found that hypothermia does not significantly increase the incidence of PPHN.[133]

Preterm Birth

After birth, PVR decreases at a slower rate in very or extremely preterm neonates compared with term neonates.[55] Echocardiographic markers of early pulmonary vascular dysfunction can be found in the first week of life in up to 40% of extremely preterm infants, and these findings are a strong risk factor for BPD and late PH.[134] In that same time frame, abnormalities of a number of circulating proteins related to extracellular matrix, growth factors, and angiogenesis were found.[135]

Chronic PH complicates the course of 10T to 14% of extremely preterm infants at 36 weeks postmenstrual age, and it is even more common in infants with moderate to severe BPD. The severity of BPD, but also antenatal findings of fetal growth restriction and oligohydramnios, are risk factors associated with development of PH.[94] BPD is associated with reduced cross-sectional perfusion area with decreased arterial density and abnormal muscularization of peripheral pulmonary arteries. The pathophysiology of PH in these infants is a combination of simplified lung parenchyma and impaired vascular development.

Pulmonary Vein Stenosis

Pulmonary vein stenosis is a complication of severe BPD that can contribute to severe and progressive PH. The left-sided pulmonary veins (particularly the left upper vein) are most often affected, and severe PH can result after stenosis of only one vein. The mechanisms producing pulmonary vein stenosis are not yet known. A number of findings, including a median age of diagnosis of 6 months, a lack of concordance in twins, and association with necrotizing enterocolitis, indicate that the disease is postnatally acquired.[136,137] The disease tends to be progressive and is associated with high mortality (30%–50%) in the first 2 years after diagnosis.

Hypoxia

Acute alveolar hypoxia and hypoxemia increase PVR and contribute to the pathophysiology of PPHN. Chronic hypoxia is a known trigger for lung vascular remodeling, in part through increasing activity of HIFs. Stretch induces HIF-1α activity in fetal pulmonary vessels, which can drive a sustained vasoconstrictor response and remodeling in response to hypoxia.[138] This rise in HIF activity could partly explain the vigorous myogenic response of fetal lung vessels and why the vasoconstrictor response in PPHN vessels is dramatically enhanced in response to hypoxia.[139] In neonatal piglets, PH develops after 3 days of hypoxia and worsens when the hypoxic exposure is extended to 10 days.[140] The underlying mechanisms are complex and appear to include "uncoupling" of endothelial NOS, possibly owing to impaired availability of its substrate, arginine. NOS uncoupling not only impairs NO signaling, but also diverts electrons to produce superoxide instead of NO.

Hyperoxia

Oxygen is a potent pulmonary vasodilator, and increased oxygen tension from fetal to ambient air levels is a key mediator of the fall in PVR at birth. The use of hyperoxia (100% oxygen) in the initial resuscitation of newborn lambs slightly enhances the rate of drop in PVR compared with normoxia,[141,142] although within minutes PVR falls to similar levels in hyperoxic and normoxic groups. Moreover, after even brief hyperoxic ventilation, formation of reactive oxygen species (ROS, e.g., hydrogen peroxide, superoxide, and peroxynitrite) occurs that impairs relaxation to endogenous or inhaled NO. Increased ROS can be generated as the result of immature or dysfunctional antioxidant defense mechanisms (e.g., superoxide dismutase, catalase) and/or increased activity of prooxidant enzymes such as reduced nicotinamide adenine dinucleotide phosphate oxidase.[143,144] These ROS can cause pulmonary vasoconstriction and trigger vascular remodeling as seen in PPHN.[144,145] In addition to disruption of NO signaling,[146] ROS generated by hyperoxia can decrease eNOS expression and activity, sGC activity, and increase PDE5 activity, resulting in decreased cGMP levels.[92,147]

Preterm birth exposes the lung to ambient oxygen concentrations that are severalfold higher than fetal levels, and supplemental oxygen is frequently required to treat respiratory failure. The preterm lung is ill equipped to cope with increased ambient oxygen concentrations, and exposure to hyperoxia during this developmentally sensitive period increases lipid and protein oxidation products and disrupts normal parenchymal and vascular lung development.[148] Because newborn rodents are born at an immature saccular phase of lung development, chronic exposure to hyperoxia (7–21 days) is commonly used to generate a rodent model of BPD and PH. However, recent studies indicate that just 24 hours of hyperoxic exposure shortly after birth is sufficient to cause PH and right ventricular hypertrophy that persists to day 14, which is associated with persistently diminished sGC and increased cGMP phosphodiesterase activity.[149] In preterm lambs, early exposure to brief hyperoxic ventilation increases expression of prolyl hydroxlase, which rapidly degrades HIF-1α and HIF2-α.[150] These events can trigger abnormal lung development after preterm birth through disrupting expression of downstream targets such as VEGF (see Fig. 3.4). Other stresses common to the sick preterm infant, such as nutritional deficiency, appear to amplify the effect of hyperoxia on the pulmonary vasculature, in part by reducing VEGR and NO synthase activity.[151]

Conclusions

In summary, lung vascular development is a dynamic process that begins in fetal life and continues through postnatal life. An increased understanding of the physiology of the fetal and neonatal pulmonary circulation has led to improved identification and management of early and chronic PH in term and preterm infants. Stresses during fetal life, such as placental insufficiency, can cause vascular dysfunction and trigger chronic PH in preterm infants. A number of open questions and controversies remain, including the role of cardiac dysfunction in CDH and the causes of PH in the premature infant. Further research to evaluate and develop appropriate strategies to ameliorate pulmonary vascular disease in these conditions is warranted.

REFERENCES

1. Thebaud B, Abman SH. Bronchopulmonary dysplasia: where have all the vessels gone? Roles of angiogenic growth factors in chronic lung disease. *Am J Respir Crit Care Med.* 2007;175(10):978–985.
2. Roth-Kleiner M, Post M. Similarities and dissimilaries of branching and septation during lung development. *Pediatr Pulmonol.* 2005;40(2):113–134.
3. Schwarz MAL, Caldwell D, Cafasso, et al. Emerging pulmonary vasculature lacks fate specification. *Am J Physiol Lung Cell Mol Physiol.* 2009;296(1):L71–L81.
4. Rudolph AM. Aortopulmonary transposition in the fetus: speculation on pathophysiology and therapy. *Pediatr Res.* 2007;61(3):375–380.
5. Rasanen J, Wood DC, Weiner S, et al. Role of the pulmonary circulation in the distribution of human fetal cardiac output during the second half of pregnancy. *Circulation.* 1996;94(5):1068–1073.
6. Morin FC 3rd, Egan EA, Ferguson W, et al. Development of pulmonary vascular response to oxygen. *Am J Physiol.* 1988;254(3 Pt 2):H542–H546.
7. Lewis AB, Heymann MA, Rudolph AM. Gestational changes in pulmonary vascular responses in fetal lambs in utero. *Circ Res.* 1976;39(4):536–541.
8. Rasanen J, Wood DC, Debbs RH, et al. Reactivity of the human fetal pulmonary circulation to maternal hyperoxygenation increases during the second half of pregnancy: a randomized study. *Circulation.* 1998;97(3):257–262.
9. Kumar VH, Hutchison AA, Lakshminrusimha S, et al. Characteristics of pulmonary hypertension in preterm neonates. *J Perinatol.* 2007;27(4):214–219.
10. Aikio O, Metsola J, Vuolteenaho R, et al. Transient defect in nitric oxide generation after rupture of fetal membranes and responsiveness to inhaled nitric oxide in very preterm infants with hypoxic respiratory failure. *J Pediatr.* 2012;161(3):397–403.e1.
11. Stenger MR, Slaughter JL, Kelleher K, et al. Hospital variation in nitric oxide use for premature infants. *Pediatrics.* 2012;129(4):e945–e951.
12. *Report of the Australian and New Zealand Neonatal Network 2012.* 2014.
13. Handley SC, Steinhorn RH, Hooper AO, et al. Patterns of inhaled nitric oxide use in California NICUs. *Pediatric Academic Societies. Abstract.* 2015.
14. Done E, Allegaert K, Lewi P, et al. Maternal hyperoxygenation test in fetuses undergoing FETO for severe isolated congenital diaphragmatic hernia. *Ultrasound Obstet Gynecol.* 2011;37(3):264–271.
15. Arraut AM, Frias AE, Hobbs TR, et al. Fetal pulmonary arterial vascular impedance reflects changes in fetal oxygenation at near-term gestation in a nonhuman primate model. *Reprod Sci.* 2013;20(1):33–38.
16. Konduri GG, Gervasio CT, Theodorou AA. Role of adenosine triphosphate and adenosine in oxygen-induced pulmonary vasodilation in fetal lambs. *Pediatr Res.* 1993;33(5):533–539.
17. Schwartz SM, Vermilion RP, Hirschl RB. Evaluation of left ventricular mass in children with left-sided congenital diaphragmatic hernia. *J Pediatr.* 1994;125(3):447–451.
18. Siebert JR, Haas JE, Beckwith JB. Left ventricular hypoplasia in congenital diaphragmatic hernia. *J Pediatr Surg.* 1984;19(5):567–571.
19. Gao Y, Raj JU. Role of veins in regulation of pulmonary circulation. *Am J Physiol.* 2005;288(2):L213–L226.
20. Steinhorn RH, Morin FC 3rd, Gugino SF, et al. Developmental differences in endothelium-dependent responses in isolated ovine pulmonary arteries and veins. *Am J Physiol.* 1993;264(6 Pt 2):H2162–H2167.
21. Gao Y, Dhanakoti S, Tolsa JF, et al. Role of protein kinase G in nitric oxide and cGMP induced relaxation of newborn ovine pulmonary veins. *J Appl Physiol.* 1999;87:993–998.

22. Semenza GL. Oxygen sensing, hypoxia-inducible factors, and disease pathophysiology. *Annu Rev Pathol.* 2014;9:47–71.

23. Yu AY, Frid MG, Shimoda LA, et al. Temporal, spatial, and oxygen-regulated expression of hypoxia-inducible factor-1 in the lung. *Am J Physiol.* 1998;275(4 Pt 1):L818–L826.

24. Compernolle V, Brusselmans K, Acker T, et al. Loss of HIF-2alpha and inhibition of VEGF impair fetal lung maturation, whereas treatment with VEGF prevents fatal respiratory distress in premature mice. *Nat Med.* 2002;8(7):702–710. Epub 2002 Jun 10.

25. Parker TA, Le Cras TD, Kinsella JP, et al. Developmental changes in endothelial NO synthase expression in the ovine fetal lung. *Am J Physiol.* 2000;266:L202–L208.

26. North AJ, Star RA, Brannon TS, et al. NO synthase type I and type III gene expression are developmentally regulated in rat lung. *Am J Physiol.* 1994;266:L635–L641.

27. Han RN, Babaei S, Robb M, et al. Defective lung vascular development and fatal respiratory distress in endothelial NO synthase-deficient mice: a model of alveolar capillary dysplasia? *Circ Res.* 2004;94(8):1115–1123.

28. Balasubramaniam V, Tang JR, Maxey A, et al. Mild hypoxia impairs alveolarization in the endothelial nitric oxide synthase (eNOS) deficient mouse. *Am J Physiol.* 2003;284(6):L964–L971.

29. Ng YS, Rohan R, Sunday ME, et al. Differential expression of VEGF isoforms in mouse during development and in the adult. *Dev Dyn.* 2001;220(2):112–121.

30. Kasahara Y, Tuder RM, Taraseviciene-Stewart L, et al. Inhibition of VEGF receptors causes lung cell apoptosis and emphysema. *J Clin Invest.* 2000;106(11):1311–1319.

31. Gao Y, Cornfield DN, Stenmark KR, et al. Unique aspects of the developing lung circulation: structural development and regulation of vasomotor tone. *Pulm Circ.* 2016;6(4):407–425.

32. Kalinichenko VV, Lim L, Stolz DB, et al. Defects in pulmonary vasculature and perinatal lung hemorrhage in mice heterozygous null for the Forkhead Box f1 transcription factor. *Dev Biol.* 2001;235(2):489–506.

33. Ren X, Ustiyan V, Pradhan A, et al. FOXF1 transcription factor is required for formation of embryonic vasculature by regulating VEGF signaling in endothelial cells. *Circ Res.* 2014;115(8):709–720.

34. Bishop NB, Stankiewicz P, Steinhorn RH. Alveolar capillary dysplasia. *Am J Respir Crit Care Med.* 2011;184(2):172–179.

35. Iosef C, Alastalo TP, Hou Y, et al. Inhibiting NF-kappaB in the developing lung disrupts angiogenesis and alveolarization. *Am J Physiol Lung Cell Mol Physiol.* 2012;302(10):L1023–L1036.

36. Solodushko V, Fouty B. Proproliferative phenotype of pulmonary microvascular endothelial cells. *Am J Physiol Lung Cell Mol Physiol.* 2007;292(3):L671–L677.

37. Alvarez DF, Huang L, King JA, et al. Lung microvascular endothelium is enriched with progenitor cells that exhibit vasculogenic capacity. *Am J Physiol Lung Cell Mol Physiol.* 2008;294(3):L419–L430.

38. Grover TR, Parker TA, Zenge JP, et al. Intrauterine hypertension decreases lung VEGF expression and VEGF inhibition causes pulmonary hypertension in the ovine fetus. *Am J Physiol Lung Cell Mol Physiol.* 2003;284(3):L508–L517.

39. Mensah E, Morin FC 3rd, Russell JA, et al. Soluble guanylate cyclase mRNA expression change during ovine lung development. *Pediatr Res.* 1998;43:290.

40. Wang Y, Coceani F. Isolated pulmonary resistance vessels from fetal lambs. Contractile behavior and responses to indomethacin and endothelin-1. *Circ Res.* 1992;71(2):320–330.

41. Zenge JP, Rairigh RL, Grover TR, et al. NO and prostaglandin interactions during hemodynamic stress in the fetal ovine pulmonary circulation. *Am J Physiol Lung Cell Mol Physiol.* 2001;281(5):L1157–L1163.

42. Delaney C, Gien J, Grover TR, et al. Pulmonary vascular effects of serotonin and selective serotonin reuptake inhibitors in the late-gestation ovine fetus. *Am J Physiol Lung Cell Mol Physiol.* 2011;301(6):L937–L944.

43. Delaney C, Gien J, Roe G, et al. Serotonin contributes to high pulmonary vascular tone in a sheep model of persistent pulmonary hypertension of the newborn. *Am J Physiol Lung Cell Mol Physiol.* 2013;304(12):L894–L901.

44. Teitel DF, Iwamoto HS, Rudolph AM. Changes in the pulmonary circulation during birth-related events. *Pediatr Res.* 1990;27(4 Pt 1):372–378.

45. Lakshminrusimha S. The pulmonary circulation in neonatal respiratory failure. *Clin Perinatol.* 2012;39(3):655–683.

46. Abman SH, Chatfield BA, Hall SL, et al. Role of endothelium-derived relaxing factor during transition of pulmonary circulation at birth. *Am J Physiol.* 1990;259(6 Pt 2):H1921–H1927.

47. Fineman JR, Heymann MA, Soifer SJ. N omega-nitro-L-arginine attenuates endothelium-dependent pulmonary vasodilation in lambs. *Am J Physiol.* 1991;260(4 Pt 2):H1299–H1306.

48. Tiktinsky MH, Morin III FC. Increasing oxygen tension dilates fetal pulmonary circulation via endothelium-derived relaxing factor. *Am J Physiol Heart Circ Physiol.* 1993;265:H376–H380.

49. Fagan KA, Fouty BW, Tyler RC, et al. The pulmonary circulation of homozygous or heterozygous eNos-null mice is hyperresponsive to mild hypoxia. *J Clin Invest.* 1999;103:291–299.

50. Balasubramaniam V, Maxey AM, Morgan DB, et al. Inhaled NO restores lung structure in eNOS-deficient mice recovering from neonatal hypoxia. *Am J Physiol Lung Cell Mol Physiol.* 2006;291(1):L119–L127.

51. Bloch KD, Filippov G, Sanchez LS, et al. Pulmonary soluble guanylate cyclase, a nitric oxide receptor, is increased during the perinatal period. *Am J Physiol Lung Cell Mol Physiol.* 1997;272(Lung Cell Mol Physiol):L400–L406.

52. Hanson KA, Ziegler JW, Rybalkin SD, et al. Chronic pulmonary hypertension increases fetal lung cGMP phosphodiesterase activity. *Am J Physiol.* 1998;275(5 Pt 1):L931–L941.

53. Sanchez LS, de la Monte SM, Filippov G, et al. Cyclic-GMP-binding, cyclic-GMP-specific phosphodiesterase (PDE5) gene expression is regulated during rat pulmonary development. *Pediatric Res*. 1998;43(2):163–168.

54. Kinsella JP, McQueston JA, Rosenberg AA, et al. Hemodynamic effects of exogenous nitric oxide in ovine transitional pulmonary circulation. *Am J Physiol*. 1992;263(3 Pt 2):H875–H880.

55. Randala M, Eronen M, Andersson S, et al. Pulmonary artery pressure in term and preterm neonates. *Acta Paediatr*. 1996;85(11):1344–1347.

56. Evans NJ, Archer LN. Doppler assessment of pulmonary artery pressure during recovery from hyaline membrane disease. *Arch Dis Child*. 1991;66(7 Spec No):802–804.

57. Evans NJ, Archer LN. Doppler assessment of pulmonary artery pressure and extrapulmonary shunting in the acute phase of hyaline membrane disease. *Arch Dis Child*. 1991;66(1 Spec No):6–11.

58. Skimming JW, Bender KA, Hutchison AA, et al. Nitric oxide inhalation in infants with respiratory distress syndrome. *J Pediatr*. 1997;130(2):225–230.

59. Mourani PM, Sontag MK, Younoszai, et al. Early pulmonary vascular disease in preterm infants at risk for bronchopulmonary dysplasia. *Am J Respir Crit Care Med*. 2014.

60. Murphy JD, Rabinovitch M, Goldstein JD, et al. The structural basis of persistent pulmonary hypertension of the newborn infant. *J Pediatr*. 1981;98(6):962–967.

61. Ohara T, Ogata H, Tezuka F. Histological study of pulmonary vasculature in fatal cases of persistent pulmonary hypertension of the newborn. *Tohoku J Exp Med*. 1991;164(1):59–66.

62. Murphy JD, Vawter GF, Reid LM. Pulmonary vascular disease in fatal meconium aspiration. *J Pediatr*. 1984;104(5):758–762.

63. Wild LM, Nickerson PA, Morin FC 3rd. Ligating the ductus arteriosus before birth remodels the pulmonary vasculature of the lamb. *Pediatr Res*. 1989;25(3):251–257.

64. Dodson RB, Morgan M, Galambos C, et al. Chronic intrauterine pulmonary hypertension increases main pulmonary artery stiffness and adventitial remodeling in fetal sheep. *Am J Physiol Lung Cell Mol Physiol*. 2014. http://dx.doi.org/ajplung 00256 2014.

65. Stenmark KR, Davie N, Frid M, et al. Role of the adventitia in pulmonary vascular remodeling. *Physiology (Bethesda)*. 2006;21:134–145.

66. Stenmark KR, Yeager ME, El Kasmi KC, et al. The adventitia: essential regulator of vascular wall structure and function. *Annu Rev Physiol*. 2013;75:23–47.

67. Galambos C, Sims-Lucas S, Abman SH. Histologic evidence of intrapulmonary anastomoses by three-dimensional reconstruction in severe bronchopulmonary dysplasia. *Ann Am Thorac Soc*. 2013;10(5):474–481.

68. Mourani PM, Abman SH. Pulmonary hypertension and vascular abnormalities in bronchopulmonary dysplasia. *Clin Perinatol*. 2015;42(4):839–855.

69. Villanueva ME, Zaher FM, Svinarich DM, et al. Decreased gene expression of endothelial nitric oxide synthase in newborns with persistent pulmonary hypertension. *Pediatr Res*. 1998;44(3):338–343.

70. Pearson DL, Dawling S, Walsh WF, et al. Neonatal pulmonary hypertension–urea-cycle intermediates, nitric oxide production, and carbamoyl-phosphate synthetase function. *N Engl J Med*. 2001;344(24):1832–1838.

71. Steinhorn RH, Russell JA, Morin FC 3rd. Disruption of cGMP production in pulmonary arteries isolated from fetal lambs with pulmonary hypertension. *Am J Physiol*. 1995;268(4 Pt 2):H1483–H4189.

72. de Buys Roessingh A, Fouquet V, Aigrain Y, et al. Nitric oxide activity through guanylate cyclase and phosphodiesterase modulation is impaired in fetal lambs with congenital diaphragmatic hernia. *J Pediatr Surg*. 2011;46(8):1516–1522.

73. Chester M, Seedorf G, Tourneux P, et al. Cinaciguat, a soluble guanylate cyclase activator, augments cGMP after oxidative stress and causes pulmonary vasodilation in neonatal pulmonary hypertension. *Am J Physiol Lung Cell Mol Physiol*. 2011;301(5):L755–L764.

74. Farrow KN, Lakshminrusimha S, Czech L, et al. SOD and inhaled nitric oxide normalize phosphodiesterase 5 expression and activity in neonatal lambs with persistent pulmonary hypertension. *Am J Physiol Lung Cell Mol Physiol*. 2010;299(1):L109–L116.

75. Farrow KN, Groh BS, Schumacker PT, et al. Hyperoxia increases phosphodiesterase 5 expression and activity in ovine fetal pulmonary artery smooth muscle cells. *Circ Res*. 2008;102(2):226–233.

76. Lakshminrusimha S, Porta NF, Farrow KN, et al. Milrinone enhances relaxation to prostacyclin and iloprost in pulmonary arteries isolated from lambs with persistent pulmonary hypertension of the newborn. *Pediatr Crit Care Med*. 2009;10(1):106–112.

77. Christou H, Adatia I, Van Marter LJ, et al. Effect of inhaled nitric oxide on endothelin-1 and cyclic guanosine 5′-monophosphate plasma concentrations in newborn infants with persistent pulmonary hypertension. *J Pediatr*. 1997;130(4):603–611.

78. Ivy DD, Le Cras TD, Horan MP, et al. Chronic intrauterine pulmonary hypertension increases preproendothelin-1 and decreases endothelin B receptor mRNA expression in the ovine fetal lung. *Chest*. 1998;114(suppl 1):65S.

79. Gien J, Tseng N, Seedorf G, et al. Endothelin-1 impairs angiogenesis in vitro through Rho-kinase activation after chronic intrauterine pulmonary hypertension in fetal sheep. *Pediatr Res*. 2013;73(3):252–262.

80. Keller RL, Tacy TA, Hendricks-Munoz K, et al. Congenital diaphragmatic hernia: endothelin-1, pulmonary hypertension, and disease severity. *Am J Respir Crit Care Med*. 2010;182(4):555–561.

81. Fagan KA, Oka M, Bauer NR, et al. Attenuation of acute hypoxic pulmonary vasoconstriction and hypoxic pulmonary hypertension in mice by inhibition of Rho-kinase. *Am J Physiol Lung Cell Mol Physiol*. 2004;287(4):L656–L664.

82. Parker TA, Roe G, Grover TR, et al. Rho kinase activation maintains high pulmonary vascular resistance in the ovine fetal lung. *Am J Physiol Lung Cell Mol Physiol.* 2006;291(5):L976–L982.

83. Byers HM, Dagle JM, Klein JM, et al. Variations in CRHR1 are associated with persistent pulmonary hypertension of the newborn. *Pediatr Res.* 2012;71(2):162–167.

84. Weijerman ME, van Furth AM, van der Mooren MD, et al. Prevalence of congenital heart defects and persistent pulmonary hypertension of the neonate with Down syndrome. *Eur J Pediatr.* 2010;169(10):1195–1199.

85. Southgate WM, Annibale DJ, Hulsey TC, et al. International experience with trisomy 21 infants placed on extracorporeal membrane oxygenation. *Pediatrics.* 2001;107(3):549–552.

86. Bush D, Abman SH, Galambos C. Prominent intrapulmonary bronchopulmonary anastomoses and abnormal lung development in infants and children with down syndrome. *J Pediatr.* 2017;180:156–162.e1.

87. Galambos C, Minic AD, Bush D, et al. Increased lung expression of anti-angiogenic factors in down syndrome: potential role in abnormal lung vascular growth and the risk for pulmonary hypertension. *PLoS One.* 2016;11(8):e0159005.

88. Abman SH, Accurso FJ. Acute effects of partial compression of ductus arteriosus on fetal pulmonary circulation. *Am J Physiol.* 1989;257(2 Pt 2):H626–H634.

89. Abman SH, Shanley PF, Accurso FJ. Failure of postnatal adaptation of the pulmonary circulation after chronic intrauterine pulmonary hypertension in fetal lambs. *J Clin Invest.* 1989;83(6):1849–1858.

90. Shaul PW, Yuhanna IS, German Z, et al. Pulmonary endothelial NO synthase gene expression is decreased in fetal lambs with pulmonary hypertension. *Am J Physiol.* 1997;272(5 Pt 1):L1005–L1012.

91. Tourneux P, Chester M, Grover T, et al. Fasudil inhibits the myogenic response in the fetal pulmonary circulation. *Am J Physiol Heart Circ Physiol.* 2008;295(4):H1505–H1513.

92. Farrow KN, Wedgwood S, Lee KJ, et al. Mitochondrial oxidant stress increases PDE5 activity in persistent pulmonary hypertension of the newborn. *Respir Physiol Neurobiol.* 2010;174(3):272–281.

93. Zayek M, Cleveland D, Morin FC 3rd. Treatment of persistent pulmonary hypertension in the newborn lamb by inhaled nitric oxide. *J Pediatr.* 1993;122(5 Pt 1):743–750.

94. Check J, Gotteiner N, Liu X, et al. Fetal growth restriction and pulmonary hypertension in premature infants with bronchopulmonary dysplasia. *J Perinatol.* 2013;33(7):553–557.

95. Turan S, Turan OM, Salim M, et al. Cardiovascular transition to extrauterine life in growth-restricted neonates: relationship with prenatal Doppler findings. *Fetal Diagn Ther.* 2013;33(2):103–109.

96. Rozance PJ, Seedorf GJ, Brown A, et al. Intrauterine growth restriction decreases pulmonary alveolar and vessel growth and causes pulmonary artery endothelial cell dysfunction in vitro in fetal sheep. *Am J Physiol Lung Cell Mol Physiol.* 2011;301(6):L860–L871.

97. Mestan KK, Check J, Minturn L, et al. Placental pathologic changes of maternal vascular underperfusion in bronchopulmonary dysplasia and pulmonary hypertension. *Placenta.* 2014;35(8):570–574.

98. Yallapragada SG, Mestan KK, Palac H, et al. Placental villous vascularity is decreased in premature infants with bronchopulmonary dysplasia-associated pulmonary hypertension. *Pediatr Dev Pathol.* 2016;19(2):101–107.

99. Mestan KK, Gotteiner N, Porta N, et al. Cord blood biomarkers of placental maternal vascular underperfusion predict bronchopulmonary dysplasia-associated pulmonary hypertension. *J Pediatr.* 2017;185:33–41.

100. Mandell EW, Abman SH. Fetal vascular origins of bronchopulmonary dysplasia. *J Pediatr.* 2017;185:7–10.e1.

101. Ball MK, Steinhorn RH. Inhaled nitric oxide for preterm infants: a Marksman's approach. *J Pediatr.* 2012;161(3):379–380.

102. de Waal K, Kluckow M. Prolonged rupture of membranes and pulmonary hypoplasia in very preterm infants: pathophysiology and guided treatment. *J Pediatr.* 2015;166(5):1113–1120.

103. Suzuki K, Hooper SB, Cock ML, et al. Effect of lung hypoplasia on birth-related changes in the pulmonary circulation in sheep. *Pediatr Res.* 2005;57(4):530–536.

104. Thibeault DW, Kilbride HK. Increased acinar arterial wall muscle in preterm infants with PROM and pulmonary hypoplasia. *Am J Perinatol.* 1997;14(8):457–460.

105. Talati AJ, Salim MA, Korones SB. Persistent pulmonary hypertension after maternal naproxen ingestion in a term newborn: a case report. *Am J Perinatol.* 2000;17(2):69–71.

106. Alano MA, Ngougmna E, Ostrea EM Jr, et al. Analysis of nonsteroidal antiinflammatory drugs in meconium and its relation to persistent pulmonary hypertension of the newborn. *Pediatrics.* 2001;107(3):519–523.

107. Van Marter LJ, Hernandez-Diaz S, Werler MM, et al. Nonsteroidal antiinflammatory drugs in late pregnancy and persistent pulmonary hypertension of the newborn. *Pediatrics.* 2013;131(1):79–87.

108. Belik J. Fetal and neonatal effects of maternal drug treatment for depression. *Semin Perinatol.* 2008;32(5):350–354.

109. Fornaro E, Li D, Pan J, et al. Prenatal exposure to fluoxetine induces fetal pulmonary hypertension in the rat. *Am J Respir Crit Care Med.* 2007;176(10):1035–1040.

110. Chambers CD, Hernandez-Diaz S, Van Marter LJ, et al. Selective serotonin-reuptake inhibitors and risk of persistent pulmonary hypertension of the newborn. *N Engl J Med.* 2006;354(6):579–587.

111. Kieler H, Artama M, Engeland A, et al. Selective serotonin reuptake inhibitors during pregnancy and risk of persistent pulmonary hypertension in the newborn: population based cohort study from the five Nordic countries. *BMJ.* 2012;344:d8012.

112. Reis M, Kallen B. Delivery outcome after maternal use of antidepressant drugs in pregnancy: an update using Swedish data. *Psychol Med.* 2010;40(10):1723–1733.

113. Grigoriadis S, Vonderporten EH, Mamisashvili L, et al. Prenatal exposure to antidepressants and persistent pulmonary hypertension of the newborn: systematic review and meta-analysis. *BMJ.* 2014;348:f6932.

114. Huybrechts KF, Bateman BT, Palmsten K, et al. Antidepressant use late in pregnancy and risk of persistent pulmonary hypertension of the newborn. *JAMA.* 2015;313(21):2142–2151.

115. Norby U, Forsberg L, Wide K, et al. Neonatal morbidity after maternal use of antidepressant drugs during pregnancy. *Pediatrics.* 2016;138(5).

116. Hooper CW, Delaney C, Streeter T, et al. Selective serotonin reuptake inhibitor exposure constricts the mouse ductus arteriosus in utero. *Am J Physiol Heart Circ Physiol.* 2016;311(3):H572–H581.

117. Chandrasekar I, Eis A, Konduri GG. Betamethasone attenuates oxidant stress in endothelial cells from fetal lambs with persistent pulmonary hypertension. *Pediatr Res.* 2008;63(1):67–72.

118. Gyamfi-Bannerman C, Thom EA, Blackwell SC, et al. Antenatal betamethasone for women at risk for late preterm delivery. *N Engl J Med.* 2016;374(14):1311–1320.

119. Luong C, Rey-Perra J, Vadivel A, et al. Antenatal sildenafil treatment attenuates pulmonary hypertension in experimental congenital diaphragmatic hernia. *Circulation.* 2011;123(19):2120–2131.

120. Oyston C, Stanley JL, Oliver MH, et al. Maternal administration of sildenafil citrate alters fetal and placental growth and fetal-placental vascular resistance in the growth-restricted ovine fetus. *Hypertension.* 2016;68(3):760–767.

121. Derderian SC, Jayme CM, Cheng LS, et al. Mass effect alone may not explain pulmonary vascular pathology in severe congenital diaphragmatic hernia. *Fetal Diagn Ther.* 2016;39(2):117–1124.

122. Tajchman UW, Tuder RM, Horan M, et al. Persistent eNOS in lung hypoplasia caused by left pulmonary artery ligation in the ovine fetus. *Am J Physiol.* 1997;272(5 Pt 1):L969–L978.

123. Gien J, Kinsella JP. Management of pulmonary hypertension in infants with congenital diaphragmatic hernia. *J Perinatol.* 2016;36(suppl 2):S28–S31.

124. Pierro M, Thebaud B. Understanding and treating pulmonary hypertension in congenital diaphragmatic hernia. *Semin Fetal Neonatal Med.* 2014;19(6):357–363.

125. Altit G, Bhombal S, Van Meurs KP, et al. Ventricular performance is associated with need for ECMO in newborns with CDH. *J Pediatr.* 2017; in press.

126. Galambos C, Sims-Lucas S, Ali N, et al. Intrapulmonary vascular shunt pathways in alveolar capillary dysplasia with misalignment of pulmonary veins. *Thorax.* 2015;70(1):84–85.

127. Towe CT, White FV, Grady RM, et al. Clinical and histopathologic characterization of infants with atypical presentations of alveolar capillary dysplasia with misalignment of the pulmonary veins who underwent bilateral lung transplantation. *J Pediatr.* 2017; in press.

128. Stankiewicz P, Sen P, Bhatt SS, et al. Genomic and genic deletions of the FOX gene cluster on 16q24.1 and inactivating mutations of FOXF1 cause alveolar capillary dysplasia and other malformations. *Am J Hum Genet.* 2009;84(6):780–791.

129. Lapointe A, Barrington KJ. Pulmonary hypertension and the asphyxiated newborn. *J Pediatr.* 2011;158(suppl 2):e19–e24.

130. Rudolph AM, Yuan S. Response of the pulmonary vasculature to hypoxia and H+ ion concentration changes. *J Clin Invest.* 1966;45(3):399–411.

131. Cornish JD, Dreyer GL, Snyder GE, et al. Failure of acute perinatal asphyxia or meconium aspiration to produce persistent pulmonary hypertension in a neonatal baboon model. *Am J Obstet Gynecol.* 1994;171(1):43–49.

132. Toubas PL, Hof RP, Heymann MA, et al. Effects of hypothermia and rewarming on the neonatal circulation. *Arch Fr Pediatr.* 1978;35(suppl 10):84–92.

133. Thoresen M. Hypothermia after perinatal asphyxia: selection for treatment and cooling protocol. *J Pediatr.* 2011;158(suppl 2):e45–e49.

134. Mourani PM, Sontag MK, Younoszai A, et al. Early pulmonary vascular disease in preterm infants at risk for bronchopulmonary dysplasia. *Am J Respir Crit Care Med.* 2015;191(1):87–95.

135. Wagner BD, Babinec AE, Carpenter C, et al. Proteomic profiles associated with early echocardiogram evidence of pulmonary vascular disease in preterm infants. *Am J Respir Crit Care Med.* 2017.

136. Mahgoub L, Kaddoura T, Kameny AR, et al. Pulmonary vein stenosis of ex-premature infants with pulmonary hypertension and bronchopulmonary dysplasia, epidemiology, and survival from a multicenter cohort. *Pediatr Pulmonol.* 2017;52(8):1063–1070.

137. Heching HJ, Turner M, Farkouh-Karoleski C, et al. Pulmonary vein stenosis and necrotising enterocolitis: is there a possible link with necrotising enterocolitis? *Arch Dis Child Fetal Neonatal Ed.* 2014;99(4):F282–F285.

138. Wedgwood S, Lakshminrusimha S, Schumacker PT, et al. Hypoxia inducible factor signaling and experimental persistent pulmonary hypertension of the newborn. *Front Pharmacol.* 2015;6:47.

139. Lakshminrusimha S, Swartz DD, Gugino SF, et al. Oxygen concentration and pulmonary hemodynamics in newborn lambs with pulmonary hypertension. *Pediatr Res.* 2009;66(5):539–544.

140. Fike CD, Dikalova A, Kaplowitz MR, et al. Rescue treatment with L-citrulline inhibits hypoxia-induced pulmonary hypertension in newborn pigs. *Am J Respir Cell Mol Biol.* 2015;53(2):255–264.

141. Lakshminrusimha S, Russell JA, Steinhorn RH, et al. Pulmonary hemodynamics in neonatal lambs resuscitated with 21%, 50%, and 100% oxygen. *Pediatr Res.* 2007;62(3):313–318.

142. Lakshminrusimha S, Steinhorn RH, Wedgwood S, et al. Pulmonary hemodynamics and vascular reactivity in asphyxiated term lambs resuscitated with 21 and 100% oxygen. *J Appl Physiol (1985).* 2011;111(5):1441–1447.

143. Auten RL, Davis JM. Oxygen toxicity and reactive oxygen species: the devil is in the details. *Pediatr Res.* 2009;66(2):121–127.

144. Brennan LA, Steinhorn RH, Wedgwood S, et al. Increased superoxide generation is associated with pulmonary hypertension in fetal lambs: a role for NADPH oxidase. *Circ Res*. 2003;92(6):683–691.

145. Konduri GG, Bakhutashvili I, Eis A, et al. Oxidant stress from uncoupled nitric oxide synthase impairs vasodilation in fetal lambs with persistent pulmonary hypertension. *Am J Physiol Heart Circ Physiol*. 2007;292(4):H1812–H1820.

146. Faraci FM, Didion SP. Vascular protection: superoxide dismutase isoforms in the vessel wall. *Arterioscler Thromb Vasc Biol*. 2004;24(8):1367–1373.

147. Farrow KN, Lakshminrusimha S, Reda WJ, et al. Superoxide dismutase restores eNOS expression and function in resistance pulmonary arteries from neonatal lambs with persistent pulmonary hypertension. *Am J Physiol Lung Cell Mol Physiol*. 2008;295(6):L979–L987.

148. Saugstad OD. Oxygen and oxidative stress in bronchopulmonary dysplasia. *J Perinat Med*. 2010;38(6):571–577.

149. Lee KJ, Berkelhamer SK, Kim GA, et al. Disrupted pulmonary artery cyclic guanosine monophosphate signaling in mice with hyperoxia-induced pulmonary hypertension. *Am J Respir Cell Mol Biol*. 2014;50(2):369–378.

150. Grover TR, Asikainen TM, Kinsella JP, et al. Hypoxia-inducible factors HIF-1alpha and HIF-2alpha are decreased in an experimental model of severe respiratory distress syndrome in preterm lambs. *Am J Physiol Lung Cell Mol Physiol*. 2007;292(6):L1345–L1351.

151. Wedgwood S, Warford C, Agvateesiri SC, et al. Postnatal growth restriction augments oxygen-induced pulmonary hypertension in a neonatal rat model of bronchopulmonary dysplasia. *Pediatr Res*. 2016;80(6):894–902.

152. Busch CJ, Graveline AR, Jiramongkolchai K, et al. Phosphodiesterase 3A expression is modulated by nitric oxide in rat pulmonary artery smooth muscle cells. *J Physiol Pharmacol*. 2010;61(6):663–669.

153. Chen B, Lakshminrusimha S, Czech L, et al. Regulation of phosphodiesterase 3 in the pulmonary arteries during the perinatal period in sheep. *Pediatr Res*. 2009.

3

CHAPTER 4

The "-Omics" of the New Bronchopulmonary Dysplasia

Charitharth Vivek Lal, Namasivayam Ambalavanan, and Vineet Bhandari

4

- Traditional biomarkers are not very useful in bronchopulmonary dysplasia (BPD) as the pathogenesis of BPD is multifactorial and the clinical phenotype is variable.

- Novel systems biology–based "-omic" approaches (genomics, proteomics, metabolomics, and microbiomics) may help determine biomarkers associated with abnormal lung development in BPD.

- Identification of the genomic determinants of BPD has proven difficult, despite genomewide analyses of single-nucleotide polymorphisms and whole-exome sequencing as well as analyses of the epigenome, perhaps owing to clinical heterogeneity as well as differences in ancestry.

- Analyses of transcriptomic differences associated with BPD require evaluation of differences in messenger ribonucleic acid (RNA), microRNA, and long noncoding RNA, although changes observed in the peripheral blood may not necessarily reflect those in tracheal aspirates or lung tissue.

- Proteomic differences in the tracheal aspirate and urine have been found to be associated with gestational age at birth and severity of BPD.

- Metabolomic differences in the amniotic fluid and tracheal aspirates have been reported among infants who did or did not develop BPD. Metabolomic differences in exhaled breath condensates of long-term survivors of BPD, compared with healthy individuals, suggest persistence of metabolic abnormalities.

- All infants, whether born at term or extremely preterm, have a diverse airway microbiome at birth that is dysregulated (e.g., reduced lactobacilli) in infants who later develop BPD.

- Detailed data collection of clinical variables for improved disease phenotyping, in addition to careful determination of unbiased, specific, temporal, "-omic" biomarkers may be necessary for a personalized medicine approach to BPD.

Since the original description of bronchopulmonary dysplasia (BPD) in late preterm infants by Northway et al.,[1] advances in neonatal care have occurred[2] and BPD is now mostly seen in extremely premature infants.[3] Although the definition of BPD has evolved over the past few decades,[4–6] it remains an operational definition, with some functional indication of the actual magnitude of lung disease, but with limited correlation to the underlying structural or molecular cardiopulmonary pathophysiology. For example, severe BPD markedly differs from that of mild or moderate

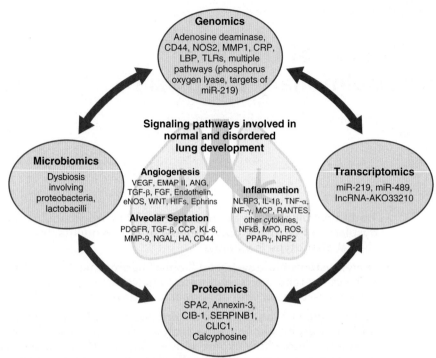

Fig. 4.1 The -omics of the new bronchopulmonary dysplasia. The figure depicts various signaling pathways impli-cated in normal and disordered lung development, along with possible gen*omic*, transcript*omic*, prote*omic*, and microbi*omic* contributors. *ANG*, Angiopoietins; *CCP*, cyclic citrullinated peptide; *CIB 1*, calcium and integrin-binding protein 1; *CLIC1*, chloride intracellular channel protein 1; *CRP*, C-reactive protein; *EMAP II*, endothelial monocyte-activating peptide; *eNOS*, endothelial nitric oxide synthase; *FGF*, fibroblast growth factor; *HA*, hyaluronic acid; *HIFs*, hypoxia-inducible factors; *IFN-γ*, interferon gamma; *IL-1β*, interleukin 1 beta; *KL-6*, Krebs von den Lungen-6; *LBP*, lipopolysaccharide-binding protein; *lncRNA*, long noncoding RNA; *MCP*, monocyte chemoattractant protein; *miR*, microRNA; *MMP1*, matrix metallopeptidase 1; *MPO*, myeloperoxidase; *NF-κB*, nuclear factor kappa B; *NGAL*, neu-trophil gelatinase-associated lipocalin; *NLRP3*, NLR family pyrin domain containing 3; *NOS2*, nitric oxide synthase; *NRF2*, nuclear factor erythroid 2 (NF-E2) related factor 2; *PDGFR*, platelet-derived growth factor receptor; *PPARγ*, peroxisome proliferator-activated receptor-gamma; *RANTES*, regulated on activation; normal T-cell expressed and secreted; *ROS*, reactive oxygen species; *SERPINB1*, leukocyte elastase inhibitor; *SPA2*, surfactant protein A2; *TGF-β*, transforming growth factor beta; *TLRs*, toll-like receptors; *TNF-α*, tumor necrosis factor alpha; *VEGF*, vascular endo-thelial growth factor.

disease, both in terms of clinical phenotype as well as in terms of genetic predis-position, rather than just being on the extreme end of the spectrum of the clinical operational definition.[7,8]

A focus on specific genes, proteins, or metabolites does not necessarily enable a deeper understanding of the "holistic" nature of normal lung development in which many different cell types have specific patterns of expression and regulation of mul-tiple genes, proteins, and metabolites, nor does it indicate how these processes are impaired during BPD. The use of newer systems biology approaches is warranted, as they allow an understanding of the phenotypes (the type of "forest") emerging from various components (trees, and so on) and interactions (of the biological community with the environment) that constitute the (eco)system.[9] This chapter discusses the various new "-omic" system biology approaches that may be available in the future for evaluating the diagnosis, prognosis, and treatment responses of BPD (Fig. 4.1).

-Omics of Disease Processes

Newer technologies have facilitated the gathering of large data sets, often through high-throughput assays, with subsequent analyses of these data sets through bio-informatic methods. In these studies, the researcher obtains a very highly detailed dataset of the changes that occur in response to a defined perturbation, such as the induction of a normal or diseased state. These large-scale data sets on the genome, proteome, metabolome, microbiome, and so forth are often referred to as -omic data sets.[9] An advantage of these technologies is that they can be used with samples (blood, tracheal aspirates [TA], urine, and so on) that can be collected using minimally invasive or noninvasive methods, which enables serial sampling for longitudinal analyses for evaluation of normal or abnormal growth and development. The analytical approaches involved are not driven by any a priori hypotheses, thus permitting unbiased -omic pattern characteristics of a given pathologic condition to be identified, followed by recognition of potential targets in the disease profile, and eventually to formulate hypothesis for diagnostics or therapy development. We have described the utility of these newer -omic methods in relation to BPD in some of our previous publications.[10–12] A better understanding of the -omic data related to BPD may provide insight not only into the predisposition to BPD (e.g., from genomic data) but also into the pathogenesis of disease (e.g., gene expression, proteomic, or metabolomic data from TA, blood, or lung tissue from individuals with and without BPD), and prediction of therapeutic response (e.g., change in -omic biomarkers with initiation of specific therapies).

Genomics

Advances in the understanding of the human genome sequence and the large-scale generation of data sets have added a new dimension to biomedical research. The role of genetics in BPD was initially proposed by Parker et al.,[13] who found a high concordance in 108 twin pairs with birth weights less than 1500 g. This first study confirming and quantifying the genetic contribution to BPD[13] has been independently ratified.[14] We recently published a detailed review summarizing the studies on genetic predisposition to BPD.[11] Genomic variants predisposing to BPD may be single-nucleotide polymorphisms (SNPs), which may increase susceptibility to the disease. Hadchouel et al.[14] conducted a genome-wide analysis and identified *SPOCK2* as a new possible candidate susceptibility gene for BPD, but this target was not confirmed in a recent study by Wang et al.[15] or Ambalavanan et al.[7] Multivariate logistic regression showed that the polymorphism vascular endothelial growth factor (VEGF)-634G>C allele was an independent risk factor for BPD in a Japanese cohort of infants.[16] However, polymorphisms in the VEGF and VEGF receptor 2 (VEGFR2) genes have not been consistently associated with BPD in other populations.[17]

Because single-marker approaches might not explain more than a small fraction of heritability of BPD, an integrated genomic analysis was recently conducted by the Eunice Kennedy Shriver National Institutes of Child Health and Human Development Neonatal Research Network (NICHD NRN).[18] Using a DNA repository of extremely low-birth-weight infants, a genome-wide scan was conducted of 1.2 million genotyped SNPs and an additional 7 million imputed SNPs followed by genome-wide association and gene set analysis for BPD or death, severe BPD or death, and severe BPD in survivors. Known pathways of lung development and repair (the cell-surface glycoprotein CD44, phosphorus oxygen lyase activity) and novel molecules and pathways (adenosine deaminase, targets of micro–ribonucleic acid [RNA; miR-219] were found to be involved in the genetic predisposition to BPD. The racial and ethnic differences found in the pathways involved in BPD further highlighted the underlying genetic predisposition of the disease. Other studies using gene expression profiling, such as those by Bhattacharya et al.[19] and Pietrzyk et al.[20] also identified different pathways associated with the genetic origins of BPD. In a recent study, whole-exome sequencing was performed to identify uncommon variants in patients with BPD.[21] The top candidate genes highlighted in this study were nitric oxide synthase 2, matrix metalloproteinase 1, C-reactive protein, lipopolysaccharide-binding protein, and the toll-like receptor family. In another study, authors performed exome sequencing on 50 BPD-affected and unaffected twin pairs using DNA isolated from neonatal blood spots and identified genes affected by extremely rare nonsynonymous mutations.[22] The genes identified were highly enriched for processes involved in pulmonary structure and function, including collagen fibril organization, morphogenesis of embryonic epithelium, and regulation of the *Wnt* signaling pathway.

In addition to the genome, major epigenetic mechanisms such as DNA methylation may regulate coordinated temporal expression of multiple genes during lung development. Cuna et al.[23] recently conducted a study to identify genes regulated by methylation during normal septation in mice and during disordered septation in BPD. Microarray analysis of gene expression and immunoprecipitation of methylated DNA followed by sequencing was done in mouse lungs, and microarray gene expression data were integrated with genome-wide DNA methylation data from human lungs (BPD vs. preterm or term lung). The authors found that changes in methylation corresponded to altered expression of several genes associated with lung development, suggesting that DNA methylation of these genes may regulate normal and abnormal alveolar septation. Genes known to be important in lung development (*Wnt* signaling, *Angpt2*, *Sox9*, and so on) and its extracellular matrix (*Tnc*, *Eln*, and so on), and genes involved with immune and antioxidant defense (*Stat4*, *Sod3*, *Prdx6*, and so on) were observed to be differentially methylated in mice. In humans, genes including detoxifying enzymes (*Gstm3*) and transforming growth factor beta signaling (bone morphogenetic protein 7 [*Bmp7*]) were differentially methylated with reciprocal changes in expression in BPD compared with preterm or term lung. Significant overlap in genes methylated during mouse and human lung development and with development of BPD strongly suggests the role of DNA methylation in normal and abnormal alveolar septation.[23]

It still remains to be ascertained how different patient characteristics and clinical practices modulate the genetic or epigenetic influences on BPD across different populations. More multicenter human studies are needed to account for clinical heterogeneity, as well as center differences in the incidence of BPD.

Transcriptomics

Transcriptomics is the study of the transcriptome, the complete set of RNA transcripts produced by the genome, using high-throughput methods. High-throughput transcriptomics became possible with microarrays, which are particularly useful for analyzing large mammalian transcriptomes, but they detect only known sequences included on the array. In recent years, RNA sequencing methods have been developed that can evaluate protein-coding mRNA, long noncoding RNA (lncRNA), transcripts of pseudogenes, and miRNA. Bhattacharya et al.[24] conducted an RNA sequencing study using the rodent model of BPD in which expression patterns for selected genes were validated by quantitative polymerase chain reaction followed by mechanistic testing. In this study, the canonical pathways dysregulated in hyperoxia included nuclear factor (erythryoid-derived 2)-like 2 (Nrf2)-mediated oxidative stress signaling, p53 signaling, endothelial nitric oxide synthase signaling, and aryl hydrocarbon receptor (Ahr) pathways. Further cluster analysis identified cyclin D1, cyclin-dependent kinase inhibitor 1A, and Ahr as critical regulatory nodes in the response to hyperoxia, with Ahr serving as the major effector node. Other investigators have used hyperoxia-exposed Nrf2-null mutant newborn mice, along with transcriptomic analyses, to identify the effector molecules of lung injury.[25] Salaets et al.[26] conducted RNA sequencing of preterm rabbit lungs after 7 days of hyperoxia exposure and identified changes in inflammatory, oxidative stress, and lung developmental pathways. In a recent study using human lung tissue, Kho et al.[27] analyzed whole-lung transcriptome profiles of 61 females and 78 males at 54 to 127 days after conception from nonsmoking mothers, using unsupervised principal component analysis and supervised linear regression models. This study using banked human fetal lung tissue found postmenstrual age to be a more dominant factor than sex on the effects of early fetal lung development or disease risk. A limitation of this study was the inability to adjust for differences in race and potential confounders such as in utero exposures owing to limited availability of phenotypic information.

Recently investigators, using a model of mouse lung injury that mimicked human BPD, noted that 882 lncRNAs were upregulated and 887 lncRNAs were downregulated in BPD lung tissues. Further analyses revealed that a downregulated lncRNA—namely, AK033210—associated with tenascin C may be involved in the pathogenesis of BPD.[28]

MicroRNAs have been seen to be dysregulated in multiple disorders and are now being studied in lung biology.[29,30] Several miRs have been shown to play a role in branching morphogenesis, a key step in early lung development.[31] The current evidence of the role of miRs in late lung development and BPD has been summarized by Nardiello and Morty.[31] We recently highlighted the role of miR-489 in guiding alveolar septation by modulation of its target genes insulin-like growth factor and tenascin C.[32] As mentioned earlier, in the integrated genomic analyses conducted by the NICHD NRN, the pathway with the lowest false discovery rate for BPD/death was the one targeting miR-219. Efforts are needed to develop sophisticated computational methods for the integration of microRNA, microRNA targets, transcription factors, and other important components of the transcriptome into biologically relevant networks, in the context of BPD.

Proteomics

Proteomics is the large-scale study of the structure and function of various proteins of a cell or organism. Several individual proteins have been implicated in the pathogenesis of BPD and are described in detail in our previous publications,[12,33] although studies using unbiased proteomic analysis for BPD are lacking to date. Some enzyme-linked immunosorbent assay–based approaches have been applied to the study of pediatric respiratory diseases[34] but not for BPD. Proteomic analysis may help define the networks of proteins that provide a real-time status of disease state and modulation of protein function.[35] In the first such pulmonary study in preterm infants, Magagnotti et al.[36] conducted proteomic analysis of TA fluids from infants with BPD and controls using mass spectroscopy. The results were further validated by Western blotting. The authors found a clear differential expression in the proteome of the 23- to 25-week group and the 26- to 29-week group. Surfactant protein A2 (↑), annexin 3 (↑), calcium and integrin-binding protein 1 (↓), leukocyte elastase inhibitor (↓), chloride intracellular channel protein 1 (↓) and calcyphosine (↓) were differentially expressed in patients with severe BPD who were of lower gestational age (23- to 25-weeks' gestation). After adjusting for severity of disease, calcyphosine, calcium and integrin-binding protein-1, and chloride intracellular channel protein 1 were found to differentiate between mild and severe BPD; annexin 3 was found to be more related to development. A limitation of this study was the small sample size and marked heterogeneity in the clinical phenotype of the patients.

Analyzing TA fluid for proteomics analysis is hampered by the limitation of defining an appropriate control. Serum sample analysis is considered low risk, making it ideal for biomarker discovery studies; however, changes within serum are often very small, and moreover, pinpointing changes specific to the lung can be difficult. Hence despite the limitations, TA fluids are probably the best option available to analyze local effects in the lungs of mechanically ventilated preterm infants.[12] Because many preterm infants are managed with noninvasive support, such as continuous positive airway pressure or oxygen supplementation by nasal cannula, evaluation of TA in these infants is not possible. However, infants who do not require mechanical ventilation may generally be considered to be at lower risk of BPD or death. Urine proteomic analysis has been used to discover novel biomarkers for BPD.[37] In a recent study, after controlling for specific clinical variables (gestational age, small-for-gestational age, and intubation status), a novel biomarker clusterin was found to be independently predictive of BPD/mortality.[37] Clusterin is a ubiquitously expressed protein and potential sensor of oxidative stress and is known to be associated with lung function in patients with asthma.

Metabolomics

Metabolomics is an emerging -omics science involving the comprehensive characterization of metabolites and metabolism in biologic systems.[38] It includes analysis of low-molecular-weight metabolites created by cellular metabolic pathways through the use of mass spectrometry or nuclear magnetic resonance spectroscopy. Extremely preterm infants are very different from other patient populations from a developmental standpoint and may have a markedly different metabolic signature in different organ systems even at baseline. In addition, factors such as oxygen exposure, mechanical ventilation, diet, drugs, antibiotics, resident microbiome, and so on, may further alter the metabolic profiles and hence affect disease pathogenesis. Recently Baraldi et al.[39] performed metabolic profiling of amniotic fluid (AF) in women with symptoms of preterm labor to predict the risk of spontaneous preterm birth and BPD development in the offspring. Twenty-four of the 32 AF samples were obtained from transabdominal amniocentesis; the other 8 were obtained by amniocentesis at the time of cesarean delivery. In this study, the AF from mothers in the preterm delivery group with BPD showed higher levels of leucinic acid, hydroxy fatty acids (putative metabolite: 4-hydroxy-3-methylbenzoic acid and 2-hydroxy caprylic acid), oxy fatty acids (putative metabolite: 3-oxododecanoic acid), and a metabolite ascribable to a sulfated steroid. The group without BPD was characterized by higher levels of S-adenosylmethionine and amino acid chains and 3b,16a-dihydroxyandrostenone sulfate compared with the BPD group. This study suggests that the onset of BPD may be associated with a perturbed AF metabolic pattern during intrauterine life. Although the authors performed internal cross-validation, the absence of external validation and small sample size were limitations of this study.

Organic volatile metabolites may also be detected by portable devices such as electronic noses.[40] In a recent study by Rogosch et al.,[41] the smellprints of volatile organic compounds measured with an electronic nose (Cyranose 320; Smiths Detection Group Ltd, Watford, United Kingdom) differed between TA from preterm infants with or without subsequent development of BPD.[41] In a study of adolescents, Carraro et al.[42] found that the metabolomic analysis of exhaled breath condensates distinguishes children who have had BPD from healthy individuals, suggesting that the lungs of survivors of BPD are characterized by long-term metabolic abnormalities. These studies emphasize the importance of conducting longitudinal studies to monitor changes in the airway metabolome among premature infants. Systems biology approaches identifying complex metabolomic dysregulation in the setting of multifactorial diseases such as BPD provide a unique opportunity to develop new diagnostic or therapeutic strategies as the metabolites may serve as a biomarker of, or mediate, lung function.

Microbiomics

It has been speculated that the development of BPD is mediated, at least in part, by inflammation secondary to airway infections,[43–46] but the direction of causality between airway injury or protection and respiratory colonization with microorganisms remains unsettled. High-throughput sequencing of 16S ribosomal RNA gene generated from bacteria-containing samples yields a large number of short sequences that can be subsequently aligned and sorted according to a predefined level of homology. These can then be classified according to publicly available taxonomic databases to provide a comprehensive view of the "microbiome."[47,48] The study of the human lung microbiome is still in its nascent phases,[49] and until recently there were no studies relating the neonatal pulmonary microbiome to BPD. Data from lung diseases indicate that airways and lungs harbor a commensal microbiota, which induce activation of an inflammatory response.[50–52] Historically, the fetus and fetal lungs were considered sterile, but we have recently discovered that the airways of infants at birth harbor a distinct microbial signature.[53] In this study, 16S sequencing microbiome analysis was conducted on TA obtained from preterm and term intubated infants at birth or shortly thereafter, longitudinally, and after the diagnosis of severe BPD. The airways of infants with BPD showed increased abundance of *Proteobacteria* and decreased *Lactobacillus*. Serial longitudinal sampling in preterm infants in whom severe BDP developed showed a temporal dysbiosis, with an increase in *Proteobacteria* and decrease in *Lactobacillus* on the way to development of severe BPD at 36 weeks postmenstrual age. In addition, an early microbial dysbiosis—decreased *Lactobacillus* at birth—was predictive for the development of severe BPD. In the past, Lohmann et al.[54] demonstrated that reduced diversity of the microbiome may be an associated factor in the development of BPD. In a study that included 10 infants, Abman et al.[55] used 16S techniques to demonstrate that early bacterial colonization with diverse species is present in the airways of intubated preterm infants and can be characterized by bacterial load and species diversity.[55] Genus *Lactobacillus* has been known to have strong antiinflammatory properties[56–58] and has been shown to regulate alveolar development in animal models.[59] Hence, favorable bacteria inoculation as "respiratory probiotics" may be further studied as a potential therapeutic strategy for BPD and other pulmonary disorders. The early airway microbiome may prime the developing pulmonary immune system, thus setting the stage and predisposing to subsequent pulmonary disease.

Economics

The emergence of personalized medicine for the preterm population using these -omic technologies may be the future of neonatal medicine, but they may still not take place as quickly as the scientific community may hope. Systems biology research requires investments in infrastructure with cutting-edge -omics facilities and analytical tools, advanced high computing and storage resources, and highly qualified multidisciplinary teams of clinicians, epidemiologists, and bioinformatics specialists. In addition, investments in security and privacy are needed. Thus the expense of operating research centers that use -omic analyses to design diagnostics and therapeutics is substantial and may remain so for many years to come.[60] Hence larger collaborative studies and industry involvement in multicenter consortia to assess -omic variables in the context of research as well as practice are needed. Once the field is more mature and -omic variables that are useful biomarkers have been identified, it is possible that commercialization of "lab-on-a-chip" techniques may enable these biomarkers to be identified at the bedside, rapidly, and at much lower cost.

Conclusion

More detailed data collection of clinical variables for improved disease phenotyping, in addition to careful determination of unbiased, specific, temporal, -omic biomarkers, are necessary for BPD prediction and management.[61,62] With the discovery of the presence and role of the neonatal airway microbiome in BPD,[53] the study of environmental pathogens and host responses is required, in addition to strategies evaluating genomic, proteomic, and metabolomics data. The economics of these technologies will decide the pace of making personalized medicine accessible to the preterm neonate at risk of developing BPD.

Acknowledgments

Supported in part by funding from the National Institutes of Health (NIH) (grant numbers U01 HL122626; R01 HD067126; R01 HD066982; and U10 HD34216).

REFERENCES

1. Northway WH Jr, Rosan RC, Porter DY. Pulmonary disease following respirator therapy of hyaline-membrane disease. Bronchopulmonary dysplasia. *N Eng J Med.* 1967;276(7):357–368.
2. Jobe AJ. The new BPD: an arrest of lung development. *Pediatr Res.* 1999;46(6):641–643.
3. Rojas MA, Gonzalez A, Bancalari E, Claure N, Poole C, Silva-Neto G. Changing trends in the epidemiology and pathogenesis of neonatal chronic lung disease. *J Pediatr.* 1995;126(4):605–610.
4. Bancalari E, Abdenour GE, Feller R, Gannon J. Bronchopulmonary dysplasia: clinical presentation. *J Pediatr.* 1979;95(5 Pt 2):819–823.
5. Jobe AH, Bancalari E. Bronchopulmonary dysplasia. *Am J Respir Crit Care Med.* 2001;163(7): 1723–1729.
6. Walsh MC, Yao Q, Gettner P, et al. Impact of a physiologic definition on bronchopulmonary dysplasia rates. *Pediatrics.* 2004;114(5):1305–1311.
7. Ambalavanan N, Cotten CM, Page GP, et al. Integrated genomic analyses in bronchopulmonary dysplasia. *J Pediatr.* 2015;166(3):531–537.e13.
8. Day CL, Ryan RM. Bronchopulmonary dysplasia: new becomes old again! *Pediatr Res.* 2016.
9. Sobie EA, Lee YS, Jenkins SL, Iyengar R. Systems biology–biomedical modeling. *Sci Signal.* 2011;4(190):tr2.

10. Piersigilli F, Bhandari V. Biomarkers in neonatology: the new "omics" of bronchopulmonary dysplasia. *J Maternal-Fetal Neonatal Med.* 2016;29(11):1758–1764.

11. Lal CV, Ambalavanan N. Genetic predisposition to bronchopulmonary dysplasia. *Semin Perinatol.* 2015;39(8):584–591.

12. Lal CV, Ambalavanan N. Biomarkers, early diagnosis, and clinical predictors of bronchopulmonary dysplasia. *Clin Perinatol.* 2015;42(4):739–754.

13. Parker RA, Lindstrom DP, Cotton RB. Evidence from twin study implies possible genetic susceptibility to bronchopulmonary dysplasia. *Semin Perinatol.* 1996;20(3):206–219.

14. Hadchouel A, Durrmeyer X, Bouzigon E, et al. Identification of SPOCK2 as a susceptibility gene for bronchopulmonary dysplasia. *Am J Respir Crit Care Med.* 2011;184(10):1164–1170.

15. Wang H, St Julien KR, Stevenson DK, et al. A genome-wide association study (GWAS) for bronchopulmonary dysplasia. *Pediatrics.* 2013;132(2):290–297.

16. Fujioka K, Shibata A, Yokota T, et al. Association of a vascular endothelial growth factor polymorphism with the development of bronchopulmonary dysplasia in Japanese premature newborns. *Sci Rep.* 2014;4(4459).

17. Mahlman M, Huusko JM, Karjalainen MK, et al. Genes encoding vascular endothelial growth factor A (VEGF-A) and VEGF receptor 2 (VEGFR-2) and risk for bronchopulmonary dysplasia. *Neonatology.* 2015;108(1):53–59.

18. Ambalavanan N, Cotten CM, Page GP, et al. Integrated genomic analyses in bronchopulmonary dysplasia. *J Pediatr.* 2014.

19. Bhattacharya S, Go D, Krenitsky DL, et al. Genome-wide transcriptional profiling reveals connective tissue mast cell accumulation in bronchopulmonary dysplasia. *Am J Respir Crit Care Med.* 2012;186(4):349–358.

20. Pietrzyk JJ, Kwinta P, Wollen EJ, et al. Gene expression profiling in preterm infants: new aspects of bronchopulmonary dysplasia development. *PLoS One.* 2013;8(10):e78585.

21. Carrera P, Di Resta C, Volonteri C, et al. Exome sequencing and pathway analysis for identification of genetic variability relevant for bronchopulmonary dysplasia (BPD) in preterm newborns: a pilot study. *Clin Chim Acta.* 2015;451(Pt A):39–45.

22. Li J, Yu KH, Oehlert J, et al. Exome sequencing of neonatal blood spots and the identification of genes implicated in bronchopulmonary dysplasia. *Am J Respir Crit Care Med.* 2015;192(5):589–596.

23. Cuna A, Halloran B, Faye-Petersen O, et al. Alterations in gene expression and DNA methylation during murine and human lung alveolar septation. *Am J Respir Cell Mol Biol.* 2015;53(1):60–73.

24. Bhattacharya S, Zhou Z, Yee M, et al. The genome-wide transcriptional response to neonatal hyperoxia identifies Ahr as a key regulator. *Am J Physiol Lung Cell Mol Physiol.* 2014;307(7):L516–L523.

25. Cho HY, van Houten B, Wang X, et al. Targeted deletion of nrf2 impairs lung development and oxidant injury in neonatal mice. *Antioxid Redox Signal.* 2012;17(8):1066–1082.

26. Salaets T, Richter J, Brady P, et al. Transcriptome analysis of the preterm rabbit lung after seven days of hyperoxic exposure. *PloS one.* 2015;10(8):e0136569.

27. Kho AT, Chhabra D, Sharma S, et al. Age, sexual dimorphism, and disease associations in the developing human fetal lung transcriptome. *Am J Respir Cell Mol Biol.* 2016;54(6):814–821.

28. Bao TP, Wu R, Cheng HP, Cui XW, Tian ZF. Differential expression of long non-coding RNAs in hyperoxia-induced bronchopulmonary dysplasia. *Cell Biochem Funct.* 2016;34(5):299–309.

29. Stoll BJ, Hansen NI, Bell EF, et al. Neonatal outcomes of extremely preterm infants from the NICHD Neonatal Research Network. *Pediatrics.* 2010;126(3):443–456.

30. Yoder BA, Harrison M, Clark RH. Time-related changes in steroid use and bronchopulmonary dysplasia in preterm infants. *Pediatrics.* 2009;124(2):673–679.

31. Nardiello C, Morty RE. MicroRNA in late lung development and bronchopulmonary dysplasia: the need to demonstrate causality. *Mol Cell Pediatr.* 2016;3(1):19.

32. Olave N, Lal CV, Halloran B, et al. Regulation of alveolar septation by microRNA-489. *Am J Physiol Lung Cell Mol Physiol.* 2016;310(5):L476–L487.

33. Lal CV, Schwarz MA. Vascular mediators in chronic lung disease of infancy: role of endothelial monocyte activating polypeptide II (EMAP II). *Birth Defects Res A, Clin Mol Teratol.* 2014;100(3):180–188.

34. Pereira-Fantini PM, Tingay DG. The proteomics of lung injury in childhood: challenges and opportunities. *Clin Proteomics.* 2016;13(5).

35. Hamvas A, Deterding R, Balch WE, et al. Diffuse lung disease in children: summary of a scientific conference. *Pediatr Pulmonol.* 2014;49(4):400–409.

36. Magagnotti C, Matassa PG, Bachi A, et al. Calcium signaling-related proteins are associated with broncho-pulmonary dysplasia progression. *J Proteomics.* 2013;94:401–412.

37. Balena-Borneman J, Ambalavanan N, Tiwari HK, Griffin RL, Halloran B, Askenazi D. Biomarkers associated with bronchopulmonary dysplasia/mortality in premature infants. *Pediatr Res.* 2016.

38. Wishart DS. Emerging applications of metabolomics in drug discovery and precision medicine. *Nat Rev Drug Discov.* 2016;15(7):473–484.

39. Baraldi E, Giordano G, Stocchero M, et al. Untargeted metabolomic analysis of amniotic fluid in the prediction of preterm delivery and bronchopulmonary dysplasia. *PloS one.* 2016;11(10):e0164211.

40. Shaw JG, Vaughan A, Dent AG, et al. Biomarkers of progression of chronic obstructive pulmonary disease (COPD). *J Thorac Dis.* 2014;6(11):1532–1547.

41. Rogosch T, Herrmann N, Maier RF, et al. Detection of bloodstream infections and prediction of bronchopulmonary dysplasia in preterm neonates with an electronic nose. *J Pediatr.* 2014;165(3):622–624.

42. Carraro S, Giordano G, Pirillo P, et al. Airway metabolic anomalies in adolescents with bronchopulmonary dysplasia: new insights from the metabolomic approach. *J Pediatr.* 2015;166(2):234–239.e1.

43. D'Angio CT, Basavegowda K, Avissar NE, Finkelstein JN, Sinkin RA. Comparison of tracheal aspirate and bronchoalveolar lavage specimens from premature infants. *Biol Neonate*. 2002;82(3):145–149.

44. Ramsay PL, DeMayo FJ, Hegemier SE, Wearden ME, Smith CV, Welty SE. Clara cell secretory protein oxidation and expression in premature infants who develop bronchopulmonary dysplasia. *Am J Respir Crit Care Med*. 2001;164(1):155–161.

45. Watterberg KL, Demers LM, Scott SM, Murphy S. Chorioamnionitis and early lung inflammation in infants in whom bronchopulmonary dysplasia develops. *Pediatrics*. 1996;97(2):210–215.

46. Viscardi RM, Muhumuza CK, Rodriguez A, et al. Inflammatory markers in intrauterine and fetal blood and cerebrospinal fluid compartments are associated with adverse pulmonary and neurologic outcomes in preterm infants. *Pediatr Res*. 2004;55(6):1009–10017.

47. Liu Z, DeSantis TZ, Andersen GL, Knight R. Accurate taxonomy assignments from 16S rRNA sequences produced by highly parallel pyrosequencers. *Nucleic Acids Res*. 2008;36(18):e120.

48. Schloss PD, Westcott SL, Ryabin T, et al. Introducing mothur: open-source, platform-independent, community-supported software for describing and comparing microbial communities. *Appl Environ Microbiol*. 2009;75(23):7537–7541.

49. Mu J, Pang Q, Guo YH, et al. Functional implications of microRNA-215 in TGF-beta1-induced phenotypic transition of mesangial cells by targeting CTNNBIP1. *PloS one*. 2013;8(3):e58622.

50. Rogers GB, Carroll MP, Serisier DJ, Hockey PM, Jones G, Bruce KD. Characterization of bacterial community diversity in cystic fibrosis lung infections by use of 16s ribosomal DNA terminal restriction fragment length polymorphism profiling. *J Clin Microbiol*. 2004;42(11):5176–5183.

51. Tunney MM, Field TR, Moriarty TF, et al. Detection of anaerobic bacteria in high numbers in sputum from patients with cystic fibrosis. *Am J Respir Crit Care Med*. 2008;177(9):995–1001.

52. Rogers GB, Zain NM, Bruce KD, et al. A novel microbiota stratification system predicts future exacerbations in bronchiectasis. *Ann Am Thorac Soc*. 2014;11(4):496–503.

53. Lal CV, Travers C, Aghai ZH, et al. The Airway microbiome at birth. *Scientific Rep*. 2016;6:31023.

54. Lohmann P, Luna RA, Hollister EB, et al. The airway microbiome of intubated premature infants: characteristics and changes that predict the development of bronchopulmonary dysplasia. *Pediatr Res*. 2014;76(3):294–301.

55. Mourani PM, Harris JK, Sontag MK, Robertson CE, Abman SH. Molecular identification of bacteria in tracheal aspirate fluid from mechanically ventilated preterm infants. *PloS One*. 2011;6(10):e25959.

56. Sagar S, Morgan ME, Chen S, et al. Bifidobacterium breve and Lactobacillus rhamnosus treatment is as effective as budesonide at reducing inflammation in a murine model for chronic asthma. *Respir Res*. 2014;15(46).

57. Simeoli R, Mattace Raso G, Lama A, et al. Preventive and therapeutic effects of Lactobacillus paracasei B21060-based synbiotic treatment on gut inflammation and barrier integrity in colitic mice. *J Nutr*. 2015;145(6):1202–1210.

58. Justino PF, Melo LF, Nogueira AF, et al. Regulatory role of Lactobacillus acidophilus on inflammation and gastric dysmotility in intestinal mucositis induced by 5-fluorouracil in mice. *Cancer Chemother Pharmacol*. 2015;75(3):559–567.

59. Yun Y, Srinivas G, Kuenzel S, et al. Environmentally determined differences in the murine lung microbiota and their relation to alveolar architecture. *PloS one*. 2014;9(12):e113466.

60. Tremblay-Servier M. Personalized medicine: the medicine of tomorrow. *Foreword Metabolism*. 2013;62(suppl 1):S1.

61. Hagood JS, Ambalavanan N. Systems biology of lung development and regeneration: current knowledge and recommendations for future research. *Wiley Interdiscip Rev Syst Biol Med*. 2013;5(2):125–133.

62. Sheppard D. Aspen Lung Conference 2010: systems biology of lung diseases—progress in the omics era. *Proc Am Thorac Soc*. 2011;8(2):199–202.

CHAPTER 5

Role of Microbiome in Lung Injury

Rose M. Viscardi and Namasivayam Ambalavanan

5

- Contrary to conventional teaching, culture-independent molecular techniques have confirmed that the healthy lung is not sterile, and the lung microbiome is likely established in early life and influences the development of immune responses and pulmonary function and is altered in disease states.

- Although the major pathway that microorganisms colonize the uterine cavity is vertical ascension from the vagina, there is emerging evidence suggesting transplacental transfer of microbiota as a route of infection.

- The airway microbiome of the newborn lung of term and preterm infants is similar in composition and diversity at birth, but the lung microbiome of infants with bronchopulmonary dysplasia (BPD) differs in composition and is less diverse compared with term and preterm infants without BPD.

- The genus *Lactobacillus* is decreased at birth in infants exposed to chorioamnionitis and in preterm infants in whom BPD develops.

- The mycoplasmas *Ureaplasma parvum* and *Ureaplasma urealyticum* are commensals in the genital tract, but have been associated with intrauterine infection, preterm birth, and adverse neonatal outcomes, including BPD. Current evidence indicates that these organisms modulate host immune responses.

In 1676, Antonie van Leeuwenhoek discovered bacteria.[1] Subsequently, work by Louis Pasteur and Robert Koch in the 19th century linked specific bacterial species to particular diseases. The development of Koch's postulates improved identification of the etiology of many infectious diseases and strengthened the approach to microbiologic diagnosis. However, it has become apparent that a reliance on culture prevents the identification of microbial species that are difficult to culture. It has been determined that only 1% of all bacteria can be cultured,[2] and many of the microbial species that normally (or abnormally) inhabit the human body are not identified by culture.

Joshua Lederberg coined the term "microbiome" to signify "the ecological community of commensal, symbiotic, and pathogenic microorganisms that literally share our body space."[3] The term "microbiota" refers specifically to the community of microorganisms living in a particular environment, while the microbiome refers to the communities of microorganisms and their encoded genes.[4] Microbial diversity measures how much variety exists in a microbial community and is characterized by richness (the number of different bacterial species present) and evenness (the relative abundance of the various species with the microbial community), while the term "dysbiosis" describes a microbial pattern associated with disease states.[5] Culture-independent molecular methods show that the microbiota of humans is far greater than previously recognized.[6] The Human Microbiome Project focused particularly on the normal microbiome of the skin, mouth, nose, digestive tract, and vagina[7] and found that even healthy individuals differ remarkably in the diversity and abundance of the microbiome at the different sites. The relative abundance of members of a microbiome are most often determined by sequencing of the variable regions (V1–3 or V4–6) of the bacterial 16S ribosomal ribonucleic acid (rRNA), but more extensive metagenomic and metatranscriptomic sequencing provide more in-depth data on microbial gene function and possible host interactions.[8]

Because of the relative inaccessibility of the lower airways and the lungs, there has been less research on the airway and pulmonary microbiome compared with the gastrointestinal or oral microbiome. Hilty et al.[9] found that lower airways are not sterile, with approximately 2000 bacterial genomes per square centimeter of surface sampled. They also found that the tracheobronchial tree contained a characteristic microbial flora that differs from the nares and oropharynx and between health and disease.[9,10] The major colonists in healthy people are anaerobes such as Bacteroidetes (e.g., *Prevotella* spp.) grown with difficulty in culture, while Proteobacteria (e.g., *Haemophilus, Moraxella, Neisseria* spp.) are strongly associated with airway disease in chronic obstructive pulmonary disease and asthma.[9] It is possible that microbial immigration from the oral cavity contributes to the lung microbiome during health, although the lungs selectively eliminate *Prevotella* bacteria derived from the upper airways.[10] In healthy lungs, spatial variation in microbiota within an individual is significantly less than variation across individuals, and bronchoalveolar lavage (BAL) of a single lung segment is probably acceptable for sampling the healthy lung microbiome.[11] A limitation of bronchoscopic sampling of the airways is the possible contamination from the oral or nasal flora.[12] However, direct sampling of lung tissue derived from nonmalignant lung tissue samples from patients with cancer determined that Proteobacteria is the dominant phylum and other common phyla include Firmicutes, Bacteroidetes, and Actinobacteria.[13] Microbiota taxonomic alpha diversity increased with environmental exposures to air particulates, residency in high-density population areas, and smoking pack-years.[13]

The newborn lung microbiome is even more technologically challenging to sample because available sampling is limited to intubated infants with upper airways sampled by tracheal aspirates of the endotracheal tube and distal airways sampled by tracheal lavage. Despite this significant limitation, some recent studies have evaluated the airway microbiome in preterm infants, specifically in relation to development of bronchopulmonary dysplasia (BPD). Mourani et al.[14] evaluated serial tracheal aspirates (at <72 hours, 7 days, 14 days, and 21 days) from 10 preterm infants who required mechanical ventilation for at least 21 days. Samples were analyzed by quantitative real-time polymerase chain-reaction (PCR) assays for total bacterial load and by pyrosequencing for bacterial identification. Seventy-two organisms were observed in total. Seven organisms represented the dominant organism (>50% of total sequences) in 31 of 32 samples with positive sequences. *Staphylococcus* and the genital mycoplasmas *Ureaplasma parvum* and *Ureaplasma urealyticum* were the most frequently identified dominant organisms, but *Pseudomonas, Enterococcus,* and *Escherichia* were also identified. Most infants in this series established either *Staphylococcus* spp. (Firmicutes) or *Ureaplasma* spp. (Tenericutes) as the predominant organism by 7 days of age. Lohmann et al.[15] evaluated tracheal aspirates of 25 preterm infants obtained at birth and on days 3, 7, and 28. Bacterial DNA was extracted, and 16S rRNA genes were amplified and sequenced. It was found that *Acinetobacter* was the predominant genus in the airways of all infants at birth. Infants in whom BPD later developed had reduced bacterial diversity at birth.

Recently we evaluated the airway microbiome of extremely preterm and term infants soon after birth and in preterm infants with established BPD.[16] Tracheal aspirates were collected from a discovery cohort of 23 extremely low-birth-weight (ELBW) infants and 10 full-term (FT) infants (with no respiratory disease) at birth or within 6 hours of birth at the time of intubation, as well as from 18 infants with established BPD in whom samples were obtained at 36 weeks postmenstrual age (PMA) at the time of endotracheal tube change. A validation cohort was used, consisting of tracheal aspirates from extremely preterm infants at a different institution. 16S rRNA sequencing was performed followed by bioinformatics analysis. We were

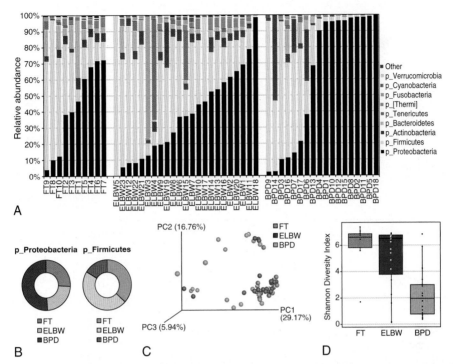

Fig. 5.1 Comparison of the lung microbiome of full-term *(FT)* infants at birth, extremely low-birth-weight infants *(ELBW)* infants at birth, and ELBW patients with established bronchopulmonary dysplasia *(BPD)*. A, Bar graph depicting the relative abundance of commonly encountered bacterial phyla between FT, ELBW, and BPD infants. B, Compared with newborn postmenstrual age–matched FT infants and ELBW infants, infants with BPD had increased Proteobacteria and decreased Firmicutes and Fusobacteria. C, Principal coordinates analysis plot (beta diversity) demonstrating unweighted UniFrac distance between samples with sample points colored for ELBW, FT, or BPD infants. Samples that are clustered closely together share a larger proportion of the phylogenetic tree comparison with samples that are more loosely separated. ELBW and FT infants have similar beta diversity, which is very different from the beta diversity of BPD infants. D, Shannon diversity index depicting decreased microbial alpha diversity in infants with BPD compared with FT and ELBW infants. (From Lal CV, Travers C, Aghai ZH, et al. The airway microbiome at birth. *Sci Rep.* 2016;6:31023.)

able to detect and characterize bacterial DNA in tracheal aspirates of all ELBW and FT infants soon after birth. The lung microbiome was similar at birth in ELBW and FT infants irrespective of gestational age. Both ELBW and FT infants had a predominance of Firmicutes and Proteobacteria on the first day of life, in addition to Actinobacteria, Bacteroidetes, Tenericutes, *Fusobacterium,* Cyanobacteria, and Verrucomicrobia (Fig. 5.1). The relative abundance of bacterial phyla and Shannon alpha diversity did not differ between ELBW and FT infants. Compared with FT newborns matched for PMA, the airway microbiome of infants after diagnosis of BPD was characterized by increased phylum Proteobacteria and decreased phyla Firmicutes and Fusobacteria (see Fig. 5.1). At the genus level, the most abundant Proteobacteria in BPD patients were Enterobacteriaceae. To confirm the presence of Proteobacteria in the samples from patients with BPD, we also performed specific endotoxin assays. Endotoxin concentrations in the airway were similar between term and preterm infants at birth, but endotoxin levels were increased in infants with established BPD compared with concentrations at birth.[16] Serial samples in five ELBW infants in whom BPD later developed demonstrated a distinct temporal dysbiotic change with decreases in Firmicutes and increases in Proteobacteria over time. It was observed both in the discovery cohort as well as the validation cohort that genus *Lactobacillus* was less abundant even as early as birth in infants in whom BPD later developed, compared with the infants without BPD (Fig. 5.2). Interestingly, preterm birth was associated with alterations in the vaginal microbial community with decreased relative abundance of *Lactobacillus.*[17]

As both extremely preterm and term infants had a similar diverse microbiome at birth, it is probable that the airway and lung microbiomes are established before

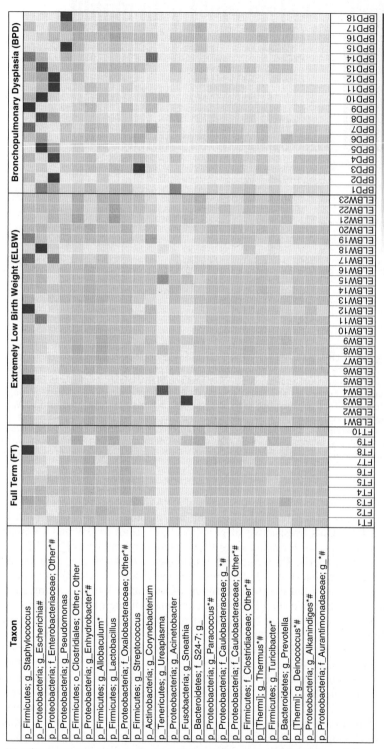

Fig. 5.2 Microbiome at genus level of extremely low-birth-weight *(ELBW)* infants, full-term infants, and patients with bronchopulmonary dysplasia *(BPD)*. Heatmap depicting the relative abundance of common bacterial families at the genus level. Statistically significant difference in microbial abundance is seen between lung microbiome of ELBW infants and infants with BPD (indicated by *asterisk*) and between FT infants and infants with BPD (indicated by *number sign*). (From Lal CV, Travers C, Aghai ZH, et al. The airway microbiome at birth. *Sci Rep.* 2016;6:31023.)

birth, potentially through transplacental passage of bacterial products. This contention is supported by culture-independent studies of the uterine microbiome demonstrating the presence of bacteria in the placenta,[18] fetal membranes,[19] and amniotic fluid[20] of healthy pregnancies that have challenged the notion that the fetus develops in a sterile environment and have increased our understanding of infection-related preterm birth as a polymicrobial diease.[20] Using next-generation sequencing and metagenomic analyses, Aagaard et al.[18] identified a low-abundance microbiota in the placenta of term and preterm placentas including *Escherichia coli*, *Prevotella tannerae*, *Bacteroides* species, and *Fusobacterium* species. Using 16S rDNA pyrosequencing to identify bacteria in placental membranes from term and preterm deliveries, Doyle et al.[19] found six genera (*Fusobacterium*, *Streptococcus*, *Mycoplasma*, *Aerococcus*, *Gardnerella*, and *Ureaplasma*) and one family (Enterobacteriaceae) that were more abundant in preterm membranes or absent in term membranes. There was reduced abundance of genus *Lactobacillus* and increased abundance of genera *Streptococcus*, *Aerococcus*, and *Ureaplasma* in membranes from preterm infants delivered vaginally.[19]

It is not currently known what proportion of the transferred bacterial DNA from the placenta is from live bacteria and what proportion is from "processed" bacterial products (DNA fragments, cell wall fragments, and so on). Our recent study indicated the presence of both bacterial DNA and bacterial lipopolysaccharide in neonatal airways at the time of birth.[16] Microbiome analysis evaluates bacterial DNA but does not indicate if the DNA is from live bacteria. It has been suggested that evaluation of susceptibility of the bacterial DNA to DNAse I may indicate the proportion of DNA from live bacteria, as live bacterial DNA is DNAse I–resistant, but bacterial DNA from dead bacteria is DNAse I–sensitive; 63% of DNA in porcine bronchoalveolar lavage fluid (BALF) is DNAse I–sensitive, suggesting the majority of airway bacterial DNA is from dead bacteria.[21]

It may be speculated that the establishment of the lung microbiome during fetal life enables the priming of the immune system in the fetus and later recognition of, and response to, bacterial flora encountered after birth. Alterations in the airway microbiome are associated with childhood pulmonary disorders such as asthma.[22,23] It is also likely that the lung microbiome contributes to normal alveolar development. Yun et al.[24] studied microbiota of sterilely excised lungs from mice of different origin including outbred wild mice caught in the natural environment or kept under non-specific pathogen–free (SPF) conditions as well as inbred mice maintained in non-SPF, SPF, or germ-free (GF) facilities. Metabolically active murine lung microbiota were found in all but GF mice.[24] Bacteria were detectable by fluorescent in situ hybridization on alveolar epithelia in the absence of inflammation. A higher bacterial abundance in non-SPF mice correlated with more and smaller size alveoli (consistent with better alveolarization), which was corroborated by transplanting *Lactobacillus* spp. lung isolates into GF mice.[24]

There are many potential mechanisms by which the microbiome may modulate lung injury and repair. It is known that manipulation of the gut microbiota may influence lung pathology via the gut-lung axis,[25] but it is not clear if the manipulation of the gut microbiome also simultaneously alters the lung microbiome or if the effects in the lung can be due solely to alterations of the microbiome in the gut. It is possible that bacteria or bacterial products from the gut may be translocated to the systemic circulation and filtered from the pulmonary circulation into the lungs. It is known that the lung microbiome is enriched with gut bacteria in sepsis and the acute respiratory distress syndrome.[26]

In the next section we review the human and experimental evidence that the low-virulence pathogens *Ureaplasma parvum* and *U. urealyticum* that are commonly members of the amniotic fluid and placental microbiota contribute to preterm birth and lung injury owing to an augmented dysregulated inflammatory response that contributes to the development of BPD. Recent studies provide new insights into how these organisms evade the host immune response to establish colonization in the intrauterine cavity and fetal/newborn lung and identify these mechanisms as potential therapeutic targets.

Role of Genital Mycoplasmas in Intrauterine Infection and Neonatal Lung Injury

The Mollicute class consists of at least 200 species, of which humans are the primary hosts for at least 17. Mollicutes are primarily associated with the mucosal surfaces of the urogenital and respiratory tracts. The four urogenital species belong to two different phylogenetic groups within the Mollicute class. *Mycoplasma hominis* belongs to the Hominis group, while *Ureaplasma* spp. and *M. genitalium* belong to the pneumoniae group.[27] *Ureaplasma* consists of 2 species and 14 serovars. *U. parvum* contains serovars 1, 3, 6, and 14, and *U. urealyticum* contains the remaining serovars.[28] The mycoplasma species are the smallest self-replicating, free-living organisms. The *M. genitalium* genome is the smallest with 580 kilobase pairs (kbp) while *U. parvum* serovar 3 genome is the second smallest known genome with 751 kbp and the recently sequenced *M. hominis* genome is 665 kbp.[27,29] Because of their small genome size, the genital mycoplasma species have limited biosynthetic capacities, requiring a parasitic relationship with a host. These species all lack cell walls and share 247 coding sequences,[27] but they have distinct energy-generating pathways and pathogenic roles in human disease. *M. genitalium* uses glycolysis, but the *Ureaplasma* spp. and *M. hominis* hydrolyze urea and arginine, respectively, to generate adenosine triphosphate.[27,28] *M. genitalium* is associated with cervicitis and male urethritis. It has been detected in 9% of BAL fluids of children who had bronchoscopy for chronic respiratory conditions such as asthma.[30] *M. hominis* is associated with pyelonephritis, bacterial vaginosis, pelvic inflammatory disease, and postpartum endometritis, but it has not been consistently associated with histologic chorioamnionitis or BPD.[28,31] It is much less commonly isolated as a single organism from amniotic fluid, chorioamnion, or neonatal tracheal or gastric aspirates than are the *Ureaplasma* spp.[28,31] The following section focuses on the evidence implicating the *Ureaplasma* spp. in neonatal lung disease.

Ureaplasma Species: Are There Species- or Serovar-Specific Virulence Factors?

U. parvum is more commonly isolated from clinical vaginal,[32] amniotic fluid,[33] and infant respiratory specimens[34–36] and is the predominant species in newborn serum and/or cerebrospinal fluid samples detected by PCR.[37] It has been proposed that some serovars have greater association with adverse pregnancy outcomes than others.[32,34,38] Abele-Horn et al.[32] reported a higher rate of BPD in infants whose respiratory tracts were colonized with *U. urealyticum.* In contrast, Katz et al.[39] observed no difference in prevalence of either species detected by PCR between infants with and without BPD. In a recent prospective study of respiratory secretions in infants less than 33 weeks' gestation, the distribution of *Ureaplasma* species and serovars was determined by real-time PCR using species- and serovar-specific primers/probes.[36,40] *U. parvum* was the predominant species (63%), compared with *U. urealyticum* (33%). Serovars 3 and 6 alone and in combination accounted for 96% *U. parvum* isolates. *U. urealyticum* isolates were commonly a mixture of multiple serovars with serovar 11 alone or combined with other serovars (59%) as the most common serovar. No individual species/ serovars or serovar mixtures were associated with moderate to severe BPD. This supports the contention that *Ureaplasma* virulence is species- and serovar-independent with regard to neonatal lung disease, but this needs to be confirmed. Recent research has shown that clinical isolates often have DNA hybrid genomes, proving that serovar-specific markers have been transferred horizontally.[41] These findings suggest that there could be innumerable serovars or strains based on different combinations of horizontally transferred genes. Thus serotyping for diagnostic purposes or in an attempt to correlate pathogenicity at the serovar level is unlikely to be useful, and host factors are more likely responsible for different outcomes following *Ureaplasma* infection.[41]

Previously proposed ureaplasmal virulence factors include immunoglobulin A (IgA) protease, urease, phospholipases A and C, and production of hydrogen peroxide.[29] These factors may allow the organism to evade mucosal immune defenses by degrading IgA and injuring mucosal cells through the local generation of ammonia, membrane phospholipid degradation and prostaglandin synthesis, and membrane peroxidation, respectively. Although functionally active IgA protease and phospholipases A and C were found in *Ureaplasma* spp., the genes that code for these proteins have not been identified in the *U. parvum* serovar 3 genome.[29] The ureaplasmal enzymes may have unique sequences compared with analogous genes in other species.

The ureaplasmal MB antigen that contains both serovar-specific and cross-reactive epitopes is the predominant antigen recognized during ureaplasmal infections in humans. It exhibits highly variable size in vitro,[42] clinical isolates in vivo,[43] and in an experimental ovine intraamniotic infection model,[44] suggesting that antigen size variation may be another mechanism through which the organism evades host defenses.[28] Ureaplasmas have multiple other host immune response avoidance mechanisms that facilitate establishing a chronic infection in the amniotic cavity and the neonatal respiratory tract. These include the ability to form biofilms,[45] the presence of multiple nucleases that may degrade neutrophil extracellular traps formed when activated neutrophils release granule proteins and chromatin that kill bacteria,[46,47] and downregulation of various endogenous antimicrobial peptides by ureaplasmal-mediated chromatin modification alterations, including significantly decreased histone H3K9 acetylation.[48] Because neutrophil extracellular traps are abundant in chorioamniotic membranes with acute chorioamnionitis,[49] *Ureaplasma*-induced nuclease degradation may explain in part the prolonged subclinical intrauterine infection with these organisms. Further genetic studies of the ureaplasmal genome are likely to identify other virulence factors that may be novel therapeutic targets.

Potential Role of *Ureaplasma* Species in Preterm Birth and Intrauterine Inflammation

Because *Ureaplasma* is a commensal in the adult female genital tract, it has been considered of low virulence. However, it has been associated with multiple obstetric complications, including infertility, stillbirth, chorioamnionitis,[50–52] and preterm delivery.[28] *Ureaplasma* spp. are the most common organisms isolated from amniotic fluid obtained from women who present with preterm labor (POL) with intact membranes,[53,54] preterm premature rupture of membranes (pPROM),[55] short cervix associated with microbial invasion of the amniotic cavity,[56] and from infected placentas.[55] The prevalence of infected amniotic fluid with cultivated *Ureaplasma* as the only microbe ranges from 6% to 9% for pregnancies complicated by POL with intact membranes[54,57] to 22% for a cohort of women with POL or pPROM.[58] Detection of cultivated *Ureaplasma* in placental chorion in pregnancies producing VLBW infants ranges from 6% to 10% in homogenized frozen tissue[59,60] to 28% in fresh tissue and is inversely related to gestational age.[61] Recovery of *Ureaplasma* from the chorion increased with duration of rupture membranes, suggesting an ascending route of infection.[61] However, *Ureaplasma* has also been detected in 31% of infected placentas with duration of rupture of membranes less than 1 hour,[62] suggesting the possibility of a preexisting infection. Indeed, *Ureaplasma* species have been detected in amniotic fluid as early as the time of genetic amniocentesis (16–20 weeks) in up to 13% asymptomatic women.[63–66] Placentas with the lowest rate of *Ureaplasma* recovery were from women delivered for preeclampsia or intrauterine growth restriction.[61]

The presence of *Ureaplasma* as the only identified microbial isolate in the upper genital tract is significantly associated with chorioamnionitis and adverse pregnancy outcomes, including premature delivery, neonatal morbidity, and perinatal death.[54,55,58,61,67] Placentas colonized with *Ureaplasma* exhibit a characteristic bistriate inflammatory pattern with maternal-derived neutrophils accumulating in the subchorion and amnion.[68] Experimental models of intrauterine *Ureaplasma* infection in mice,[69] sheep,[70,71] and nonhuman primates[72] have been described. Intraamniotic inoculation of *U. parvum* did not stimulate preterm labor in mice or sheep, but it did stimulate progressive uterine contractions and preterm delivery in rhesus macaques inoculated at 136 days of gestation (80% term),[72] suggesting species differences in the host response or serovar differences in virulence. The rhesus macaque model is the first experimental model to definitely show a causal link between *Ureaplasma* intrauterine infection and preterm labor.

In the presence of pPROM, cultivated *Ureaplasma* as the sole microbe was associated with increased leukocytes and proinflammatory cytokines (interleukin [IL]-6, IL-1β, and tumor necrosis factor α [TNF-α]) in amniotic fluid and increased cord blood IL-6 concentrations, indicating a robust inflammatory response to this infection.[73] However, amniotic fluid IL-8 levels were higher and the amniocentesis-to-delivery interval was shorter when preterm labor was caused by a combination of *Mycoplasma/Ureaplasma* and other bacteria than *Mycoplasma/Ureaplasma* alone.[52] Ureaplasmal bacterial load determined by quantitative PCR in amniotic fluid of women who delivered preterm was associated with histologic chorioamnionitis, preterm labor, PROM, and BPD.[33] The bacterial load correlated with amniotic fluid IL-8 concentrations. Although the majority of women in whom subclinical *Ureaplasma* amniotic cavity infection is detected midtrimester deliver at term,[66] those with elevated amniotic fluid IL-6 levels have increased risk for an adverse pregnancy outcome, including fetal loss and preterm delivery.[74] In the rhesus monkey *U. parvum* intrauterine infection model, uterine activity was preceded by a rise in amniotic fluid leukocytes, inflammatory cytokines, prostaglandins (PGs) PGE_2 and $PGF_{2\alpha}$, and matrix metalloproteinase-9, demonstrating that *Ureaplasma* alone stimulates the mediators of preterm labor.[72] Recently Lal and coworkers[75] demonstrated that *Ureaplasma* spp. stimulate neutrophil matrix metalloproteinase-9 release and express the serine protease prolyl endopeptidase that together induce collagen fragmentation, resulting in release of the tripeptide PGP (proline-glycine-proline), a neutrophil chemoattractant. These findings implicate *Ureaplasma* spp. in the causal pathway of preterm rupture of membranes and neutrophil influx causing chorioamnionitis.

In vitro studies have provided additional evidence supporting the contention that *Ureaplasma* spp. stimulate inflammation in the intrauterine compartment. Plasma from placental whole blood (source of maternal circulating leukocytes) that had been preincubated with *U. parvum* serovar 3 clinical isolate stimulated IL-1β and PGE_2 secretion by chorioamnion explants.[76] High inoculum (10^6 color changing units [CCU]/mL), but not low inoculum (10^2–10^4 CCU/mL), heat-killed *U. urealyticum* serotype 8 stimulated TNF-α, IL-10, and PGE_2 production by choriodecidual explants in vitro. In contrast, heat-killed *U. parvum* serovar 1 laboratory reference strain failed to stimulate a significant increase in cytokine and PGE_2 response in fetal membrane explants derived from term placentas. The apparent low virulence of *Ureaplasma* in these in vitro studies may be due, in part, to the use of a laboratory reference strain rather than more virulent clinical isolates, or killed rather than live organisms. Alternatively, a decreased capacity to stimulate an inflammatory response in the intrauterine compartment may allow *Ureaplasma* infections to persist for long periods of time.

Ureaplasma spp. and Neonatal Lung Injury

Ureaplasma respiratory tract colonization in the newborn has been associated with higher incidence of pneumonia[77,78] and BPD.[28,34,79,80] The rate of *Ureaplasma* respiratory tract colonization in infants with birth weights less than 1500 g ranges from 20% to 45%, depending on study entry criteria and frequency of sampling and detection methods.[79,81] In a recent cohort of infants at 33 weeks' gestation, *Ureaplasma* spp. were detected by combined culture/PCR during the first week of life in tracheal aspirates or nasopharyngeal specimens in 35% of infants.[37] *Ureaplasma*-colonized infants are more likely to be born extremely preterm (<28 weeks' gestation) and to be delivered by spontaneous vaginal delivery following preterm labor or preterm premature rupture of membranes.[82] Typically they experience less respiratory distress in the first week of life with clinical deterioration in the second week, requiring increased oxygen and ventilatory support.[34,82] *Ureaplasma* respiratory tract colonization is associated with a peripheral blood leukocytosis[78] and early radiographic emphysematous changes of BPD.[77,82,83] These findings may be explained, in part, by an in utero onset of the inflammatory response and lung injury. Indeed, neonatal *Ureaplasma* respiratory colonization was associated with BPD in infants exposed to antenatal histological chorioamnionitis.[84] Clinical, radiographic, and laboratory characteristics of neonatal *Ureaplasma* respiratory tract colonization are summarized in Box 5.1.

The contribution of *Ureaplasma* respiratory tract colonization to the development of BPD has been debated; however, three meta-analyses of more than 40

Box 5.1   CHARACTERISTIC CLINICAL AND LABORATORY FINDINGS IN
UREAPLASMA-POSITIVE PRETERM INFANTS

Clinical Presentation	Laboratory/Radiographic Findings
Preterm onset of labor or preterm premature rupture of membranes[82]	Bistriate inflammatory pattern chorioamnionitis[68]
Gestational age <28 weeks[36]	Leukocytosis at birth[78,84,132]
Mild respiratory distress syndrome, but worsening gas exchange requiring increased respiratory support in second week of life[34,82]	Early radiographic emphysematous changes[77,82,83]

studies over the past 30 years have confirmed that *Ureaplasma* respiratory colonization is an independent risk factor for BPD.[79,81,85] Overall, *Ureaplasma* respiratory tract colonization increased the risk for BPD at 28 days threefold and BPD at 36 weeks PMA twofold.[85,86] Despite changes in neonatal care over the past three decades, this association has remained unchanged. Recently we observed that in infants who had been mechanically ventilated for any duration and had a positive tracheal aspirate with or without a paired positive nasopharyngeal sample had a 7.9-fold increased risk (odds ratio = 7.86, 95% confidence interval 1.31 to 47) to develop moderate-severe BPD than mechanically ventilated infants with a positive nasopharyngeal sample alone.[36] This suggests that lower tract infection, but not nasopharyngeal colonization, augments lung injury in mechanically ventilated infants.

Human and Experimental Evidence for Role of *Ureaplasma* spp. in BPD

Evidence from studies of human preterm infants[87–89] and intrauterine infection models in mice,[69] sheep,[70,71] and nonhuman primates[72,90] support that *Ureaplasma* infection is proinflammatory and profibrotic and results in a BPD phenotype. In a review of lung pathology of archived autopsy specimens from preterm infants infected with *Ureaplasma,* the most striking findings were (1) the presence of moderate to severe fibrosis, (2) increased myofibroblasts, (3) disordered elastin accumulation, and (4) increased numbers of TNF-α and transforming growth factor beta 1 (TGF-β_1)-immunoreactive cells in all *Ureaplasma*-infected infants compared with gestational controls and infants who died with pneumonia from other causes.[88,89] The increase in fibrosis and elastic fiber accumulation in the distal lung correlated spatially and temporally with the presence of macrophages positive for TGF-β_1, suggesting that these are closely linked. Severity of fibrosis score and elastic fiber density exhibited strong correlation with duration of ventilation in *Ureaplasma*-positive infants, suggesting that *Ureaplasma* infection augments the inflammatory response to volutrauma.[88,89] Preterm infants with *Ureaplasma* respiratory colonization have elevated tracheal aspirate IL-1β, TNF-α, and monocyte chemoattractant protein-1 (MCP-1) concentrations and neutrophil chemotactic activity during the first weeks of life compared with noncolonized infants.[87,91,92]

Experimental pneumonia models demonstrate the inflammatory response to *Ureaplasma* pulmonary infection. Intratracheal *Ureaplasma* inoculation caused an acute bronchiolitis in 140-day-old preterm baboons[93] and an acute interstitial pneumonia in newborn, but not 14-day-old, mice.[94] Hyperoxia exposure increased mortality, lung inflammation, and delayed pathogen clearance in *Ureaplasma*-inoculated newborn mice,[95] consistent with the hypothesis that *Ureaplasma* augments the inflammatory response to secondary stimuli. In a mouse *Ureaplasma* pneumonia model, intratracheal inoculation with *Ureaplasma* induced a prolonged inflammatory response as indicated by a sustained recruitment of neutrophils and macrophages into the lung.[96]

Antenatal infection models provide insights into the effects of *Ureaplasma* on lung development. Experimental murine intrauterine *U. parvum* exposure stimulated fetal lung cytokine expression and augmented hyperoxia-induced lung injury.[69]

Intraamniotic *Ureaplasma* (serovar 1) inoculation 2 days before delivery at 125 days (67% of term gestation) in the baboon caused an inflammatory response in the amniotic and fetal lung compartments and vertical transmission to the fetal lung that persisted up to 2 weeks postnatally in half of the antenatally exposed animals.[97] We observed extensive fibrosis, an increase in the myofibroblast phenotype, increased expression of proinflammatory (TNF-α, IL-1β) and pro-fibrotic cytokines (TGF-β_1, oncostatin M), and presence of macrophages as the predominant recruited leukocyte in lungs of *Ureaplasma*-exposed immature baboons, compared with gestational controls or noninfected ventilated animals.[90] After 14 days of ventilation, active TGF-β_1– and TGF-β_1–induced Smad signaling was increased in lung homogenates of *Ureaplasma*-infected animals compared with gestational and ventilated controls. Similarly, fetal sheep exposed to intraamniotic *U. parvum* serovar 3 for 3 to 14 days before delivery at 124 days demonstrated increased fetal lung neutrophils after 3 days and decreased alveolar septa and elastin foci, and increased α-smooth muscle actin in arteries and bronchioli after 14 days of exposure.[98] This demonstrated that short-term intrauterine exposure to *Ureaplasma* induces an inflammatory response and altered structural lung development. This may mimic the exposure with an ascending infection after rupture of membranes in the human condition.

Because subclinical *Ureaplasma* intrauterine infection has been detected early in human pregnancy, the effects of prolonged intrauterine exposure to this infection have been examined. In fetal sheep exposed to intraamniotic *Ureaplasma* for periods up to 10 weeks, long-term exposure was associated with improvement in lung function, but poor fetal growth, fetal acidemia, and evidence of fetal pulmonary inflammation.[70] Intraamniotic inoculation of *U. parvum* serovar 3 or 6 at midgestation in fetal sheep did not result in preterm labor, but did cause placental and fetal pulmonary inflammation and altered lung development whether delivery occurred preterm or at term.[71] However, after intraamniotic inoculation of these serovars at 50 days' gestation, there was evidence of persistent infection, lung inflammation, increased surfactant, and improved lung volumes but no significant effects on indices of air space and vascular morphology in fetuses delivered preterm at 125 days' gestation.[99] This suggests that effects on lung development are not sustained after prolonged exposure to *Ureaplasma* in utero in the sheep model. In contrast, in a nonhuman primate study of rhesus macaques, histologic changes in the fetal lungs depended on the duration of intrauterine exposure to *U. parvum*.[72] Infection exposure duration less than 136 hours resulted in neutrophil infiltration without epithelial injury. With progressive duration of exposure there was an influx of neutrophils and macrophages, epithelial necrosis, and type II cell proliferation. For exposure duration longer than 10 days, increased collagen and thickened alveolar walls were evident. These observations suggest that an early and prolonged exposure to *Ureaplasma*-mediated inflammation may be necessary to adversely affect lung development. Discrepancies among the experimental models may be due to species differences. Overall, the experimental models confirm that intraamniotic *Ureaplasma* mimics many of the clinical features of the human disease.

The stimulatory effect of *Ureaplasma* on cytokine release has been confirmed in vitro. *Ureaplasma* stimulated TNF-α and IL-6 release by alveolar macrophages from preterm infant tracheal aspirates,[100] and cytokine, nitric oxide production, and upregulation of inducible nitric oxide synthase, nuclear factor kappa B (NF-κB) activation, and vascular endothelial growth factor and soluble and cell-associated intracellular adhesion molecule 1 expression by human and murine-derived monocytic cells.[100–102] *Ureaplasma* induced apoptosis in A549 cells, a human type II cell line, and in THP-1 human monocytic cells.[103] These effects could be partially blocked by anti–TNF-α monoclonal antibody,[102,103] implicating TNF-α as a mediator of the host immune response to this infection that contributes to altered lung development. In cultured human monocytes, *Ureaplasma* stimulated release of TNF-α and IL-8.[104] Moreover, in the presence of bacterial endotoxic lipopolysaccharide (LPS), *Ureaplasma* greatly augmented monocyte production of proinflammatory cytokines while blocking expression of antiinflammatory cytokines (IL-6 and IL-10).

These data confirm that *Ureaplasma* infection contributes to chronic inflammation in the preterm lung. We propose that *Ureaplasma* infection initiated in utero and augmented postnatally by exposure to volutrauma and oxygen elicits a sustained, dysregulated inflammatory response in the immature lung that (1) impairs alveolarization and (2) stimulates myofibroblast proliferation and excessive collagen and elastin deposition.

Developmental Deficiencies in Innate Immunity Contribute to Susceptibility to *Ureaplasma* Infection and Dysregulated Inflammation

Immaturity of fetal host defense mechanisms may increase the susceptibility of the preterm lung to *Ureaplasma* infection and dysregulated inflammation. Surfactant protein A (SP-A), a product of the alveolar type II cell that is an important component of the lung's innate immune response, is deficient in the preterm lung. SP-A is critical for clearance of infection and limiting inflammation in the lung.[105,106] We have shown that SP-A binds to *Ureaplasma* isolates in a calcium-dependent manner and enhances phagocytosis and bacterial killing by RAW264.7 cells, a murine macrophage cell line.[107,108] Furthermore, bacterial clearance was delayed and inflammatory response exaggerated in SP-A–deficient mice compared with wild-type mice inoculated intratracheally with *U. parvum*. Coadministration of purified human SP-A with the *Ureaplasma* inoculum to SP-A$^{-/-}$ mice reduced the inflammatory response to the infection but did not improve the rate of bacterial clearance. SP-A deficiency of the preterm lung may contribute to the prolonged inflammatory response, lung injury, and risk for fibrosis in *Ureaplasma*-infected infants contributing to the pathogenesis of BPD.

Other important components of the innate immune response are toll-like receptors (TLRs) that respond to a broad range of pathogen-associated molecular patterns, including LPS, viral coat proteins, bacterial lipoproteins and glycolipids, viral RNA, and 5′-cytosine—phosphate—guanine—3′ (CpG)-containing bacterial DNA.[109] Engagement of TLR proteins activates the expression of proinflammatory mediators by macrophages, neutrophils, dendritic cells, B cells, endothelial cells, and epithelial cells. TLR signaling activates the transcription factor NF-κB and subsequent upregulation of gene expression. Peltier et al.[110] and Shimizu et al.[111] demonstrated that Triton X-114 detergent extracted lipoproteins from *U. urealyticum* serovar 4 and *U. parvum* serovar 3 are responsible for NF-κB activation. Active lipoproteins identified for serovar 3 included the MB antigen.[111] The serovar 3 detergent extracts activated NF-κB through TLR2 cooperatively with TLR1 and TLR6,[111] whereas serovar 4 extracts activated both TLR2 and TLR4.[110] Further studies are needed to determine if the different *Ureaplasma* species or serovars interact with different TLRs. If so, this could explain, in part, differences in host responses to the different serovars.

Little is known concerning TLR expression during human lung development. In mice, TLR2 and TLR4 mRNA levels were barely detectable early in gestation, increasing thereafter during late gestation and postnatally.[112] In fetal sheep lung, TLR2 and TLR4 mRNA levels increased throughout late gestation to reach half of adult levels at term but were induced by intraamniotic LPS exposure.[113] In the immature baboon model, TLR2 and TLR4 mRNA and protein expression were low in 125-day and 140-day nonventilated gestational controls, reached adult levels near term, and were increased in 125-day preterm baboons ventilated with oxygen for 21 days.[114] These data may explain, in part, the developmental susceptibility to *Ureaplasma* infection and interaction with other stimuli. Low TLR2 and 4 expression early in gestation may increase the susceptibility of the fetal lung to *Ureaplasma* infection and delay clearance, but postnatal exposures to mechanical ventilation, oxygen and other infections may stimulate pulmonary TLR expression and enhance *Ureaplasma*-mediated inflammatory signaling. Single-nucleotide polymorphisms in relevant TLRs may affect both the susceptibility to *Ureaplasma* respiratory infection and the risk of developing BPD in infected preterm infants.[115]

Can BPD Be Prevented by *Ureaplasma* Eradication?

Despite in vitro susceptibility of *Ureaplasma* to erythromycin,[116] trials of erythromycin therapy in the first few weeks of life in *Ureaplasma*-colonized preterm infants failed to demonstrate efficacy to prevent BPD[117,118] or eradicate respiratory tract colonization.[119] The failure to prevent BPD in these studies may have been due to the small sample size of each study or to the initiation of erythromycin therapy too late to prevent the lung inflammation and injury that contribute to the pathogenesis of BPD.

The 14-membered macrolides that are derivatives of erythromycin and the related 15-member azalides have immunomodulatory effects, including effects on neutrophil function (e.g., chemotaxis, cell adhesion, oxidative burst, and phagocytosis) and inhibition of cytokine release[120] and nitric oxide production in vitro.[121] Macrolide antibiotics may exert immunomodulatory antiinflammatory effects in the setting of infection, and these may occur independently of a direct bactericidal effect.[122] Recently Segal et al.[123] studied the effect of azithromycin on the lung microbiome and bacterial metabolites in adults with chronic obstructive pulmonary disease in a placebo, double-blind, randomized trial. Although azithromycin did not alter bacterial abundance, it reduced alpha diversity and increased antiinflammatory bacterial metabolites glycolic acid and indol-3-acetate. In addition, azithromycin exhibits higher potency than erythromycin against clinical *Ureaplasma* isolates in vitro.[124] Pharmacokinetic studies in mice and humans have shown that azithromycin is preferentially concentrated in pulmonary epithelial lining fluid and alveolar macrophages.[125–127] Since neutrophil recruitment and activation has been implicated in BPD pathogenesis,[128,129] the experimental effects observed with azithromycin in vitro and in vivo indicate that this drug may be beneficial in the treatment of *Ureaplasma* infection and the prevention of BPD in preterm infants.

Because *Ureaplasma*-mediated lung injury may be initiated in utero and augmented postnatally by exposure to mechanical ventilation and hyperoxia, therapy to prevent BPD should be initiated as soon as possible after birth in infants at risk. Recently Walls et al.[130] demonstrated that azithromycin, but not erythromycin, prophylaxis improved outcomes and reduced inflammation in a murine neonatal *Ureaplasma* infection model. This suggests that azithromycin may be effective if administered immediately after birth. An initial single-dose pharmacokinetic study of 10 mg/kg azithromycin in infants 24 to 28 weeks' gestation suggested that this dose was well tolerated but likely insufficient to maintain azithromycin concentrations above the MIC_{50} (minimum concentration that inhibits 50% of organisms) for *Ureaplasma*.[131] However, until additional pharmacokinetics and efficacy trials are conducted, a dosing regimen for azithromycin in neonates cannot be recommended.

Acknowledgment

This work was supported by National Institutes of Health grants nos. HL071113, HL087166, HL129907, HL122626, and HL133536.

REFERENCES

1. Bardell D. The roles of the sense of taste and clean teeth in the discovery of bacteria by Antoni van Leeuwenhoek. *Microbiol Rev.* 1983;47(1):121–126.
2. Staley JT, Konopka A. Measurement of in situ activities of nonphotosynthetic microorganisms in aquatic and terrestrial habitats. *Annu Rev Microbiol.* 1985;39:321–346.
3. Lederberg J, McCray AT. 'Ome sweet' omics—a genealogical treasury for words. *Scientist.* 2001;15:8.
4. Lynch SV. The lung microbiome and airway disease. *Ann Am Thorac Soc.* 2016;13(suppl 5):S462–S465.
5. Gallacher DJ, Kotecha S. Respiratory microbiome of new-born infants. *Front Pediatr.* 2016;4:10.
6. Turnbaugh PJ, Ley RE, Hamady M, Fraser-Liggett CM, Knight R, Gordon JI. The human microbiome project. *Nature.* 2007;449(7164):804–810.
7. Human Microbiome Project Consortium. Structure, function and diversity of the healthy human microbiome. *Nature.* 2012;486(7402):207–214.
8. Warner BB, Hamvas A. Lungs, microbes and the developing neonate. *Neonatology.* 2015;107(4):337–343.
9. Hilty M, Burke C, Pedro H, et al. Disordered microbial communities in asthmatic airways. *PLoS One.* 2010;5(1):e8578.
10. Bassis CM, Erb-Downward JR, Dickson RP, et al. Analysis of the upper respiratory tract microbiotas as the source of the lung and gastric microbiotas in healthy individuals. *MBio.* 2015;6(2):e00037.
11. Dickson RP, Erb-Downward JR, Freeman CM, et al. Spatial variation in the healthy human lung microbiome and the adapted island model of lung biogeography. *Ann Am Thorac Soc.* 2015;12(6):821–830.
12. Beck JM, Young VB, Huffnagle GB. The microbiome of the lung. *Transl Res.* 2012;160(4):258–266.

13. Yu G, Gail MH, Consonni D, et al. Characterizing human lung tissue microbiota and its relationship to epidemiological and clinical features. *Genome Biol.* 2016;17(1):163.

14. Mourani PM, Harris JK, Sontag MK, Robertson CE, Abman SH. Molecular identification of bacteria in tracheal aspirate fluid from mechanically ventilated preterm infants. *PLoS One.* 2011;6(10):e25959.

15. Lohmann P, Luna RA, Hollister EB, et al. The airway microbiome of intubated premature infants: characteristics and changes that predict the development of bronchopulmonary dysplasia. *Pediatr Res.* 2014;76(3):294–301.

16. Lal CV, Travers C, Aghai ZH, et al. The airway microbiome at birth. *Sci Rep.* 2016;6:31023.

17. DiGiulio DB, Callahan BJ, McMurdie PJ, et al. Temporal and spatial variation of the human microbiota during pregnancy. *Proc Natl Acad Sci U S A.* 2015;112(35):11060–11065.

18. Aagaard K, Ma J, Antony KM, Ganu R, Petrosino J, Versalovic J. The placenta harbors a unique microbiome. *Sci Transl Med.* 2014;6(237):237ra265.

19. Doyle RM, Alber DG, Jones HE, et al. Term and preterm labour are associated with distinct microbial community structures in placental membranes which are independent of mode of delivery. *Placenta.* 2014;35(12):1099–1101.

20. Payne MS, Bayatibojakhi S. Exploring preterm birth as a polymicrobial disease: an overview of the uterine microbiome. *Front Immunol.* 2014;5:595.

21. Pezzulo AA, Kelly PH, Nassar BS, et al. Abundant DNase I-sensitive bacterial DNA in healthy porcine lungs and its implications for the lung microbiome. *Appl Environ Microbiol.* 2013;79(19):5936–5941.

22. Singanayagam A, Ritchie AI, Johnston SL. Role of microbiome in the pathophysiology and disease course of asthma. *Curr Opin Pulm Med.* 2017;23(1):41–47.

23. Huang YJ. The respiratory microbiome and innate immunity in asthma. *Curr Opin Pulm Med.* 2015;21(1):27–32.

24. Yun Y, Srinivas G, Kuenzel S, et al. Environmentally determined differences in the murine lung microbiota and their relation to alveolar architecture. *PLoS One.* 2014;9(12):e113466.

25. Budden KF, Gellatly SL, Wood DL, et al. Emerging pathogenic links between microbiota and the gut-lung axis. *Nat Rev Microbiol.* 2017;15(1):55–63.

26. Dickson RP, Singer BH, Newstead MW, et al. Enrichment of the lung microbiome with gut bacteria in sepsis and the acute respiratory distress syndrome. *Nat Microbiol.* 2016;1(10):16113.

27. Pereyre S, Sirand-Pugnet P, Beven L, et al. Life on arginine for *Mycoplasma hominis*: clues from its minimal genome and comparison with other human urogenital mycoplasmas. *PLoS Genet.* 2009;5(10):e1000677.

28. Waites KB, Katz B, Schelonka RL. Mycoplasmas and ureaplasmas as neonatal pathogens. *Clin Microbiol Rev.* 2005;18(4):757–789.

29. Glass JI, Lefkowitz EJ, Glass JS, Heiner CR, Chen EY, Cassell GH. The complete sequence of the mucosal pathogen *Ureaplasma urealyticum. Nature.* 2000;407(6805):757–762.

30. Patel KK, Salva PS, Webley WC. Colonization of paediatric lower respiratory tract with genital *Mycoplasma* species. *Respirology.* 2011;16(7):1081–1087.

31. Payne MS, Goss KC, Connett GJ, et al. Molecular microbiological characterization of preterm neonates at risk of bronchopulmonary dysplasia. *Pediatr Res.* 2010;67(4):412–418.

32. Abele-Horn M, Wolff C, Dressel P, Pfaff F, Zimmermann A. Association of *Ureaplasma urealyticum* biovars with clinical outcome for neonates, obstetric patients, and gynecological patients with pelvic inflammatory disease. *J Clin Microbiol.* 1997;35:1199–1202.

33. Kasper DC, Mechtler TP, Reischer GH, et al. The bacterial load of *Ureaplasma parvum* in amniotic fluid is correlated with an increased intrauterine inflammatory response. *Diagn Microbiol Infect Dis.* 2010;67(2):117–121.

34. Hannaford K, Todd DA, Jeffrey H, John E, Byth K, Gilbert GL. Role of *Ureaplasma urealyticum* in lung disease of prematurity. *Arch Dis Child Fetal Neonatal Ed.* 1999;81:F162–F167.

35. Beeton ML, Maxwell NC, Davies PL, et al. Role of pulmonary infection in the development of chronic lung disease of prematurity. *Eur Respir J.* 2010.

36. Sung TJ, Xiao L, Duffy L, Waites KB, Chesko KL, Viscardi RM. Frequency of *Ureaplasma* serovars in respiratory secretions of preterm infants at risk for bronchopulmonary dysplasia. *Pediatr Infect Dis J.* 2010, in press.

37. Viscardi RM, Hashmi N, Gross GW, Sun CC, Rodriguez A, Fairchild KD. Incidence of invasive *Ureaplasma* in VLBW infants: relationship to severe intraventricular hemorrhage. *J Perinatol.* 2008.

38. Grattard F, Soleihac B, De Barbeyrac B, Bebear C, Seffert P, Pozzetto B. Epidemiologic and molecular investigations of genital mycoplasmas from women and neonates at delivery. *Pediatr Infect Dis J.* 1995;14:853–858.

39. Katz B, Patel P, Duffy L, Schelonka RL, Dimmitt RA, Waites KB. Characterization of ureaplasmas isolated from preterm infants with and without bronchopulmonary dysplasia. *J Clin Microbiol.* 2005;43(9):4852–4854.

40. Xiao L, Glass JI, Paralanov V, et al. Detection and characterization of human *Ureaplasma* species and serovars by real-time PCR. *J Clin Microbiol.* 2010;48(8):2715–2723.

41. Xiao L, Paralanov V, Glass JI, et al. Extensive horizontal gene transfer in ureaplasmas from humans questions the utility of serotyping for diagnostic purposes. *J Clin Microbiol.* 2011;49(8):2818–2826.

42. Zimmerman CU, Stiedl T, Rosengarten R, Spergser J. Alternate phase variation in expression of two major surface membrane proteins (MBA and UU376) of *Ureaplasma parvum* serovar 3. *FEMS Microbiol Lett.* 2009;292(2):187–193.

43. Zheng X, Watson HL, Waites KB, Cassell GH. Serotype diversity and antigen variation among invasive isolates of *Ureaplasma urealyticum* from neonates. *Infect Immun.* 1992;60:3472–3474.

44. Knox CL, Dando SJ, Nitsos I, et al. The severity of chorioamnionitis in pregnant sheep is associated with in vivo variation of the surface-exposed multiple-banded antigen/gene of *Ureaplasma parvum.* *Biol Reprod.* 2010;83(3):415–426.

45. Pandelidis K, McCarthy A, Chesko KL, Viscardi RM. Role of biofilm formation in *Ureaplasma* antibiotic susceptibility and development of bronchopulmonary dysplasia in preterm neonates. *Pediatr Infect Dis J.* 2013;32(4):394–398.

46. Paralanov V, Lu J, Duffy LB, et al. Comparative genome analysis of 19 *Ureaplasma urealyticum* and *Ureaplasma parvum* strains. *BMC Microbiol.* 2012;12(1):88.

47. Yamamoto T, Kida Y, Sakamoto Y, Kuwano K. Mpn491, a secreted nuclease of *Mycoplasma pneumoniae*, plays a critical role in evading killing by neutrophil extracellular traps. *Cell Microbiol.* 2016.

48. Xiao L, Crabb DM, Dai Y, Chen Y, Waites KB, Atkinson TP. Suppression of antimicrobial peptide expression by *Ureaplasma* species. *Infect Immun.* 2014;82(4):1657–1665.

49. Gomez-Lopez N, Romero R, Leng Y, et al. Neutrophil extracellular traps in acute chorioamnionitis: a mechanism of host defense. *Am J Reprod Immunol.* 2017.

50. Sweeney EL, Dando SJ, Kallapur SG, Knox CL. The human *Ureaplasma* species as causative agents of chorioamnionitis. *Clin Microbiol Rev.* 2017;30(1):349–379.

51. Kikhney J, von Schoning D, Steding I, et al. Is *Ureaplasma* spp. the leading causative agent of acute chorioamnionitis in women with preterm birth? *Clin Microbiol Infect.* 2016.

52. Yoneda N, Yoneda S, Niimi H, et al. Polymicrobial amniotic fluid infection with *Mycoplasma/Ureaplasma* and other bacteria induces severe intra-amniotic inflammation associated with poor perinatal prognosis in preterm labor. *Am J Reprod Immunol.* 2016;75(2):112–125.

53. Gomez R, Ghezzi F, Romero R, Munoz H, Tolosa JE, Rojas I. Premature labor and intra-amniotic infection. *Clin Perinatol.* 1995;22:281–342.

54. Yoon BH, Chang JW, Romero R. Isolation of *Ureaplasma urealyticum* from the amniotic cavity and adverse outcome in preterm labor. *Obstet Gynecol.* 1998;92:77–82.

55. Romero R, Yoon BH, Mazor M, et al. A comparative study of the diagnostic performance of amniotic fluid glucose, white blood cell count, interleukin-6, and gram stain in the detection of microbial invasion in patients with preterm premature rupture of membranes. *Am J Obstet Gynecol.* 1993;169:839–851.

56. Hassan S, Romero R, Hendler I, et al. A sonographic short cervix as the only clinical manifestation of intra-amniotic infection. *J Perinat Med.* 2006;34(1):13–19.

57. Yoon BH, Romero R, Lim JH, et al. The clinical significance of detecting *Ureaplasma urealyticum* by the polymerase chain reaction in the amniotic fluid of patients with preterm labor. *Am J Obstet Gynecol.* 2003;189:919–924.

58. Kirchner L, Helmer H, Heinze G, et al. Amnionitis with *Ureaplasma urealyticum* or other microbes leads to increased morbidity and prolonged hospitalization in very low birth weight infants. *Eur J Obstet Gynecol Reprod Biol.* 2007;134(1):44–50.

59. Onderdonk AB, Delaney ML, DuBois AM, Allred EN, Leviton A. Detection of bacteria in placental tissues obtained from extremely low gestational age neonates. *Am J Obstet Gynecol.* 2008;198(1):110.e111–e117.

60. Olomu IN, Hecht JL, Onderdonk AO, Allred EN, Leviton A. Perinatal correlates of *Ureaplasma urealyticum* in placenta parenchyma of singleton pregnancies that end before 28 weeks of gestation. *Pediatrics.* 2009;123(5):1329–1336.

61. Kundsin RB, Leviton A, Allred EN, Poulin SA. *Ureaplasma urealyticum* infection of the placenta in pregnancies that ended prematurely. *Obstet Gynecol.* 1996;87:122–127.

62. Dammann O, Allred EN, Genest DR, Kundsin RB, Leviton A. Antenatal *Mycoplasma* infection, the fetal inflammatory response and cerebral white matter damage in very-low-birthweight infants. *Paediatr Perinat Epidemiol.* 2003;17(1):49–57.

63. Gray DJ, Robinson HB, Malone J, Thomson RB Jr. Adverse outcome in pregnancy following amniotic fluid isolation of *Ureaplasma urealyticum.* *Prenat Diagn.* 1992;12(2):111–117.

64. Horowitz S, Mazor M, Romero R, Horowitz J, Glezerman M. Infection of the amniotic cavity with *Ureaplasma urealyticum* in the midtrimester of pregnancy. *J Reprod Med.* 1995;40(5):375–379.

65. Berg TG, Philpot KL, Welsh MS, Sanger WG, Smith CV. *Ureaplasma/Mycoplasma*-infected amniotic fluid: pregnancy outcome in treated and nontreated patients. *J Perinatol.* 1999;19(4):275–277.

66. Perni SC, Vardhana S, Korneeva I, et al. *Mycoplasma hominis* and *Ureaplasma urealyticum* in midtrimester amniotic fluid: association with amniotic fluid cytokine levels and pregnancy outcome. *Am J Obstet Gynecol.* 2004;191(4):1382–1386.

67. Witt A, Berger A, Gruber CJ, et al. Increased intrauterine frequency of *Ureaplasma urealyticum* in women with preterm labor and preterm premature rupture of the membranes and subsequent cesarean delivery. *Am J Obstet Gynecol.* 2005;193(5):1663–1669.

68. Namba F, Hasegawa T, Nakayama M, et al. Placental features of chorioamnionitis colonized with *Ureaplasma* species in preterm delivery. *Pediatr Res.* 2010;67(2):166–172.

69. Normann E, Lacaze-Masmonteil T, Eaton F, Schwendimann L, Gressens P, Thebaud B. A novel mouse model of *Ureaplasma*-induced perinatal inflammation: effects on lung and brain injury. *Pediatr Res.* 2009;65(4):430–436.

70. Moss TJ, Nitsos I, Ikegami M, Jobe AH, Newnham JP. Experimental intrauterine *Ureaplasma* infection in sheep. *Am J Obstet Gynecol.* 2005;192(4):1179–1186.

71. Moss TJ, Knox CL, Kallapur SG, et al. Experimental amniotic fluid infection in sheep: effects of *Ureaplasma parvum* serovars 3 and 6 on preterm or term fetal sheep. *Am J Obstet Gynecol.* 2008;198(1). 122 e121–128.

72. Novy MJ, Duffy L, Axthelm MK, et al. *Ureaplasma parvum* or *Mycoplasma hominis* as sole pathogens cause chorioamnionitis, preterm delivery, and fetal pneumonia in rhesus macaques. *Reprod Sci.* 2009;16(1):56–70.

73. Yoon BH, Romero R, Chang JW, et al. Microbial invasion of the amniotic cavity with *Ureaplasma urealyticum* is associated with a robust host response in fetal, amniotic, and maternal compartments. *Am J Obstet Gynecol.* 1998;179:1254–1260.

74. Bashiri A, Horowitz S, Huleihel M, Hackmon R, Dukler D, Mazor M. Elevated concentrations of interleukin-6 in intra-amniotic infection with *Ureaplasma urealyticum* in asymptomatic women during genetic amniocentesis. *Acta Obstet Gynecol Scand.* 1999;78(5):379–382.

75. Lal CV, Xu X, Jackson P, et al. *Ureaplasma* infection-mediated release of matrix metalloproteinase-9 and PGP: a novel mechanism of preterm rupture of membranes and chorioamnionitis. *Pediatr Res.* 2017;81(1-1):75–79.

76. Estrada-Gutierrez G, Gomez-Lopez N, Zaga-Clavellina V, et al. Interaction between pathogenic bacteria and intrauterine leukocytes triggers alternative molecular signaling cascades leading to labor in women. *Infect Immun.* 2010;78(11):4792–4799.

77. Crouse DT, Odrezin GT, Cutter GR, et al. Radiographic changes associated with tracheal isolation of *Ureaplasma urealyticum* from neonates. *Clin Infect Dis.* 1993;17(suppl 1):S122–S130.

78. Panero A, Pacifico L, Roggini M, Chiesa C. *Ureaplasma urealyticum* as a cause of pneumonia in preterm infants: analysis of the white cell response. *Arch Dis Child.* 1995;73:F37–F40.

79. Wang EL, Ohlsson A, Kellner JD. Association of *Ureaplasma urealyticum* colonization with chronic lung disease of prematurity: results of a metaanalysis. *J Pediatr.* 1995;127:640–644.

80. Castro-Alcaraz S, Greenberg EM, Bateman DA, Regan JA. Patterns of colonization with *Ureaplasma urealyticum* during neonatal intensive care unit hospitalizations of very low birth weight infants and the development of chronic lung disease. *Pediatrics.* 2002;110(4):E45.

81. Schelonka RL, Katz B, Waites KB, Benjamin DK Jr. Critical appraisal of the role of *Ureaplasma* in the development of bronchopulmonary dysplasia with metaanalytic techniques. *Pediatr Infect Dis J.* 2005;24(12):1033–1039.

82. Theilen U, Lyon AJ, Fitzgerald T, Hendry GM, Keeling JW. Infection with *Ureaplasma urealyticum*: is there a specific clinical and radiological course in the preterm infant? *Arch Dis Child Fetal Neonatal Ed.* 2004;89(2):F163–F167.

83. Pacifico L, Panero A, Roggini M, Rossi N, Bucci G, Chiesa C. *Ureaplasma urealyticum* and pulmonary outcome in a neonatal intensive care population. *Pediatr Infect Dis.* 1997;16:579–586.

84. Honma Y, Yada Y, Takahashi N, Momoi MY, Nakamura Y. Certain type of chronic lung disease of newborns is associated with *Ureaplasma urealyticum* infection in utero. *Pediatr Int.* 2007;49(4):479–484.

85. Lowe J, Watkins WJ, Edwards MO, et al. Association between pulmonary *Ureaplasma* colonization and bronchopulmonary dysplasia in preterm infants: updated systematic review and meta-analysis. *Pediatr Infect Dis J.* 2014;33(7):697–702.

86. Viscardi RM, Kallapur SG. Role of *Ureaplasma* respiratory tract colonization in bronchopulmonary dysplasia pathogenesis: current concepts and update. *Clin Perinatol.* 2015;42(4):719–738.

87. Patterson AM, Taciak V, Lovchik J, Fox RE, Campbell AB, Viscardi RM. *Ureaplasma urealyticum* respiratory tract colonization is associated with an increase in IL-1β and TNF-α relative to IL-6 in tracheal aspirates of preterm infants. *Pediatr Infect Dis J.* 1998;17:321–328.

88. Viscardi RM, Manimtim WM, Sun CCJ, Duffy L, Cassell GH. Lung pathology in premature infants with *Ureaplasma urealyticum* infection. *Pediatr Devel Pathol.* 2002;5:141–150.

89. Viscardi R, Manimtim W, He JR, et al. Disordered pulmonary myofibroblast distribution and elastin expression in preterm infants with *Ureaplasma urealyticum* pneumonitis. *Pediatr Dev Pathol.* 2006;9(2):143–151.

90. Viscardi RM, Atamas SP, Luzina IG, et al. Antenatal *Ureaplasma urealyticum* respiratory tract infection stimulates proinflammatory, profibrotic responses in the preterm baboon lung. *Pediatr Res.* 2006;60(2):141–146.

91. Groneck P, Goetze-Speer B, Speer CP. Inflammatory bronchopulmonary response of preterm infants with microbial colonisation of the airways at birth. *Arch Dis Child Fetal Neonatal Ed.* 1996;74:F51–F55.

92. Baier RJ, Loggins J, Kruger TE. Monocyte chemoattractant protein-1 and interleukin-8 are increased in bronchopulmonary dysplasia: relation to isolation of *Ureaplasma urealyticum*. *J Invest Med.* 2001;49(4):362–369.

93. Walsh WF, Butler J, Coalson J, Hensley D, Cassell GH, deLemos RA. A primate model of *Ureaplasma urealyticum* infection in the premature infant with hyaline membrane disease. *Clin Infect Dis.* 1993;17(suppl 1):S158–S162.

94. Rudd PT, Cassell GH, Waites KB, Davis JK, Duffy LB. *Ureaplasma urealyticum* pneumonia: experimental production and demonstration of age-related susceptibility. *Infect Immun.* 1989;57:918–925.

95. Crouse DT, Cassell GH, Waites KB, Foster JM, Cassady G. Hyeroxia potentiates *Ureaplasma urealyticum* pneumonia in newborn mice. *Infect Immun.* 1990;58:3487–3493.

96. Viscardi RM, Kaplan J, Lovchik JC, et al. Characterization of a murine model of *Ureaplasma urealyticum* pneumonia. *Infect Immun.* 2002;70:5721–5729.

97. Yoder BA, Coalson JJ, Winter VT, Siler-Khodr T, Duffy LB, Cassell GH. Effects of antenatal colonization with *Ureaplasma urealyticum* on pulmonary disease in the immature baboon. *Pediatr Res.* 2003;54:797–807.

98. Collins JJ, Kallapur SG, Knox CL, et al. Inflammation in fetal sheep from intra-amniotic injection of *Ureaplasma parvum. Am J Physiol Lung Cell Mol Physiol.* 2010;299(6):L852–L860.

99. Polglase GR, Dalton RG, Nitsos I, et al. Pulmonary vascular and alveolar development in preterm lambs chronically colonized with *Ureaplasma parvum. Am J Physiol Lung Cell Mol Physiol.* 2010;299(2):L232–L241.

100. Li YH, Brauner A, Jonsson B, et al. *Ureaplasma urealyticum*-induced production of proinflammatory cytokines by macrophages. *Pediatr Res.* 2000;48:114–119.

101. Li YH, Yan ZQ, Jensen JS, Tullus K, Brauner A. Activation of nuclear factor kappaB and induction of inducible nitric oxide synthase by *Ureaplasma urealyticum* in macrophages. *Infect Immun.* 2000;68(12):7087–7093.

102. Li YH, Brauner A, Jensen JS, Tullus K. Induction of human macrophage vascular endothelial growth factor and intercellular adhesion molecule-1 by *Ureaplasma urealyticum* and downregulation by steroids. *Biol Neonate.* 2002;82(1):22–28.

103. Li YH, Chen M, Brauner A, Zheng C, Skov Jensen J, Tullus K. *Ureaplasma urealyticum* induces apoptosis in human lung epithelial cells and macrophages. *Biol Neonate.* 2002;82(3):166–173.

104. Manimtim WM, Hasday JD, Hester L, Fairchild KD, Lovchik JC, Viscardi RM. *Ureaplasma urealyticum* modulates endotoxin-induced cytokine release by human monocytes derived from preterm and term newborns and adults. *Infect Immun.* 2001;69(6):3906–3915.

105. LeVine AM, Kurak KE, Bruno MD, Stark JM, Whitsett JA, Korfhagen TR. Surfactant protein-A-deficient mice are susceptible to *Pseudomonas aeruginosa* infection. *Am J Respir Cell Mol Biol.* 1998;19(4):700–708.

106. LeVine AM, Kurak KE, Wright JR, et al. Surfactant protein-A binds group B streptococcus enhancing phagocytosis and clearance from lungs of surfactant protein-A-deficient mice. *Am J Respir Cell Mol Biol.* 1999;20(2):279–286.

107. Famuyide ME, Hasday JD, Carter HC, Chesko KL, He JR, Viscardi RM. Surfactant protein-A limits *Ureaplasma*-mediated lung inflammation in a murine pneumonia model. *Pediatr Res.* 2009;66(2):162–167.

108. Okogbule-Wonodi AC, Chesko KL, Famuyide ME, Viscardi RM. Surfactant protein-A enhances ureaplasmacidal activity in vitro. *Innate Immun.* 2011;17(2):145–151.

109. Kaisho T, Akira S. Pleiotropic function of toll-like receptors. *Microbes Infect.* 2004;6(15):1388–1394.

110. Peltier MR, Freeman AJ, Mu HH, Cole BC. Characterization of the macrophage-stimulating activity from *Ureaplasma urealyticum. Am J Reprod Immunol.* 2007;57(3):186–192.

111. Shimizu T, Kida Y, Kuwano K. *Ureaplasma parvum* lipoproteins, including MB antigen, activate NF-κB through TLR1, TLR2 and TLR6. *Microbiology.* 2008;154(Pt 5):1318–1325.

112. Harju K, Glumoff V, Hallman M. Ontogeny of toll-like receptors Tlr2 and Tlr4 in mice. *Pediatr Res.* 2001;49(1):81–83.

113. Hillman NH, Moss TJ, Nitsos I, et al. Toll-like receptors and agonist responses in the developing fetal sheep lung. *Pediatr Res.* 2008;63(4):388–393.

114. Awasthi S, Cropper J, Brown KM. Developmental expression of toll-like receptors-2 and -4 in preterm baboon lung. *Dev Comp Immunol.* 2008;32(9):1088–1098.

115. Winters AH, Levan TD, Vogel SN, Chesko KL, Pollin TI, Viscardi RM. Single nucleotide polymorphism in toll-like receptor 6 is associated with a decreased risk for *Ureaplasma* respiratory tract colonization and bronchopulmonary dysplasia in preterm infants. *Pediatr Infect Dis J.* 2013;32(8):898–904.

116. Renaudin H, Bebear C. Comparative in vitro activity of azithromycin, clarithromycin, erythromycin and lomefloxacin against *Mycoplasma pneumoniae, Mycoplasma hominis* and *Ureaplasma urealyticum. Eur J Clin Microbiol Infect Dis.* 1990;9(11):838–841.

117. Bowman ED, Dharmalingam A, Fan WQ, Brown F, Garland SM. Impact of erythromycin on respiratory colonization of *Ureaplasma urealyticum* and the development of chronic lung disease in extremely low birth weight infants. *Pediatr Infect Dis J.* 1998;17:615–620.

118. Jonsson B, Rylander M, Faxelius G. *Ureaplasma urealyticum*, erythromycin and respiratory morbidity in high-risk preterm neonates. *Acta Paediatr.* 1998;87:1079–1084.

119. Baier RJ, Loggins J, Kruger TE. Failure of erythromycin to eliminate airway colonization with *Ureaplasma urealyticum* in very low birth weight infants. *BMC Pediatr.* 2003;3:10.

120. Rubin BK. Macrolides as biologic response modifiers. *J Respir Dis.* 2002;23:S31–S38.

121. Ianaro A, Ialenti A, Maffia P, et al. Anti-inflammatory activity of macrolide antibiotics. *J Pharmacol Exp Ther.* 2000;292(1):156–163.

122. Tsai WC, Standiford TJ. Immunomodulatory effects of macrolides in the lung: lessons from in-vitro and in-vivo models. *Curr Pharm Des.* 2004;10(25):3081–3093.

123. Segal LN, Clemente JC, Wu BG, et al. Randomised, double-blind, placebo-controlled trial with azithromycin selects for anti-inflammatory microbial metabolites in the emphysematous lung. *Thorax.* 2017;72(1):13–22.

124. Duffy LB, Crabb D, Searcey K, Kempf MC. Comparative potency of gemifloxacin, new quinolones, macrolides, tetracycline and clindamycin against *Mycoplasma* spp. *J Antimicrob Chemother.* 2000;45(suppl 1):29–33.

125. Girard AE, Cimochowski CR, Faiella JA. Correlation of increased azithromycin concentrations with phagocyte infiltration into sites of localized infection. *J Antimicrob Chemother.* 1996;37(suppl C):9–19.

126. Patel KB, Xuan D, Tessier PR, Russomanno JH, Quintiliani R, Nightingale CH. Comparison of bronchopulmonary pharmacokinetics of clarithromycin and azithromycin. *Antimicrob Agents Chemother*. 1996;40(10):2375–2379.

127. Capitano B, Mattoes HM, Shore E, et al. Steady-state intrapulmonary concentrations of moxifloxacin, levofloxacin, and azithromycin in older adults. *Chest*. 2004;125(3):965–973.

128. Auten RL, Ekekezie II. Blocking leukocyte influx and function to prevent chronic lung disease of prematurity. *Pediatr Pulmonol*. 2003;35(5):335–341.

129. Liao L, Ning Q, Li Y, et al. CXCR2 blockade reduces radical formation in hyperoxia-exposed newborn rat lung. *Pediatr Res*. 2006;60(3):299–303.

130. Walls SA, Kong L, Leeming HA, Placencia FX, Popek EJ, Weisman LE. Antibiotic prophylaxis improves *Ureaplasma*-associated lung disease in suckling mice. *Pediatr Res*. 2009;66(2):197–202.

131. Hassan HE, Othman AA, Eddington ND, et al. Pharmacokinetics, safety, and biologic effects of azithromycin in extremely preterm infants at risk for *Ureaplasma* colonization and bronchopulmonary dysplasia. *J Clin Pharmacol*. 2011;51(9):1264–1275.

132. Ohlsson A, Wang E, Vearncombe M. Leukocyte counts and colonization with *Ureaplasma urealyticum* in preterm neonates. *Clin Infect Dis*. 1993;17(suppl 1):S144–S147.

5

Definitions and Diagnostic Criteria of Bronchopulmonary Dysplasia: Clinical and Research Implications

Eduardo Bancalari, Nelson Claure, Alan H. Jobe, and Matthew M. Laughon

6

- Bronchopulmonary dysplasia (BPD) is a common complication of prematurity that results from abnormal lung development that leads to chronic impairment of lung function.
- Use of standard diagnostic classifications of BPD and its severity is important in clinical trials that evaluate therapeutic strategies, in epidemiologic cohorts, and to benchmark respiratory outcomes in neonatal centers.
- Standard criteria to diagnose BPD do not consistently predict long-term lung health. This is because postdischarge events can positively or negatively affect lung structure and function.
- Better markers of lung injury that may predict more precisely long-term lung health in this population are needed.

Bronchopulmonary dysplasia (BPD) results from abnormal lung development after premature birth and prolonged respiratory support. BPD progresses from initial respiratory failure that evolves into more chronic forms of lung disease. The impaired lung function associated with BPD frequently persists through childhood and into adulthood. Therefore it is important that the diagnostic criteria define the severity of the pulmonary dysfunction and provide prognostic indicators of the degree of respiratory impairment after the initial hospital discharge. Standard BPD diagnostic and severity criteria are also important to compare outcomes in infants included in clinical trials, for epidemiologic identification of risk factors, and to compare outcomes between centers or within centers for quality improvement activities.

We provide a brief update of the epidemiology of BPD, describe the most frequent diagnostic criteria of BPD, and discuss their possible advantages and limitations with the changing presentation and management.

Clinical Presentation of BPD

The term "bronchopulmonary dysplasia" was introduced by Northway and collaborators to describe a clinical, radiographic, and pathologic entity that occurred in preterm infants who survived severe respiratory distress syndrome (RDS) after aggressive mechanical ventilation and exposure to high concentrations of inspired oxygen.[1] These infants had severe respiratory failure shortly after birth and required mechanical ventilation and supplemental oxygen for long periods. The severity of the respiratory failure and the radiographic images from these infants were clear evidence of their serious lung derangement that resulted in poor short- and long-term outcomes. This presentation of BPD changed over the years with the introduction of prenatal steroid therapy, postnatal surfactant treatments, and the many advances in respiratory support.[2] The severe forms of BPD are less common and have been replaced by milder forms that occur more frequently as the survival of extremely premature infants has markedly increased.

The underlying abnormality in the lungs of the premature infant with BPD is a disruption of the normal process of alveolar and capillary development.[3] The more severe cases are also associated with airway and vascular remodeling, leading to airway obstruction and pulmonary hypertension that can be accompanied by interstitial edema and fibrous tissue proliferation.[4]

Although the classic severe forms of BPD are less common today, some infants still have a severe clinical course with a prolonged need for respiratory support resulting in significant respiratory failure, pulmonary hypertension, and marked alterations in the chest radiographs. These infants offer minimal diagnostic or prognostic dilemma. The difficulty lies with the diagnosis of the less severe forms of BPD that have a mild initial respiratory course and require only low levels of respiratory support. The clinical and radiographic evidence in these infants is less conclusive than that in infants with severe BPD. The radiographs show mainly diffuse haziness, indicating loss of gas volume or fluid accumulation. Dense areas of segmental or lobar atelectasis or pneumonic infiltrates are occasionally observed but there are no areas of severe overinflation typical of the severe forms of BPD.

Lethal, severe cases of BPD were characterized by morphologic alterations, including emphysema, atelectasis, and fibrosis, and marked epithelial squamous metaplasia and smooth muscle hypertrophy in the airways and in the pulmonary vasculature.[5] These alterations were associated with airway obstruction, pulmonary hypertension, and cor pulmonale that resulted from prolonged respiratory failure. Infants developing BPD today are considerably more immature than the earlier cases of severe BPD, and the incidence of BPD among infants born after 32 weeks' gestation has become negligible in modern neonatal centers. Today, BPD predominantly occurs in infants of less than 29 weeks' gestation. The incidence of BPD in infants of less than 29 weeks' gestational age (GA) in the centers of the Eunice Kennedy Shriver National Institute of Child Health and Human Development (NICHD) Neonatal Research Network (NRN) was 42% during the years 2003 to 2007.[6] According to a recent report from stratified samples of nearly one-fifth of U.S. hospitals, the incidence of BPD among surviving infants of birth weights below 1500 g has declined from 50% to 60% in the 1990s to nearly 40% in the years 2000 to 2006.[7] However, in the past 10 years the incidence of BPD in infants born before 28 weeks in the centers of the NICHD-NRN has slightly increased.[8]

The initial presentation of the infants who develop BPD, even when they are more premature, is more heterogeneous than in earlier years. Most infants who had BPD in earlier years had severe RDS, and it is likely that the incidence of BPD would have been even higher absent the relatively high early mortality resulting from severe respiratory failure in those years. At present, many premature infants who develop BPD present with no or only mild RDS after birth. Based on autopsy and animal models the BPD cases today probably have a reduction in alveolar septation and vascular development,[2,3,5,9–11] suggesting that the underlying lung immaturity contributes to the pathogenesis and the clinical presentation of BPD.

BPD Diagnosis

Clinicians are confident with a diagnosis of severe BPD because there are not diagnostic ambiguities. These infants have persistent severe respiratory failure and require supplemental oxygen and respiratory support for prolonged periods, which indicates severe chronic lung injury and conveys a poor long-term prognosis. In contrast, most infants who develop BPD today have mild or transient initial respiratory distress.[12–14] Although these infants receive prolonged respiratory support, they do not require high levels of assistance and the support is not always continuous, which results in inconsistencies in the diagnosis of BPD based on the levels of respiratory support.[15]

Because diagnostic criteria for BPD are intended not only for use by clinicians to diagnose individual infants but also for benchmarking clinical outcomes and as endpoints for clinical and epidemiologic studies, such criteria are expected to fulfill several requirements:

1. They should capture the severity of lung damage. This is particularly important because the lung dysfunction associated with BPD is a continuum from mild to severe disease rather than a categorical presence or absence of disease.

2. They must provide meaningful information to clinicians, serve as a reliable outcome to researchers, and, ideally, predict long-term lung function and health.
3. They must be based on objective and verifiable data that can be easily obtained from the medical record. This is necessary for standardization purposes for benchmarking clinical outcomes within and between neonatal centers and in epidemiologic or interventional studies.
4. They should not be affected by confounding pathologies that can produce respiratory failure or by therapies that may acutely but transiently improve lung function at the time of assessment.

While some of the current diagnostic criteria of BPD fulfill most of these requirements, none fulfills all of them. This is in part because current criteria rely on treatments for the respiratory failure rather than on assessments of lung structure or function. Until now, the diagnostic criteria have been primarily based on the need for supplemental oxygen as the marker of respiratory failure with the duration of supplemental oxygen and the fraction of inspired oxygen (FIO_2) needed for adequate arterial oxygen levels used as surrogates of the severity of BPD. There are some important caveats in using oxygen supplementation as the main criterion to diagnose BPD. Although the need for oxygen is a simple variable to assess, oxygen is also linked to the pathogenesis of BPD and is the main therapy used to maintain adequate oxygenation in respiratory failure from any cause.

The indications for supplemental oxygen can vary from center to center because there is no consensus among clinicians on the optimal arterial oxygen level for these infants. In addition, there are interventions, such as steroids, diuretics, and respiratory stimulants, that can change oxygen requirement. The use of different forms of respiratory support can also influence the need for supplemental oxygen and the diagnosis of BPD. Application of positive airway pressure in any form can improve gas exchange and oxygenation, thereby reducing the need for oxygen. For this reason, most diagnostic criteria of BPD must also include the use of positive airway pressure.

Diagnosis Based on Various Supplemental Oxygen Criteria

Continuous Oxygen Use for the First 28 Days

A workshop sponsored by the National Institutes of Health in 1979 proposed the diagnosis of BPD based on a continued use of supplemental oxygen during the first 28 days plus clinical and radiographic findings compatible with chronic lung disease.[16] These criteria are not suitable for today's preterm infants who develop chronic lung disease because many of them do not receive continuous supplemental oxygen for the first month after birth. Fig. 6.1 illustrates a declining proportion of premature infants who require supplemental oxygen during the first week after birth. As shown in Fig. 6.2 this results in a small proportion of premature infants who require continuous supplemental oxygen during the first 28 days after birth. Nevertheless, many infants who initially need oxygen for only a few days will subsequently have prolonged oxygen dependency and chronic respiratory failure. This is also illustrated in the increasing proportion of infants who require oxygen after the first and second week shown in Fig. 6.1. These infants present a diagnostic dilemma because they have an early relatively mild but persistent respiratory insufficiency that cannot be directly attributed to their initial RDS but they do have persistent chronic lung changes.[17]

Supplemental Oxygen at Day 28

To simplify the diagnosis of BPD some clinicians and investigators have classified as BPD infants who require supplemental oxygen *at* day 28.[18] This approach simplifies the diagnosis of BPD by eliminating the need to count days of oxygen supplementation. However, this single time point criterion lacks specificity and has important limitations. Some infants may require supplemental oxygen around day 28 because of a transient deterioration and not because of chronic lung damage. On the other hand, in the smaller infants the 4-week postnatal age assessment time may be too early to be a reliable indicator of chronic lung disease, whereas in the older infants it may be too late (see Fig. 6.1).

Oxygen at 36 Weeks Postmenstrual Corrected Age

The use of supplemental oxygen at 36 weeks postmenstrual age (PMA) has become the most frequent criterion to diagnose BPD.[18] This criterion was introduced to

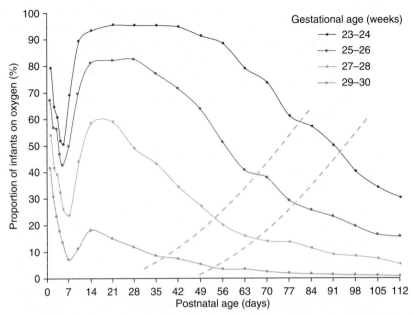

Fig. 6.1 The figure shows the proportion of infants who require supplemental oxygen during the first 16 weeks for each stratum of gestational age (GA). Varying proportions of infants require oxygen supplementation at different time points during the first 4 weeks after birth with increasing proportions at lower gestations. Most infants have an initial decline in the need for supplemental oxygen, but the proportion of infants requiring supplemental oxygen increases after the first week, peaks between weeks 2 and 4, and remains elevated for several weeks. This is more evident among infants of lower GA. *Dashed lines* show the proportion of infants classified as having bronchopulmonary dysplasia (BPD) based on their need for oxygen at 36 weeks PMA for each 2-week GA stratum. (Data from 1735 infants of 23–30 weeks GA admitted to the neonatal intensive care unit of Holtz Children's Hospital of the Jackson Health System/University of Miami during the years 2005–2015. The proportion of infants receiving supplemental oxygen is calculated from the infants alive at each postnatal age.)

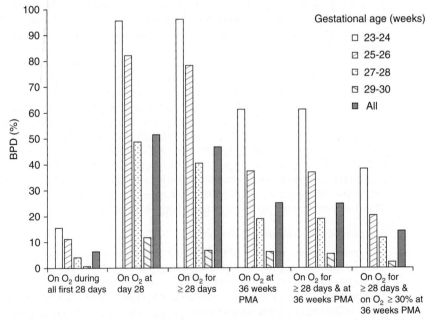

Fig. 6.2 The figure shows the incidence of bronchopulmonary dysplasia *(BPD)* according to each diagnostic criteria of BPD across different gestational ages. A small proportion of infants require oxygen continuously during the first 28 days. A considerably greater proportion of infants need oxygen at day 28 or longer than 28 days. This is particularly evident in the lower GA groups. Nearly two-thirds of those infants remain oxygen-dependent at 36 weeks postmenstrual age *(PMA)* and about one-third of them need an oxygen concentration of 30% or higher. (Data from 1735 infants of 23–30 weeks GA admitted to the neonatal intensive care unit of Holtz Children's Hospital of the Jackson Health System/University of Miami during the years 2005–2015 who were alive at 36 weeks postmenstrual age.)

Table 6.1 NATIONAL INSTITUTES OF HEALTH WORKSHOP DEFINITION OF BRONCHOPULMONARY DYSPLASIA

Gestational Age	<32 Weeks	≥32 Weeks
Time point of assessment	36 Weeks PMA or discharge to home, whichever comes first	>28 days but <56 days postnatal age or discharge to home, whichever comes first
Treatment With Oxygen Concentration >21% for At Least 28 Days *Plus*		
Mild BPD	Breathing room air at 36 weeks PMA or discharge, whichever comes first	Breathing room air by 56 days postnatal age or discharge, whichever comes first
Moderate BPD	Need for <30% oxygen at 36 weeks PMA or discharge, whichever comes first	Need for <30% oxygen at 56 days postnatal age or discharge, whichever comes first
Severe BPD	Need for ≥30% oxygen and/or positive pressure (PPV or NCPAP) at 36 weeks PMA or discharge, whichever comes first	Need for ≥30% oxygen and/or positive pressure (PPV or NCPAP) at 56 days postnatal age or discharge, whichever comes first

BPD, Bronchopulmonary dysplasia; *NCPAP*, nasal continuous positive airway pressure; *PMA*, postmenstrual age; *PPV*, positive-pressure ventilation.
Reprinted with permission of the American Thoracic Society. Copyright © 2018 American Thoracic Society. Adapted from Jobe AH, Bancalari E. Bronchopulmonary dysplasia. *Am J Respir Crit Care Med.* 2001;163(7):1723–1729. The American Journal of Respiratory and Critical Care Medicine is an official journal of the American Thoracic Society.

define the abnormal respiratory status at near-term corrected age and to better predict poor long-term outcome.

By adjusting for GA oxygen use at 36 weeks requires longer times of supplemental oxygen for the more immature infants. An infant born at 24 weeks of gestation must be receiving oxygen at 12 weeks after birth to meet criteria, whereas one born at 30 weeks is labeled as having BPD if receiving supplemental oxygen at 6 weeks of age. Fig. 6.1 illustrates the relatively longer oxygen supplementation in infants in the lower GA stratum who are still oxygen dependent at 36 weeks PMA. A serious limitation of BPD diagnosed only by the need for oxygen at a specific time point is that it will capture infants without chronic lung disease who may be receiving oxygen only briefly for other reasons.

Cumulative Oxygen Supplementation Combined With Oxygen Requirement at 36 Weeks PMA

The diagnostic classification of BPD based on the cumulative need for oxygen longer than 28 days and at 36 weeks PMA as recommended by the NIH workshop in 2001[19] addressed the limitations of using oxygen requirement at a single time point or the duration of oxygen dependency as the only indicators of BPD. The recommendations included a cumulative duration of oxygen supplementation of at least 28 days to indicate the chronicity of the lung damage plus the concentration of inspired oxygen at 36 weeks PMA to define the severity of the chronic lung damage at near-term corrected age before discharge. These criteria classify BPD as mild, moderate, and severe based on the F_{IO_2} or the need for positive pressure support at 36 weeks PMA (Table 6.1).

The cumulative oxygen supplementation allows classification of infants with a mild initial respiratory course who may have only intermittent oxygen needs during the first weeks but still have a protracted respiratory course and prolonged oxygen supplementation (see Fig. 6.1). Alternatively, infants with more severe lung damage could be classified using a combination of duration and concentration of inspired oxygen—for example, the area under the curve or mean oxygen exposure over time. Calculating the cumulative supplemental oxygen to assess severity of lung disease can be time-consuming but now this information may be abstracted from electronic medical records.

The striking effect of using different diagnostic criteria for BPD in the same population of infants is illustrated in Fig. 6.2. The proportion of infants who require continuous supplemental oxygen for the first 28 days is much smaller than the

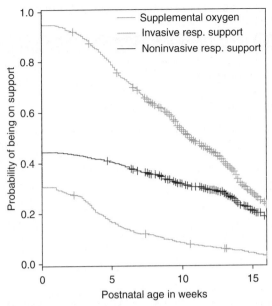

Fig. 6.3 Proportion of infants receiving supplemental oxygen, invasive respiratory *(resp.)* support, and noninvasive respiratory support with advancing postnatal age. (Data from 765 infants of 23–28 weeks gestational age from the centers of the Prematurity and Respiratory Outcomes Program of the National Heart, Lung, and Blood Institute show that about one-fourth of the infants who receive supplemental oxygen also require invasive mechanical ventilation. This proportion remains relatively constant with advancing postnatal age. In contrast, the proportion of infants receiving noninvasive respiratory support among infants who remain oxygen-dependent increases with postnatal age. (Reprinted with permission of the American Thoracic Society. Copyright © 2018 American Thoracic Society. Poindexter BB, Feng R, Schmidt B, et al/2015/Annals of the American Thoracic Society/Comparisons and Limitations of Current Definitions of Bronchopulmonary Dysplasia for the Prematurity and Respiratory Outcomes Program/12/1822–1830. The American Journal of Respiratory and Critical Care Medicine is an official journal of the American Thoracic Society.)

proportion of infants requiring oxygen at 36 weeks PMA. Although most infants who require oxygen continuously during the first 28 days remain oxygen-dependent at 36 weeks PMA, these infants account only for a small fraction of the infants who develop BPD. The proportion of infants who require oxygen at 36 weeks PMA is nearly half of those who are require oxygen at day 28 or those with a cumulative duration of at least 28 days. Thus there is relatively low specificity of using the need for oxygen at an early age or even the cumulative duration of oxygen use to determine the need for oxygen at a later age or at discharge.

The NIH workshop criteria recommended classifying cases as severe BPD in infants who require supplemental oxygen at 30% or higher or receive any form of positive-pressure respiratory support at 36 weeks PMA. Nearly half of the infants who need supplemental oxygen at 36 weeks PMA meet this definition of severe BPD (Fig. 6.2). Most infants meet these criteria based on their need for oxygen and few because of the need for positive-pressure respiratory support. However, this is likely to vary significantly among institutions depending on respiratory support practices. Fig. 6.3, based on data from the centers of the Prematurity and Respiratory Outcomes Program (PROP) of the National Heart, Lung, and Blood Institute,[20] shows that the proportion of infants who receive invasive mechanical ventilation is about one-fourth of the infants who receive supplemental oxygen. This proportion remains relatively constant with postnatal age. In contrast, the proportion of infants receiving noninvasive respiratory support out of the infants who remain oxygen-dependent increases with postnatal age.

In recent years the use of nasal cannulas (NCs) has increased considerably. As evidenced in the data from PROP centers, 47% of infants younger than 29 weeks of gestation received oxygen via NC at 36 weeks PMA.[20] Because the effective F_{IO_2} and airway pressure vary widely and are not measured, NC therapy has introduced a new variable to the diagnosis of BPD. This is particularly evident among infants who receive low flows or low oxygen concentrations.

The use of a higher concentration of supplemental oxygen as a criterion to diagnose BPD severity reduces the ambiguity resulting from the use of low supplemental oxygen, nasal continuous positive airway pressure (NCPAP), or NCs as indicators of lung disease.

Some clinicians have suggested using 40 weeks corrected age as the time point to establish the diagnosis of BPD.[21] The advantage of using term corrected age is that a later diagnosis selects a group of infants with more severe disease and may better predict later outcomes. Recent data from the Canadian Neonatal Network (CNN),[22] applying the diagnostic criteria of BPD at 40 weeks PMA, show that BPD diagnosed at this later point is better correlated with long-term respiratory and neurosensory outcomes than when the diagnosis is made at 36 weeks. The main limitation of this later time point is that a larger number of infants are transferred or discharged from the hospital before that time, thus excluding them from this classification. In the cohort reported by the CNN the BPD rate declined from 46% at 36 weeks PMA to 28% at 40 weeks, but more than a third of the decline resulted from attrition in the cohort. This limitation can be addressed by classifying these infants at the time of discharge or transfer.

Impact of the Arterial Oxygenation Targets

The need for oxygen supplementation is influenced by the saturation target used in each center. Centers that target higher oxygen saturation levels keep infants in the hospital longer and receiving higher supplemental oxygen and vice versa.[23] To minimize the influence of different oxygen targets on the incidence of BPD, Walsh et al. developed a test to standardize the need for oxygen at 36 weeks PMA as part of the BPD assessment.[24] Infants receiving oxygen at a concentration less than 30% are challenged by decreasing the inspired oxygen to 21%. Only infants who are unable to maintain arterial oxygen saturation at or above 90% while breathing room air are classified as BPD cases. Applying this test to a cohort of premature infants from the NICHD-NRN reduced the BPD incidence from 35% based on the clinical use of oxygen to 25% with the standardized test.[24] As the saturation targets are better maintained in recent years the impact of this test on the diagnosis of BPD has become less relevant. The test also does not accommodate the high NC flows used today, without a more complex testing scheme that includes both oxygen and flow reduction. In practice, oxygen and/or flow reduction tests are difficult to perform even for clinical trials.[20]

Competing Outcomes

Differences in mortality rates before 36 weeks PMA can influence the incidence of BPD in surviving infants. A composite outcome such as "BPD or death before 36 weeks PMA" can be used to adjust for the effect of mortality.[25] With this approach, one assumes that if the infants had survived they would have developed BPD. Although this is a valid statistical approach, it is important that the rates of the individual components—death and BPD—are also reported separately because of the obvious difference in importance. In addition, the cause of death may differ in trials in the BPD population. For example, a therapy may shift deaths from BPD to sepsis by immune suppression without changing the death rate. Any change in the death rate is more important than the possible effects of an intervention on BPD. The same concept applies to other major outcomes such as neurologic development in the preterm infant. As an example, the effects of high-dose postnatal steroids that improve the short-term respiratory outcomes may increase the risk of cerebral palsy.[26] Deaths before 36 weeks will include the majority of infants with respiratory failure from severe progressive lung injury.[20] These infants most likely would have had BPD had they survived. This population of infants with respiratory deaths before 36 weeks should also be considered for the most innovative and high-risk therapies for BPD.

Predicting BPD

Predictors of disease are more commonly known as risk factors. In general, risk is used to mean probability of disease occurrence; however, risk may represent a wide variety of statistical measures that include incidence, prevalence, rates, or odds.

A risk factor generally implies an increase in the outcome of interest with exposure, though risk measures may also represent protective effects.[27] A risk factor does not imply that all participants will develop the disease. For example, infants born at 23 weeks have a high risk of death (about 50%), but clearly there will be survivors. When compared with infants born at 24 weeks, the risk of death decreases greatly to about 25%. Thus the relative risk of death increases by 100% (from 25% to 50% in this example). The relative terms that are often used need to be put into perspective using the incidence of the risk factor and the incidence of the outcome of interest.

Risk Factors for BPD Before Birth

Antenatal Steroids, Chorioamnionitis, and Fetal Growth Restriction

Antenatal steroids decrease the severity of RDS and decrease mortality[28,29] and thus were thought to decrease the risk of BPD.[30] In a Cochrane analysis that included 818 infants from 6 studies, the risk of BPD (defined as oxygen use at 36 weeks PMA) was not significantly different between infants who were exposed to antenatal steroids compared to controls (relative risk [RR] 0.86, 95% confidence interval [CI] 0.61–1.22).[31] This suggests that antenatal steroids do not decrease the risk of BPD per se and that this may be due to an increase in survival of the most immature infants at highest risk for BPD.

Chorioamnionitis is a frequent cause of preterm delivery. The clinical diagnosis of chorioamnionitis based on maternal symptoms is subject to significant variability among providers and may not reflect acute inflammatory changes. Histologic evidence of chorioamnionitis is the gold standard, may reflect chronic infection, and is not often available in a timely fashion for infant management. Antenatal inflammation, including chorioamnionitis, is associated with an increased rate of lung maturation[32] and a significant decrease in the incidence of RDS.[33,34] Chorioamnionitis is also associated with a disturbance in the normal lung maturation and growth process that may affect the development of BPD.[35–37] A recent meta-analysis suggested that even when adjusted for other confounding factors, an association between chorioamnionitis and an increased risk for BPD still remains.[38] However, other studies aimed at identifying the role of chorioamnionitis in the development of BPD using clinical or histologic diagnosis have not shown a clear association with BPD.[39,40] The association between chorioamnionitis and BPD may include less RDS because of induced lung maturation, severe RDS with inflammation/pneumonia leading to BPD, and confounding of RDS from postnatal interventions that change the association between chorioamnionitis and BPD.[41]

Fetal growth restriction, defined as a birth weight less than 1 standard deviation below the median, is associated with an increased risk of BPD among premature infants. Bose et al. evaluated the characteristics and potential risk factors for BPD among 1241 infants. For infants born before 28 weeks' GA, growth restriction was highly predictive of the development of BPD in all GAs except the lowest stratum (23–24 weeks) after adjustment for preeclampsia and fetal indications for delivery, chorioamnionitis, and neonatal characteristics.[42]

Infant Demographics

GA, Birth Weight, and Gender

Extreme prematurity and extremely low birth weight are well-established risk factors for BPD. GA and birth weight are inversely proportional to the incidence and severity of BPD (see Figs. 6.1 and 6.2). Among infants meeting the physiologic definition of BPD at 36 weeks postmenstrual age (PMA), 95% have very low birth weights.[24] In 2003–2007, the incidence of BPD at 23 weeks PMA (as defined as oxygen at 36 weeks PMA) in the centers of the NICHD-NRN was 73%, and 56% of those had severe BPD.[6] In contrast, at 28 weeks PMA, the incidence of BPD was 23% with only 8% of infants with severe BPD. Male infants have a higher risk of developing BPD compared with females.[43]

Postnatal Risk Factors

Mechanical Ventilation, Patent Ductus Arteriosus, and Oxygen Use

Mechanical ventilation is lifesaving but uses positive pressure that can produce ventilator-induced lung injury.[44,45] With the availability of surfactant therapy since 1990, many extremely premature infants received surfactant followed by mechanical ventilation. However, reports emerged about substantial differences in BPD rates showing that centers that used more mechanical ventilation had more cases of BPD.[46,47] For example, the risk of BPD ranges from less than 10% to more than 40% among the NRN centers in the Benchmarking Trial in infants with birth weights less than 1250 g.[48] This variation was not explained by differences in birth weight, GA, race, frequency of prenatal steroid use, or incidence of RDS.

Avoidance of mechanical ventilation might decrease the risk of injury and BPD and might also explain some of the center differences in BPD rates.[47] Mechanical ventilation often begins shortly after birth; therefore delivery room management strategies might influence the risk of BPD.[49,50] The use of NCPAP is a successful strategy for avoiding the need for mechanical ventilation in some infants, with the benefit of decreasing the risk of BPD.[51] Although mechanical ventilation can be avoided by using NCPAP in the delivery room, this means that some of these infants will receive delayed surfactant treatments or do not need surfactant.

The role of the patent ductus arteriosus (PDA) in the development of BPD in preterm infants remains controversial. A PDA has been associated with the need for prolonged mechanical ventilation, increased mortality, and a higher risk of BPD.[52,53] However, the relationship between PDA and BPD is often distorted by confounding factors such as GA and illness severity and may not be causal. Studies to assess the role of ductal closure in the prevention of BPD have small sample sizes. Meta-analyses have not consistently shown a decrease in the risk of BPD with closing the PDA.[54–56] In a systematic review, Benitz compiled all available randomized controlled trials to create a pooled point estimate for the associations between PDA closure and multiple morbidities. The pooled estimate showed a strong effect of pharmacologic therapies (OR 0.23, 95% CI 0.20–0.26) to close the duct; however, the effects on the incidence of BPD and BPD or death were inconsistent.[57] It is possible that the presence of a PDA is only a marker for an increased risk of BPD.[58] However, the large rate of crossover and the design of the studies limits assessments of the risks and benefits of strategies designed to close the PDA.

The use of supplemental oxygen therapy in infants is used to diagnose BPD, but oxygen use has also been implicated as a potential toxin for the developing lung and brain.[59] Infants who require high amounts of oxygen exposure may represent a sicker group of infants for whom gas exchange is already impaired at the alveolar level. However, oxygen can also produce oxidative injury to capillary, endothelial, and alveolar membranes. Prior studies have indicated that high levels of oxygen exposure result in increased polymorphonuclear cell migration, increased proteolysis, and elevated levels of inflammatory cytokines.[60,61] Yet oxygen therapy is often necessary in premature infants to prevent hypoxemia, and oxygen may be important for cell growth and development. In the Benefits of Oxygen Saturation Targeting (BOOST)-1 trial, infants younger than 30 weeks who were randomly assigned to receive higher oxygen saturations (95%–98%) compared with standard oxygen saturations (92%–94%) at 32 weeks corrected gestation were still receiving oxygen therapy at 36 weeks corrected gestation more often (odds risk [OR] 1.40, 95% CI 1.15–1.70). However, there was no difference in the growth or development at 12 months between groups.[62]

The need for supplemental oxygen therapy can be a marker of severe illness and is therefore associated with an increased risk of BPD. In the Surfactant, Positive Pressure, and Oxygenation Randomized Trial (SUPPORT), one arm of the study examined the effect of different target ranges of oxygen saturation in extremely preterm infants. Infants who were randomly assigned to receive lower oxygen saturations (85%–89%) compared with infants who were randomly assigned to receive higher oxygen saturations (91%–95%) had similar rates of BPD among survivors (48.5% vs. 54.2%; RR 0.91, 95% CI 0.83–1.01).[63] This would suggest that the role of oxygen in the development of BPD for preterm infants might be due more to the severity of illness than to direct oxygen toxicity. The combined meta-analysis of the oxygen saturation targets may provide additional insight into the risks and benefits of oxygen therapy.

Predictive Models of BPD

Clinicians, parents, and researchers would benefit from an accurate predictive model of BPD risk based on readily available clinical information. Prediction scoring systems for BPD that included birth weight, GA, sex, PDA, sepsis, and exposure to mechanical ventilation have been available but not widely adopted. Problems with these scoring systems include the limitations of the BPD definition used, oxygen therapy at 28 days of life, and the fact that death was not included in all models as a competing outcome for BPD.[64–66] Some models included radiographs as part of the scoring system, which introduces subjectivity and reduces generalizability.[67–70] Several models used respiratory variables that are not readily available to clinicians.[71,72] Despite generally good negative predictive values, the range of the best positive predictive values of these models is low: from 65% to 75%.[67–74] Other significant problems were the absence of a contemporary cohort that included infants who received antenatal corticosteroids, surfactant therapy, or noninvasive respiratory support strategies. None examined the risk of BPD based on the NICHD severity definitions.

An additional problem with previously reported analyses is a lack of detail regarding the change in BPD risk with advancing postnatal age.[64–66,68] Prior multivariate models included risk factors identifiable at birth, as well as exposures up to the time of diagnosis of BPD, but they did not include postnatal age. The inclusion of postnatal age allows for variable contribution of risk factors over time as potential preventative or therapeutic strategies that may be used to decrease the risk of BPD.

A predictive model that overcomes many of these problems using data from the NICHD-NRN Benchmarking Trial is available online at https://neonatal.rti.org.[75] This model includes GA, birth weight, race and ethnicity, sex, respiratory support, and F_{IO_2} in a parsimonious model, providing estimates of severity of BPD or death by postnatal day. In addition, several previously described risk factors—PDA, necrotizing enterocolitis, sepsis, and postnatal corticosteroids—did not significantly improve the prediction of BPD after the other six factors are adjusted for. For example, a white male infant born at 26 weeks (birth weight 750 g) who at day 7 of life is receiving continuous positive airway pressure with an oxygen requirement of 35% has a 19.9% probability of having severe BPD, 34.2% probability of moderate BPD, 28.6% probability of mild BPD, and 10.2% probability of no BPD. An important feature of this model is that the relative contribution of each predicting factor changes with increasing postnatal age. In postnatal day 1 and 3 models, GA provides the most information, whereas in later models, mechanical ventilation conveys the most information. A recent secondary analysis of the Trial of Late Surfactant found that cumulative supplemental oxygen during the first 14 days was independently associated with BPD or death at 36 weeks corrected age.[76]

Defining the Populations at Risk

An important aspect to consider when interpreting data that use a BPD diagnostic classification for benchmarking purposes or in clinical trials is the baseline characteristic of the cohort or population from which the incidence of BPD is being reported. Benchmarking comparisons should also account for differences in mortality between populations. The reported incidence per total admissions is likely to be lower than the incidence among premature infants surviving the neonatal period, at 36 weeks PMA, or at discharge.

Because BPD is greatly influenced by the degree of prematurity, the stratification by GA or birth weight is very important for comparative interpretations between trials or cohorts. Also important is the approach used to define the ranges of birth weight or GA for inclusion in a trial or a cohort. For instance, a cohort that includes only infants born within a specific range of birth weight (e.g., <1000 g) may inadvertently include a high proportion of growth-restricted infants of more advanced GA who meet the birth weight cutoff for inclusion. The risk for BPD in these more mature infants may differ from that of other infants in the same weight strata born at lower GA. A better approach would be to use a given range of GA for eligibility regardless of birth weight.

When interpreting the findings of clinical trials or epidemiologic cohorts, other entry criteria that could change the basal risk for BPD should be considered. For example, studies that include only ventilated preterm infants would have higher BPD rates than studies that include all infants. This is also true for studies that deliberately enroll infants at higher risk of BPD based on their initial respiratory course. The findings from those studies may not be directly applicable to infants of lesser risk or comparable to other studies with different entry criteria. Trials of infants for whom consent for randomization was obtained before birth will differ from those with infants for whom later consent is obtained.

Application of any BPD diagnostic criterion and interpretation of the results should also consider the use of oxygen or other forms of respiratory support for conditions other than parenchymal lung disease. Transient conditions such as abnormal control of breathing, concomitant respiratory illness, and the use of medications such as caffeine, diuretics, or steroids can acutely influence the need for oxygen and thereby the classification of BPD.

Center-specific characteristics such as the target range of arterial oxygen saturation and the center's altitude above sea level can also influence the need for supplemental oxygen. More importantly, there may be interactions between these cofactors that further increase the need for oxygen supplementation. A recent study showed that nearly half of the infants with failing oxygen weaning challenge test results developed periodic breathing that led to decreases in arterial oxygen saturation.[77] Some premature infants may need to be maintained at oxygen saturation levels above 90% to stabilize their respiratory control function.

The use of positive-pressure respiratory support in infants with respiratory control issues or airway problems who have minimal parenchymal involvement should also be accounted for when diagnosing BPD. This is particularly important in view of the definition of severity of BPD recommended by the NIH workshop. Based on that definition, infants who do not need or need low supplemental oxygen levels would be classified as severe BPD if they receive positive-pressure support at 36 weeks PMA. If the control of breathing problems eventually subsides, these infants may have normal long-term pulmonary outcomes. This has become a particularly important issue resulting from the increased use of NC flow. When used at higher flows than those required for oxygen supplementation alone, flow can generate positive airway pressure that can stabilize lung volume. On the other hand, when the NC flow is insufficient to meet the infant's inspiratory demand, the cannula itself can produce an obstructive effect and increase the need for inspired oxygen. In addition, with NCs there is uncertainty of the actual F_{IO_2} oxygen and classification of BPD severity becomes difficult to assess. The use of low flow with high oxygen concentrations or high flow with 21% oxygen are major confounders in the diagnosis of BPD and explains the increased incidence of BPD reported in some centers recently.[20] Many of the smaller infants are supported for long periods of NCPAP or NCs because of frequent hypoxemic episodes that are more related to unstable respiratory patterns than to lung parenchymal disease. This is not the case in infants who need high oxygen concentrations at high flow rates that reflect more severe lung damage and predict worse long-term outcome.

Prognosis for Long-Term Impairment

One of the purposes of having diagnostic criteria for BPD is to provide a prognosis for long-term respiratory outcome. BPD at 36 weeks PMA is often associated with adverse health outcomes in infancy and into adulthood. The costs of BPD are both social and economic and are measured in impaired childhood health and quality of life, family stress and economic hardship, and increased health care costs.[78–80] Premature infants with BPD have a longer initial hospitalization than their peers without BPD. The sensitivity and specificity of the different diagnostic criteria of BPD based on the cumulative duration of oxygen for at least 28 days, the need for oxygen at 36 weeks PMA, and the NIH workshop criteria were evaluated in a cohort of infants from the NICHD-NRN at 18 to 22 months corrected age.[81] The criteria including oxygen supplementation for at least 28 days were more sensitive in detecting postdischarge respiratory complications than oxygen dependency at 36 weeks PMA, but the specificity was considerably lower. Both criteria using oxygen dependency at 36 weeks PMA were more specific but at a cost of not classifying some infants as having BPD that may later require additional respiratory care. This was in agreement with a report showing discontinuation of supplemental oxygen after day 28 was a more sensitive test (although less specific) than after 36 weeks PMA in predicting poor long-term pulmonary outcome.[82]

The higher specificity of the severe BPD classification (oxygen use of ≥30% at 36 weeks PMA) on long-term respiratory prognosis clearly showed how this indicator of severity avoided some of the limitations of the milder classifications of BPD. This finding underscores the importance of analyzing not only for the incidence of BPD but also for its severity when conducting clinical trials or epidemiologic studies. Despite this, very few studies report the incidence of severe BPD. Data from the cohort of the NICHD-NRN indicate that the BPD criterion of oxygen at 36 weeks PMA was a better predictor of mental and psychomotor developmental impairment than other criteria.[81] However, the association between poor neurologic outcome and BPD can be confounded by many coexisting morbidities.

The intended use of these diagnostic criteria of BPD has been to characterize the severity of the chronic lung disease and to predict respiratory course later in life. However, it is important to consider that these diagnostic criteria of BPD do not indicate that infants who do not meet these criteria will have normal lung development and function. Multiple studies have shown that long-term lung function in former premature infants is often abnormal compared with term infants.[83,84] These alterations occur in many preterm infants but are more common and severe among infants with BPD. Therefore these working diagnostic criteria of BPD can differentiate patients with more severe lung damage from those less affected, but its absence does not ensure normal lung function. Most preterm infants can maintain adequate arterial oxygen levels without supplemental oxygen at 36 weeks PMA, but this does not rule out underlying alterations in lung structure and function that could manifest later in life or when exposed to higher demands.

The fact that many premature infants have altered respiratory function later in life, irrespective of their BPD classification, suggests that the lung damage associated with premature birth and the impact of the many factors that can interfere with lung development cannot be defined as a simple dichotomized outcome, presence, or absence. Like most biologic processes, BPD may be more appropriately represented by a continuum across the spectrum between normal lung development and the alterations observed in the more severe cases.

The correlation between the diagnosis of BPD and lung function later in life can be affected by many events that can positively or negatively influence lung development and function after discharge from the hospital.[85] While an early diagnostic criterion of BPD that reliably predicts long-term outcome is desirable, it is not realistic. For this reason, it is important to use short- and long-term endpoints in the assessment of BPD. The first should reflect the neonatal respiratory evolution and shorter-term outcome, whereas the second would account for the postnatal respiratory course and longer-term outcome.

Arterial oxygenation or the need for supplemental oxygen to maintain oxygen saturation in the prescribed range provides a practical but relatively crude measure of lung function. Supplemental oxygen alone does not fully reflect the complex alterations in respiratory function that can be at play in these infants. Tests measuring the different aspects of lung function, including lung volumes, pulmonary mechanics, gas distribution, diffusion capacity, and ventilation/perfusion abnormalities that can be used individually or as a battery, could lead to more specific and sensitive ways to predict lung function later in life. Unfortunately, most of these tests are too complex for clinical use and their interpretation is not simple. Until there are more practical and simpler tests to evaluate lung structure and function, the only tools available are basic indicators of gas exchange to classify BPD in these infants and to predict their long-term lung function.

In summary, the use of standard diagnostic classifications of BPD and its severity is important to define the predischarge respiratory condition of the infants at near-term corrected age. These standard criteria should be used to select endpoints for clinical trials that evaluate therapeutic strategies and to monitor clinical outcomes among centers and within centers over time. Most diagnostic criteria of BPD are based on the need for supplemental oxygen and respiratory support to identify the degree of chronic lung dysfunction. Although the need for supplemental oxygen largely reflects the severity of the lung damage at near-term corrected age, a clear need exists for more precise markers of lung injury and function and better predictors of long-term pulmonary health.

REFERENCES

1. Northway WH Jr, Rosan RC, Porter DY. Pulmonary disease following respirator therapy of hyaline-membrane disease. Bronchopulmonary dysplasia. *N Engl J Med.* 1967;276(7):357–368.
2. Jobe AJ. The new BPD: an arrest of lung development. *Pediatr Res.* 1999;46(6):641–643.
3. Husain AN, Siddiqui NH, Stocker JT. Pathology of arrested acinar development in postsurfactant bronchopulmonary dysplasia. *Hum Pathol.* 1998;29(7):710–717.
4. McEvoy CT, Jain L, Schmidt B, Abman S, Bancalari E, Aschner JL. Bronchopulmonary dysplasia: NHLBI Workshop on the Primary Prevention of Chronic Lung Diseases. *Ann Am Thorac Soc.* 2014;11(suppl 3):S146–S153.
5. Margraf LR, Tomashefski JF Jr, Bruce MC, Dahms BB. Morphometric analysis of the lung in bronchopulmonary dysplasia. *Am Rev Respir Dis.* 1991;143(2):391–400.
6. Stoll BJ, Hansen NI, Bell EF, et al. Neonatal outcomes of extremely preterm infants from the NICHD Neonatal Research Network. *Pediatrics.* 2010;126(3):443–456.
7. Stroustrup A, Trasande L. Epidemiological characteristics and resource use in neonates with bronchopulmonary dysplasia: 1993–2006. *Pediatrics.* 2010;126(2):291–297.
8. Stoll BJ, Hansen NI, Bell EF, et al. Trends in care practices, morbidity, and mortality of extremely preterm neonates, 1993–2012. *JAMA.* 2015;314(10):1039–1051.
9. Thibeault DW, Mabry SM, Ekekezie II, Zhang X, Truog WE. Collagen scaffolding during development and its deformation with chronic lung disease. *Pediatrics.* 2003;111(4 Pt 1):766–776.
10. Coalson JJ, Winter V, deLemos RA. Decreased alveolarization in baboon survivors with bronchopulmonary dysplasia. *Am J Respir Crit Care Med.* 1995;152(2):640–646.
11. Abman S. *Pulmonary Hypertension in Chronic Lung Disease of Infancy. Pathogenesis, Pathophysiology and Treatment.* New York: Dekker; 2000.
12. Parker RA, Lindstrom DP, Cotton RB. Improved survival accounts for most, but not all, of the increase in bronchopulmonary dysplasia. *Pediatrics.* 1992;90(5):663–668.
13. Rojas MA, Gonzalez A, Bancalari E, Claure N, Poole C, Silva-Neto G. Changing trends in the epidemiology and pathogenesis of neonatal chronic lung disease. *J Pediatr.* 1995;126(4):605–610.
14. Charafeddine L, D'Angio CT, Phelps DL. Atypical chronic lung disease patterns in neonates. *Pediatrics.* 1999;103(4 Pt 1):759–765.
15. Bancalari E, Claure N, Sosenko IR. Bronchopulmonary dysplasia: changes in pathogenesis, epidemiology and definition. *Semin Neonatal.* 2003;8(1):63–71.
16. Bancalari E, Abdenour GE, Feller R, Gannon J. Bronchopulmonary dysplasia: clinical presentation. *J Pediatr.* 1979;95(5 Pt 2):819–823.
17. Bancalari EH, Jobe AH. The respiratory course of extremely preterm infants: a dilemma for diagnosis and terminology. *J Pediatr.* 2012;161(4):585–588.
18. Shennan AT, Dunn MS, Ohlsson A, Lennox K, Hoskins EM. Abnormal pulmonary outcomes in premature infants: prediction from oxygen requirement in the neonatal period. *Pediatrics.* 1988;82(4):527–532.
19. Jobe AH, Bancalari E. Bronchopulmonary dysplasia. *Am J Respir Crit Care Med.* 2001;163(7): 1723–1729.
20. Poindexter BB, Feng R, Schmidt B, et al. Comparisons and limitations of current definitions of bronchopulmonary dysplasia for the prematurity and respiratory outcomes program. *Ann Am Thorac Soc.* 2015;12(12):1822–1830.
21. Ballard RA, Keller RL, Black DM, et al. Randomized trial of late surfactant treatment in ventilated preterm infants receiving inhaled nitric oxide. *J Pediatr.* 2016;168:23–29.e24.
22. Isayama T, Lee SK, Yang J, et al. Revisiting the definition of bronchopulmonary dysplasia: effect of changing panoply of respiratory support for preterm neonates. *JAMA Pediatr.* 2017;171(3):271–279.
23. Ellsbury DL, Acarregui MJ, McGuinness GA, Klein JM. Variability in the use of supplemental oxygen for bronchopulmonary dysplasia. *J Pediatr.* 2002;140(2):247–249.
24. Walsh MC, Yao Q, Gettner P, et al. Impact of a physiologic definition on bronchopulmonary dysplasia rates. *Pediatrics.* 2004;114(5):1305–1311.
25. Parekh SA, Field DJ, Johnson S, Juszczak E. Accounting for deaths in neonatal trials: is there a correct approach? *Arch Dis Child Fetal Neonatal Ed.* 2015;100(3):F193–F197.
26. Doyle LW, Ehrenkranz RA, Halliday HL. Dexamethasone treatment in the first week of life for preventing bronchopulmonary dysplasia in preterm infants: a systematic review. *Neonatology.* 2010;98(3):217–224.
27. Fletcher RFS. *Clinical Epidemiology.* 4th ed. Philadelphia: Lippincott Williams & Wilkins; 2005.

28. Crowley P. The effects of corticosteroid administration before preterm delivery: an overview of the evidence from controlled trials. *BJOG*. 1990;97(1):11–25.

29. Gilstrap LC, Christensen R, Clewell WH, et al. Effect of corticosteroids for fetal maturation on perinatal outcomes. *JAMA*. 1995;273(5):413–418.

30. Van Marter LJ. Maternal glucocorticoid therapy and reduced risk of bronchopulmonary dysplasia. *Pediatrics (Evanston)*. 1990;86(3):331–336.

31. Roberts D, Dalziel S. Antenatal corticosteroids for accelerating fetal lung maturation for women at risk of preterm birth. *Cochrane Database Syst Rev*. 2006;(3):CD004454.

32. Been JV, Zimmermann LJ. Histological chorioamnionitis and respiratory outcome in preterm infants. *Arch Dis Child Fetal Neonatal Ed*. 2009;94(3):F218–F225.

33. Dempsey E, Chen MF, Kokottis T, Vallerand D, Usher R. Outcome of neonates less than 30 weeks gestation with histologic chorioamnionitis. *Am J Perinatol*. 2005;22(3):155–159.

34. Meredith KS, deLemos RA, Coalson JJ, et al. Role of lung injury in the pathogenesis of hyaline membrane disease in premature baboons. *J Appl Physiol*. 1989;66(5):2150–2158.

35. Richardson BS. Preterm histologic chorioamnionitis: impact on cord gas and pH values and neonatal outcome. *Am J Obstet Gynecol*. 2006;195(5):1357–1365.

36. Mu S-C. Impact on neonatal outcome and anthropometric growth in very low birth weight infants with histological chorioamnionitis. *J Formos Med Assoc*. 2008;107(4):304–310.

37. De Felice C. Histologic chorioamnionitis and severity of illness in very low birth weight newborns. *Pediatr Crit Care Med*. 2005;6(3):298–302.

38. Hartling L, Liang Y, Lacaze-Masmonteil T. Chorioamnionitis as a risk factor for bronchopulmonary dysplasia: a systematic review and meta-analysis. *Arch Dis Child Fetal Neonatal Ed*. 2012;97(1):F8–F17.

39. Prendergast M, May C, Broughton S, et al. Chorioamnionitis, lung function and bronchopulmonary dysplasia in prematurely born infants. *Arch Dis Child Fetal Neonatal Ed*. 2011;96(4):F270–F274.

40. Ahn HM, Park EA, Cho SJ, Kim YJ, Park HS. The association of histological chorioamnionitis and antenatal steroids on neonatal outcome in preterm infants born at less than thirty-four weeks' gestation. *Neonatology*. 2012;102(4):259–264.

41. Van Marter LJ, Dammann O, Allred EN, et al. Chorioamnionitis, mechanical ventilation, and postnatal sepsis as modulators of chronic lung disease in preterm infants. *J Pediatr*. 2002;140(2):171–176.

42. Bose C, Van Marter LJ, Laughon M, et al. Fetal growth restriction and chronic lung disease among infants born before the 28th week of gestation. *Pediatrics*. 2009;124(3):e450–e458.

43. Farstad T, Bratlid D, Medbo S, Markestad T. Bronchopulmonary dysplasia—prevalence, severity and predictive factors in a national cohort of extremely premature infants. *Acta Paediatr*. 2011;100(1):53–58.

44. Muscedere JG, Mullen JB, Gan K, Slutsky AS. Tidal ventilation at low airway pressures can augment lung injury. *Am J Respir Crit Care Med*. 1994;149(5):1327–1334.

45. Meredith KS, deLemos RA, Coalson JJ, et al. Role of lung injury in the pathogenesis of hyaline membrane disease in premature baboons. *J Appl Physiol*. 1989;66(5):2150–2158.

46. Avery ME, Tooley WH, Keller JB, et al. Is chronic lung disease in low birth weight infants preventable? A survey of eight centers. *Pediatrics*. 1987;79(1):26–30.

47. Van Marter LJ, Allred EN, Pagano M, et al. Do clinical markers of barotrauma and oxygen toxicity explain interhospital variation in rates of chronic lung disease? The Neonatology Committee for the Developmental Network. *Pediatrics*. 2000;105(6):1194–1201.

48. Walsh M, Laptook A, Kazzi SN, et al. A cluster-randomized trial of benchmarking and multimodal quality improvement to improve rates of survival free of bronchopulmonary dysplasia for infants with birth weights of less than 1250 grams. *Pediatrics*. 2007;119(5):876–890.

49. Leone TA, Rich W, Finer NN. A survey of delivery room resuscitation practices in the United States. *Pediatrics*. 2006;117(2):e164–e175.

50. Morley CJ, Davis PG, Doyle LW, Brion LP, Hascoet JM, Carlin JB. Nasal CPAP or intubation at birth for very preterm infants. *N Engl J Med*. 2008;358(7):700–708.

51. Finer NN, Carlo WA, Walsh MC, et al. Early CPAP versus surfactant in extremely preterm infants. *N Engl J Med*. 2010;362(21):1970–1979.

52. Schmidt B, Davis P, Moddemann D, et al. Long-term effects of indomethacin prophylaxis in extremely-low-birth-weight infants. *N Engl J Med*. 2001;344(26):1966–1972.

53. Brown ER. Increased risk of bronchopulmonary dysplasia in infants with patent ductus arteriosus. *J Pediatr*. 1979;95(5 Pt 2):865–866.

54. Fowlie PW, Davis PG. Prophylactic intravenous indomethacin for preventing mortality and morbidity in preterm infants. *Cochrane Database Syst Rev*. 2002;(3):CD000174.

55. Cooke L, Steer P, Woodgate P. Indomethacin for asymptomatic patent ductus arteriosus in preterm infants. *Cochrane Database Syst Rev*. 2003;(2):CD003745.

56. Shah SS, Ohlsson A. Ibuprofen for the prevention of patent ductus arteriosus in preterm and/or low birth weight infants. *Cochrane Database Syst Rev*. 2006;(1):CD004213.

57. Benitz WE. Treatment of persistent patent ductus arteriosus in preterm infants: time to accept the null hypothesis? *J Perinatol*. 2010;30(4):241–252.

58. Benitz WE. Patent ductus arteriosus: to treat or not to treat? *Arch Dis Child Fetal Neonatal Ed*. 2012;97(2):F80–F82.

59. Saugstad OD. Chronic lung disease: the role of oxidative stress. *Biol Neonate*. 1998;74(suppl 1):21–28.

60. Ogihara T, Hirano K, Morinobu T, et al. Raised concentrations of aldehyde lipid peroxidation products in premature infants with chronic lung disease. *Arch Dis Child Fetal Neonatal Ed*. 1999;80(1):F21–F25.

61. Delacourt C, d'Ortho MP, Macquin-Mavier I, et al. Oxidant-antioxidant balance in alveolar macrophages from newborn rats. *Eur Respir J.* 1996;9(12):2517–2524.
62. Askie LM, Henderson-Smart DJ, Irwig L, Simpson JM. Oxygen-saturation targets and outcomes in extremely preterm infants. *N Engl J Med.* 2003;349(10):959–967.
63. Carlo WA, Finer NN, Walsh MC, et al. Target ranges of oxygen saturation in extremely preterm infants. *N Engl J Med.* 2010;362(21):1959–1969.
64. Ryan SW, Nycyk J, Shaw BN. Prediction of chronic neonatal lung disease on day 4 of life. *Eur J Pediatr.* 1996;155(8):668–671.
65. Subhedar NV, Hamdan AH, Ryan SW, Shaw NJ. Pulmonary artery pressure: early predictor of chronic lung disease in preterm infants. *Arch Dis Child.* 1998;78(1):F20–F24.
66. Romagnoli C, Zecca E, Tortorolo L, Vento G, Tortorolo G. A scoring system to predict the evolution of respiratory distress syndrome into chronic lung disease in preterm infants. *Intensive Care Med.* 1998;24(5):476–480.
67. Toce SS, Farrell PM, Leavitt LA, Samuels DP, Edwards DK. Clinical and roentgenographic scoring systems for assessing bronchopulmonary dysplasia. *Am J Dis Chil (1960).* 1984;138(6):581–585.
68. Corcoran JD, Patterson CC, Thomas PS, Halliday HL. Reduction in the risk of bronchopulmonary dysplasia from 1980–1990: results of a multivariate logistic regression analysis. *Eur J Pediatr.* 1993;152(8):677–681.
69. Noack G, Mortensson W, Robertson B, Nilsson R. Correlations between radiological and cytological findings in early development of bronchopulmonary dysplasia. *Eur J Pediatr.* 1993;152(12):1024–1029.
70. Yuksel B, Greenough A, Karani J. Prediction of chronic lung disease from the chest radiograph appearance at seven days of age. *Acta Paediatr.* 1993;82(11):944–947.
71. Bhutani VK, Abbasi S. Relative likelihood of bronchopulmonary dysplasia based on pulmonary mechanics measured in preterm neonates during the first week of life. *J Pediatr.* 1992;120(4 Pt 1):605–613.
72. Kim YD, Kim EA, Kim KS, Pi SY, Kang W. Scoring method for early prediction of neonatal chronic lung disease using modified respiratory parameters. *J Korean Med Sci.* 2005;20(3):397–401.
73. Sinkin RA, Cox C, Phelps DL. Predicting risk for bronchopulmonary dysplasia: selection criteria for clinical trials. *Pediatrics.* 1990;86(5):728–736.
74. Rozycki HJ, Narla L. Early versus late identification of infants at high risk of developing moderate to severe bronchopulmonary dysplasia. *Pediatr Pulmonol.* 1996;21(6):345–352.
75. Laughon MM, Langer JC, Bose CL, et al. Prediction of bronchopulmonary dysplasia by postnatal age in extremely premature infants. *Am J Respir Crit Care Med.* 2011;183(12):1715–1722.
76. Wai KC, Kohn MA, Ballard RA, et al. Early cumulative supplemental oxygen predicts bronchopulmonary dysplasia in high risk extremely low gestational age newborns. *J Pediatr.* 2016;177:97–102.e102.
77. Coste F, Ferkol T, Hamvas A, et al. Ventilatory control and supplemental oxygen in premature infants with apparent chronic lung disease. *Arch Dis Child Fetal Neonatal Ed.* 2015;100(3):F233–F237.
78. Vohr BR, Wright LL, Dusick AM, et al. Neurodevelopmental and functional outcomes of extremely low birth weight infants in the National Institute of Child Health and Human Development Neonatal Research Network, 1993–1994. *Pediatrics.* 2000;105(6):1216–1226.
79. Wood NS, Costeloe K, Gibson AT, Hennessy EM, Marlow N, Wilkinson AR. The EPICure study: associations and antecedents of neurological and developmental disability at 30 months of age following extremely preterm birth. *Arch Dis Child Fetal Neonatal Ed.* 2005;90(2):F134–F140.
80. Fily A, Pierrat V, Delporte V, Breart G, Truffert P, EPIPAGE Nord-Pas-de-Calais Study Group. Factors associated with neurodevelopmental outcome at 2 years after very preterm birth: the population-based Nord-Pas-de-Calais EPIPAGE cohort. *Pediatrics.* 2006;117(2):357–366.
81. Ehrenkranz RA, Walsh MC, Vohr BR, et al. Validation of the National Institutes of Health consensus definition of bronchopulmonary dysplasia. *Pediatrics.* 2005;116(6):1353–1360.
82. Davis PG, Thorpe K, Roberts R, et al. Evaluating "old" definitions for the "new" bronchopulmonary dysplasia. *J Pediatr.* 2002;140(5):555–560.
83. Fawke J, Lum S, Kirkby J, et al. Lung function and respiratory symptoms at 11 years in children born extremely preterm: the EPICure study. *Am J Respir Crit Care Med.* 2010;182(2):237–245.
84. Hjalmarson O, Sandberg K. Abnormal lung function in healthy preterm infants. *Am J Respir Crit Care Med.* 2002;165(1):83–87.
85. Stevens TP, Dylag A, Panthagani I, Pryhuber G, Halterman J. Effect of cumulative oxygen exposure on respiratory symptoms during infancy among VLBW infants without bronchopulmonary dysplasia. *Pediatr Pulmonol.* 2010;45(4):371–379.

CHAPTER 7

Patent Ductus Arteriosus and the Lung: Acute Effects and Long-Term Consequences

Martin Kluckow, Eduardo Bancalari, Ilene R.S. Sosenko, and Nelson Claure

- The ductus arteriosus plays a vital role in fetal life but failure to constrict and close postnatally, particularly in a premature infant, can result in systemic to pulmonary shunting.

- A significant patent ductus arteriosus (PDA) can have both systemic consequences with reduced systemic blood flow and pulmonary consequences with increased pulmonary blood flow and potential for lung injury.

- Despite the experimental and epidemiologic evidence supporting the role of the PDA in the pathogenesis of chronic lung injury, there are scarce data from more recent prospective clinical trials to confirm this association or demonstrate that treatment of the PDA has any effect on chronic lung injury.

- The need for treatment of the PDA is increasingly controversial because of a high rate of spontaneous closure, only moderate efficacy of the treatment options, and a risk of adverse effects.

- Until further evidence becomes available, the decision on management of PDA must balance the consequences of ductal patency that are closely related to its hemodynamic significance versus the side effects of the interventions to close it.

- More data are needed to define the impact of a more conservative approach toward the PDA on respiratory, cardiovascular, and neurologic outcomes.

During fetal development the ductus arteriosus plays a critical role by allowing most of the blood returning to the right heart to bypass the pulmonary circulation while maintaining fetal systemic blood flow. In the term infant the ductus closes during the first hours after birth. However, in the very premature infant the ductus frequently remains open for longer periods and as the pulmonary vascular resistance falls, there is an increasing systemic-to-pulmonary shunt that can result in a significant rise in pulmonary blood flow and a fall in systemic blood flow. This pressure difference appears earlier in infants with less severe initial lung disease because of a more rapid drop in pulmonary vascular resistance in the first days.[1,2] The increase in pulmonary blood flow through an immature pulmonary vascular bed can have a number of immediate and long-term consequences on the structure and function of the still developing cardiovascular and respiratory systems. This chapter addresses some of the short- and long-term respiratory consequences of a persistent ductus arteriosus (PDA) in preterm infants and the controversies regarding which infants with PDA require treatment as well as when and how to treat it.

Why Does the Ductus Arteriosus Remain Open in Preterm Infants?

The ductus arteriosus closes in most term infants within hours after birth, but in the very premature infant the ductus frequently closes considerably later or fails to undergo spontaneous closure. This is in part due to the elevated sensitivity of the immature ductal tissue to the dilating effects of prostaglandins (PG) and the low sensitivity to the constrictive effects of oxygen.[3] The ductus of the smaller preterm infant can remain open for days or weeks and in many cases, even when it may constrict initially, it can reopen later. This reopening is frequently associated with clinical deterioration induced by episodes of systemic infection or other events associated with a systemic inflammatory response, such as pneumonia or necrotizing enterocolitis. The incidence of a PDA is also increased in infants who are exposed to antenatal magnesium sulfate administered to the mother,[4] while persistence of ductal patency after indomethacin therapy was observed in infants exposed to infection and inflammatory mediators before birth.[5]

The incidence of a PDA is inversely related to gestational age and this is even more striking in preterm infants with respiratory failure. Some statistics indicate that more than 70% of preterm infants born before 28 weeks of gestation historically have been exposed to therapeutic interventions to close the PDA, with decreased efficacy of medical treatment at earlier gestational ages that had led to an increased need for surgical ligation.[6] However, as a consequence of results of recent trials showing lack of prevention of bronchopulmonary dysplasia (BPD) with early PDA treatment, the substantial rate of spontaneous PDA closure, and the increasing use of noninvasive forms of respiratory support with less mechanical ventilation, fewer PDAs are being diagnosed and treated.

Despite multiple studies evaluating the effects of antenatal corticosteroids on neonatal outcomes, only a few evaluated their effect on the PDA. Evidence in experimental animals demonstrates a constrictive effect of glucocorticoids on the ductus and an increased responsiveness of the ductal muscle to oxygen.[7,8] When premature infants were exposed to corticosteroids at least 24 hours before preterm delivery, the incidence of symptomatic PDA and PDA requiring treatment was significantly reduced.[9–11] This effect was not observed when the steroids were administered to the mother less than 24 hours before delivery. There is also an association between lower cortisol levels in preterm infants during the first week after birth and a higher incidence of PDA.[12] This may be explained by the fact that cortisol decreases the sensitivity of the ductal tissue to the dilatory effects of PGs.

With the introduction of exogenous surfactant therapy, the clinical presentation and incidence of patent ductus arteriosus in premature infants with respiratory distress syndrome (RDS) has been modified. Whereas surfactant itself has no effect on ductal contractility, the rapid improvement in the arterial partial pressure of oxygen (Pao_2) observed after surfactant administration can result in a rapid fall in pulmonary vascular resistance, producing an earlier clinical presentation of the ductus in preterm infants and in experimental animals.[2,13–15] This may explain the results shown in a meta-analysis of several randomized trials that prophylactic administration of synthetic surfactant seems to increase the incidence of symptomatic PDA,[16] as well as the possible association between surfactant administration and the development of pulmonary hemorrhage in infants with left-to-right ductal shunting.[2,14,17] There is also a relationship between a large ductal diameter with significant shunting and pulmonary hemorrhage[18,19] and early treatment (first 24 hours) with indomethacin in infants with a large PDA that shows significant reduction of pulmonary hemorrhage.[20,21] Data from exogenous surfactant trials, when pooled, demonstrate an increased rate of symptomatic PDA and an increased risk of pulmonary hemorrhage, a serious complication associated with significant mortality and an increased risk of chronic respiratory morbidity.[22,23] This is one clear pathway wherein a symptomatic PDA can result in lung injury and longer-term respiratory morbidity.

Systemic Consequences of a PDA

The consequences of a PDA in preterm infants depend on the size of the ductus and the magnitude of left-to-right shunting. This is determined by the difference in pressures between the systemic and pulmonary circulations. The left-to-right shunting

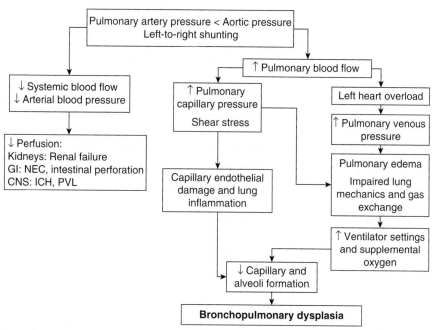

Fig. 7.1 Hemodynamic and respiratory consequences of patent ductus arteriosus. *CNS,* Central nervous system; *GI,* gastrointestinal; *ICH,* intracranial hemorrhage; *NEC,* necrotizing enterocolitis; *PVL,* periventricular leukomalacia.

results in increased pulmonary blood flow, volume overload of the left heart chambers, and decreased systemic flow and perfusion. While the left ventricle has the ability to increase its output, systemic blood flow distribution may be compromised by the decline in diastolic blood pressure and local vasoconstriction in different organs, resulting in decreased organ perfusion.[24] This may explain many of the systemic manifestations of a significant PDA, such as renal dysfunction, poor gastrointestinal function, and increased risk of necrotizing enterocolitis.[25,26] A significant PDA can also compromise cerebral blood flow, thus producing ischemia and contributing to the development of brain injury.[27–29] The hemodynamic consequences of PDA are summarized in Fig. 7.1.

Pulmonary Consequences of a PDA

Acute Effects

Premature birth is frequently complicated by respiratory failure resulting from inadequate surfactant treatment and/or pneumonia. The increased pulmonary blood flow from ductal shunting can have a significant negative impact on the underlying disease process; in fact, delayed recovery from the initial respiratory failure has been reported in infants with PDA.[30,31] Because low plasma oncotic pressure and increased capillary permeability are common in premature infants with respiratory distress, the increase in pulmonary blood flow and microvascular pressure can lead to increased interstitial and alveolar edema.[32] The edema and leakage of plasma proteins into the alveoli can inhibit surfactant function and worsen the effects of surfactant deficiency. As the ductal flow increases because of the falling pulmonary vascular resistance, the likelihood of pulmonary edema increases significantly along with alterations in lung mechanics and gas exchange.[33] Mechanical ventilation can worsen this by disturbing the balance between hydraulic fluid filtration and lung lymphatic drainage,[34,35] resulting in later presentation of a hemodynamically significant PDA.

A rapid improvement in lung compliance was reported after PDA ligation and was more striking among those infants with worse baseline lung mechanics.[36] A similar improvement in lung mechanics was also reported in infants with respiratory distress when the ductus was closed with indomethacin.[37–39] In contrast, critically ill infants often demonstrate a significant deterioration in pulmonary and cardiovascular function after PDA ligation.[40] Compared with infants with asymptomatic PDA and those with spontaneous ductal closure, infants requiring treatment for symptomatic

PDA had lower dynamic lung compliance and required respiratory support with higher mean airway pressures.[41] The lower compliance and increased pulmonary resistance in infants with a significant PDA explain why many of these infants present with hypercarbia and require increased ventilator settings to maintain arterial blood gas levels.

Infants with PDA and a significant increase in pulmonary blood flow often develop pulmonary edema that in the more severe cases can manifest as frank pulmonary hemorrhage, frequently resulting in a dramatic deterioration in respiratory function and gas exchange. This is exacerbated by the lack of distensibility of the immature left ventricle,[42] such that as the left-to-right shunt increases there is increased pulmonary venous pressure and pulmonary congestion.

Long-Term Consequences

Effects of Increased Pulmonary Blood Flow on Vascular and Alveolar Development

Although the patency of the ductus in the fetus protects the developing pulmonary circulation from overflow, the persistence of ductal patency after birth exposes the pulmonary vessels to higher driving pressures and excessive blood flow that can negatively affect the development of the pulmonary vasculature. Lung injury in the premature infant is limited not only to air spaces and conducting airways but also includes the immature pulmonary vasculature. In fact, inadequate structural development and function of the pulmonary vessels is a major feature of BPD.[43] This likely explains why a longer duration of systemic pulmonary shunt through a PDA increases the risk of BPD.[44]

Constriction of the ductus arteriosus in utero results in an increase in blood flow through the pulmonary vessels and exposure to higher vascular pressure. This can be a consequence of antenatal exposure to PG inhibitors.[45,46] Vascular remodeling resulting in a postnatal increase in pulmonary vascular resistance[47,48] and alterations in alveolar development can be caused by elevated blood flow through an immature pulmonary bed.[49–51] In experimental animal models of surgical aortopulmonary shunts, significant postnatal pulmonary hypertension and increased reactivity of the pulmonary vessels were found.[52]

When fetuses were exposed to indomethacin in utero, the result was a decreased effectiveness of PG inhibitor therapy for ductal closure after birth.[53,54] In fact, an increase in respiratory morbidity and BPD has been reported after maternal indomethacin administration for tocolysis.[55–59] It is important to note that these studies included not only extremely low birth weight infants, but also infants born at more advanced gestations. Whereas more mature infants have a lower risk of respiratory morbidity, the fetal ductus in infants of more advanced gestations is actually more sensitive to the effects of in utero PG inhibition.[60,61] Therefore the increased pulmonary blood flow in the more mature fetus produced by antenatal indomethacin may increase the risk of respiratory morbidity among these infants who would otherwise not have significant respiratory disease.

The presence of a systemic-to-pulmonary communication after birth results in an increase in blood flow through an immature pulmonary vascular bed that can produce marked vascular lesions with intimal fibrosis and medial hypertrophy.[62,63] Significant anatomic changes in the small pulmonary arteries are observed in experimental animals after exposure to high inspired oxygen and increased pulmonary blood flow that result in an increase in pulmonary vascular resistance and abnormal vasoreactivity.[64,65] Similar features are commonly observed in infants with severe BPD who have experienced prolonged supplemental oxygen exposure and a hemodynamically significant PDA.[66–68]

In addition, examination of the lung vasculature that has been exposed to increased shear and stretch has shown profound alterations in pulmonary vascular bed structure and cellular function. Endothelial injury occurs secondary to the increased blood flow or pressure and results in a disruption of the regulation of pulmonary vascular tone and growth. When experimental animals were exposed to increased pulmonary blood flow and hypertension, they showed alteration of the genetic regulatory cascade of endothelin-1 (ET-1).[69] In fact, preterm infants who developed BPD had elevated levels of ET-1 in tracheoalveolar fluid early after birth,[70] which correlated with an increase of the proinflammatory cytokine interleukin 8. Of note, infants with severe pulmonary hypertension have also been found to have elevated ET-1 levels.[71]

Both vascular endothelial growth factor (VEGF) and transforming growth factor beta (TGF-β) are key to lung development and function. Whereas VEGF is a cell-specific mediator of angiogenesis and vasculogenesis, TGF-β regulates cell growth and differentiation in the airways and pulmonary vasculature. Fetal lambs with increased pulmonary blood flow and hypertension show decreased VEGF expression shortly after birth.[72] Decreased expression of VEGF is also seen in preterm infants with severe RDS and in infants with BPD.[73,74] Unlike the decrease in VEGF expression, TGF-β expression is increased in animals exposed to increased pulmonary blood flow and in infants with BPD.[75–77] Thus both VEGF and TGF-β expression are affected by increased pulmonary blood flow and intravascular pressure, which may play a significant role in lung morphologic and functional alterations.

Studies in preterm baboons support the deleterious effect of increased pulmonary blood flow on lung development. Preterm baboons that had early pharmacologic closure of the PDA with ibuprofen at day 3 were found to have better alveolar development and improved alveolar surface area than animals in which the PDA remained open.[78] Interestingly, and perhaps paradoxically, this advantage in lung development was not observed in animals in which the PDA was closed surgically on day 6.[79] The acute and long-term respiratory consequences of PDA are summarized in Fig. 7.1.

PDA and BPD

Despite the strong experimental evidence that increased flow and pressure in the developing pulmonary vasculature can produce severe morphologic and functional alterations in the immature lung, there is still no conclusive evidence regarding the role of the PDA in the pathogenesis of BPD. The respiratory morbidity associated with a PDA is caused not only by the increase in pulmonary blood flow, edema, and pulmonary inflammation; many premature infants presenting with symptomatic PDA require mechanical ventilation and/or supplemental oxygen. The need for increased mean airway pressure and fraction of inspired oxygen (F_{IO_2}) in the setting of increased left-to-right shunt may also be one of the factors in the causal pathway of BPD. Infants with PDA are exposed to multiple factors that increase the risk of lung injury, and these become important confounders in the reported association between PDA and increased risk for BPD.[44,80–82] The negative effects of PDA on lung function were documented many years ago by Cotton et al. with the demonstration of a longer duration of mechanical ventilation among infants with symptomatic PDA compared with those without PDA.[83] In addition, they reported a decreased duration of mechanical ventilation with early surgical PDA closure.[84] The opposite was found when Clyman and colleagues reanalyzed the results of an earlier randomized, controlled clinical trial comparing early PDA ligation with expectant management and showed that infants who underwent early PDA ligation had a higher risk of developing BPD compared with the controls.[85] A subsequent small trial of early pharmacologic PDA closure with indomethacin also revealed a reduction in BPD.[86] It is important to note that these studies were conducted in the era before antenatal steroids and surfactant therapy.

From an epidemiologic standpoint, several studies since therapy with surfactant and antenatal steroids became available have found an increasing incidence of BPD with increased survival of extremely preterm infants, many of whom actually had mild or no initial RDS.[87–91] In these populations multivariate logistic analysis showed an increased risk of BPD in infants with a symptomatic PDA and episodes of sepsis.[80,82,92,93] The BPD risk was even greater when the PDA and sepsis occurred simultaneously, suggesting an interaction between these two events (Fig. 7.2). Late reopening of a PDA was more frequent in infected infants, and failed PDA closure was more common when sepsis and PDA were temporally related.[80] Moreover, infants with infection and those with PDA have higher levels of 6-keto-PGF$_{1\alpha}$ and elevated levels of tumor necrosis factor α (TNF-α). Elevated levels of 6-keto-PGF$_{1\alpha}$ in infected infants were found to be associated with an increased rate of late PDA and unresponsiveness to treatment with indomethacin.[94] These data explain the association between infection and PDA outcome by increasing the risk of ductal reopening and closure failure.[95–97]

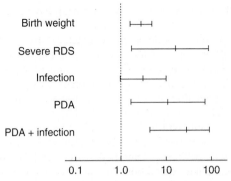

Fig. 7.2 Risk for development of bronchopulmonary dysplasia. Adjusted odds ratios and 95% confidence intervals obtained by multivariate logistic regression analysis show increased risk of developing bronchopulmonary dysplasia with the occurrence of patent ductus arteriosus *(PDA)* and when PDA is temporally related with sepsis. *RDS*, Respiratory distress syndrome. (Modified from Gonzalez A, Sosenko IR, Chandar J, et al. Influence of infection on patent ductus arteriosus and chronic lung disease in premature infants weighing 1000 grams or less. *J Pediatr.* 1996;128:470–478.)

Despite the experimental and epidemiologic evidence supporting the role of the PDA in the pathogenesis of chronic lung injury, there are scarce data from more recent prospective clinical trials to confirm this association or demonstrate that treatment of the PDA has any effect on chronic lung injury.

Management of the PDA and Respiratory Outcome

Different strategies to close the PDA have been investigated in an attempt to reduce its adverse consequences. Closure of the PDA by surgical or pharmacologic means is generally associated with rapid improvement in lung mechanics, although it is uncertain whether this translates into improvement in clinical course.[36–39] Several randomized trials conducted in the pre-surfactant era have compared early PDA closure with delayed treatment—that is, at a time when the PDA was deemed hemodynamically significant (by various definitions). In these trials, even when the time difference between early and late closure was relatively small, many studies demonstrated that early PDA closure was associated with decreased pulmonary morbidity.[86,98–104] When Clyman conducted a meta-analysis of these earlier studies, results indicated that infants who received early PDA treatment were at lower risk for BPD and had a reduction in the duration of mechanical ventilation compared with those receiving delayed treatment.[105] More recent trials, including the trial of Van Overmeire et al., did not find significant differences in respiratory outcome between infants with RDS and PDA who received indomethacin "early" (on day 3 ± 0.5) compared to "late" (on day 7 ± 1.7).[106] However, in this study infants were relatively mature and half of the patients in the "late" treatment group had spontaneous PDA closure by day 9, suggesting that even the infants who were treated late were not exposed to the effects of the PDA for very long. Similarly, in a group of smaller and less mature infants, Sosenko and coworkers demonstrated lack of benefit from "early" PDA closure, compared with expectant management, with closure only when the PDA became hemodynamically significant.[107] This study did not include infants with significant hemodynamic PDA at the time of enrollment.

Prophylactic indomethacin for the prevention of PDA has been extensively investigated.[108–114] In most of these studies prophylactic indomethacin was started on the first day after birth, even before the onset of PDA symptoms. As expected, most of these reports found a significant reduction in the incidence of PDA and need for surgical ligation with indomethacin prophylaxis. Surprisingly, the most dramatic effect of prophylactic indomethacin was a reduction in the incidence of severe intracranial hemorrhage. However, in terms of pulmonary outcome, pooled data from two meta-analyses failed to demonstrate a decrease in long-term pulmonary morbidity when prophylactic indomethacin treatment (given before PDA symptoms) was compared with later treatment after the PDA became symptomatic.[105,115] It is important to note that most infants randomly assigned to the control arm of these trials were exposed to a relatively short period of increased pulmonary blood flow because indomethacin was administered soon after the symptoms of PDA appeared.[116] Another explanation for these findings is that the potential benefits of early PDA closure may have been negated by the detrimental effects of indomethacin on renal function and fluid retention,[117] contributing to deterioration in lung function, particularly in those infants who did not have a PDA but still received prophylactic indomethacin.[118]

Most recently published randomized controlled trials (RCTs) were not designed to assess the association between PDA and BPD as they are essentially early versus later treatment trials with little or no exposure of the untreated group to a prolonged systemic to pulmonary shunt. From these trials there is little evidence that a short-term exposure to a PDA leads to BPD.[21,111,112,114,119] Newer studies have attempted to differentiate the effects of larger and more hemodynamically significant PDA by the use of scoring systems to delineate the magnitude of the left-to-right shunt. Larger PDA shunts were more predictive of subsequent death or chronic lung disease.[120] Furthermore, the risk of BPD has been found to increase with the duration of exposure to a hemodynamically significant PDA.[44]

When ibuprofen was compared with indomethacin for PDA closure in a meta-analysis of 6 randomized control trials, PDA treatment with intravenous ibuprofen after 24 hours was associated with an increased risk of BPD compared to treatment using indomethacin, RR 1.28, CI 1.03–1.60. However, no significant difference in BPD incidence was found in infants who received indomethacin versus placebo.[121]

Paracetamol is a new option for medical treatment of the PDA with some apparent efficacy, especially for early treatment. It appears to have a less adverse vasoconstrictive effect and therefore may cause less fluid retention/impaired renal function.[122] There is only one published placebo-controlled RCT of paracetamol for PDA treatment, which showed no associations with BPD either way.[123]

In a recent extensive analysis of the literature, Benitz concluded that there was no clear evidence that routine medical or surgical closure of the ductus was beneficial in preterm infants.[124] However, this conclusion is not entirely supported by the results of the review that showed a significant decrease in death or chronic lung disease in infants who received early treatment compared with those treated late for symptomatic PDA. Another important issue regarding this systematic review is the variation in the studies included. Many were performed more than 20 years ago, with poorly defined diagnosis and enrolment criteria, in more mature infants than are treated today, and with high rates of open-label treatment.[125] Other large retrospective studies of different treatment approaches to PDA in extremely low-birth-weight infants have shown higher mortality in the conservative group and more BPD in the surgical closure group versus pharmacologic treatment that was protective for death/ BPD at 36 weeks,[85,126] although not all cohort trials have found these results.[127]

The main argument of those proposing a conservative approach to interventions to close the PDA is the fact that many will close spontaneously, and waiting for spontaneous closure prevents the unnecessary use of drugs or surgery, both of which are associated with significant complications. However, the rate of spontaneous PDA closure is dependent on gestational age and is much lower in an infant with a birth weight less than 1000 g who has severe lung disease and is already at higher risk of severe BPD. There is no experimental or clinical evidence that the persistence of an open ductus (especially one causing hemodynamic compromise) confers any benefit in the clinical course of premature infants. Therefore the risk/benefit ratio must be measured in each individual case (i.e., the possible negative consequences of a persistent open ductus vs. the complications associated with the interventions to close it). Without definitive data, the approach to PDA treatment must be individualized to each infant, taking into account the gestational age, clinical course, size, and hemodynamic consequences of the ductal shunt and the potential side effects of the interventions to close the PDA (Fig. 7.3). The relatively low and unpredictable efficacy of the available medical treatments compounds the problem and provides an area in which research to predict which infants would benefit from therapy, as well as the optimal dosing and timing of treatment, would be useful.

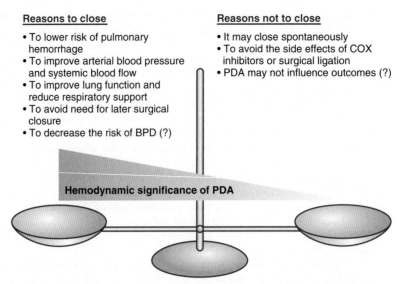

Reasons to close

- To lower risk of pulmonary hemorrhage
- To improve arterial blood pressure and systemic blood flow
- To improve lung function and reduce respiratory support
- To avoid need for later surgical closure
- To decrease the risk of BPD (?)

Reasons not to close

- It may close spontaneously
- To avoid the side effects of COX inhibitors or surgical ligation
- PDA may not influence outcomes (?)

Hemodynamic significance of PDA

Fig. 7.3 Clinical considerations in the management of patent ductus arteriosus *(PDA)*. *BPD*, Bronchopulmonary dysplasia; *COX*, cyclooxygenase.

Most infants who have a PDA and develop BPD are extremely premature, but surprisingly few studies have focused an analysis on this population. When Mahony et al. compared the effects of early versus late medical treatment of PDA, early treatment did not reduce oxygen dependency in the overall population.[101,104] However, stratified birth weight analysis showed early treatment was associated with a significantly shorter duration of oxygen need in infants with birth weights less than 1000 g. This finding was not seen in the more recent study of Kluckow and coworkers,[21] who were unable to demonstrate a decrease in BPD with early indomethacin in infants less than 29 weeks of GA, or in the study by Sosenko et al.[107] in which early administration of ibuprofen in infants with birth weights less than 800 g actually resulted in an increased need for oxygen at concentrations greater than 30% at 36 weeks postmenstrual age compared with the control group. One of the major obstacles in deciding whether early treatment is superior to a conservative approach is that a large proportion of infants assigned to the conservative arms (placebo) in the various trials eventually received open-label treatment when the PDA became significant. In these cases, open-label treatment reduced the exposure of the infants to the negative effects of the PDA. Thus when the treatment strategy of one arm of the trial becomes the rescue therapy for the other, it poses a significant challenge to those designing clinical trials to balance ethical and scientific standards.

Studies that evaluated the effect of short versus prolonged indomethacin therapy did not show consistent effects on PDA closure or on respiratory outcome, but the strategies that have led to more effective PDA closure have also resulted in lower respiratory morbidity.[127–129]

When pharmacologic treatment is contraindicated or fails, surgical ligation of the PDA is generally used as a second alternative. As with medical treatment, the potential benefits of surgical closure must be weighed against the potential side effects of the surgical procedure. The effect of surgical PDA closure on lung mechanics is an immediate improvement, with a rapid increase in compliance,[36] most likely due to the sudden reduction in pulmonary blood flow, blood volume, and interstitial lung fluid. Despite these positive hemodynamic and pulmonary changes from surgical PDA ligation, the clinical condition of a significant number of infants deteriorates after surgery.[40,130] This deterioration, manifested by higher inspired oxygen requirement and arterial hypotension, occurs mostly in smaller infants who had a prolonged left to right shunt via the PDA.[131–133] The mechanisms for this may be related to surgical trauma, to left ventricular dysfunction caused by an immediate increase in afterload, or a sudden reduction in pulmonary blood flow after ductal closure.[134–136] The early use of milrinone in this population appears to improve cardiovascular function.[130] Studies of surgical ligation in a baboon model have demonstrated a significant upregulation of genes involved with pulmonary inflammation (cyclooxygenase 2-2, TNF-α, and CD14), which may explain deterioration in some infants, or why postligation pulmonary mechanics fail to improve.[137]

Because no trials have compared surgical closure of a hemodynamically significant PDA with continued medical management when this has been ineffective, the benefits or side effects of surgical ligation on respiratory function remain unclear. However, recent reports have suggested significantly worse neurologic and pulmonary outcomes in infants who had PDA ligation versus those who had successful pharmacologic closure or needed no treatment.[138,139] Several other complications have been associated with PDA ligation, all of which can be associated with an increase in respiratory morbidity, including compromised cerebral oxygen supply, diaphragmatic paralysis owing to phrenic nerve injury, chylothorax, scoliosis, and vocal cord paralysis.[140–142] As previously mentioned, Clyman et al. reanalyzed data from a previous RCT of early PDA ligation during the first days of life and found a threefold increase in risk of developing BPD with early PDA ligation compared with the controls.[85] Most recently Janz-Robinson et al. found that both medical and surgical PDA treatment were independent risk factors associated with poor neurodevelopmental outcomes in 29-week-old preterm infants.[143]

In another interesting finding, Schmidt and coworkers showed that caffeine, administered to decrease apnea and favor successful weaning from mechanical ventilation in premature infants, lowered the incidence of PDA, decreased the need for PDA ligation, and also decreased the incidence of BPD compared with infants who received placebo.[144] The mechanisms for these beneficial effects are not clear but besides favoring weaning from mechanical ventilation by stimulating central respiratory activity, caffeine may function through its weak diuretic effect or through its antiinflammatory properties.

The persistence of a PDA in critically ill preterm infants can be associated with acute deleterious effects and an increased risk of BPD.[44] Although the effects of the ductus on lung development and function are likely related to the size of the ductus and duration and magnitude of left-to-right shunting, more data are needed to define the impact of a more conservative approach toward the PDA on respiratory, cardiovascular, and neurologic outcomes. These trials should clearly separate treatment from nontreatment arms by increasing drug efficacy, choosing patients likely to have a high treatment effect, and avoiding open-label treatment in the placebo group. Until further evidence becomes available, the decision on management of PDA must balance the consequences of ductal patency that are closely related to its hemodynamic significance versus the side effects of the interventions to close it (see Fig. 7.3).

Respiratory Management of Infants With PDA

Although ductal patency does not appear to have a significant effect on the respiratory system shortly after birth, as the pulmonary vascular resistance declines during the first hours, left-to-right shunting increases; it is at this time that infants often show deterioration in lung function requiring increased levels of respiratory support. A very common finding in these infants is an increase in arterial carbon dioxide tension requiring increased ventilator settings. A possible mechanism for this observation is that elevated levels of circulating PGE_2 that induce ductal patency may also lead to inhibition of the respiratory center, contributing to the hypoventilation.[145,146]

A common strategy used to attempt to reduce the left-to-right ductal shunting consists of an increase in the level of positive end-expiratory pressure (PEEP). In animal models of hyaline membrane disease, institution of PEEP reduced the left-to-right ductal flow.[147] In addition, higher PEEP is thought to prevent alveolar and small airway closure and severe pulmonary edema, although actual data on the effects of this intervention are lacking and the possible benefits of a higher PEEP in preterm infants could be offset by the negative effects on cardiac function, venous return, and respiratory mechanics. A recent study to evaluate the hemodynamic effects of different levels of PEEP in infants with a symptomatic PDA it showed that the application of higher levels of PEEP did not consistently reduce ductal left-to-right shunting.[148]

Regarding oxygenation, there are opposite effects of increased or decreased oxygen tension on the ductus and the pulmonary vasculature. Ductal patency is to some extent the result of a reduced sensitivity of the ductal tissue to oxygen. Although an increase in alveolar oxygen tension can produce constriction of the ductus arteriosus and reduce the shunt, it can also increase left-to-right ductal shunting owing to a reduction in pulmonary vascular resistance.[149]

In summary, a persistent ductus arteriosus is very common in preterm infants, although spontaneous PDA closure in the first 7 to 10 days occurs with higher frequency as gestational age increases. When the ductus fails to close, the increased pulmonary blood flow caused by systemic-to-pulmonary shunting that occurs as the pulmonary vascular resistance decreases after birth can have significant negative cardiovascular and respiratory consequences. Acute pulmonary effects include pulmonary edema and occasionally pulmonary hemorrhage, worsening lung mechanics, and deterioration in gas exchange with hypoxemia and hypercapnia.

The increased pulmonary blood flow can also produce damage to the immature pulmonary vasculature and trigger an inflammatory cascade that can lead to decreased alveolar and capillary formation and to pulmonary hypertension. These pathologic effects, plus the need for longer and more aggressive mechanical ventilation as well as possible effects on the lung from both medical and surgical treatment of the PDA, may explain the reported association between a hemodynamically significant PDA and an increased risk for BPD in extremely premature infants. Despite this association, there is no consistent evidence that early therapeutic interventions to close the PDA substantially improve long-term respiratory outcome.

REFERENCES

1. Fujii A, Allen R, Doros G, O'Brien S. Patent ductus arteriosus hemodynamics in very premature infants treated with poractant alfa or beractant for respiratory distress syndrome. *J Perinatol.* 2010;30:671–676.
2. Kaapa P, Seppanen M, Kero P, Saraste M. Pulmonary hemodynamics after synthetic surfactant replacement in neonatal respiratory distress syndrome. *J Pediatr.* 1993;123:115–119.
3. Clyman RI. Mechanisms regulating the ductus arteriosus. *Biol Neonate.* 2006;89:330–335.
4. del moral T, Gonzalez-Quintero VH, Claure N, Vanbuskirk S, Bancalari E. Antenatal exposure to magnesium sulfate and the incidence of patent ductus arteriosus in extremely low birth weight infants. *J Perinatol.* 2007;27:154–157.
5. Kim ES, Kim EK, Choi CW, Kim HS, Kim BI, Choi JH, et al. Intrauterine inflammation as a risk factor for persistent ductus arteriosus patency after cyclooxygenase inhibition in extremely low birth weight infants. *J Pediatr.* 2010;157:745–750.e1.
6. Stoll BJ, Hansen NI, Bell EF, Shankaran S, Laptook AR, Walsh MC, et al. Neonatal outcomes of extremely preterm infants from the NICHD Neonatal Research Network. *Pediatrics.* 2010;126:443–456.
7. Momma K, Nishihara S, Ota Y. Constriction of the fetal ductus arteriosus by glucocorticoid hormones. *Pediatr Res.* 1981;15:19–21.
8. Clyman RI, Mauray F, Roman C, Rudolph AM, Heymann MA. Glucocorticoids alter the sensitivity of the lamb ductus arteriosus to prostaglandin E2. *J Pediatr.* 1981;98:126–128.
9. Clyman RI, Ballard PL, Sniderman S, Ballard RA, Roth R, Heymann MA, et al. Prenatal administration of betamethasone for prevention of patient ductus arteriosus. *J Pediatr.* 1981;98:123–126.
10. Morales WJ, Angel JL, O'Brien WF, Knuppel RA. Use of ampicillin and corticosteroids in premature rupture of membranes: a randomized study. *Obstet Gynecol.* 1989;73:721–726.
11. Waffarn F, Siassi B, Cabal LA, Schmidt PL. Effect of antenatal glucocorticoids on clinical closure of the ductus arteriosus. *Am J Dis Child.* 1983;137:336–338.
12. Watterberg KL, Scott SM, Backstrom C, Gifford KL, Cook KL. Links between early adrenal function and respiratory outcome in preterm infants: airway inflammation and patent ductus arteriosus. *Pediatrics.* 2000;105:320–324.
13. Shimada S, Raju TN, Bhat R, Maeta H, Vidyasagar D. Treatment of patent ductus arteriosus after exogenous surfactant in baboons with hyaline membrane disease. *Pediatr Res.* 1989;26:565–569.
14. Clyman RI, Jobe A, Heymann M, Ikegami M, Roman C, Payne B, et al. Increased shunt through the patent ductus arteriosus after surfactant replacement therapy. *J Pediatr.* 1982;100:101–107.
15. Reller MD, Buffkin DC, Colasurdo MA, Rice MJ, McDonald RW. Ductal patency in neonates with respiratory distress syndrome. A randomized surfactant trial. *Am J Dis Child.* 1991;145:1017–1020.
16. Soll R, Ozek E. Prophylactic protein free synthetic surfactant for preventing morbidity and mortality in preterm infants. *Cochrane Database Syst Rev.* 2010:CD001079.

17. Garland J, Buck R, Weinberg M. Pulmonary hemorrhage risk in infants with a clinically diagnosed patent ductus arteriosus: a retrospective cohort study. *Pediatrics*. 1994;94:719–723.
18. Kluckow M, Evans N. Ductal shunting, high pulmonary blood flow, and pulmonary hemorrhage. *J Pediatr*. 2000;137:68–72.
19. Gonzalez AHH, Sosenko I, Chandar J, Goldberg R, Bancalari E. Surfactant administration, patent ductus arteriosus and pulmonary hemorrhage in premature infants <1000 g. *Pediatr Res*. 1994;35:227A.
20. Alfaleh K, Smyth JA, Roberts RS, Solimano A, Asztalos EV, Schmidt B, et al. Prevention and 18-month outcomes of serious pulmonary hemorrhage in extremely low birth weight infants: results from the trial of indomethacin prophylaxis in preterms. *Pediatrics*. 2008;121:e233–e238.
21. Kluckow M, Jeffery M, Gill A, Evans N. A randomised placebo-controlled trial of early treatment of the patent ductus arteriosus. *Arch Dis Child Fetal Neonatal Ed*. 2014;99:F99–F104.
22. Raju TN, Langenberg P. Pulmonary hemorrhage and exogenous surfactant therapy: a metaanalysis. *J Pediatr*. 1993;123:603–610.
23. Pandit PB, O'Brien K, Asztalos E, Colucci E, Dunn MS. Outcome following pulmonary haemorrhage in very low birthweight neonates treated with surfactant. *Arch Dis Child Fetal Neonatal Ed*. 1999;81:F40–F44.
24. Shimada S, Kasai T, Hoshi A, Murata A, Chida S. Cardiocirculatory effects of patent ductus arteriosus in extremely low-birth-weight infants with respiratory distress syndrome. *Pediatr Int*. 2003;45:255–262.
25. Shimada S, Kasai T, Konishi M, Fujiwara T. Effects of patent ductus arteriosus on left ventricular output and organ blood flows in preterm infants with respiratory distress syndrome treated with surfactant. *J Pediatr*. 1994;125:270–277.
26. Meyers RL, Alpan G, Lin E, Clyman RI. Patent ductus arteriosus, indomethacin, and intestinal distension: effects on intestinal blood flow and oxygen consumption. *Pediatr Res*. 1991;29:569–574.
27. Martin CG, Snider AR, Katz SM, Peabody JL, Brady JP. Abnormal cerebral blood flow patterns in preterm infants with a large patent ductus arteriosus. *J Pediatr*. 1982;101:587–593.
28. Perlman JM, Hill A, Volpe JJ. The effect of patent ductus arteriosus on flow velocity in the anterior cerebral arteries: ductal steal in the premature newborn infant. *J Pediatr*. 1981;99:767–771.
29. Weir FJ, Ohlsson A, Myhr TL, Fong K, Ryan ML. A patent ductus arteriosus is associated with reduced middle cerebral artery blood flow velocity. *Eur J Pediatr*. 1999;158:484–487.
30. Kitterman JA, Edmunds LH Jr, Gregory GA, Heymann MA, Tooley WH, Rudolph AM. Patent ducts arteriosus in premature infants. Incidence, relation to pulmonary disease and management. *N Engl J Med*. 1972;287:473–477.
31. Neal WA, Bessinger Jr FB, Hunt CE, Lucas Jr RV. Patent ductus arteriosus complicating respiratory distress syndrome. *J Pediatr*. 1975;86:127–132.
32. Alpan G, Scheerer R, Bland R, Clyman R. Patent ductus arteriosus increases lung fluid filtration in preterm lambs. *Pediatr Res*. 1991;30:616–621.
33. Alpan G, Mauray F, Clyman RI. Effect of patent ductus arteriosus on water accumulation and protein permeability in the lungs of mechanically ventilated premature lambs. *Pediatr Res*. 1989;26:570–575.
34. Perez Fontan JJ, Clyman RI, Mauray F, Heymann MA, Roman C. Respiratory effects of a patent ductus arteriosus in premature newborn lambs. *J Appl Physiol*. 1987;63:2315–2324.
35. Clyman RI. The role of patent ductus arteriosus and its treatments in the development of bronchopulmonary dysplasia. *Semin Perinatol*. 2013;37:102–107.
36. Gerhardt T, Bancalari E. Lung compliance in newborns with patent ductus arteriosus before and after surgical ligation. *Biol Neonate*. 1980;38:96–105.
37. Krauss AN, Fatica N, Lewis BS, Cooper R, Thaler HT, Cirrincione C, et al. Pulmonary function in preterm infants following treatment with intravenous indomethacin. *Am J Dis Child*. 1989;143:78–81.
38. Yeh TF, Thalji A, Luken L, Lilien L, Carr I, Pildes RS. Improved lung compliance followoing indomethacin therapy in premature infants with persistent ductus arteriosus. *Chest*. 1981;80:698–700.
39. Stefano JL, Abbasi S, Pearlman SA, Spear ML, Esterly KL, Bhutani VK. Closure of the ductus arteriosus with indomethacin in ventilated neonates with respiratory distress syndrome. Effects of pulmonary compliance and ventilation. *Am Rev Respir Dis*. 1991;143:236–239.
40. Ting JY, Resende M, More K, et al. Predictors of respiratory instability in neonates undergoing patient ductus arteriosus ligation after the introduction of targeted milrinone treatment. *J Thorac Cardiovasc Surg*. 2016;152:498–504.
41. Heldt GP, Pesonen E, Merritt TA, Elias W, Sahn DJ. Closure of the ductus arteriosus and mechanics of breathing in preterm infants after surfactant replacement therapy. *Pediatr Res*. 1989;25:305–310.
42. Friedman WF. Intrinsic physiological properties of the developing heart. *Prog Cardiovasc Dis*. 1972;15:87–111.
43. Abman SH. *Pulmonary Hypertension in Chronic Lung Disease of Infancy. Pathogenesis, Pathophysiology and Treatment*. New York: Dekker; 2000.
44. Schena F, Francescato G, Cappelleri A, Picciolli I, Mayer A, Mosca F, et al. Association between hemodynamically significant patent ductus arteriosus and bronchopulmonary dysplasia. *J Pediatr*. 2015;166:1488–1492.
45. Heymann MA, Rudolph AM. Effects of acetylsalicylic acid on the ductus arteriosus and circulation in fetal lambs in utero. *Circ Res*. 1976;38:418–422.
46. Levin DL, Fixler DE, Morriss FC, Tyson J. Morphologic analysis of the pulmonary vascular bed in infants exposed in utero to prostaglandin synthetase inhibitors. *J Pediatr*. 1978;92:478–483.

47. Levin DL, Hyman AI, Heymann MA, Rudolph AM. Fetal hypertension and the development of increased pulmonary vascular smooth muscle: a possible mechanism for persistent pulmonary hypertension of the newborn infant. *J Pediatr.* 1978;92:265–269.

48. Morin 3rd FC. Ligating the ductus arteriosus before birth causes persistent pulmonary hypertension in the newborn lamb. *Pediatr Res.* 1989;25:245–250.

49. Demello DE, Murphy JD, Aronovitz MJ, Davies P, Reid LM. Effects of indomethacin in utero on the pulmonary vasculature of the newborn guinea pig. *Pediatr Res.* 1987;22:693–697.

50. Herget J, Hampl V, Povysilova V, Slavik Z. Long-term effects of prenatal indomethacin administration on the pulmonary circulation in rats. *Eur Respir J.* 1995;8:209–215.

51. Bustos R, Ballejo G, Giussi G, Rosas R, Isa JC. Inhibition of fetal lung maturation by indomethacin in pregnant rabbits. *J Perinat Med.* 1978;6:240–245.

52. Reddy VM, Meyrick B, Wong J, Khoor A, Liddicoat JR, Hanley FL, et al. In utero placement of aortopulmonary shunts. A model of postnatal pulmonary hypertension with increased pulmonary blood flow in lambs. *Circulation.* 1995;92:606–613.

53. Norton ME, Merrill J, Cooper BA, Kuller JA, Clyman RI. Neonatal complications after the administration of indomethacin for preterm labor. *N Engl J Med.* 1993;329:1602–1607.

54. Dungan WT, Norton Jr JB, Readinger RI, Sotomora RF. Prostaglandin E1 in neonates with critical congenital heart disease. *J Ark Med Soc.* 1982;79:167–170.

55. Major CA, Lewis DF, Harding JA, Porto MA, Garite TJ. Tocolysis with indomethacin increases the incidence of necrotizing enterocolitis in the low-birth-weight neonate. *Am J Obstet Gynecol.* 1994;170:102–106.

56. Hammerman C, Glaser J, Kaplan M, Schimmel MS, Ferber B, Eidelman AI. Indomethacin tocolysis increases postnatal patent ductus arteriosus severity. *Pediatrics.* 1998;102:E56.

57. Eronen M, Pesonen E, Kurki T, Teramo K, Ylikorkala O, Hallman M. Increased incidence of bronchopulmonary dysplasia after antenatal administration of indomethacin to prevent preterm labor. *J Pediatr.* 1994;124:782–788.

58. Van Overmeire B, Slootmaekers V, De Loor J, Buytaert P, Hagendorens M, Sys SU, et al. The addition of indomethacin to betamimetics for tocolysis: any benefit for the neonate? *Eur J Obstet Gynecol Reprod Biol.* 1998;77:41–45.

59. Panter KR, Hannah ME, Amankwah KS, Ohlsson A, Jefferies AL, Farine D. The effect of indomethacin tocolysis in preterm labour on perinatal outcome: a randomised placebo-controlled trial. *Br J Obstet Gynaecol.* 1999;106:467–473.

60. Moise Jr KJ. Effect of advancing gestational age on the frequency of fetal ductal constriction in association with maternal indomethacin use. *Am J Obstet Gynecol.* 1993;168:1350–1353.

61. Van den Veyver IB, Moise Jr KJ, Ou CN, Carpenter Jr RJ. The effect of gestational age and fetal indomethacin levels on the incidence of constriction of the fetal ductus arteriosus. *Obstet Gynecol.* 1993;82:500–503.

62. Broccard AF, Hotchkiss JR, Kuwayama N, Olson DA, Jamal S, Wangensteen DO, et al. Consequences of vascular flow on lung injury induced by mechanical ventilation. *Am J Respir Crit Care Med.* 1998;157:1935–1942.

63. Corno AF, Tozzi P, Genton CY, von Segesser LK. Surgically induced unilateral pulmonary hypertension: time-related analysis of a new experimental model. *Eur J Cardiothorac Surg.* 2003;23:513–517.

64. Jones R, Zapol WM, Reid L. Pulmonary artery remodeling and pulmonary hypertension after exposure to hyperoxia for 7 days. A morphometric and hemodynamic study. *Am J Pathol.* 1984;117:273–285.

65. Jones R, Jacobson M, Steudel W. Alpha-smooth-muscle actin and microvascular precursor smooth-muscle cells in pulmonary hypertension. *Am J Respir Cell Mol Biol.* 1999;20:582–594.

66. Hislop AA, Haworth SG. Pulmonary vascular damage and the development of cor pulmonale following hyaline membrane disease. *Pediatr Pulmonol.* 1990;9:152–161.

67. Abman SH, Wolfe RR, Accurso FJ, Koops BL, Bowman CM, Wiggins Jr JW. Pulmonary vascular response to oxygen in infants with severe bronchopulmonary dysplasia. *Pediatrics.* 1985;75:80–84.

68. Halliday HL, Dumpit FM, Brady JP. Effects of inspired oxygen on echocardiographic assessment of pulmonary vascular resistance and myocardial contractility in bronchopulmonary dysplasia. *Pediatrics.* 1980;65:536–540.

69. Black SM, Bekker JM, Johengen MJ, Parry AJ, Soifer SJ, Fineman JR. Altered regulation of the ET-1 cascade in lambs with increased pulmonary blood flow and pulmonary hypertension. *Pediatr Res.* 2000;47:97–106.

70. Niu JO, Munshi UK, Siddiq MM, Parton LA. Early increase in endothelin-1 in tracheal aspirates of preterm infants: correlation with bronchopulmonary dysplasia. *J Pediatr.* 1998;132:965–970.

71. Rosenberg AA, Kennaugh J, Koppenhafer SL, Loomis M, Chatfield BA, Abman, et al. Elevated immunoreactive endothelin-1 levels in newborn infants with persistent pulmonary hypertension. *J Pediatr.* 1993;123:109–114.

72. Grover TR, Parker TA, Zenge JP, Markham NE, Kinsella JP, Abman SH. Intrauterine hypertension decreases lung VEGF expression and VEGF inhibition causes pulmonary hypertension in the ovine fetus. *Am J Physiol Lung Cell Mol Physiol.* 2003;284:L508–L517.

73. Bhatt AJ, Pryhuber GS, Huyck H, Watkins RH, Metlay LA, Maniscalco WM. Disrupted pulmonary vasculature and decreased vascular endothelial growth factor, Flt-1, and TIE-2 in human infants dying with bronchopulmonary dysplasia. *Am J Respir Crit Care Med.* 2001;164:1971–1980.

74. Lassus P, Turanlahti M, Heikkila P, Andersson LC, Nupponen I, Sarnesto A, et al. Pulmonary vascular endothelial growth factor and Flt-1 in fetuses, in acute and chronic lung disease, and in persistent pulmonary hypertension of the newborn. *Am J Respir Crit Care Med.* 2001;164:1981–1987.

75. Mata-Greenwood E, Meyrick B, Steinhorn RH, Fineman JR, Black SM. Alterations in TGF-beta1 expression in lambs with increased pulmonary blood flow and pulmonary hypertension. *Am J Physiol Lung Cell Mol Physiol*. 2003;285:L209–L221.

76. Kotecha S, Wangoo A, Silverman M, Shaw RJ. Increase in the concentration of transforming growth factor beta-1 in bronchoalveolar lavage fluid before development of chronic lung disease of prematurity. *J Pediatr*. 1996;128:464–469.

77. Lecart C, Cayabyab R, Buckley S, Morrison J, Kwong KY, Warburton D, et al. Bioactive transforming growth factor-beta in the lungs of extremely low birthweight neonates predicts the need for home oxygen supplementation. *Biol Neonate*. 2000;77:217–223.

78. McCurnin D, Seidner S, Chang LY, Waleh N, Ikegami M, Petershack J, et al. Ibuprofen-induced patent ductus arteriosus closure: physiologic, histologic, and biochemical effects on the premature lung. *Pediatrics*. 2008;121:945–956.

79. Chang LY, McCurnin D, Yoder B, Shaul PW, Clyman RI. Ductus arteriosus ligation and alveolar growth in preterm baboons with a patent ductus arteriosus. *Pediatr Res*. 2008;63:299–302.

80. Gonzalez A, Sosenko IR, Chandar J, Hummler H, Claure N, Bancalari E. Influence of infection on patent ductus arteriosus and chronic lung disease in premature infants weighing 1000 grams or less. *J Pediatr*. 1996;128:470–478.

81. Brown ER. Increased risk of bronchopulmonary dysplasia in infants with patent ductus arteriosus. *J Pediatr*. 1979;95:865–866.

82. Rojas MA, Gonzalez A, Bancalari E, Claure N, Poole C, Silva-Neto G. Changing trends in the epidemiology and pathogenesis of neonatal chronic lung disease. *J Pediatr*. 1995;126:605–610.

83. Cotton RB, Stahlman MT, Kovar I, Catterton WZ. Medical management of small preterm infants with symptomatic patent ductus arteriosus. *J Pediatr*. 1978;92:467–473.

84. Cotton RB, Stahlman MT, Bender HW, Graham TP, Catterton WZ, Kovar I. Randomized trial of early closure of symptomatic patent ductus arteriosus in small preterm infants. *J Pediatr*. 1978;93:647–651.

85. Clyman R, Cassady G, Kirklin JK, Collins M, Philips 3rd JB. The role of patent ductus arteriosus ligation in bronchopulmonary dysplasia: reexamining a randomized controlled trial. *J Pediatr*. 2009;154:873–876.

86. Merritt TA, Harris JP, Roghmann K, Wood B, Campanella V, Alexson C, et al. Early closure of the patent ductus arteriosus in very low-birth-weight infants: a controlled trial. *J Pediatr*. 1981;99:281–286.

87. Wung JT, Koons AH, Driscoll Jr JM, James LS. Changing incidence of bronchopulmonary dysplasia. *J Pediatr*. 1979;95:845–847.

88. O'Brodovich HM, Mellins RB. Bronchopulmonary dysplasia. Unresolved neonatal acute lung injury. *Am Rev Respir Dis*. 1985;132:694–709.

89. Heneghan MA, Sosulski R, Baquero JM. Persistent pulmonary abnormalities in newborns: the changing picture of bronchopulmonary dysplasia. *Pediatr Radiol*. 1986;16:180–184.

90. Parker RA, Lindstrom DP, Cotton RB. Improved survival accounts for most, but not all, of the increase in bronchopulmonary dysplasia. *Pediatrics*. 1992;90:663–668.

91. Charafeddine L, D'Angio CT, Phelps DL. Atypical chronic lung disease patterns in neonates. *Pediatrics*. 1999;103:759–765.

92. Marshall DD, Kotelchuck M, Young TE, Bose CL, Kruyer L, O'Shea TM. Risk factors for chronic lung disease in the surfactant era: a North Carolina population-based study of very low birth weight infants. North Carolina Neonatologists Association. *Pediatrics*. 1999;104:1345–1350.

93. Cavazza ATP, Fedeli T. Investigators of the Italian Group of Neonatal Pneumology. Impact of chronic lung disease on very low birth weight infants: a collaborative study of the Italian Group of Neonatal Pneumology. *Ital J Pediatr*. 2004;30:393–400.

94. Hutchison AA, Ogletree ML, Palme CJ, Leheup BP, Barrett JM, Fleischer AC, et al. Plasma 6-keto prostaglandin F1 alpha and thromboxane B2 in sick preterm neonates. *Prostaglandins Leukot Med*. 1985;18:163–181.

95. Lucas A, Mitchell MD. Plasma-prostaglandins in pre-term neonates before and after treatment for patient ductus arteriosus. *Lancet*. 1978;2:130–132.

96. Hammerman C, Zaia W, Berger S, Strates E, Aldousany A. Prostaglandin levels: predictors of indomethacin responsiveness. *Pediatr Cardiol*. 1986;7:61–65.

97. Lamont RF, Rose M, Elder MG. Effect of bacterial products on prostaglandin E production by amnion cells. *Lancet*. 1985;2:1331–1333.

98. Gersony WM, Peckham GJ, Ellison RC, Miettinen OS, Nadas AS. Effects of indomethacin in premature infants with patent ductus arteriosus: results of a national collaborative study. *J Pediatr*. 1983;102:895–906.

99. Cotton RB, Hickey DE, Graham TP, Stahlman MT. Effect of early indomethacin on ventilatory status of preterm infants with symptomatic patent ductus arteriosus. *Pediatr Res*. 1980;14:442.

100. Kaapa P, Lanning P, Koivisto M. Early closure of patent ductus arteriosus with indomethacin in preterm infants with idiopathic respiratory distress syndrome. *Acta Paediatr Scand*. 1983;72:179–184.

101. Mahony L, Carnero V, Brett C, Heymann MA, Clyman RI. Prophylactic indomethacin therapy for patent ductus arteriosus in very-low-birth-weight infants. *N Engl J Med*. 1982;306:506–510.

102. Weesner KM, Dillard RG, Boyle RJ, Block SM. Prophylactic treatment of asymptomatic patent ductus arteriosus in premature infants with respiratory distress syndrome. *South Med J*. 1987;80:706–708.

103. Pongiglione G, Marasini M, Silvestri G, Tuo P, Ribaldone D, Bertolini A, et al. Early treatment of patent ductus arteriosus in premature infants with severe respiratory distress syndrome. *Pediatr Card*. 1988;9:91–94.

104. Mahony L, Caldwell RL, Girod DA, Hurwitz RA, Jansen RD, Lemons JA, et al. Indomethacin therapy on the first day of life in infants with very low birth weight. *J Pediatr.* 1985;106:801–805.

105. Clyman RI. Recommendations for the postnatal use of indomethacin: an analysis of four separate treatment strategies. *J Pediatr.* 1996;128:601–607.

106. Van Overmeire B, Van de Broek H, Van Laer P, Weyler J, Vanhaesebrouck P. Early versus late indomethacin treatment for patent ductus arteriosus in premature infants with respiratory distress syndrome. *J Pediatr.* 2001;138:205–211.

107. Sosenko IR, Fajardo M, Claure N, Bancalari E. Timing of patent ductus arteriosus treatment and respiratory outcome in premature infants: a double blind randomized control trial. *J Pediatr.* 2016;160:929–935.

108. Rennie JM, Doyle J, Cooke RW. Early administration of indomethacin to preterm infants. *Arch Dis Child.* 1986;61:233–238.

109. Vincer M, Allen A, Evans J, Nwaesei C, Stinson D, Rees E, et al. Early intravenous indomethacin prolongs respiratory support in very low birth weight infants. *Acta Paediatr Scand.* 1987;76:894–897.

110. Krueger E, Mellander M, Bratton D, Cotton R. Prevention of symptomatic patent ductus arteriosus with a single dose of indomethacin. *J Pediatr.* 1987;111:749–754.

111. Bandstra ES, Montalvo BM, Goldberg RN, Pacheco I, Ferrer PL, Flynn J, et al. Prophylactic indomethacin for prevention of intraventricular hemorrhage in premature infants. *Pediatrics.* 1988;82:533–542.

112. Bada HS, Green RS, Pourcyrous M, Leffler CW, Korones SB, Magill HL, et al. Indomethacin reduces the risks of severe intraventricular hemorrhage. *J Pediatr.* 1989;115:631–637.

113. Ment LR, Oh W, Ehrenkranz RA, Philip AG, Vohr B, Allan W, et al. Low-dose indomethacin and prevention of intraventricular hemorrhage: a multicenter randomized trial. *Pediatrics.* 1994;93:543–550.

114. Schmidt B, Davis P, Moddemann D, Ohlsson A, Roberts RS, Saigal S, et al. Long-term effects of indomethacin prophylaxis in extremely-low-birth-weight infants. *N Engl J Med.* 2001;344:1966–1972.

115. Fowlie PW, Davis PG, McGuire W. Prophylactic intravenous indomethacin for preventing mortality and morbidity in preterm infants. *Cochrane Database Syst Rev.* 2010;(7):CD000174.

116. Evans N. Preterm patent ductus arteriosus: are we any closer to knowing when to treat? *Paediatr Child Health.* 2015;25.

117. Cifuentes RF, Olley PM, Balfe JW, Radde IC, Soldin SJ. Indomethacin and renal function in premature infants with persistent patent ductus arteriosus. *J Pediatr.* 1979;95:583–587.

118. Schmidt B, Roberts RS, Fanaroff A, Davis P, Kirpalani HM, Nwaesei C, et al. Indomethacin prophylaxis, patent ductus arteriosus, and the risk of bronchopulmonary dysplasia: further analyses from the Trial of Indomethacin Prophylaxis in Preterms (TIPP). *J Pediatr.* 2006;148:730–734.

119. Aranda JV, Clyman R, Cox B, Van Overmeire B, Wozniak P, Sosenko I, et al. A randomized, double-blind, placebo-controlled trial on intravenous ibuprofen L-lysine for the early closure of nonsymptomatic patent ductus arteriosus within 72 hours of birth in extremely-low-birth-weight infants. *Am J Perinatol.* 2009;26:235–245.

120. El-Khuffash A, James AT, Corcoran JD, Dicker P, Franklin O, Elsayed YN, et al. A patent ductus arteriosus severity score predicts chronic lung disease or death before discharge. *J Pediatr.* 2015;167:1354–1361.e2.

121. Jones LJ, Craven PD, Attia J, Thakkinstian A, Wright I. Network meta-analysis of indomethacin versus ibuprofen versus placebo for PDA in preterm infants. *Arch Dis Child Fetal Neonatal Ed.* 2011;96:F45–F52.

122. Terrin G, Conte F, Oncel MY, Scipione A, McNamara PJ, Simons S, et al. Paracetamol for the treatment of patent ductus arteriosus in preterm neonates: a systematic review and meta-analysis. *Arch Dis Child Fetal Neonatal Ed.* 2016;101:F127–F136.

123. Härkin P, Harma A, Aikio O, Valkama M, Leskinen M, Saarela T, et al. Paracetamol accelerates closure of the ductus arteriosus after premature birth: a randomized trial. *J Pediatr.* 2016.

124. Benitz WE. Treatment of persistent patent ductus arteriosus in preterm infants: time to accept the null hypothesis? *J Perinatol.* 2010;30:241–252.

125. Zonnenberg I, de Waal K. The definition of a haemodynamic significant duct in randomized controlled trials: a systematic literature review. *Acta Paediatr.* 2012;101:247–251.

126. Sadeck LS, Leone CR, Procianoy RS, Guinsburg R, Marba ST, Martinez FE, et al. Effects of therapeutic approach on the neonatal evolution of very low birth weight infants with patent ductus arteriosus. *J Pediatr (Rio J).* 2014;90:616–623.

127. Hammerman C, Aramburo MJ. Prolonged indomethacin therapy for the prevention of recurrences of patent ductus arteriosus. *J Pediatr.* 1990;117:771–776.

128. Tammela O, Ojala R, Iivainen T, Lautamatti V, Pokela ML, Janas M, et al. Short versus prolonged indomethacin therapy for patent ductus arteriosus in preterm infants. *J Pediatr.* 1999;134:552–557.

129. Lee J, Rajadurai VS, Tan KW, Wong KY, Wong EH, Leong JY. Randomized trial of prolonged low-dose versus conventional-dose indomethacin for treating patent ductus arteriosus in very low birth weight infants. *Pediatrics.* 2003;112:345–350.

130. El-Khuffash AF, Jain A, Weisz D, Mertens L, McNamara PJ. Assessment and treatment of post patent ductus arteriosus ligation syndrome. *J Perinatol.* 2014;165:46–52.e1.

131. Nagle MG, Peyton MD, Harrison Jr LH, Elkins RC. Ligation of patent ductus arteriosus in very low birth weight infants. *Am J Surg.* 1981;142:681–686.

132. Moin F, Kennedy KA, Moya FR. Risk factors predicting vasopressor use after patent ductus arteriosus ligation. *Am J Perinatol.* 2003;20:313–320.

133. El-Khuffash AF, Jain A, Dragulescu A, McNamara PJ, Mertens L. Acute changes in myocardial systolic function in preterm infants undergoing patent ductus arteriosus ligation: a tissue Doppler and myocardial deformation study. *J Am Soc Echocardiogr*. 2012;25:1058–1067.

134. Taylor AF, Morrow WR, Lally KP, Kinsella JP, Gerstmann DR, deLemos RA. Left ventricular dysfunction following ligation of the ductus arteriosus in the preterm baboon. *J Surg Res*. 1990;48:590–596.

135. El-Khuffash AF, Jain A, McNamara PJ. Ligation of the patent ductus arteriosus in preterm infants: understanding the physiology. *J Pediatr*. 2013;162:1100–1106.

136. Noori S, McNamara P, Jain A, Lavoie PM, Wickremasinghe A, Merritt TA, et al. Catecholamine-resistant hypotension and myocardial performance following patent ductus arteriosus ligation. *J Perinatol*. 2015;35:123–127.

137. Waleh N, McCurnin DC, Yoder BA, Shaul PW, Clyman RI. Patent ductus arteriosus ligation alters pulmonary gene expression in preterm baboons. *Pediatr Res*. 2011;69:212–216.

138. Kabra NS, Schmidt B, Roberts RS, Doyle LW, Papile L, Fanaroff A, et al. Neurosensory impairment after surgical closure of patent ductus arteriosus in extremely low birth weight infants: results from the trial of indomethacin prophylaxis in preterms. *J Pediatr*. 2007;150:229–234.

139. Madan JC, Kendrick D, Hagadorn JI, Frantz ID 3rd. National Institute of Child Health and Human Development Neonatal Research Network. Patent ductus arteriosus therapy: impact on neonatal and 18-month outcome. *Pediatrics*. 2009;123:674–681.

140. Lemmers PM, Molenschot MC, Evens J, Toet MC, van Bel F. Is cerebral oxygen supply compromised in preterm infants undergoing surgical closure for patent ductus arteriosus? *Arch Dis Child Fetal Neonatal Ed*. 2010;95:F429–F434.

141. Roclawski M, Sabiniewicz R, Potaz P, Smoczynski A, Pankowski R, Mazurek T, et al. Scoliosis in patients with aortic coarctation and patent ductus arteriosus: does standard posterolateral thoracotomy play a role in the development of the lateral curve of the spine? *Pediatr Cardiol*. 2009;30:941–945.

142. Benjamin JR, Smith PB, Cotten CM, Jaggers J, Goldstein RF, Malcolm WF. Long-term morbidities associated with vocal cord paralysis after surgical closure of a patent ductus arteriosus in extremely low birth weight infants. *J Perinatol*. 2010;30:408–413.

143. Janz-Robinson EM, Badawi N, Walker K, Bajuk B, Abdel-Latif ME. Neonatal Intensive Care Units Network. Neurodevelopmental outcomes of premature infants treated for patent ductus arteriosus: a population-based cohort study. *J Pediatr*. 2015;167:1025–1032.e3.

144. Schmidt B, Roberts RS, Davis P, Doyle LW, Barrington KJ, Ohlsson A, et al. Caffeine therapy for apnea of prematurity. *N Engl J Med*. 2006;354:2112–2121.

145. Guerra FA, Savich RD, Wallen LD, Lee CH, Clyman RI, Mauray FE, et al. Prostaglandin E2 causes hypoventilation and apnea in newborn lambs. *J Appl Physiol (1985)*. 1988;64:2160–2166.

146. Hoch B, Bernhard M. Central apnoea and endogenous prostaglandins in neonates. *Acta Paediatr*. 2000;89:1364–1368.

147. Cotton RB, Lindstrom DP, Kanarek KS, Sundell H, Stahlman MT. Effect of positive-end-expiratory-pressure on right ventricular output in lambs with hyaline membrane disease. *Acta Paediatr Scand*. 1980;69:603–606.

148. Fajardo MF, Claure N, Swaminathan S, Sattar S, Vasquez A, D'Ugard C, et al. Effect of positive end-expiratory pressure on ductal shunting and systemic blood flow in preterm infants with patent ductus arteriosus. *Neonatology*. 2014;105:9–13.

149. Skinner JR, Hunter S, Poets CF, Milligan DW, Southall D, Hey EN. Haemodynamic effects of altering arterial oxygen saturation in preterm infants with respiratory failure. *Arch Dis Child Fetal Neonatal Ed*. 1999;80:F81–F87.

CHAPTER 8

Ventilator-Associated Pneumonia

Thomas A. Hooven and Richard A. Polin

- Invasive mechanical ventilation of neonates increases their risk of developing bacterial infection of the lower airways and lung parenchyma, which is termed "ventilator-associated pneumonia" (VAP).
- VAP is diagnosed on the basis of defined clinical, radiographic, and laboratory criteria.
- Unlike other neonatal bacterial infections, culture isolation of a single, causative organism is unusual in VAP.
- Suspected VAP should initially be treated with broad-spectrum antibiotics with coverage against common drug-resistant bacteria.
- As treatment progresses, empiric antibiotic coverage should be narrowed—as possible—based on available data.
- VAP is associated with prolonged hospitalization and poor clinical outcomes, including death.
- VAP "bundles," consisting of standard practices universally applied to prevent pneumonia among intubated patients, are accruing strong evidence and are now in widespread use.

Introduction

Infants in the neonatal intensive care unit (NICU) requiring mechanical ventilation (MV) can develop superimposed bacterial infection of the small airways and lung parenchyma, which is termed "ventilator-associated pneumonia" (VAP). VAP is classified as a type of health care–associated infection (also known as nosocomial infection). Health care–associated infections have come under increasing scrutiny as potentially preventable contributors to poor hospitalization outcomes and ballooning costs of inpatient care.

VAP is difficult to diagnose in the neonate and therefore requires a high index of suspicion. The concept of VAP first emerged in literature from adult ICUs, where a specific etiologic diagnosis can be aided by invasive airway sampling through bronchial brushings or lavage—techniques that are rarely used in the NICU. Adding further challenge to identifying VAP in the neonate is the fact that affected infants often have chronic pulmonary inflammation and dysfunction related to prematurity and respiratory support, which can complicate the diagnostic impression and make infection difficult to detect. Finally, as is the case with neonatal infection in general, infants with VAP show fewer localizing signs and symptoms than older children and adults, often presenting with general deterioration that may not immediately be attributed to VAP.

Nevertheless, with increasing awareness of VAP as a contributor to poor NICU outcomes, guidelines for diagnosis, management, and prevention have been developed and refined. This chapter reviews VAP epidemiology, pathogenesis, and the latest recommendations for limiting its impact on neonatal health.

Definition

The Centers for Disease Control (CDC)/National Nosocomial Infections Surveillance (NNIS) define VAP as pneumonia occurring in the setting of at least 2 days of MV through an endotracheal tube (ETT). Noninvasive forms of ventilation such as nasal continuous positive airway pressure or intermittent positive pressure through nasal prongs do not qualify. Formal criteria for diagnosing pneumonia are based on a combination of radiographic, laboratory, and clinical findings.

When there is underlying respiratory or cardiac disease (such as respiratory distress syndrome, chronic lung disease, or a patent ductus arteriosus), at least two serial chest radiographs demonstrating a new or progressive focal infiltrate, consolidation, cavitation, or pneumatocele are required to meet the radiographic diagnostic criteria for pneumonia. For an infant with no preexisting pulmonary or cardiac disease, a single chest radiograph demonstrating one or more of the above features is sufficient.

The clinical and laboratory findings required to diagnose pneumonia in patients younger than 1 year of age include worsening gas exchange (manifesting as desaturations, need for increasing ventilator settings, and/or a rising fraction of inspired oxygen requirement) *and* at least three of the following:

- Temperature instability
- Leukopenia ($\leq$4000 white blood cells/mm^3) or leukocytosis ($\geq$15,000 white blood cells/mm^3) and left shift (>10% band forms)
- New onset of purulent sputum, change in character of sputum, or increased respiratory secretions requiring increased suctioning frequency
- Apnea, tachypnea, or retractions of the chest wall
- Wheezing, rales, or rhonchi
- Bradycardia (<100 beats/min) or tachycardia (>170 beats/min)

In studies of VAP that have reported on the frequency of different clinical signs in newborns, the need for increased ventilator settings, increased airway secretions, and a new radiographic infiltrate have been described as the most common.[1]

Some authors have argued for inclusion of microbiologic criteria in the definition of VAP, and positive culture results from suctioned sputum, bronchoscopy, blind bronchoalveolar lavage (BAL), or pleural fluid have sometimes been included as diagnostic criteria in clinical studies. However, there are several downsides to relying on microbiologic evidence of VAP in neonates. For example, suctioned secretion samples are frequently contaminated with bacteria colonizing the oropharynx and upper airway. The use of BAL may reduce this contamination. Comparisons between concurrent cultures of secretions suctioned from an endotracheal tube and BAL have shown that BAL samples are less likely to yield polymicrobial growth, suggesting less oropharyngeal and upper airway commensal contamination. However, BAL can be technically challenging in smaller patients and may not be feasible in an unstable infant. Bronchoscopy poses the same, if not greater, risks as BAL. Large infectious pleural effusions are unusual in neonatal VAP; therefore pleurocentesis should be reserved for cases when an effusion is hindering respiratory mechanics. Blood cultures are not reliable for diagnosing VAP.

Although not required to diagnose VAP, Gram stain and culture of a tracheal aspirate sample can provide valuable supplemental evidence. A Gram stain of tracheal secretions that shows a significant leukocytic infiltrate and a high bacterial load is consistent with VAP, and the bacterial morphology can potentially help inform antibiotic selection (see the "Treatment" section). Serial cultures and microscopic assessments of tracheal aspirate samples during treatment can be useful gauges of the patient's response to antibiotics. Results from tracheal suction samples should not be considered definitive, however, and the diagnosis of VAP can be made solely based on radiographic, clinical, and laboratory criteria described previously and summarized in Box 8.1.

Epidemiology

While the reported incidence of VAP varies depending on the source, neonatal VAP is common, accounting for 6.8% to 32.2% of health care–associated infections in level II and III NICUs in the United States.[2] VAP rates appear to be decreasing. Sequential reports from the National Healthcare Safety Network, published in 2009 and 2013,

Box 8.1   CENTERS FOR DISEASE CONTROL/NATIONAL NOSOCOMIAL INFECTIONS SURVEILLANCE DEFINITION OF VAP[a]

Radiographic	Worsening Gas Exchange	Clinical/Laboratory Evidence
If there is underlying pulmonary or cardiac disease, two serial x-rays demonstrating at least one of the following: • New or progressive infiltrate • Consolidation • Cavitation • Pneumatocele If there is no underlying pulmonary or cardiac disease, *one definitive imaging test result is acceptable*	Any of the following: • Oxygen desaturation • Increased oxygen requirement • Increased ventilator demand	Must have *at least three* of the following: • Temperature instability • Leukopenia ($\leq$4000 WBC/mm^3) or leukocytosis ($\geq$15000 WBC/mm^3) and left shift ($\geq$10% band forms) • New onset of purulent sputum or change in character of sputum, or increased respiratory secretions or increased suctioning requirements • Apnea, tachypnea, nasal flaring with retractions of the chest wall or nasal flaring with grunting • Wheezing, rales, or rhonchi • Cough • Bradycardia (<100 beats/min) or tachycardia (>170 beats/min)

[a]Infants receiving mechanical ventilation through an endotracheal tube for at least 48 hours must meet criteria in *all three columns.*
VAP, Ventilator-associated pneumonia; *WBC,* white blood cell.

show a drop from 1.9 to 1.2 cases of VAP per thousand ventilator days in level II and III NICUs.[3,4]

Prematurity, low birth weight, and duration of MV have all been identified as major risk factors for VAP in multiple studies. Since smaller, sicker patients tend to require longer treatment with MV, it is difficult to conclusively establish which of these variables are independent risks. Several authors have shown statistically significant differences in VAP incidence per thousand ventilator days based on gestational age, but this analytical approach could be confounded by an uneven distribution of MV duration within preterm and term populations.

Cernada et al. published a prospective study of VAP in 198 neonates (gestational age range 27–37 weeks) intubated for more than 48 hours; VAP developed in 18 of the infants. In a multivariate regression model, only duration of MV emerged as an independent risk factor for VAP.[1] In contrast, Apisarnthanarak et al. performed logistical regression on data from 19 extremely premature infants with VAP and found no significant independent risk from each additional week of MV.[5] Instead, that group identified prior bloodstream infection as an independent risk factor for preterm VAP, although there was no significant relationship between the organism causing the prior bloodstream infection and the isolate (if any) responsible for pneumonia. One possibility is that treatment of an earlier infection with antibiotics may alter the microbiome of the neonate and allow colonization with pathogens more likely to cause VAP.

The infection control infrastructure of the NICU may also significantly affect local rates of VAP. An observational study by Goldmann et al. reported a 16-fold decrease in VAP after relocation of their nursery to a new facility with 50% more staffing, improved isolation and cohorting capacity, more sinks, and better air filtration.[6] Other potential risk factors for VAP include administration of opiates for sedation during intubation, frequent suctioning (>8 times per day), and reintubation.[7]

Pathogenesis

The most common organisms cultured from respiratory cultures in the setting of neonatal VAP are *Pseudomonas aeruginosa, Enterobacter* spp., *Klebsiella* spp., and

> **Box 8.2**   VAP PATHOGENS RANKED FROM MOST COMMON TO LEAST COMMON[a]
>
> **Pathogen**
> *Pseudomonas aeruginosa*
> *Enterobacter* spp.
> *Klebsiella* spp.
> *Staphylococcus aureus*
> *Escherichia coli*
> *Enterococcus* spp.
> *Acinetobacter* spp.
> *Proteus* spp.
> *Citrobacter* spp.
> *Stenotrophomonas maltophilia*
> Group B *Streptococcus*
>
> [a]Based on multiple studies; the exact order may vary depending on local factors.

Staphylococcus aureus (Box 8.2). Tracheal aspirates from the ETT almost always yield polymicrobial growth owing to commensal contamination. BAL samples have a higher likelihood of growing a single isolate, but Cernada et al. still reported that 16% of BAL samples from neonates with VAP grew multiple organisms.[8] Therefore it is likely that VAP often results from polymicrobial overgrowth rather than a single pathogen.

Immature innate immunity in the neonate increases the risk of VAP. Low immunoglobin levels (particularly in the premature population) and functionally impaired alveolar neutrophils and macrophages limit opsonization and phagocytosis of bacteria in the lower airways. Tissue damage from chronic inflammation, atelectasis, and pulmonary edema create potential niduses of infection and impede normal mucosal barrier functions and ciliary clearance of debris.

Although intubation can be lifesaving, the ETT itself contributes to VAP in multiple ways. It creates a physical barrier to ciliary action, prevents effective coughing, and provides a protected milieu for high-density bacterial colonization and biofilm formation. Zur et al. used electron microscopy to demonstrate progressive biofilm growth on the inner luminal and outer surfaces of ETTs from neonates intubated for at least 12 hours (Fig. 8.1).[9] Adair et al. performed within-patient comparisons of bacterial culture results from respiratory secretions and ETT biofilm swabs in 40 intubated patients and used genotyping to confirm clonal matches.[10] Patients with VAP showed high correlation between ETT and sputum isolates, whereas controls without VAP showed no statistical correlation, suggesting that the ETT serves as a reservoir for pathogenic organisms once infection is established.

VAP develops from overgrowth of bacteria colonizing the oropharynx, which may have been present before intubation or may become introduced afterward from contaminated oral or gastric secretions. Through alterations in the tracheobronchial milieu described earlier, MV leads to positive selection for these organisms, followed by tracheal colonization and population expansion in the lower airways (Fig. 8.2).

Patient positioning may influence pooling of orogastric secretions and the propensity of oropharyngeal commensals to be drawn into the trachea. Aly et al. performed a randomized controlled trial to test the hypothesis that gravity contributes to tracheal colonization, which may progress to VAP.[11] They compared tracheal cultures among 60 intubated infants who were maintained in either supine or side-lying positions and showed that after 5 days of intubation, there was significantly more tracheal colonization among the supine group, which also had higher tracheal bacterial density and greater introduction of new species over the observation period.

The contribution of gastric bacteria to VAP pathogenesis is uncertain. Some experimental evidence supports the hypothesis that the stomach serves as a reservoir for potential VAP pathogens. Gastric pepsin has been shown to be present in the lungs of intubated neonates, indicating that gastric secretions become aspirated in this population. One study measured tracheal pepsin among intubated neonates and

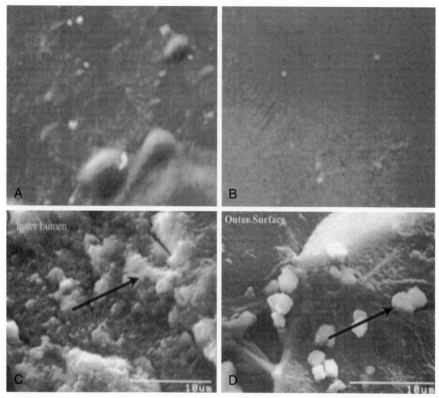

Fig. 8.1 Electron micrographs of the inner (A) and outer (B) surfaces of a sterile endotracheal tube before use and the inner (C) and outer (D) surfaces after 8 days of intubation. The 8-day micrographs demonstrate individual cocci *(arrows)* within a thick biofilm. (Adapted from Zur KB, Mandell DL, Gordon RE, et al. Electron microscopic analysis of biofilm on endotracheal tubes removed from intubated neonates. *Otolaryngol Head Neck Surg.* 2004;130(4):407–414. Reprinted with permission.)

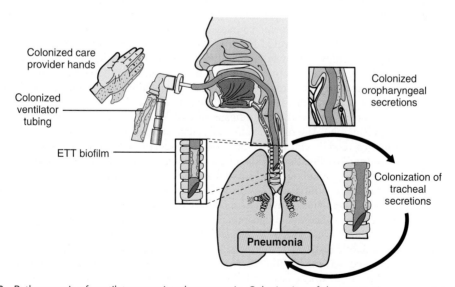

Fig. 8.2 Pathogenesis of ventilator-associated pneumonia. Colonization of the upper airway can originate from care provider hands, ventilator equipment, oropharyngeal secretions or a biofilm within the endotracheal tube *(ETT)*. Ultimately, pathogenic organisms spread into the trachea, where the population expands and moves downward into the small airways and lung parenchyma, causing pneumonia. (Adapted from illustrations by Walter Earhart from Garland JS. Strategies to prevent ventilator-associated pneumonia in neonates. *Clin Perinatol.* 2010;37(3):629–643. Reprinted with permission.)

identified a reliable inverse relationship with the degree of head of bed elevation.[12] In a study on 19 intubated adults in a medical ICU, technetium labeling of gastric contents was followed by scintigraphy of endotracheal suctioning samples to assess for migration of gastric bacteria to the lungs. Radioactivity counts were compared between patients maintained in supine and semi-recumbent positions. Migration occurred in both groups but happened faster among patients in the supine position, again indicating a role of patient positioning in the pathogenesis of VAP.[13]

Other studies have cast doubt on the theory that gastric bacteria are a major cause of VAP. Cardeñosa Cendrero et al. performed daily, simultaneous sampling of the trachea, pharynx, and stomach in 123 adults receiving mechanical ventilation to study temporal patterns of colonization and invasion. Nineteen patients in whom VAP developed subsequently underwent bronchoscopy with BAL and protected brush sampling. There was no evidence of primary gastric colonization for any of the VAP isolates, which generally matched preceding tracheal colonizers.[14] A smaller study by Feldman et al. with a similar design also did not reveal any evidence of primary gastric colonization with eventual VAP pathogens.[15]

In summary, VAP pathogenesis data are limited and—in some regard—contradictory. The current model is also derived largely from adult research, which may limit its generalizability to the neonatal population. Based on the available evidence, the key steps of VAP pathogenesis seem to be initial tracheal colonization by one or more potentially virulent microorganisms, followed by progressive distal airway colonization and population expansion. This process is aided by the ETT itself, which offers a protected niche for potential pathogens; alterations in innate pulmonary immunity stemming from prematurity and chronic disease; and possibly from supine positioning that favors bacterial spread from the upper airways into the lungs.

Treatment

The central pillar of VAP treatment is an appropriate course of intravenous antibiotics. However, there are no consensus guidelines for specific antibiotics that should be used to treat VAP. Instead, several general principles should guide therapy.

When VAP is suspected, empiric broad-spectrum antibiotics should be initiated promptly. The empiric regimen should be tailored, if possible, to antibiotic resistance patterns of pathogens commonly isolated in the unit and to any bacteria—particularly drug-resistant strains—previously cultured from the patient. Consideration should also be given to any prior courses of antibiotic therapy the patient has received, which might have selected for drug-resistant organisms. Whenever possible, initial empiric therapy should subsequently be narrowed on the basis of culture results and sensitivity testing. Microbiologic data that can inform rational narrowing of empiric antibiotics can come from respiratory secretion cultures from the current illness and any prior cultures that revealed specific colonizers.

For patients with a significant risk of VAP from one or more drug-resistant organisms, the American Thoracic Society and the Infectious Diseases Society of America recommend a three-antibiotic combination as initial therapy (Box 8.3).[16] Two-drug combinations with broad coverage of gram-positive and gram-negative pathogens—including a substantial fraction of drug-resistant organisms—may be appropriate as initial therapy in milder cases or when the concern for multidrug-resistant organisms is lower. Acceptable examples of two-drug combinations include linezolid or vancomycin plus piperacillin/tazobactam or gentamicin.

Methicillin-resistant *S. aureus* (MRSA) is a common cause of VAP. In a study on antibiotic resistance patterns in VAP isolates from adult patients, 62% of *S. aureus* recovered was methicillin-resistant.[17] Vancomycin or linezolid can be used to treat MRSA. Both drugs have been studied as monotherapy for nosocomial pneumonia (not necessarily ventilator-associated) caused by MRSA in adult and pediatric populations, although they have never been subject to head-to-head comparison in treatment of neonatal VAP. Meta-analysis of data from two prospective studies in adults with nosocomial pneumonia showed better cure rates and improved overall survival among patients treated with linezolid compared with those treated with

**Box 8.3 INITIAL EMPIRIC THERAPY FOR VAP IN PATIENTS WITH
SIGNIFICANT RISK FACTORS FOR MULTIDRUG-RESISTANT
PATHOGENS**

Potential Pathogens	Combination Antibiotic Therapy
Multidrug-resistant pathogens • *Pseudomonas aeruginosa* • *Klebsiella* spp. • *Acinetobacter* spp. Methicillin-resistant *Staphylococcus aureus*	Antipseudomonal cephalosporin (cefepime, ceftazidime) *or* Antipseudomonal carbapenem (imipenem or meropenem) *or* β-Lactam/β-lactamase inhibitor (piperacillin-tazobactam) *plus* Antipseudomonal fluoroquinolone (ciprofloxacin or levofloxacin) *or* Aminoglycoside (amikacin, gentamicin, or tobramycin) *plus* Linezolid or vancomycin

Adapted from American Thoracic Society, Infectious Diseases Society of America. Guidelines for the management of adults with hospital-acquired, ventilator-associated, and healthcare-associated pneumonia. *Am J Respir Crit Care Med.* 2005;171(4):388–416.

vancomycin.[18] In a prospective study of 39 children with nosocomial pneumonia treated with either linezolid or vancomycin, Jantausch et al. found no significant difference in overall cure rates.[19] However, the group treated with linezolid may have been more severely ill—with higher rates of multilobar pneumonia and longer duration of MV—at treatment initiation. Furthermore, the linezolid group experienced faster resolution of symptoms and shorter treatment durations compared with the vancomycin group.

Neonatal VAP caused by carbapenem-resistant *Acinetobacter* species is associated with high mortality and morbidity. A Thai case-case-control study reported outcomes for 76 neonates with VAP, 63 of who had carbapenem-resistant *Acinetobacter baumannii* (CRAB) isolated from ETT secretion samples during their illness. In-hospital mortality was approximately twofold among the VAP patients with CRAB compared with those with cabapenem-sensitive *A. baumannii*, and there was a higher rate of bronchopulmonary dysplasia (BPD) among CRAB survivors.[20] In their 2005 guidelines for management of adult patients with VAP, the American Thoracic Society recommended consideration of colistin as therapy for patients with VAP proven or suspected to be caused by carbapenem-resistant *Acinetobacter* species.[16] Several case series have reported on the safety profile of intravenous colistin in neonates. The main side effect is transient renal injury among some patients; therefore urine output, creatinine, and serum electrolytes should be carefully monitored during therapy.

While prompt initiation of broad-spectrum antibiotics to cover potential drug-resistant pathogens is important, prolonged or repeated treatment with empiric antibiotics increases the risk of a drug-resistant infection in the future and is associated with considerable cost. A Swiss study of antibiotic use among over 450 patients admitted to a combined pediatric and neonatal intensive care unit between 1998 and 1999 identified suspected pneumonia as the most common reason for initiation of antibiotics (probably reflecting the pediatric population more than the neonates, for whom rule-out sepsis episodes are more common). When the illnesses that prompted antibiotics were subjected to retrospective review, only 41% of antibiotic courses corresponded to a proven bacterial infection.[21]

Given the challenges associated with isolating a VAP etiologic pathogen described earlier, rationally narrowing antibiotic coverage based on microbiologic evidence can be difficult. One approach is to wait 24 to 48 hours after starting empiric therapy before obtaining a suctioned ETT sample for culture. The rationale is that after exposure to a broad-spectrum regimen, much of the microbiome colonizing the airway will have been eliminated, increasing the chances of isolating any drug-resistant strains that might be causing disease. Obviously if the causative organism is actually sensitive to the empiric treatment, it will likely not be recovered and—in this circumstance—any cultured organism is probably a nonpathogenic colonizer. In navigating these uncertainties, physicians are advised to incorporate multiple forms of evidence when planning therapy for suspected VAP. The patient's history and clinical response to empiric treatment, laboratory data, and caution regarding overuse of broad-spectrum antibiotics must all be included in the calculus.

Antibiotic treatment of VAP should continue for 7 to 14 days, but there is no consensus on the best antibiotic course duration. One study in adults with VAP compared outcomes after either 8 or 15 days of therapy and found no overall difference in mortality or relapse rates. The subset of patients with VAP caused by gram-negative, nonfermenting bacilli (such as *P. aeruginosa*) did experience higher relapse rates when treated for only 8 days, suggesting that gram-negative infections may warrant a longer treatment course. On the other hand, patients in the 8-day treatment group were less likely to develop a multidrug-resistant infection in the future.[22] When deciding on treatment duration for a neonate with suspected VAP, 10 days is a reasonable standard course, which can be adjusted based on clinical response.

Inhaled antimicrobials, which have proven benefit in cystic fibrosis, represent an area of potential innovation in neonatal VAP management. In a small pilot study, aerosolized colistin was investigated as a potential adjunctive therapy in cases of neonatal VAP caused by certain multidrug-resistant strains of *A. baumannii*.[23] This form of treatment was effective in the seven infants who received it, all of whom recovered from VAP with no serious adverse effects (one died later of apparently unrelated sepsis).

Prevention

The Centers for Disease Control and Prevention and the American Thoracic Society have published guidelines for reducing the incidence of hospital-acquired pneumonia, including VAP.[16,24] Recommendations for preventing VAP are generally aimed at limiting opportunities for cross-contamination between caregivers and patients, decreasing tissue damage from prolonged or recurrent intubation, avoiding unnecessary medication that may promote infection and/or antibiotic resistance, and maximizing oral hygiene and pulmonary toilet.

Many hospitals have implemented VAP "bundles," which are based on published guidelines and consist of multiple, simultaneous practices—applied universally to intubated patients—intended to ensure quality care and to minimize the risk of infection. VAP bundles have been shown in several studies to effectively reduce VAP rates among adult patients. Some bundle components that are standard in adult units—such as using cuffed ETTs—are generally inapplicable to neonates, but other components are feasible in the NICU, and an emerging literature indicates that neonatal VAP bundles are also effective. Box 8.4 summarizes VAP bundle elements that are generally believed to help prevent neonatal VAP, several of which are discussed later.

Proper hand hygiene is likely the single most important defense against VAP. Potential pathogens on caregivers' hands can be passed to patients during examination, routine care, or through contamination of medical equipment. An observational study of nosocomial infection rates before and after an intensive hospital-wide hand hygiene improvement initiative documented a decrease in neonatal VAP rates from 16.9 to 6.4 per 1000 ventilator days.[25] A similar Taiwanese study performed during hospital quality reforms that nearly doubled local handwashing rates documented a simultaneous threefold decrease in neonatal respiratory infections.[26]

Several studies have investigated possible approaches to limiting introduction of VAP pathogens from contaminated equipment. One well-examined strategy involves scheduled exchanges of ventilators, tubing, and suctioning equipment. The rationale for this approach is that regular substitution of sterilized equipment might decrease accumulation of bacterial contamination. This hypothesis, however, has not been borne out in clinical trials. Routine disconnection and replacement of ventilator circuits probably actually creates unnecessary opportunities for

Box 8.4   POSSIBLE COMPONENTS OF A NEONATAL VAP PREVENTION BUNDLE[a]

Hand Hygiene

Meticulous hand hygiene before and after patient contact and handling respiratory equipment

Wear gloves when handling ventilator condensate and other respiratory/oral secretions

Intubation

Use a new, sterile ETT for each intubation attempt

Ensure that the ETT does not contact environmental surfaces before insertion

Use a sterilized laryngoscope

Have at least two NICU staff members present for ETT retaping or repositioning

Suctioning Practices

Clear secretions from the posterior oropharynx before:
- ETT manipulation
- Patient repositioning
- Extubation
- Reintubation

Feeding

Prevent gastric distention

Monitor gastric residuals

Adjust feeding to prevent large residuals and/or distention

Positioning

Use side-lying position as tolerated

Keep the head of bed elevated 15 to 30 degrees as tolerated

Use left lateral positioning after feedings as tolerated

Oral Care

Provide oral care:
- Within 24 hours after intubation
- Every 3 to 4 hours
- Before reintubation as time allows
- Before orogastric tube insertion

Use sterile water, breast milk, or approved pharmaceutical oral care solution

Respiratory Equipment

Use a separate suction catheter, connection tubing, and canister for oral and tracheal suction

Drain ventilator condensate away from the patient every 2 to 4 hours and before repositioning

Avoid unnecessary disconnection of the ventilator circuit

Change ventilator equipment when visibly soiled or mechanically malfunctioning

Use heated ventilator circuits

[a]Elements have been adapted from the adult literature, and there is no consensus on a universal bundle.

ETT, Endotracheal tube; *NICU,* neonatal intensive care unit.

Adapted from Weber CD. Applying adult ventilator-associated pneumonia bundle evidence to the ventilated neonate. *Adv Neonatal Care.* 2016;16:178–190.

contamination. The consensus of multiple agencies, therefore, is that ventilator equipment—including tubing and suctioning apparatuses—should be replaced only when visibly soiled.

Another factor that has been studied—particularly among adult populations—is the type of suctioning device used. So-called in-line devices, which allow suctioning of the trachea and ETT lumen without disconnecting it from the ventilator, may prevent VAP in adults without compromising adequate clearance of salivary and mucous secretions. A Cochrane review of four studies in neonates concluded that in-line suctioning may yield improved short-term advantages—such as fewer desaturation events and improved ease of use by nursing staff—but there was no clear long-term benefit in terms of mortality or major morbidity. The included investigations did not allow strong conclusions about the effect on VAP rates.[27] A well-performed, prospective study by Cordero and colleagues (not included in the Cochrane review) demonstrated no significant difference in infectious or noninfectious complications between in-line and open suctioning systems in 175 randomly assigned premature infants, but reported a nursing preference for the convenience and ease of the in-line system.[28] While the data are arguably too limited to draw definite conclusions about in-line suctioning and neonatal VAP, there is no strong evidence that one type of suctioning apparatus has marked advantages for infection prevention over the others.

Other neonatal VAP bundle components intended to prevent infection from equipment contamination include ensuring that at least two people are present during ETT retaping or repositioning; draining ventilator condensate away from the patient every 2 to 4 hours; clearing secretions before ETT retaping or repositioning, patient repositioning, or extubation; and using only sterilized laryngoscopes and newly opened ETTs that have not touched any environmental surfaces.

As discussed previously, there is some evidence that patient positioning can affect the likelihood of tracheal contamination from gastric secretions. Intubated infants should be kept in a side-lying position as tolerated, with the head of the bed elevated 15 to 30 degrees. Other measures that can prevent gastric reflux from contributing to VAP include minimizing large gastric residuals by monitoring gastric aspirates every 4 hours and adjusting enteral feed volume and duration as needed. Although not well studied in neonatal populations, gastric antacid medications and histamine-2 receptor blockers have been shown to promote bacterial growth in the stomach and secondary tracheal colonization. These medications should be avoided in the NICU unless there is a clear indication that outweighs potential risks.

In general, excess oral secretions should be removed because pooling of saliva may create a niche for colonization by potential pathogens. There is good evidence from the adult literature that careful nursing attention to oral hygiene among intubated patients leads to decreased VAP. The evidence for a strong effect of oral hygiene is weaker in neonates, who are less susceptible to cavities and bacterial gingivitis. One small study of intubated preterm infants investigated routine oral swabbing with a pharmacologic gel containing several potentially antimicrobial compounds (e.g., lactoperoxidase, lysozyme, lactoferrin) or sterile water as a control. The authors reported a statistically nonsignificant drop in VAP rates among the experimental group, who also had lower neutrophil density in tracheal aspirates relative to controls, possibly suggesting decreased airway inflammation. The safety profile of the gel was acceptable, with no significant differences in noninfectious morbidities between the two groups.[29]

Another study tested the hypothesis that neonatal oral care with human breast milk—which is rich in antimicrobial substances—might decrease VAP rates. Using a preintervention/postintervention observational design, they reported nonsignificant drops in tracheal colonization and VAP among 138 enrolled neonates.[30] There were no concerning side effects in the treatment group and nursing compliance was high. Given the possible benefits and overall low risks of gentle oral care with breast milk or a commercial product, some NICUs currently include this practice in their VAP prevention bundles.

Outcomes

VAP undoubtedly increases mortality and morbidity, although the precise degree of risk for neonates has so far not been determined. In one study of intubated children in the pediatric ICU, VAP was shown to almost double unadjusted mortality rates (from 6.99% to 12.04%), to increase overall MV duration 2.5-fold, and to increase the duration of pediatric ICU admission.[31] Neonatal studies have demonstrated the same trends. Multiple neonatal studies have demonstrated that VAP increases hospital length of stay, but sample sizes have not been sufficient to draw firm conclusions about the degree of increased mortality risk attributable to neonatal VAP.[5,7]

Certain patterns of tracheal colonization may promote later development of BPD, although this line of inquiry has only recently been vigorously explored using culture-free microbiomic approaches. Early tracheal colonization with *Ureaplasma* has been implicated in eventual development of BPD among premature neonates, but causal links between *Ureaplasma* and the pulmonary inflammatory cascade that leads to BPD have not been proven and remain controversial.[32] Using next-generation sequencing to define the tracheal microbiome, Lohmann et al. demonstrated that, consistent with establishment of a predominant, pathogenic organism, decreased diversity among tracheal colonizing bacteria correlates with eventual BPD.[33]

Future Research Directions

Accurate diagnostic tests that allow discrimination between normal oropharyngeal colonization and true infection are needed, and work in this direction is underway. Several laboratories have investigated individual or grouped biomarkers as indicators of VAP. Harwood et al. investigated the potential of glutathione sulfonamide (GSA), a by-product of neutrophil-mediated oxidation, to detect the presence of infectious airway inflammation. They measured GSA concentrations in tracheal aspirates from intubated preterm neonates and correlated levels with culture results. GSA concentration was significantly correlated with the presence of potential pathogenic bacteria, and—importantly—did not increase in the presence of likely commensals such as *Staphylococcus epidermidis*. The study was not powered to identify a significant relationship between GSA concentration and diagnosed VAP.[34]

An emerging question in VAP research is how establishment and maintenance of a normal neonatal microbiome affects VAP pathogenesis. Early studies on this question suggest that there is a "protective" airway microbiome, whose disruption may create an opportunity for pathogenic populations to expand.[35] This possibility is indirectly supported by data linking early, prolonged antibiotic exposure with later development of BPD among very low-birth-weight neonates.[36] The existence of a microbiome structure protective against VAP, if proven, would be consistent with recent discoveries relating microbiome diversity and fluctuation with other important neonatal infectious diseases, such as necrotizing enterocolitis and sepsis.

Conclusion

Recognition of neonatal VAP as a disease with potentially serious consequences is a relatively recent development. VAP, which has been better studied in adult populations, is inherently difficult to diagnose with certainty—even more so in the NICU, where invasive airway testing is rarely feasible. Bacterial contamination of the airway is a significant challenge, which currently can be surmounted only by using multimodal clinical, laboratory, and radiographic diagnostic criteria.

Nevertheless, prompt diagnosis and evidence-based antibiotic treatment of VAP can speed extubation, decrease NICU admission duration, and save lives. Several important questions about the best approach to VAP diagnosis and management remain unanswered, making VAP an inviting topic for impactful scientific research.

REFERENCES

1. Cernada M, Aguar M, Brugada M, et al. Ventilator-associated pneumonia in newborn infants diagnosed with an invasive bronchoalveolar lavage technique. *Pediatr Crit Care Med.* 2013;14(1):55–61.
2. Dudeck MA, Edwards JR, Allen-Bridson K, et al. National Healthcare Safety Network report, data summary for 2013, device-associated module. *AJIC.* 2015;43(3):206–221.
3. Edwards JR, Peterson KD, Mu Y, et al. National Healthcare Safety Network (NHSN) report: data summary for 2006 through 2008, issued December 2009. *Am J Infect Control.* 2009;37(10):783–805.
4. Dudeck MA, Horan TC, Peterson KD, et al. National Healthcare Safety Network report, data summary for 2011, device-associated module. *Am J Infect Control.* 2013;41(4):286–300.
5. Apisarnthanarak A, Holzmann-Pazgal G, Hamvas A, Olsen MA, Fraser VJ. Ventilator-associated pneumonia in extremely preterm neonates in a neonatal intensive care unit: characteristics, risk factors, and outcomes. *Pediatrics.* 2003;112(6 Pt 1):1283–1289.
6. Goldmann DA, Freeman J, Durbin WA Jr. Nosocomial infection and death in a neonatal intensive care unit. *J Infect Dis.* 1983;147(4):635–641.
7. Singh-Naz N, Yuan T-M, Chen L-H, Sprague BM, Patel KM, Yu H-M. Risk factors and outcomes for ventilator-associated pneumonia in neonatal intensive care unit patients. *J Perinat Med.* 2007;35(4):334–338.

8. Cernada M, Aguar M, Brugada M, et al. Ventilator-associated pneumonia in newborn infants diagnosed with an invasive bronchoalveolar lavage technique. *Pediatr Crit Care Med.* 2013;14(1): 55–61.

9. Zur KB, Mandell DL, Gordon RE, Holzman I, Rothschild MA. Electron microscopic analysis of biofilm on endotracheal tubes removed from intubated neonates. *Otolaryngol Head Neck Surg.* 2004;130(4):407–414.

10. Adair CG, Gorman SP, Feron BM, et al. Implications of endotracheal tube biofilm for ventilator-associated pneumonia. *Intensive Care Med.* 1999;25(10):1072–1076.

11. Aly H, Badawy M, El-Kholy A, Nabil R, Mohamed A. Randomized, controlled trial on tracheal colonization of ventilated infants: can gravity prevent ventilator-associated pneumonia? *Pediatrics.* 2008;122(4):770–774.

12. Garland JS, Alex CP, Johnston N, Yan JC, Werlin SL. Association between tracheal pepsin, a reliable marker of gastric aspiration, and head of bed elevation among ventilated neonates. *J Neonatal Perinatal Med.* 2014;7(3):185–192.

13. Torres A, Serra-Batlles J, Ros E, et al. Pulmonary aspiration of gastric contents in patients receiving mechanical ventilation: the effect of body position. *Ann Intern Med.* 1992;116(7):540–543.

14. Cardeñosa Cendrero JA, Solé-Violán J, Bordes Benítez A, et al. Role of different routes of tracheal colonization in the development of pneumonia in patients receiving mechanical ventilation. *Chest.* 1999;116(2):462–470.

15. Feldman C, Kassel M, Cantrell J, et al. The presence and sequence of endotracheal tube colonization in patients undergoing mechanical ventilation. *Eur Respir J.* 1999;13(3):546–551.

16. American Thoracic Society, Infectious Diseases Society of America. Guidelines for the management of adults with hospital-acquired, ventilator-associated, and healthcare-associated pneumonia. *Am J Respir Crit Care Med.* 2005;171(4):388–416.

17. Trouillet JL, Chastre J, Vuagnat A, et al. Ventilator-associated pneumonia caused by potentially drug-resistant bacteria. *Am J Respir Crit Care Med.* 1998;157(2):531–539.

18. Wunderink R, Rello P, Cammarata SK, Croos-Dabrera RV, Kollef MH. Linezolid vs vancomycin: analysis of two double-blind studies of patients with methicillin-resistant *Staphylococcus aureus* nosocomial pneumonia. *Chest.* 2003;124(5):1789–1797.

19. Jantausch BA, Deville J, Adler S, et al. Linezolid for the treatment of children with bacteremia or nosocomial pneumonia caused by resistant gram-positive bacterial pathogens. *Pediatr Infect Dis J.* 2003;22(suppl 9):S164–S171.

20. Thatrimontrichai A, Techato C, Dissaneevate S, et al. Risk factors and outcomes of carbapenem-resistant *Acinetobacter baumannii* ventilator-associated pneumonia in the neonate: a case-case-control study. *J Infect Chemother.* 2016;22(7):444–449.

21. Fischer JE, Ramser M, Fanconi S. Use of antibiotics in pediatric intensive care and potential savings. *Intensive Care Med.* 2000;26(7):959–966.

22. Chastre J, Wolff M, Fagon J-Y, et al. Comparison of 8 vs 15 days of antibiotic therapy for ventilator-associated pneumonia in adults: a randomized trial. *JAMA.* 2003;290(19):2588–2598.

23. Nakwan N, Wannaro J, Thongmak T, et al. Safety in treatment of ventilator-associated pneumonia due to extensive drug-resistant *Acinetobacter baumannii* with aerosolized colistin in neonates: a preliminary report. *Pediatr Pulmonol.* 2011;46(1):60–66.

24. Tablan OC, Anderson LJ, Besser R, Bridges C. Guidelines for preventing healthcare-associated pneumonia, 2003. *MMWR.* 2004.

25. Lam BCC, Lee J, Lau YL. Hand hygiene practices in a neonatal intensive care unit: a multimodal intervention and impact on nosocomial infection. *Pediatrics.* 2004;114(5):e565–e571.

26. Won SP, Chou HC, Hsieh WS, et al. Handwashing program for the prevention of nosocomial infections in a neonatal intensive care unit. *Infect Control Hosp Epidemiol.* 2004;25(9):742–746.

27. Taylor JE, Hawley G, Flenady V, Woodgate PG. Tracheal suctioning without disconnection in intubated ventilated neonates. *Cochrane Database Syst Rev.* 2011;(12):CD003065.

28. Cordero L, Sananes M, Ayers LW. Comparison of a closed (Trach Care MAC) with an open endotracheal suction system in small premature infants. *J Perinatol.* 2000;20(3):151–156.

29. Stefanescu BM, Hétu C, Slaughter JC, O'Shea TM, Shetty AK. A pilot study of Biotene OralBalance® gel for oral care in mechanically ventilated preterm neonates. *Contemp Clin Trials.* 2013;35(2): 33–39.

30. Thibeau S, Boudreaux C. Exploring the use of mothers' own milk as oral care for mechanically ventilated very low-birth-weight preterm infants. *Adv Neonat Care.* 2013;13(3):190–197.

31. Gupta S, Boville BM, Blanton R, et al. A multicentered prospective analysis of diagnosis, risk factors, and outcomes associated with pediatric ventilator-associated pneumonia. *Pediatr Crit Care Med.* 2015;16(3):e65–e73.

32. Schelonka RL, Waites KB. Ureaplasma infection and neonatal lung disease. *Semin Perinatol.* 2007;31(1):2–9.

33. Lohmann P, Luna RA, Hollister EB, et al. The airway microbiome of intubated premature infants: characteristics and changes that predict the development of bronchopulmonary dysplasia. *Pediatr Res.* 2014;76(3):294–301.

34. Harwood DT, Darlow BA, Cheah F-C, McNeill N, Graham P, Winterbourn CC. Biomarkers of neutrophil-mediated glutathione and protein oxidation in tracheal aspirates from preterm infants: association with bacterial infection. *Pediatr Res.* 2011;69(1):28–33.

35. Lu W, Yu J, Ai Q, Liu D, Song C, Li L. Increased constituent ratios of *Klebsiella* sp., *Acinetobacter* sp., and *Streptococcus* sp. and a decrease in microflora diversity may be indicators of ventilator-associated pneumonia: a prospective study in the respiratory tracts of neonates. *PLoS One.* 2014;9(2):e87504–e87509.
36. Novitsky A, Tuttle D, Locke R, Saiman L, Mackley A, Paul D. Prolonged early antibiotic use and bronchopulmonary dysplasia in very low birth weight infants. *Am J Perinatol.* 2014;32(01):043–048.

8

CHAPTER 9

Long-Term Pulmonary Outcome of Preterm Infants

Jeanie L.Y. Cheong and Lex W. Doyle

- Both very and late preterm infants have worse respiratory health in childhood and adolescence.
- Very preterm survivors have worse lung function, particularly airway obstruction, in childhood up to young adulthood.
- BPD in the newborn period is associated with worse respiratory outcomes in childhood and later years.
- More research is required into the effects of cigarette smoking on later lung function in preterm survivors.

Preterm birth continues to be a significant problem in the developed world. Preterm birth rates peaked at 13% in 2006 in the United States and have since declined to approximately 10%.[1,2] "Late preterm" infants, with gestational ages from 34 to 36 completed weeks, represent the majority of preterm births. Moreover, survival rates for preterm neonates, particularly those born very preterm (<32 completed weeks) have increased because of technologic and therapeutic advances, such as antenatal administration of corticosteroids and postnatal administration of exogenous surfactant, combined with a greater willingness to offer intensive care before and after birth. Unfortunately, preterm infants are more susceptible to adverse sequelae than are term infants, and the lungs of preterm infants are particularly vulnerable to injury.[3] Despite advances in care, respiratory problems remain the major cause of mortality in extremely preterm (<28 completed weeks) infants in the surfactant era.[4] Of those who survive the neonatal period, some experience bronchopulmonary dysplasia (BPD), both "old"[5] and "new" forms,[3] with prolonged oxygen dependency, occasionally for years. Although most preterm survivors have no ongoing oxygen dependency or respiratory distress in early childhood, their pulmonary function should be determined, because they are more prone to respiratory ill health in late childhood and adulthood.

Controversies

Some of the controversies regarding pulmonary outcomes of preterm birth are as follows:
- What are the pulmonary outcomes for the late preterm infants, who make up the majority of preterm survivors?
- What are the pulmonary outcomes for the very preterm infants, including hospital readmissions, respiratory health problems, pulmonary function in childhood and later life, and exercise tolerance?
- What are the effects of exogenous surfactant, cigarette smoking, and BPD in the newborn period on outcomes in very preterm infants?

  This chapter reviews long-term pulmonary outcomes for preterm infants. If data by gestational age are not available, data by birth weight are substituted, with the assumption that birth weight less than 1500 g is equivalent to gestational age less than 32 weeks, and birth weight less than 1000 g to gestational age less than 28 weeks.

What Are the Long-Term Pulmonary Outcomes for Late Preterm Infants?

There are two published reviews of studies reporting long-term respiratory morbidity of late preterm infants.[6,7] Some studies have also included infants born "moderately preterm" (between 32 and 33 completed weeks of gestation). In total, there were 34 studies reporting respiratory outcomes of late preterm infants between 2000 and 2014. Rates of readmission to hospital after first discharge home were higher in the late preterm group compared with term controls. Data from the U.K. Millennium Cohort Study reported higher rates of hospital admissions for late preterm infants and children compared with term born controls (39–41 weeks).[8] In the first 9 months after birth, the mean adjusted odds ratio (OR) of three or more hospital admissions for late preterm infants was 5.1 (95% confidence interval [CI] 3.0–8.8). The hospital admission rates decreased as the children became older. However, late preterm children up to 5 years in that study were still at increased risk of hospital admissions compared with term children (adjusted OR 1.9, 99% CI 1.3–2.7). The major reason for rehospitalization was respiratory illness.[8] In a study enrolling infants born in Manitoba, Canada, during 1997 to 2001, preterm birth was a significant risk factor for readmission to the hospital in the first 6 weeks after discharge. On the basis of birth weights, gestational ages for the majority of the infants in that study would have been 32 to 36 weeks.[9] The most common cause for readmission during the 6 weeks was respiratory illness (22%), which was more than twice as common as the next leading cause. Both reviews reported substantial respiratory morbidity caused by respiratory syncytial virus (RSV). One study reported that rates of hospital admission for RSV were 57 per 1000 in late preterm infants, which exceeded that of term controls (30 per 1000) but were close to that of very preterm infants (66–70 per 1000).[10] A similar trend was noticed in a regional study of preterm children in the Netherlands, where the rates of hospitalization in the first year owing to RSV were 4% in those born between 32 and 36 weeks of gestation, compared with 3% in those born before 32 weeks and 1% in the full-term children.[11]

It has become clearer that respiratory morbidity for late preterm children persists beyond infancy. Many studies report an increased prevalence of asthma, bronchiolitis, or wheezing illnesses in this group of children compared with term controls.[8,11–13] A large retrospective study of 7925 infants using electronic health data from 31 practices affiliated with an academic center in the United States reported associations between late preterm birth and persistent asthma to 18 months (adjusted OR 1.68, 95% CI 1.20–2.29) and inhaled corticosteroid use (adjusted OR 1.66, 95% CI 1.01–2.80). A large observational study between 1989 and 2008 in Finland also reported a similar increase in asthma risk with lower gestation at birth (adjusted OR 1.7, 95% CI 1.4–2.0).[13] In the United Kingdom, the increased rates of asthma or wheezing illnesses persisted up to 5 years, with an adjusted OR of being prescribed any asthma-related medication of 2.2 (95% CI 1.6–3.1).[8] However, data from the Third National Health and Nutrition Examination Survey (NHANES III, 1988–1994) did not show a significantly increased risk of asthma in late preterm infants.[14] Data were available from 6187 singletons of gestational ages 34 to 41 weeks who were between 2 and 83 months old at the time of the survey; the 537 late preterm (34–36 weeks) children had a slightly higher rate of physician-diagnosed asthma than the 5650 children who were born at term, but the increase was not statistically significant (adjusted hazard ratio 1.3; 95% CI 0.8–2.0).

There are now several reports of pulmonary function in late preterm children, all of which report more airway obstruction in late preterm infants compared with controls. One study from Brazil reported on 26 infants born with a mean gestational age of 32.7 weeks (range 30–34 weeks) who did not have substantial respiratory distress in the neonatal period. Pulmonary function tests performed at a mean age of 10 weeks and repeated at a mean age of 64 weeks showed more airway obstruction in these infants compared with 24 term controls, with no evidence of improvement between the two tests.[15] The investigators concluded that preterm birth per se resulted in abnormal lung development, but late preterm children clearly need to be reassessed later in childhood and into adulthood to determine whether lung function abnormalities are permanent. A more recent study of a cohort of 31 infants born at 33 to 36 weeks of gestation with no clinical respiratory disease and 31 race- and sex-matched term controls also reported abnormal pulmonary function at term corrected age in the late preterm group compared with term controls.[16] The late preterm group had decreased respiratory compliance, decreased expiratory flow ratio, and increased respiratory resistance compared with term controls. A decrease in expiratory flow ratio in the newborn period is thought to be a reflection of expiratory airflow limitation and predicts subsequent wheezing. Kotecha et al. reported respiratory function at 8 to 9 years and 14 to 17 years from the Avon Longitudinal Study of Parents and Children.[17] Participants were divided into 4 gestational age groups (i.e., <32 weeks, 33–34 weeks, 35–36 weeks, and term). Of the 6705 children with lung function at 8 to 9 years, those born at 33 to 34 weeks had poorer spirometry measures (forced expiratory volume at 1 second [FEV_1], forced vital capacity [FVC], forced expiratory flow in the middle of the exhaled volume [FEF_{25-75}], and the FEV_1/FVC ratio) than term children. There was attenuation of differences in FEV_1 and FVC between those born at 33 to 34 weeks and term controls by the time the children were reassessed at 14 to 17 years. Interestingly, the spirometry measures of the "late preterm group" (35–36 weeks' gestation) were similar to term controls at all time points. In a recent study from Sweden, lung function data of 149 children born at 32 to 36 weeks were compared at 8 and 16 years of age with 2472 children born at term at 8 and 16 years of age. At 8 years of age FEV_1 was lower only in preterm girls compared with girls born at term, but by 16 years of age airflow was lower in both sexes compared with controls.[18] In addition to these studies, Northway and colleagues[19] reported respiratory function at a mean age of 18.3 years of subjects who would have mostly been late preterm; this study is discussed further in the section "Pulmonary Function in Adolescence or Early Adulthood."

What Are the Long-Term Pulmonary Outcomes for Very Preterm Infants, and What Is the Effect of BPD on These Outcomes?

Hospital Readmissions for Respiratory Illness

Rates of rehospitalization of very preterm infants are several fold higher than in term controls, and rates of hospital readmission have risen as survival rates of more very preterm infants have increased over time.[20] For example, the UK Millennium Cohort Study reported an adjusted OR of 13.7 (95% CI 6.5–29.2) for 3 or more admissions to the hospital for very preterm infants up to 9 months, which decreased with age (adjusted OR 6.0, 95% CI 3.2–11.4) between 9 months and 5 years of age.[8] Respiratory illnesses are the most common cause of rehospitalization in these early years,[21–23] and they occur more frequently in preterm survivors who had BPD, especially those who were discharged home while receiving oxygen treatment.[21] However, as the rate of hospital readmission declines later in childhood, those who had BPD are no more likely to be readmitted to the hospital for respiratory or other reasons by the time they reach mid-adolescence.[24,25]

Respiratory Health Problems

Very preterm children have more ill health than term children over the first few years of life, particularly upper and lower respiratory tract illnesses.[20,26–28] Rates of morbidity are further increased in those who had BPD.[20,29–31] Asthma or recurrent wheezing is more prevalent later in life in those born very tiny or preterm than in those not born preterm or very tiny in some[32–34] but not all studies.[24,35] Those who had BPD have even higher rates of asthma than those who did not.[36]

Pulmonary Function in Childhood

Before the widespread availability of antenatal corticosteroids and exogenous surfactant therapy in the 1990s, very preterm survivors had more abnormalities in

Table 9.1   FEATURES AND MAIN FINDINGS OF STUDIES REPORTING PULMONARY FUNCTION
TESTS IN CHILDHOOD OF VERY PRETERM CHILDREN COMPARED WITH CONTROLS

Study (Year Published)	Age Studied	Very Preterm (N) and Definition	Controls (N)	Main Findings
Children Born Before the 1990s				
Chan et al.[37] (1989)	7 yr	130; <2000 g	120	Airway obstruction
Kitchen et al.[38] (1992)	8–9 yr	240; <1000 g or <28 wk	208	Airway obstruction; worse with BPD
McLeod et al.[39] (1996)	8–9 yr	300; <1500 g	590	Airway obstruction with exercise
Kennedy et al.[40] (2000)	11 yr	102; <1501 g	82	Airway obstruction and air trapping
Anand et al.[41] (2003)	15 yr	128 <1500 g	128	Airway obstruction
Siltanen et al.[34] (2004)	10 yr	72; <1501 g	65	Airway obstruction
Children Born After 1990				
Hjalmarson and Sandberg[47] (2002)	Term corrected age	Mean 32[a] (range 25–33) wk	53	Reduced compliance; higher resistance
Thunqvist et al.[51] (2015)	6 and 18 mo	55; ≤30 wk	0	Airflow limitation (relative to published norms)
Korhonen et al.[48] (2004)	7–8 yr	34 BPD; 34 no BPD; all <1500 g	34	Airway obstruction
Doyle et al.[49] (2006)	8–9 yr	240; <1000 g or <28 wk	208	Airway obstruction; worse with BPD
Fawke et al.[50] (2010)	11 yr	182; <26 wk	161	Airway obstruction; worse with BPD
Fortuna et al.[45] (2016)	8 and 12 yr	48; <28 wk and <1000 g	27	Airway obstruction; worse with BPD, deterioration between 8 and 12 years
MacLean et al.[46] (2016)	8–12 yr	103; ≤28 wk	65	Airway obstruction; worse with BPD

[a]Minimal neonatal respiratory disease.
BPD, Bronchopulmonary dysplasia.

pulmonary function in childhood than term controls (Table 9.1).[34,37–41] Very preterm survivors with BPD had even more abnormalities in childhood pulmonary function than did very preterm survivors without BPD.[24,38,42–46]

After 1990 pulmonary function was still worse in very preterm survivors than in controls (see Table 9.1).[47–50] However, survivors from later eras of neonatal care are, on average, more immature and weigh less at birth than those in earlier eras and hence are more at risk for abnormal pulmonary function. There may have been some improvement in pulmonary function with antenatal corticosteroids and exogenous surfactant that has been offset by the survival of higher-risk survivors. Children with the new BPD[3] in later eras still have the reductions in airflow and increased gas trapping observed before the widespread availability of surfactant and antenatal corticosteroids.[45,46,48–51] Fawke and associates[50] measured lung function data with portable devices at 11 years of age in 59% of survivors born before 26 weeks of gestation from the EPICure study of births in the United Kingdom in 1995. They reported large differences in several variables reflecting airway obstruction between these very preterm survivors and term controls. However, the differences reported were wider between preterm survivors and term controls than differences reported in another study of preterm survivors born in the 1990s and evaluated at 8 to 9 years of age; this study measured pulmonary function using standard laboratory tests.[49] A more recent study reported deterioration in spirometry between age 8 and 12 years in a subgroup of children with BPD compared with controls.[45] It will be important to reassess pulmonary function later in life in such extremely immature infants, particularly to determine the effects of environmental hazards, such as cigarette smoking.

Table 9.2   FEV$_1$ FOR STUDIES WITH RESPIRATORY FUNCTION REPORTED IN LATE ADOLESCENCE/EARLY ADULTHOOD[a]

Study (Year Published)	FEV$_1$ in Preterm Groups Data are Mean (SD) Unless Otherwise Specified BPD	No BPD	FEV$_1$ in NBW Controls
Northway et al.[19] (1990)	74.8 (14.5); $n = 25$[b]	96.6 (10.2); $n = 26$	100.4 (10.9); $n = 53$
Halvorsen et al.[32] (2004)	87.8 (13.8); $n = 12$[c]	97.7 (12.9); $n = 34$	108.1 (13.8); $n = 46$
Doyle et al.[52] (2006)	81.6 (18.7); $n = 33$[b]	92.9 (12.8); $n = 114$	99.4 (9.5); $n = 37$
Vrijlandt et al.[53] (2006)	90.1 (19.8); $n = 8$[d]	99.2 (17.9); $n = 12$[e]	109.6 (13.4); $n = 48$
Wong et al.[54] (2008)	89.0 (22.6–121.9)[e]; $n = 21$		
Gough et al.[56] (2014)	81.9 (15.9); $n = 72$	97.0 (15.2); $n = 57$	101.2 (11.4); $n = 78$
Gibson et al.[57] (2015) (z scores)	−1.37 (2.21); $n = 24$	−0.47 (1.30); $n = 63$	0.38 (0.79); $n = 19$
Vollsaeter et al.[58] (2015)	84.1 (75.8–92.3)[f]; $n = 11$	93.6 (85.0–102.3); $n = 12$	100.4 (95.5–105.3); $n = 39$
Caskey et al.[59] (2016)	88.2 (15.2); $n = 25$	102.0 (14.9); $n = 24$	109.4 (11.8); $n = 25$

[a]FEV$_1$ is reported as percentage of predicted for age, height, and sex, with one exception.
[b]BPD determined by ventilator dependency, oxygen requirement for more than 28 days, and chest radiograph findings consistent with Northway stage 3 or 4 changes.[5]
[c]BPD group had oxygen requirement at 36 weeks of gestation; the remainder of preterm subjects in this study are considered to have no BPD.
[d]Males only.
[e]Range; this study had no controls, either preterm or term.
[f]Data are mean (95% confidence interval).
BPD, Bronchopulmonary dysplasia; FEV$_1$, forced expiratory volume in 1 second; NBW, normal birth weight.

Pulmonary Function in Adolescence or Early Adulthood

Several studies have reported respiratory function data in the second and third decades of life for very preterm subjects and controls.[19,32,52–59] Results for FEV$_1$, reported as percentage of predicted for age, height, and sex, are shown in Table 9.2 for those studies in which data are available separately for preterm subjects with BPD and without BPD as well as for controls. All subjects in these studies were born before exogenous surfactant was available for clinical use.

Northway and colleagues[19] reported respiratory function at a mean age of 18.3 years in 25 subjects born between 1964 and 1973 who had old BPD[5]; subjects had required assisted ventilation, were oxygen-dependent at 28 days of life, and had chest radiographic evidence of scarring or cystic changes (stages 3 or 4). Data were compared with those from 26 age-matched controls of similar birth weight and gestational age who had not undergone ventilation as infants and 53 age-matched normal subjects who were not born preterm. Most of the preterm survivors must have been late preterm because the mean gestational ages were 33.2 and 34.5 weeks for the two preterm groups, respectively. Those with BPD had reductions in variables reflecting airflow and increased gas trapping in comparison with both the preterm controls and the normal controls.

Halvorsen and coworkers[32] reported the pulmonary outcomes for 46 subjects with birth weight less than 1001 g or gestational ages less than 29 weeks at a mean age of 17.7 years from a geographically based cohort of children born between 1982 and 1985 in western Norway. Twelve (26%) of the subjects had moderate or severe BPD (oxygen requirement at postmenstrual age 36 weeks), 24 (52%) had mild BPD (oxygen requirement at 28 days but not 36 weeks), and 10 (22%) had no BPD. Compared with 46 term controls, the preterm group had reductions in variables reflecting flow, and these variables were lower with increasing severity of BPD.

In a study of 147 survivors with birth weights less than 1501 g born during 1977 through 1982 in the Royal Women's Hospital, Melbourne, Australia, who underwent respiratory function tests at a mean age of 18.9 (standard deviation [SD] 1.1) years, the 33 (22%) who had old BPD showed substantial reductions in respiratory function variables reflecting airflow; more of the subjects in this group had reductions in airflow in clinically important ranges compared with the 114 preterm survivors without BPD.[52] Compared with normal birth weight term controls, the preterm subjects without BPD also had substantially reduced variables reflecting flow.

Vrijlandt and associates[53] studied 42 children at 19 years of age who had been born either before 32 weeks of gestation or at less than 1500 g birth weight in 1983 in the Netherlands, and compared the results with those in 48 "healthy" term controls. The respiratory function of the preterm subjects was mostly in the normal range (e.g., FEV_1 mean 95.4% [SD 15.9] predicted) but that in the controls was better than expected (e.g., FEV_1 mean 109.6% [SD 13.4]), so the respiratory function in preterm subjects was significantly worse than in the controls. Results for preterm males with and without BPD were not substantially different (see Table 9.2), but the sample sizes were small and hence the power to detect differences between the groups was low.

Wong and colleagues[54] reported the outcome of 21 survivors with BPD and birth weight <1500 g who had been cared for in one hospital in Western Australia between 1980 and 1987. The subjects were between 18 and 26 years old when they were assessed; two other subjects, ages 17 and 33 years, respectively, who were referred by respiratory physicians were also included. There were no preterm or term controls in this study, and those who participated represented only 16% (21/133) of all known survivors who required oxygen treatment at 36 weeks corrected gestational age. Values for FEV_1 were similar to those for BPD subjects in the other studies (see Table 9.2). In addition, 19 of the subjects in this study underwent computed tomography of the lungs, which showed changes consistent with emphysema in 16 (84%).

A recent study from Belfast reported airway limitation in preterm adults in their mid-20s with BPD compared with those without BPD.[56] Importantly, there were more variables within abnormally low and clinically important ranges in the BPD subgroup. Of note, 40% of the BPD group compared with 6% in term controls had FEV_1 less than 80% predicted, and 50% of the BPD group compared with less than 10% of controls had FEF_{25-75} less than 60% predicted.

The overall impression from the data in Table 9.2 is that most survivors with BPD have FEV_1 values within the normal range (means >80%), with the exception of the highly selected study by Northway and colleagues,[19] but they are worse than preterm controls without BPD, and even worse relative to term controls.

In contrast with the preceding studies, one study of 58 preterm subjects born in the pre-surfactant era, compared with 48 healthy term controls, found no significant differences in measured z scores for FEV_1, maximum mid-expiratory flow (FEF_{25-75}), or FVC at 21 years of age.[55] Because the preterm subjects had a median gestational age of 31.5 weeks, the majority of them must have been very preterm (<32 weeks); some, however, must have also been late preterm and even term because the gestational age range was 27 to 37 weeks. In this study, there was a strong positive correlation for z scores for FEV_1 between childhood and adulthood even though the mean z score for FEV_1 fell from childhood to adulthood.[60] In another study, data at 8 years and 18 to 22 years of age in 129 subjects with birth weights less than 1501 g were described; 29 of the 129 subjects had BPD.[52] Compared with respiratory function variables measured at 8 years, the only variable with a statistically significant difference over time in BPD subjects was a larger drop in the FEV_1/FVC ratio between 8 and 18 years of age compared with preterm subjects who did not have BPV (mean reduction 3.4%, 95% CI 0.2%–6.7%).

Trends in Pulmonary Function With Increasing Age

It is vital to have information about how lung function in preterm survivors may change as they mature. In a regional Australian cohort of 297 extremely preterm or extremely low-birth-weight participants and 260 term controls recruited in 1991–1992 (i.e., in an era when surfactant was given liberally to extremely preterm infants with respiratory distress syndrome), Doyle et al. reported spirometry changes from age 8 to 18 years.[61] The preterm group had lower FEV_1 at both ages compared with controls (mean differences [95% CI] in z score for FEV_1; 8 years −1.02 [−1.21 to −0.82]); 18 years −0.92 [−1.14 to −0.71]). The spirometry parameters declined with increasing age and were worse in those with BPD and in those who smoked. Two other reports of survivors from the 1970s and 1980s did not find deterioration of lung function between mid-childhood and young adulthood.[55,58] This may reflect differences between pre-surfactant and post-surfactant cohorts and factors specific to the populations from different geographic regions.

Exercise Tolerance

Cardiopulmonary limitations may not be evident during standard respiratory function measurements conducted at rest, but they may become apparent during an exercise test. In one study of 10-year-old children born in 1992 through 1994 weighing less than 1000 g and before 32 weeks of gestation, the exercise capacity of the preterm group was approximately one-half that of term controls.[62] More recent studies have reported shorter walking distances using the 6-minute walk test in former preterm children with BPD compared with those without BPD.[63,64] Some other studies,[65-68] but not all,[53,69,70] have also reported diminished peak oxygen consumption with exercise testing in preterm children. Not all of these studies were limited to very preterm subjects; one evaluated only infants with birth weights less than 801 g,[67] another selected subjects of less than 32 weeks' gestational age or with birth weights less than 1500 g,[53] another included extremely preterm children born before 28 weeks' gestation,[68] and the remainder studied only subjects with BPD and not complete cohorts of preterm children. Exercise limitation has also been reported in one study of young adults (mean age 24 years) born preterm compared with term controls.[59]

What Are the Effects of Exogenous Surfactant?

The effect of exogenous surfactant administered soon after birth on later respiratory function on small numbers of children enrolled in clinical trials has been reported to be minimal[71] or possibly beneficial.[72] Several studies have reported that the effect of BPD in the surfactant era on respiratory function is similar to that before surfactant was available.[48,49] In one study the 34 subjects with BPD had lower FEV_1 at 7 to 8 years of age than 34 very low-birth-weight children without oxygen dependency and 34 term controls.[48] In a geographic study of children born in the state of Victoria, Australia, respiratory function was measured at a mean age of 8.9 years in 81% (240/298) of children born either before 28 weeks of gestation or at less than 1000 g birth weight and in 79% (208/262) of controls with normal birth weight controls.[49] Most of the preterm children had respiratory function within the expected range. However, some variables reflecting airflow were lower in preterm children with BPD than in both preterm children without BPD and normal birth weight controls, although the differences were not as marked as in the pre-surfactant era. Within this cohort, respiratory function was not substantially different between those preterm subjects who received and those who did not receive surfactant.

What Are the Effects of Cigarette Smoking?

Respiratory function in subjects with birth weights less than 1000 g who smoke in early adulthood has been reported to be worse than in those who do not smoke; Doyle and associates[73] reported the results of respiratory function at a mean age of 20.2 years in a cohort of 44 of 60 consecutive survivors born at less than 1000 g birth weight during 1977 through 1980 at the Royal Women's Hospital, Melbourne, Australia. Respiratory function had also been measured in 42 of the 44 subjects at 8 years of age. Respiratory function was compared in the 14 smokers and the 30 nonsmokers. Several respiratory function variables reflecting airflow were significantly diminished in smokers. The proportion with a clinically important reduction in airflow (FEV_1/FVC ratio <75%) was significantly higher in smokers (64%) than in nonsmokers (20%) ($\chi^2 = 8.3$; $P < .01$). There was a significantly larger decrease in the FEV_1/FVC ratio between ages 8 and 20 years in the smokers than in the nonsmokers (mean difference in rate of change: −8.2%, 95% CI −14.1% to −2.4%). Given that the rate of deterioration in respiratory function is more rapid up to age 20 years in smokers who weighed less than 1000 g at birth and the fact that cigarette smoking is detrimental to respiratory function in all subjects in adulthood,[74,75] preterm-born adults who smoke should undergo respiratory function testing well into adulthood to establish whether chronic obstructive airway disease develops more rapidly and at earlier ages. As mentioned earlier, in a more contemporary cohort of extremely preterm or extremely low-birth-weight participants born in the state of Victoria, those who smoked at 18 years of age had a decline in expiratory airflow between 8 and 18 years of age compared with nonsmokers.[61]

What Further Research Is Required?

Lower birth weight, and presumably increasing prematurity, is associated with worse respiratory health later in adulthood, including higher death rates from chronic obstructive airways disease and worse respiratory function, as reported in 1991 by Barker and coworkers[76] in a follow-up study of 5718 men born in Hertfordshire, England, from 1911 through 1930. The period of follow-up for very preterm survivors of modern perinatal/neonatal intensive care thus far has been only into the third decade and is clearly too short for accurate detection of chronic obstructive lung disease, which typically occurs much later in life. Even less is known about the late preterm group. However, given the higher rates of respiratory ill health and clear reductions in airflow in preterm survivors compared with controls up to the third decade, follow-up until much later into adulthood is required.

Summary

- Late preterm (32–36 weeks of gestation) survivors, who greatly outnumber very preterm survivors, have more respiratory ill health in early childhood than controls. However, the duration of follow-up has thus far been very short relative to total life expectancy.
- Very preterm (<32 weeks of gestation) survivors have more readmissions to the hospital in early childhood, more upper and lower respiratory tract infections, and more asthma symptoms than controls.
- Very preterm survivors have worse respiratory function than controls, particularly airway obstruction, both in childhood and in adolescence and early adulthood. They also have worse exercise tolerance than controls.
- Exogenous surfactant seems not to have altered long-term respiratory problems for preterm survivors.
- The detrimental effects of cigarette smoking on respiratory function are probably greater in preterm survivors, but more research is required.
- BPD in the newborn period generally exacerbates all of these long-term respiratory problems.
- Respiratory function and respiratory health later in adult life for preterm infants must be determined, because they are more susceptible to earlier onset of chronic obstructive airway disease than controls.

REFERENCES

1. Goldenberg RL, Culhane JF, Iams JD, Romero R. Epidemiology and causes of preterm birth. *Lancet*. 2008;371:75–84.
2. Births: preliminary data for 2015. National vital statistics reports, Vol. 65 No 3, June 2016.
3. Jobe AH, Bancalari E. Bronchopulmonary dysplasia. *Am J Respir Crit Care Med*. 2001;163:1723172–1723179.
4. Doyle LW, Gultom E, Chuang SL, et al. Changing mortality and causes of death in infants 23–27 weeks' gestational age. *J Paediatr Child Health*. 1999;35:255–259.
5. Northway Jr WH, Rosan RC, Porter DY. Pulmonary disease following respirator therapy of hyaline-membrane disease. Bronchopulmonary dysplasia. *N Engl J Med*. 1967;276:357–368.
6. Colin AA, McEvoy C, Castile RG. Respiratory morbidity and lung function in preterm infants of 32 to 36 weeks' gestational age. *Pediatrics*. 2010;126:115–128.
7. Pike KC, Lucas JS. Respiratory consequences of late preterm birth. *Paediatr Respir Rev*. 2015;16:182–188.
8. Boyle EM, Poulsen G, Field DJ, et al. Effects of gestational age at birth on health outcomes at 3 and 5 years of age: population based cohort study. *BMJ*. 2012;344:e896.
9. Martens PJ, Derksen S, Gupta S. Predictors of hospital readmission of Manitoba newborns within six weeks postbirth discharge: a population-based study. *Pediatrics*. 2004;114:708–713.
10. Boyce TG, Mellen BG, Mitchel Jr EF, Wright PF, Griffin MR. Rates of hospitalization for respiratory syncytial virus infection among children in medicaid. *J Pediatr*. 2000;137:865–870.

11. Vrijlandt EJ, Kerstjens JM, Duiverman EJ, Bos AF, Reijneveld SA. Moderately preterm children have more respiratory problems during their first 5 years of life than children born full term. *Am J Respir Crit Care Med.* 2013;187:1234–1240.

12. Goyal NK, Fiks AG, Lorch SA. Association of late-preterm birth with asthma in young children: practice-based study. *Pediatrics.* 2011;128:e830–e838.

13. Harju M, Keski-Nisula L, Georgiadis L, Raisanen S, Gissler M, Heinonen S. The burden of childhood asthma and late preterm and early term births. *J Pediatr.* 2014;164:295–299.e291.

14. Abe K, Shapiro-Mendoza CK, Hall LR, Satten GA. Late preterm birth and risk of developing asthma. *J Pediatr.* 2010;157:74–78.

15. Friedrich L, Pitrez PM, Stein RT, et al. Growth rate of lung function in healthy preterm infants. *Am J Respir Crit Care Med.* 2007;176:1269–1273.

16. McEvoy C, Venigalla S, Schilling D, Clay N, Spitale P, Nguyen T. Respiratory function in healthy late preterm infants delivered at 33–36 weeks of gestation. *J Pediatr.* 2013;162:464–469.

17. Kotecha SJ, Watkins WJ, Paranjothy S, Dunstan FD, Henderson AJ, Kotecha S. Effect of late preterm birth on longitudinal lung spirometry in school age children and adolescents. *Thorax.* 2012;67:54–61.

18. Thunqvist P, Gustafsson PM, Schultz ES, et al. Lung function at 8 and 16 years after moderate-to-late preterm birth: a prospective cohort study. *Pediatrics.* 2016;137. pii: e20152056.

19. Northway Jr WH, Moss RB, Carlisle KB, et al. Late pulmonary sequelae of bronchopulmonary dysplasia. *N Engl J Med.* 1990;323:1793–1799.

20. Doyle LW, Ford G, Davis N. Health and hospitalisations after discharge in extremely low birth weight infants. *Semin Neonatol.* 2003;8:137–145.

21. Cunningham CK, McMillan JA, Gross SJ. Rehospitalization for respiratory illness in infants of less than 32 weeks' gestation. *Pediatrics.* 1991;88:527–532.

22. Hennessy EM, Bracewell MA, Wood N, et al. Respiratory health in pre-school and school age children following extremely preterm birth. *Arch Dis Child.* 2008;93:1037–1043.

23. Kitchen WH, Ford GW, Doyle LW, et al. Health and hospital readmissions of very-low-birth-weight and normal-birth-weight children. *Am J Dis Child.* 1990;144:213–218.

24. Doyle LW, Cheung MM, Ford GW, et al. Birth weight <1501 g and respiratory health at age 14. *Arch Dis Child.* 2001;84:40–44.

25. McCormick MC, Workman-Daniels K, Brooks-Gunn J, Peckham GJ. Hospitalization of very low birth weight children at school age. *J Pediatr.* 1993;122:360–365.

26. O'Callaghan MJ, Burns Y, Gray P, et al. Extremely low birth weight and control infants at 2 years corrected age: a comparison of intellectual abilities, motor performance, growth and health. *Early Hum Dev.* 1995;40:115–128.

27. Chien YH, Tsao PN, Chou HC, Tang JR, Tsou KI. Rehospitalization of extremely-low-birth-weight infants in first 2 years of life. *Early Hum Dev.* 2002;66:33–40.

28. Skromme K, Leversen KT, Eide GE, Markestad T, Halvorsen T. Respiratory illness contributed significantly to morbidity in children born extremely premature or with extremely low birthweights in 1999–2000. *Acta Paediatr.* 2015;104:1189–1198.

29. Yu VY, Orgill AA, Lim SB, et al. Bronchopulmonary dysplasia in very low birthweight infants. *Aust Paediatr J.* 1983;19:233–236.

30. Tammela OK. First-year infections after initial hospitalization in low birth weight infants with and without bronchopulmonary dysplasia. *Scand J Infect Dis.* 1992;24:515–524.

31. Korhonen P, Koivisto AM, Ikonen S, et al. Very low birthweight, bronchopulmonary dysplasia and health in early childhood. *Acta Paediatr.* 1999;88:1385–1391.

32. Halvorsen T, Skadberg BT, Eide GE, et al. Pulmonary outcome in adolescents of extreme preterm birth: a regional cohort study. *Acta Paediatr.* 2004;93:1294–1300.

33. Vrijlandt EJ, Boezen HM, Gerritsen J, et al. Respiratory health in prematurely born preschool children with and without bronchopulmonary dysplasia. *J Pediatr.* 2007;150:256–261.

34. Siltanen M, Savilahti E, Pohjavuori M, Kajosaari M. Respiratory symptoms and lung function in relation to atopy in children born preterm. *Pediatr Pulmonol.* 2004;37:43–49.

35. Steffensen FH, Sorensen HT, Gillman MW, et al. Low birth weight and preterm delivery as risk factors for asthma and atopic dermatitis in young adult males. *Epidemiology.* 2000;11:185–188.

36. Ng DK, Lau WY, Lee SL. Pulmonary sequelae in long-term survivors of bronchopulmonary dysplasia. *Pediatr Int.* 2000;42:603–607.

37. Chan KN, Noble-Jamieson CM, Elliman A, et al. Lung function in children of low birth weight. *Arch Dis Child.* 1989;64:1284–1293.

38. Kitchen WH, Olinsky A, Doyle LW, et al. Respiratory health and lung function in 8-year-old children of very low birth weight: a cohort study. *Pediatrics.* 1992;89:1151–1158.

39. McLeod A, Ross P, Mitchell S, et al. Respiratory health in a total very low birthweight cohort and their classroom controls. *Arch Dis Child.* 1996;74:188–194.

40. Kennedy JD, Edward LJ, Bates DJ, et al. Effects of birthweight and oxygen supplementation on lung function in late childhood in children of very low birth weight. *Pediatr Pulmonol.* 2000;30:32–40.

41. Anand D, Stevenson CJ, West CR, Pharoah PO. Lung function and respiratory health in adolescents of very low birth weight. *Arch Dis Child.* 2003;88:135–138.

42. Chan KN, Wong YC, Silverman M. Relationship between infant lung mechanics and childhood lung function in children of very low birthweight. *Pediatr Pulmonol.* 1990;8:74–81.

43. Doyle LW, Kitchen WH, Ford GW, et al. Outcome to 8 years of infants less than 1000 g birthweight: relationship with neonatal ventilator and oxygen therapy. *J Paediatr Child Health.* 1991;27:184–188.

9

44. Doyle LW, Ford GW, Olinsky A, et al. Bronchopulmonary dysplasia and very low birthweight: lung function at 11 years of age. *J Paediatr Child Health*. 1996;32:339–343.
45. Fortuna M, Carraro S, Temporin E, et al. Mid-childhood lung function in a cohort of children with "new bronchopulmonary dysplasia." *Pediatr Pulmonol*. 2016;51:1057–1064.
46. MacLean JE, DeHaan K, Fuhr D, et al. Altered breathing mechanics and ventilatory response during exercise in children born extremely preterm. *Thorax*. 2016;71:1012–1019.
47. Hjalmarson O, Sandberg K. Abnormal lung function in healthy preterm infants. *Am J Respir Crit Care Med*. 2002;165:83–87.
48. Korhonen P, Laitinen J, Hyodynmaa E, Tammela O. Respiratory outcome in school-aged, very-low-birth-weight children in the surfactant era. *Acta Paediatr*. 2004;93:316–321.
49. Doyle LW, The Victorian Infant Collaborative Study Group. Respiratory function at age 8–9 years in extremely low birthweight/very preterm children born in Victoria in 1991–92. *Pediatr Pulmonol*. 2006;41:570–576.
50. Fawke J, Lum S, Kirkby J, et al. Lung function and respiratory symptoms at 11 years in children born extremely preterm: the EPICure study. *Am J Respir Crit Care Med*. 2010;182:237–245.
51. Thunqvist P, Gustafsson P, Norman M, Wickman M, Hallberg J. Lung function at 6 and 18 months after preterm birth in relation to severity of bronchopulmonary dysplasia. *Pediatr Pulmonol*. 2015;50:978–986.
52. Doyle LW, Faber B, Callanan C, et al. Bronchopulmonary dysplasia in very low birth weight subjects and lung function in late adolescence. *Pediatrics*. 2006;118:108–113.
53. Vrijlandt EJ, Gerritsen J, Boezen HM, et al. Lung function and exercise capacity in young adults born prematurely. *Am J Respir Crit Care Med*. 2006;173:890–896.
54. Wong PM, Lees AN, Louw J, et al. Emphysema in young adult survivors of moderate-to-severe bronchopulmonary dysplasia. *Eur Respir J*. 2008;32:321–328.
55. Narang I, Rosenthal M, Cremonesini D, et al. Longitudinal evaluation of airway function 21 years after preterm birth. *Am J Respir Crit Care Med*. 2008;178:74–80.
56. Gough A, Linden M, Spence D, Patterson CC, Halliday HL, McGarvey LP. Impaired lung function and health status in adult survivors of bronchopulmonary dysplasia. *Eur Respir J*. 2014;43:808–816.
57. Gibson AM, Reddington C, McBride L, Callanan C, Robertson C, Doyle LW. Lung function in adult survivors of very low birth weight, with and without bronchopulmonary dysplasia. *Pediatr Pulmonol*. 2015;50:987–994.
58. Vollsaeter M, Clemm HH, Satrell E, et al. Adult respiratory outcomes of extreme preterm birth. A regional cohort study. *Ann Am Thorac Soc*. 2015;12:313–322.
59. Caskey S, Gough A, Rowan S, et al. Structural and functional lung impairment in adult survivors of bronchopulmonary dysplasia. *Ann Am Thorac Soc*. 2016;13:1262–1270.
60. Chambers DC. Lung function in ex-preterm adults. *Am J Respir Crit Care Med*. 2009;179:517.
61. Doyle LW, Adams AM, Robertson C, et al. Increasing airway obstruction from 8 to 18 years in extremely preterm/low-birthweight survivors born in the surfactant era. *Thorax*. 2016;6.
62. Smith LJ, van Asperen PP, McKay KO, et al. Reduced exercise capacity in children born very preterm. *Pediatrics*. 2008;122:e287–e293.
63. Praprotnik M, Stucin Gantar I, Lucovnik M, Avcin T, Krivec U. Respiratory morbidity, lung function and fitness assessment after bronchopulmonary dysplasia. *J Perinatol*. 2015;35:1037–1042.
64. Vardar-Yagli N, Inal-Ince D, Saglam M, et al. Pulmonary and extrapulmonary features in bronchopulmonary dysplasia: a comparison with healthy children. *J Phys Ther Sci*. 2015;27:1761–1765.
65. Santuz P, Baraldi E, Zaramella P, et al. Factors limiting exercise performance in long-term survivors of bronchopulmonary dysplasia. *Am J Respir Crit Care Med*. 1995;152:1284–1289.
66. Pianosi PT, Fisk M. Cardiopulmonary exercise performance in prematurely born children. *Pediatr Res*. 2000;47:653–658.
67. Kilbride HW, Gelatt MC, Sabath RJ. Pulmonary function and exercise capacity for ELBW survivors in preadolescence: effect of neonatal chronic lung disease. *J Pediatr*. 2003;143:488–493.
68. MacLean JE, DeHaan K, Fuhr D, et al. Altered breathing mechanics and ventilatory response during exercise in children born extremely preterm. *Thorax*. 2016;71:1012–1019.
69. Bader D, Ramos AD, Lew CD, et al. Childhood sequelae of infant lung disease: exercise and pulmonary function abnormalities after bronchopulmonary dysplasia. *J Pediatr*. 1987;110:693–699.
70. Jacob SV, Lands LC, Coates AL, et al. Exercise ability in survivors of severe bronchopulmonary dysplasia. *Am J Respir Crit Care Med*. 1997;155:1925–1929.
71. Gappa M, Berner MM, Hohenschild S, et al. Pulmonary function at school-age in surfactant-treated preterm infants. *Pediatr Pulmonol*. 1999;27:191–198.
72. Pelkonen AS, Hakulinen AL, Turpeinen M, Hallman M. Effect of neonatal surfactant therapy on lung function at school age in children born very preterm. *Pediatr Pulmonol*. 1998;25:182–190.
73. Doyle LW, Olinsky A, Faber B, Callanan C. Adverse effects of smoking on respiratory function in young adults born weighing less than 1000 grams. *Pediatrics*. 2003;112:565–569.
74. Higgins MW, Enright PL, Kronmal RA, et al. Smoking and lung function in elderly men and women. the cardiovascular health study. *JAMA*. 1993;269:2741–2748.
75. Dockery DW, Speizer FE, Ferris BGJ, et al. Cumulative and reversible effects of lifetime smoking on simple tests of lung function in adults. *Am Rev Respir Dis*. 1988;137:286–292.
76. Barker DJ, Godfrey KM, Fall C, et al. Relation of birth weight and childhood respiratory infection to adult lung function and death from chronic obstructive airways disease. *Brit Med J*. 1991;303:671–675.

Management of Respiratory Problems

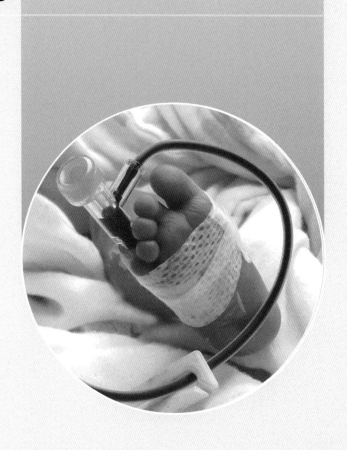

CHAPTER 10

Respiratory and Cardiovascular Support in the Delivery Room

Gary M. Weiner, Stuart B. Hooper, Peter G. Davis, and
Myra H. Wyckoff

10

- Following delivery, the processes of lung aeration and increases in pulmonary blood flow are closely linked.
- Establishing effective ventilation is the key to successful resuscitation.
- Although risk factors indicating likelihood of requiring resuscitation are identified, appropriately trained personnel should be present at all deliveries.
- Maintaining normal temperature reduces the risk of adverse outcomes.
- Routine tracheal suction for nonvigorous newborns with meconium stained amniotic fluid is no longer recommended.
- Air should be used for resuscitation of term and late preterm infants, and oxygen supplementation should be guided by pulse oximetry.
- The two-thumb technique should be used to deliver cardiac compressions.

Understanding the Transition to Newborn Life

The transition from fetal to newborn life represents one of the greatest physiologic challenges that all humans encounter. During fetal life, the lungs are liquid-filled, and at birth this liquid must be rapidly cleared from the airways to allow the entry of air and the onset of pulmonary gas exchange.[1] Pulmonary blood flow (PBF) must also markedly increase and several specialized vascular shunts must close to separate the pulmonary and systemic circulations.[2] While it is often considered that these events are independent, we now know that they are intimately linked.[3] Lung aeration is the primary trigger that not only facilitates the onset of pulmonary gas exchange but also stimulates an increase in PBF, which in turn initiates the cardiovascular changes.[3] The fact that lung aeration triggers the physiologic transition at birth underpins the well-established tenet of neonatal resuscitation. That is, establishing effective pulmonary ventilation is the key.

Recent radiographic imaging studies have demonstrated that lung aeration can occur very rapidly (in three to five breaths) and mostly occurs during inspiration or during positive-pressure inflations in ventilated neonates (Fig. 10.1).[4,5] It is thought that hydrostatic pressure gradients generated by inspiration (or positive-pressure inflations) drive liquid from the airways into the surrounding lung tissue.[4,5] However, as the interstitial tissue compartment of the lung has a fixed volume, the clearance of airway liquid into this compartment during lung aeration increases lung interstitial tissue pressures. Thus immediately following lung aeration, the neonatal lung is essentially edematous, which affects lung tissue mechanics and increases the likelihood of liquid reentering the airways during expiration.[6] Use of positive end-expiratory pressure (PEEP) opposes liquid reentry and ensures that air remains in the distal gas exchange units throughout the respiratory cycle (Fig. 10.2).[7] Thus PEEP

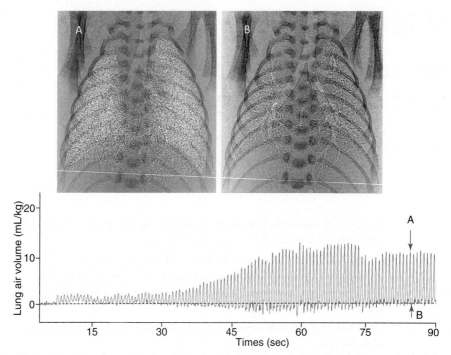

Fig. 10.1   Phase-contrast radiographic images and a plethysmograph recording of a preterm newborn rabbit immediately after birth ventilated from birth in the absence of a positive end-expiratory pressure (PEEP). In the absence of PEEP, preterm rabbits failed to develop a functional residual capacity (FRC), resulting in liquid reentry or airway collapse at end-expiration. Phase-contrast radiographic images (A and B) were recorded at each time point on the plethysmograph trace. Image A was acquired at end inspiration, whereas image B was acquired at FRC.

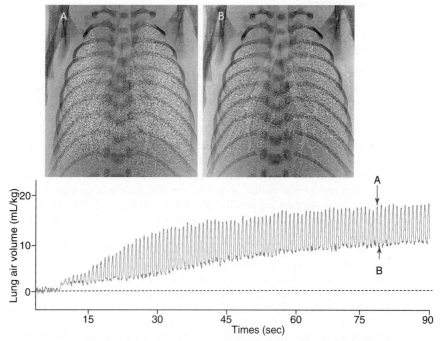

Fig. 10.2   Phase contrast radiographic images and a plethysmograph recording of a preterm newborn rabbit immediately after birth ventilated from birth with a positive end-expiratory pressure (PEEP) of 5 cm H_2O. With this level of PEEP, preterm rabbits gradually develop a significant functional residual capacity (FRC) with most distal airways (not all, see basal lung regions) remaining aerated at FRC. Phase contrast X-ray images (A and B) were recorded at each time point on the plethysmograph trace. Image A was acquired at end inspiration, whereas image B was acquired at FRC.

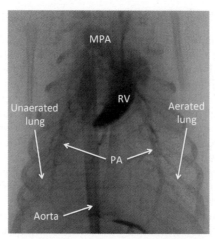

Fig. 10.3 Simultaneous phase-contrast and angiographic radiographic image of a near-term rabbit kitten following partial ventilation of the right lung. Aerated lung regions can be seen as "speckle" in the image and are due to refraction at the air/water interface. Although only part of the right lung is aerated, pulmonary blood flow is increased in both lungs equally. *MPA*, Main pulmonary artery; *PA*, pulmonary artery; *RV*, right ventricle.

not only reduces distal airway collapse at end-expiration, it also reduces airway liquid reentry and by retaining air in the distal airways allows gas exchange to continue throughout the respiratory cycle.[7]

The entry of air into the lung also triggers the cardiovascular transition at birth. Before birth, the majority of right ventricular output bypasses the lung and flows through the ductus arteriosus into the systemic circulation mainly because pulmonary vascular resistance (PVR) is high.[3] As a result, fetal PBF is low and contributes little to venous return and the supply of preload for the left ventricle. Instead, this mainly comes from umbilical venous return via the ductus venosus and foramen ovale.[2] Thus blood flow through the placenta is not only vital for oxygen and nutrient supply during fetal life, but is also vital for supplying preload for the left ventricle. Clamping the umbilical cord at birth therefore greatly reduces preload for the left ventricle, causing a large reduction in cardiac output.[8] Furthermore, cardiac output remains low until the lungs aerate and PBF increases to restore preload for the left ventricle.[8] Recognition of this shift in dependence from umbilical venous return to pulmonary venous return for sustaining ventricular preload at birth has led to the concept of physiology-based cord clamping.[9] That is, if cord clamping is delayed until after the lungs have aerated and PBF has increased, then PBF can immediately replace umbilical venous return as the major source of ventricular preload as soon as the cord is clamped, with no diminution in supply. This procedure greatly mitigates the large decreases and increases in cardiac output associated with cord clamping followed by ventilation onset.[8] It also greatly reduces the instantaneous increase in arterial blood pressure associated with cord clamping that is caused by the removal of the low-resistance placental vascular bed.[8]

Recent imaging studies have demonstrated that at birth, only partial lung aeration is required to stimulate a global increase in PBF and while increased oxygenation enhances this response, it is not oxygen dependent (Fig. 10.3).[10,11] Although partial aeration has the potential to cause large ventilation-perfusion mismatches in the lung at birth, this response arguably has an overall benefit during transition. As a redistribution of cardiac output and increased blood flow to the brain is critical for protecting the fetal brain from hypoxia, any constraint on cardiac output caused by a lack of venous return at birth is potentially catastrophic. By not limiting the increase in PBF to the degree of lung aeration, venous return and cardiac output will also not be limited by the degree of lung aeration immediately after birth.

At birth, lung aeration is important not only for establishing pulmonary gas exchange. It also triggers the increase in PBF required for facilitating pulmonary gas exchange and for replacing left ventricular preload lost following cord clamping, which is required to maintain cardiac output.

Anticipating the Need for Resuscitation

While the majority of newly born infants successfully transition from in utero to ex utero life without any intervention, approximately 4% to 10% of term and late preterm newborns require assistance to establish spontaneous respiratory effort, and a very small number require chest compressions or epinephrine during the transition period.[12] Given the nearly 131 million births per year worldwide, this means that many newborns each year require skilled assistance to support transition immediately after birth. Asphyxiation is the most common reason that newborns fail to transition successfully. *Asphyxia* is defined as a lack of gas exchange that results in simultaneous hypoxia and carbon dioxide (CO_2) elevation, leading to a mixed metabolic and respiratory acidosis. The asphyxial insult can result from either failure of placental gas exchange before birth or deficient pulmonary gas exchange once the newborn is delivered.[13]

Premature or postterm gestation, fetal hydrops, intrauterine growth restriction, gestational diabetes, multiple gestation, abnormal placentation, maternal illness, and maternal drug abuse are examples of antenatal risk factors that increase the likelihood of impaired gas exchange before delivery and increase the probability that the newborn will require resuscitation after birth. Intrapartum risk factors for impaired gas exchange include abnormal presentation (breech or transverse position), fetal bradycardia, umbilical cord compression or prolapse, placental abruption, intrapartum bleeding, meconium-stained amniotic fluid (MSAF), and chorioamnionitis. Risk factors that could affect gas exchange of the newborn include drug-induced respiratory depression (maternal magnesium exposure, opiates, and prolonged maternal general anesthesia), airway obstruction, prematurity, pneumonia, pneumothorax, and congenital malformations of the brain, airway, abdomen, heart, or lungs.

Although the likelihood of requiring resuscitation is higher in the presence of risk factors, individual risk factors and scoring systems that combine risk factors have limited discriminatory power and identify many births where no interventions are needed.[14,15] Moreover, some newborns require intervention in the absence of any risk factors. In one large cohort study, approximately 7% of newborns who received positive-pressure ventilation in the delivery room had no identifiable risk factors.[14] Thus for every delivery, the appropriate personnel must be present to immediately assess the newborn and initiate resuscitation.

After evaluating the obstetric history and known risk factors, the necessary neonatal health providers should be assembled. The number and qualifications of providers will vary depending on the specific circumstances. However, at every birth at least one person trained in neonatal resuscitation should be present whose only responsibility is to assess the infant, perform the initial steps of newborn care, and administer positive-pressure ventilation if necessary. A qualified team proficient in all resuscitation skills should be immediately available if resuscitation is required.[12] If risk factors suggest a high likelihood of the need for resuscitation, the team should be present at the time of birth to perform the necessary procedures without delay. Depending on the setting, this team may include providers from a variety of disciplines, such as respiratory therapy, anesthesiology, and emergency medicine.

Before the delivery, all members of the team should assemble to complete a briefing similar to the "time out" performed before any medical procedure. During this briefing, the team identifies a team leader, reviews the pregnancy history and risk factors, discusses the anticipated clinical scenario, delegates roles and responsibilities, considers contingency plans, and prepares the necessary supplies and equipment.

Preparation

Prior to delivery, all resuscitation supplies and equipment should be identified and checked for working order using a standardized checklist. Standardized checklists help to ensure adequate preparation by improving communication and rapidly identifying missing equipment.[16,17] The environmental temperature of the delivery room should be maintained at least 23°C (74°F) and free from drafts to help prevent hypothermia.[12,18] Warm blankets and a radiant warmer should be prepared. Depending on the circumstances, additional equipment and supplies including hats, thermal mattresses, and polyethylene plastic bags or wraps should be available.[19–24] A functioning positive-pressure ventilation (PPV) device (such as a self-inflating bag, a flow-inflating bag, or a T-piece device) and an appropriate sized face mask, manometer, and the capability to deliver blended oxygen are the most important equipment needed for newborn resuscitation. Suction devices (bulb syringe as well as wall suction and suction catheters), a functioning laryngoscope with appropriate sized blade and endotracheal tube, and a CO_2 detector for confirmation of correct tube placement should be ready for immediate use. Laryngeal masks are alternative airway devices that may provide a lifesaving airway when both face mask ventilation and endotracheal intubation are unsuccessful and should be readily available. Pulse oximetry to measure oxygen saturation and an electronic cardiac (electrocardiograph [ECG]) monitor to accurately measure the newborn's heart rate if resuscitation is required should be immediately accessible.[25] In certain high-risk circumstances, an umbilical venous line should be prepared and epinephrine drawn into a labeled syringe for rapid use.[13]

Initial Assessment

Immediately after birth, a rapid initial assessment is performed to determine if the newborn is vigorous and can remain with the mother to complete transition or should be moved to a radiant warmer for the initial steps of newborn care. This assessment can be performed during the interval between birth and umbilical cord clamping. Within 10 to 30 seconds of birth, approximately 85% of term newborns are vigorous with good muscle tone and strong respiratory effort, and an additional 10% becoming vigorous as they are dried and stimulated.[26] The healthy, term newborn's heart rate rapidly rises and remains above 100 beats/min within the first 2 minutes (median 123 beats/min at 1.5 minutes).[27] Clinical judgment of the newborn's color is notoriously difficult and is not an accurate predictor of the newborn's arterial oxygenation.[28] When measured by preductal pulse oximetry, the healthy newborn's oxygen saturation increases gradually from a median of near 60% at 1 minute of life to around 90% by 10 minutes of life.[29,30]

Vigorous term newborns with good tone and adequate respiratory effort should remain with their mother after birth to receive routine newborn care.[12] The infant may be placed on the mother's chest or abdomen and covered with a warm, dry blanket. Warmth is maintained by drying the newborn's skin and maintaining direct skin-to-skin contact with the mother. Secretions may be gently wiped from the face, mouth, and nose with a soft cloth or towel. Clearing secretions from the mouth and nose with a suction device should be reserved for those infants who have respiratory depression or cannot clear secretions on their own. If the infant is crying vigorously, there is no need for routine oral suction.[31] Additional steps of routine newborn care include drying, gentle stimulation, and continued observation during the transition period.[12]

Initial Steps for Nonvigorous and Preterm Newborns

Infants who are not vigorous after birth and those who are born preterm should be taken to a radiant warmer for assessment, the initial steps of newborn care, and possible resuscitative interventions (Fig. 10.4).[25] In some settings, this may performed on a specially designed resuscitation trolley placed immediately adjacent to the mother, allowing the steps to be performed without dividing the umbilical cord.[32]

Provide Warmth and Maintain Normal Temperature

Wet newborns rapidly lose heat and become hypothermic. For newly born, nonasphyxiated infants, the goal is to maintain normothermia (36.5°C–37.5°C) while avoiding both hypothermia and hyperthermia.[25] Cold stress in nonasphyxiated newborns is associated with multiple adverse outcomes, including hypoglycemia, metabolic acidosis, late-onset sepsis, lower arterial oxygen tension, and increased mortality.[33] Premature newborns are particularly vulnerable to hypothermia. A large cohort study including more than 5000 very low-birth-weight infants found that for every 1°C decrease in admission temperature below 36.5°C, the odds of dying

Neonatal Resuscitation Algorithm—2015 Update

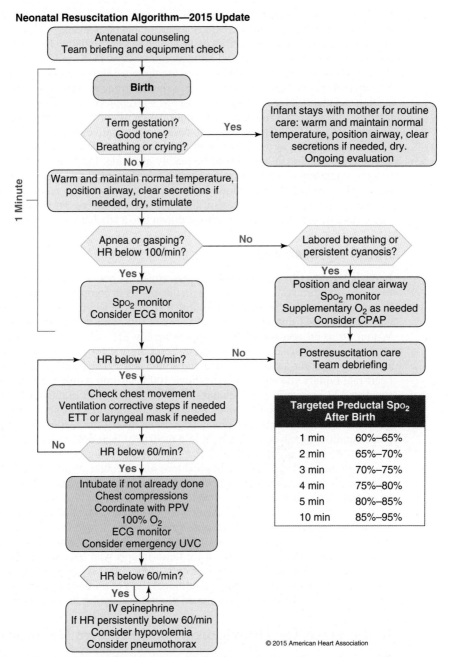

Fig. 10.4   Neonatal resuscitation algorithm. *CPAP*, Continuous positive airway pressure; *ECG*, electrocardiograph; *ETT*, endotracheal tube; *HR*, heart rate; *IV*, intravenous; *O₂*, oxygen; *PPV*, positive-pressure ventilation; *Spo₂*, oxygen saturation measured by pulse oximetry; *UVC*, umbilical venous catheter. (Reprinted with permission. From Circulation 132:S543-S560, 2015. ©2015 American Heart Association, Inc.)

increased by 28%.[34] Infants who do not qualify for routine care should be received in warm blankets and placed under a preheated radiant warmer set at 100% power. The initial wet receiving blanket should be removed while the infant is dried. Newly born preterm infants of less than 32 weeks' gestation may require a combination of interventions to maintain normothermia.[25,35,36] They should be placed immediately in a high-diathermancy food-grade polyethylene bag or wrap to the level of the shoulders without initial drying.[22,33] This maneuver allows radiant heat from the warmer to pass through to the infant while limiting convective and evaporative heat losses.

All subsequent resuscitation interventions can be performed with the polyethylene bag/wrap in place. Additional heat loss prevention strategies that may be considered for preterm infants include increasing the delivery room temperature above 25°C,[37] using a chemically activated thermal mattress in addition to the radiant warmer,[20,21] using warmed and humidified respiratory gases,[23,24,38] and covering the infant's head with a plastic bonnet.[19] It is important to monitor the newborn's temperature in the delivery room to guide these interventions because perinatal hyperthermia (>38°C) is also associated with respiratory depression and other complications.[39,40] Newborn preterm lambs exposed to initial hyperthermia have increased acidosis, inflammatory messenger ribonucleic acid, lung injury, and higher risks of pneumothoraces and death compared with normothermic animals.[41] If the newborn remains under the radiant warmer for more than a few minutes, a temperature sensor with servocontrol should be used to adjust the radiant warmer's output.

Position

The infant should be placed with the head and neck in a neutral or slightly extended position so that the airway is maximally opened. Excessive flexion or extension of the infant's neck is a common cause of airway obstruction. A shoulder roll lifts the shoulders and can help maintain correct positioning of the head, especially if there is a prominent occiput from cranial molding.

Additional Steps: Clear the Airway If Needed, Dry, and Stimulate

If the infant is apneic or is having difficulty breathing, a bulb syringe or suction catheter should be used to clear the mouth and then the nose.[12] Deep, vigorous, or prolonged suctioning is rarely needed, particularly in the early minutes of resuscitation, because it can traumatize tissues and induce vagal responses that are counterproductive during transition.

The approach to MSAF has evolved over the past several decades and remains controversial. MSAF occurs frequently, becomes more common with advancing gestational age, and may indicate fetal distress. The presence of MSAF is a risk factor that should alert the neonatal care team to the potential need for resuscitation. If meconium is aspirated into the airways either before or after birth, the newborn may develop meconium aspiration syndrome (MAS) with pulmonary hypertension and severe cardiorespiratory failure. On the basis of physiologic plausibility and nonrandomized observational studies in the 1970s, oropharyngeal suction at the perineum before delivery of the shoulders and tracheal suction immediately after birth were recommended to reduce the incidence and severity of MAS.[42–44] Although the incidence of MAS has decreased since the 1970s, it appears unlikely that these interventions were responsible for this decline. Data from single-center and population based studies suggest that the declining incidence of MAS may be attributed to contemporary obstetric practices that avoid postmaturity and prolonged fetal distress.[45–47] As the level of evidence progressed from observational studies to large randomized controlled trials, both oropharyngeal suction and routine tracheal suction of vigorous newborns were shown to be ineffective and are no longer recommended.[48,49] Intubation and tracheal suction of nonvigorous newborns with meconium-stained fluid is the delivery room intervention that has been the most difficult to study. Routine tracheal suction did not decrease the incidence or severity of MAS in either of the small randomized controlled trials enrolling nonvigorous newborns.[50,51] At present, there is no high-quality evidence supporting routine intubation and tracheal suction of nonvigorous newborns born through meconium-stained fluid. As international treatment guidelines are developed, the approach to an existing treatment recommendation that lacks robust supporting evidence can be controversial. Some prefer to continue existing recommendations until strong evidence supports the superiority of a new treatment, whereas others advocate using the same evidence standard to evaluate existing and newly proposed therapies. Based on explicit statements that the authors value, avoiding an invasive intervention without strong evidence of benefit, the 2015 International Liaison Committee on Resuscitation (ILCOR) Consensus on Science and Treatment Recommendations, American Heart Association (AHA) Guidelines, and European Resuscitation Council Guidelines no longer recommend routine tracheal suction for nonvigorous newborns with MSAF.[18,25,52] Although there may be subgroups of infants that could benefit from tracheal suction, the current consensus guidelines emphasize initiating ventilation for nonbreathing newborns and reserving tracheal suction for suspected airway obstruction.

Assessing the Infant's Response to the Initial Steps

After the initial steps of newborn care are completed, the infant's heart rate and respiratory effort are assessed. Initially, heart rate may be assessed by listening to the precordium with a stethoscope, because assessment of pulse by palpation is not as accurate.[53,54] If the infant is apneic, gasping or has a heart rate less than 100 beats/min, PPV should be promptly initiated.[12] If PPV is started, pulse oximetry is recommended and ECG monitoring should be considered.[12,55] The rapid postbirth assessment, initial steps of newborn care, reassessment of the infant's response, and initiation of PPV if indicated should be completed within approximately 60 seconds. This 1-minute interval between birth and the initiation of PPV has been referred to as "the golden minute." Audits of actual delivery room interventions suggest that this goal is infrequently attained.[56]

Effective Ventilation: The Key!

Any newborn who does not establish spontaneous respiratory effort after the initial steps or who remains bradycardic (heart rate <100 beats/min) should be given PPV.[12] Effective ventilation of the lungs is the single most important action to stabilize a newborn infant who is compromised following delivery. The goal is to provide aeration and ventilation that supports gas exchange without causing lung injury. PPV can be administered with a self-inflating bag, flow-inflating bag, T-piece resuscitator, or a neonatal ventilator. Each device has advantages and disadvantages and the choice of device may be made based on cost; availability of compressed gas; the desire to deliver sustained inflation, PEEP, and continuous positive airway pressure (CPAP); or personal preference.[57] Self-inflating bags are always ready for immediate use and reexpand without a compressed gas source. Although inadvertent high peak pressures have been demonstrated with self-inflating bags when operators use only a pop-off safety valve, if providers use an appropriately designed manometer they can accurately achieve the targeted peak inspiratory pressure.[58] Self-inflating bags are not routinely used to administer free-flow oxygen or continuous positive airway pressure (CPAP). Even when outfitted with a positive end-expiratory pressure (PEEP) valve, traditional self-inflating bags do not reliably deliver PEEP through the face mask.[59] A novel PEEP valve designed to work with a self-inflating bag in resource-limited settings without an external gas source may be effective.[60] The flow-inflating bag requires more time and practice to set up and a compressed gas source.[61] Because the bag does inflate without a tight seal, large mask leaks are easy to identify. PEEP and CPAP can be generated by balancing the gas flow into the bag and the amount of gas leaking out of a control valve; however, this adjustment requires experience. T-piece resuscitators more accurately and consistently deliver set inspiratory pressures and PEEP than the other devices, but they require a compressed gas source and changing the inflation pressures during resuscitation is more difficult.[57,62] Among infants born at 26 weeks' gestation or later requiring resuscitation, Szyld et al. found no difference between the T-piece resuscitator and self-inflating bag in achieving a heart rate of 100 beats/min or higher within 2 minutes; however, the T-piece decreased the maximum applied inspiratory pressure and the need for intubation.[63] Among extremely low-birth-weight infants, Dawson et al. found the self-inflating bag to be as effective as the T-piece resuscitator in achieving goal oxygen saturation values by 5 minutes of life.[64] If either a T-piece device or a flow-inflating bag is used, there must be a backup self-inflating bag in case compressed gas is lost. Whichever PPV device is chosen, the most important thing is to become proficient using and troubleshooting the selected device.

Ventilation can be provided via an appropriately sized face mask, endotracheal tube, or laryngeal mask. To achieve effective ventilation via face mask, the provider must first open the airway by placing the infant in the "sniffing" position.[12] To achieve a good seal, the mask should rest on the chin and snugly cover the mouth and nose, but not the eyes to avoid trauma and a vagal response.[65] Lack of appropriate airway positioning and inadequate seal are the most frequent causes of ineffective ventilation. A delivery room study of mask ventilation of premature infants documented that up to 25% of breaths had evidence of airway obstruction and 75% had mask leak.[66] Even experienced providers have difficulty identifying obstruction, leak, changes in compliance, and the tidal volume of their manual ventilations.[67,68] Simple disposable CO_2 detectors or continuous capnography may help confirm airway patency and effective lung aeration during bag-mask ventilation.[69,70] More sophisticated respiratory function monitors might also be helpful in detection of airway obstruction, mask leak, and delivered tidal volume.[71,72] Because providers have difficulty sensing changes in compliance, if the compliance suddenly improves, they may inadvertently deliver excessive tidal volumes that could lead to lung injury. When tidal volume is displayed, operator performance is markedly improved.[73] The currently available manual ventilation devices do not measure tidal volume; however, incorporating a respiratory function monitor to measure and display this information during manual ventilation may be useful.

Ventilation rates of 40 to 60 breaths/min are recommended.[12] Faster rates should be avoided to allow adequate exhalation time and to prevent stacked breaths, which could increase the risk of pneumothorax. Counting the ventilation rhythm out loud or using a metronome for pacing may be helpful.[74]

The optimal inflation pressure, inflation time, and target volume required to establish an effective functional residual capacity (FRC) have not been determined but likely vary among infants.[25] Inflation pressures should be monitored and every ventilation device should include a manometer. Guidelines suggest initial peak pressures in the range of 20 to 30 cm H_2O, but the pressure required to aerate the liquid filled lungs of an apneic infant may be as high as 30 to 40 cm H_2O. Infants without respiratory effort may require higher pressures initially, but pressures should be reduced as the lungs aerate and become more compliant. The goal is to provide the minimum inflating pressure necessary to quickly achieve and maintain a heart rate greater than 100 beats/min. The actual delivered volume varies widely depending on the newborn's spontaneous effort, lung compliance, glottic closure, face mask leak, and airway obstruction. In animal models, prolonged initial sustained inflations of 10 to 20 seconds have been shown to achieve functional residual capacity faster and to improve lung function without adverse circulatory effects.[75,76] However, randomized trials enrolling preterm newborns (25–32 weeks' gestation) with sustained inflations (20–25 cm H_2O for 10–15 seconds) compared with either CPAP or conventional ventilation have not shown a consistent benefit with regard to mortality or significant morbidities.[77]

The majority of newborns who require resuscitation improve promptly with assisted ventilation alone. The best sign that the lungs are being effectively aerated and ventilated is a rapid rise in heart rate,[78] followed by improvement in oxygen saturation and the infant's tone. If monitored, expired CO_2 levels higher than 10 mm Hg, indicating lung aeration, may be detected before the heart rate increases.[70] If the heart rate has not increased within 15 seconds of initiating PPV, the most likely reason is that the lungs are not being adequately ventilated because of an airway obstruction or large mask leak. The provider should attempt to improve the efficacy of ventilation by using the series of steps described in the **MRSOPA** mnemonic:

- **M**ask—ensure a good seal.
- **R**eposition—ensure the head and neck are in the sniffing position.
- **S**uction—clear the airway of any obstructing secretions.
- **O**pen the mouth—and reapply mask.
- **P**ressure—gradually increase the pressure until you see chest movement.
- **A**irway alternative—consider using an endotracheal tube or laryngeal mask airway.

If the heart rate remains less than 60 beats/min despite face mask ventilation that achieves chest movement, or if chest movement cannot be achieved with the basic corrective steps, insertion of an alternative airway (endotracheal tube or laryngeal mask) is strongly recommended.[12] In the unusual case when the infant does not improve with ventilation through an appropriately placed alternative airway and the heart rate remains lower than 60 beats/min, chest compressions are indicated.[25]

Continuous Positive Airway Pressure

If an infant is breathing spontaneously but has labored breathing or persistently low oxygen saturation, CPAP may help establish and maintain an FRC.[79] For premature infants, applying CPAP shortly after birth with subsequent selective surfactant administration has been recommended as an alternative to routine intubation with prophylactic surfactant administration.[80] Pooled analysis of four randomized controlled trials in preterm infants born at less than 32 weeks' gestation showed a significant benefit for the combined outcome of death or bronchopulmonary dysplasia for infants treated with nasal CPAP (risk difference –0.04, 95% confidence interval –0.08 to –0.00).[81] In one study that used CPAP levels of 8 cm H_2O in the delivery room, an increased risk of pneumothorax was observed,[82] but this higher risk was not seen in the other studies that used lower CPAP levels. For term infants there is no evidence to support or refute the use of CPAP in the delivery room, but it is frequently used in the situation of respiratory distress. Although CPAP may help establish and maintain an FRC, thus improving respiratory distress, it should not be used in place of PPV when the infant is apneic or bradycardic.

Alternative Airways: Endotracheal Tube or Laryngeal Mask Airway

Insertion of an alternative airway may be performed at various points during resuscitation and for several different indications. Examples include prolonged or ineffective face mask ventilation, heart rate remaining below 100 beats/min after 30 seconds of otherwise effective ventilation, or the need for chest compressions are needed.[12] An endotracheal tube should be inserted promptly if the infant has a congenital diaphragmatic hernia.

The equipment for endotracheal intubation should be readily available wherever infants may be born. The correct laryngoscope blade and tube size are based on the infant's estimated weight and/or gestational age (Table 10.1). An intubating stylet that stiffens the tube may be used with caution to ensure that the tip does not protrude beyond the end of the tube; however, one randomized trial showed that use of a stylet did not significantly improve the intubation success rate of pediatric trainees.[83] Once the procedure is completed, the placement of the tube within the trachea must be verified and the use of a CO_2 detector is recommended.[25] Use of a flow sensor that

Table 10.1 LARYNGOSCOPE BLADE SIZE, ENDOTRACHEAL TUBE SIZE, AND DEPTH OF INSERTION

Gestation (Weeks)	Weight (g)	Blade Size (No.)	Tube Size (mm ID)	Insertion Depth (Tip-to-Lip [cm])
23–24	500–600	0 or 00	2.5	5.5
25–26	700–800	0 or 00	2.5	6.0
27–29	900–1000	0	2.5–3.0	6.5
30–32	1100–1400	0	3.0	7.0
33–34	1500–1800	0	3.0	7.5
35–37	1900–2400	1.0	3.5	8.0
38–40	2500–3100	1.0	3.5	8.5
41–43	3200–4200	1.0	3.5	9.0

Adapted from Weiner GM, Zaichkin J, Kattwinkel J, American Academy of Pediatrics, American Heart Association. *Textbook of Neonatal Resuscitation.* ed 7. Elk Grove Village, IL: American Academy of Pediatrics; 2016; and Kempley ST, Moreiras JW, Petrone FL. Endotracheal tube length for neonatal intubation. *Resuscitation.* 2008;77(3): 369–373.

displays gas flow in and out of the tube may be a faster and more accurate method to confirm tube placement than a CO_2 detector.[84] Clinical indicators of tracheal placement include a rapid increase in heart rate, observing chest rise with PPV, auscultating air entry in both axillae, and observing condensation inside the tube during expiration; however, these signs can be misleading. Incomplete intubation attempts should be interrupted and bag mask ventilation resumed if the heart rate starts to fall or remains unstable. Limiting intubation attempts to a duration of seconds has been suggested as a reasonable goal.[12,85]

Initially, the endotracheal tube should be advanced so the printed vocal cord guide (black line on the distal end of the tube) is level with the vocal cords. At this depth, the tube is expected to be above the carina; however, the marker position varies by manufacturer and should only be used as an initial guide during the insertion procedure.[86,87] Previous recommendations suggested estimating the insertion depth (tip-to-lip) by adding 6 cm to the infant's weight in kilograms.[88] In preterm infants, this method may overestimate the insertion depth and place the tube in the infant's right mainstem bronchus, especially in extremely low-birth-weight infants.[89,90] More accurate methods for estimating the insertion depth have been validated in term and preterm newborns. One method uses the infant's estimated weight or gestational age to predict the insertion depth (see Table 10.1).[91] Another method estimates the insertion depth by measuring the distance (in centimeters) between the newborn's nasal septum and ear tragus (the nasal-tragus length). The tube is inserted to the nasal-tragus length distance + 1 cm with the appropriate centimeter mark secured at the infant's upper lip.[92] Radiographic confirmation of proper tube placement should be obtained as soon as feasible. The goal is to place the tip of the tube in the midtrachea, above the carina, with the tip aligned between the first and second thoracic vertebrae when assessed by chest radiography.[93]

Intubation is not an easy skill to acquire and requires extensive training to become proficient. Changes in practice have led to fewer infants being intubated in the delivery room and trainees having fewer opportunities to acquire this skill.[94] As a result, resident physicians take longer to complete the procedure, require multiple attempts, are successful in less than half of attempts, and repeated attempts are associated with adverse events.[85,95–97] When an alternative airway is needed, insertion of a laryngeal mask may be more successful. Laryngeal mask airways are effective for ventilating newborns who are 34 weeks or more estimated gestational age and weigh more than 2000 g at birth and may be effective for smaller and less mature newborns ($\geq$29 weeks, $\geq$1000 g).[98–102] Studies in adult models and patients suggest that placement of a laryngeal mask may be an easier task to learn than endotracheal intubation.[103–105] In addition, laryngeal masks have been used to administer surfactant and, when compared with standard endotracheal tube administration, decreased the proportion of newborns who ultimately required mechanical ventilation.[102] This technique requires further evaluation before it is widely applied. Insertion of a laryngeal mask should be considered during resuscitation if face mask ventilation is unsuccessful and intubation is either unsuccessful or not feasible, but the technique has not been evaluated for use during chest compressions or for administration of tracheal epinephrine.[18]

Oxygenation

Use of 100% oxygen was routine for newborn resuscitation until recent changes in resuscitation guidelines.[106] Oxygen tension values of the fetus are low compared with those achieved after transition. Pulse oximetry studies of healthy term infants who require no resuscitation at birth demonstrate that preductal oxygen saturation starts at around 60% and takes 5 to 10 minutes to reach 90%.[30,107] The ideal oxygen saturation range at each minute of life has not been defined, but a reasonable goal is to target a preductal oxygen saturation within the interquartile range for healthy term infants (Table 10.2). Clearly, medical providers should not expect infants to be instantaneously pink at birth and should break the old habit of routinely exposing infants to oxygen at birth. In fact, clinical judgment of color is poor and thus it is recommended that oxygen use be guided by pulse oximetry rather than clinical judgment alone.[54]

Table 10.2   PREDUCTAL OXYGEN SATURATION TARGET RANGE

Time After Birth (min)	Goal Oxygen Saturations (Interquartile Range [%])
1	60–65
2	65–70
3	70–75
4	75–80
5	80–85
>5	85–94

From Weiner GM, Zaichkin J, Kattwinkel J, American Academy of Pediatrics, American Heart Association. *Textbook of Neonatal Resuscitation.* ed 7. Elk Grove Village, IL: American Academy of Pediatrics; 2016.

Although the optimal starting concentration of oxygen is unknown, the available evidence suggests that resuscitation of late preterm and term infants should be started with air (21% oxygen).[18] There is evidence from both animal and human studies of significant oxidative tissue damage in the lung and brain following asphyxia that is exacerbated by subsequent hyperoxygenation. In one study, hyperoxemia (arterial partial pressure of oxygen >100 mm Hg) during the first hour of recovery from perinatal asphyxia was associated with a higher incidence of hypoxic-ischemia encephalopathy and abnormal findings on magnetic resonance imaging of the brain.[108] Several cohort studies reporting an association of delivery room oxygen exposure with increased risk for childhood cancer raise additional concern about the risks of hyperoxygenation in the delivery room.[109–111] Meta-analyses of trials comparing oxygen with room air for newborns during delivery room resuscitation suggest that infants resuscitated with air begin spontaneous breathing faster, reach acceptable oxygen saturation values just as quickly, have less evidence of oxidative damage, and, most importantly, lower mortality.[112,113] Preterm infants are deficient in antioxidant protection and thus face potential adverse effects of oxygen toxicity, such as chronic lung disease, retinopathy of prematurity, and necrotizing enterocolitis. A meta-analysis of eight studies in preterm infants born at less than 28 weeks' gestation demonstrated no benefit to initiating resuscitation with a high (≥60%) compared with a low (≤30%) oxygen concentration.[114] Most of the preterm infants studied did receive some supplemental oxygen during resuscitation to achieve the saturation target, regardless of their group assignment, and were frequently receiving 30% to 40% oxygen at the time of stabilization. This accumulation of data led Sola to write, "Too much oxygen in the blood is a health hazard, and health care providers are the only known cause of neonatal hyperoxemia!"[115]

Current guidelines recommend starting resuscitation with air in late preterm and term infants.[25] Based on a goal of limiting additional oxygen exposure without evidence of benefit, the current guidelines for preterm infants born at less than 35 weeks' gestation recommend starting resuscitation with 21% to 30% oxygen.[25] For all infants, oxygen supplementation should be guided by pulse oximetry and should be adjusted to meet minute-specific oxygen saturation targets. To achieve this goal, blended oxygen and pulse oximetry should be promptly available at every delivery. The pulse oximeter should be placed on the infant's right hand or wrist whenever resuscitation is anticipated, when PPV is administered, when central cyanosis persists beyond the first 5 to 10 minutes of life, and when supplemental oxygen is administered.[12] There is currently little evidence to guide how much oxygen should be administered during neonatal chest compressions (cardiopulmonary resuscitation [CPR]). There are no human studies available and those in animals have not shown any consistent advantage to the use of 100% oxygen during CPR.[116–118] Once the newborn has reached the point of requiring CPR, however, return of circulation has not occurred despite ventilation with a low oxygen concentration, and pulse oximetry may not be providing a reliable signal. With the lack of evidence in mind, the current European and AHA/American Academy of Pediatrics guidelines make the cautious recommendation to use 100% oxygen until the heart rate has recovered (>60 beats/min) and pulse oximetry is functioning.[25,52] Subsequently, the oxygen should be weaned as quickly as possible while maintaining saturation goals.

Chest Compressions During Delivery Room Resuscitation

Regardless of gestational age, most newborns requiring resuscitation have primary respiratory failure and only require effective PPV. If gas exchange is impaired for a prolonged period, myocardial energy stores may become sufficiently depleted to depress cardiac function to the point that assisted ventilation alone will not be sufficient.[119] Chest compressions increase coronary artery perfusion and help to restore cardiac function by increasing the diastolic pressure gradient between the aorta and coronary sinus. Two reports from a large, urban obstetric practice with a trained, dedicated neonatal resuscitation team consistently reported the incidence rate for chest compressions to be around 0.1% of all deliveries,[120,121] although the rate is significantly higher in infants born at less than 33 weeks' gestation.[122,123] The latest Neonatal Resuscitation Program (NRP) guidelines continue to recommend chest compressions for a newborn infant with a heart rate less than 60 beats/min despite at least 30 seconds of ventilation that aerates and ventilates the lung.[12] Because effective ventilation is the critical step in newborn resuscitation and chest compressions are likely to interfere with effective ventilation, resuscitation providers are strongly encouraged to optimize assisted ventilation via placement of an advanced airway such as endotracheal tube or laryngeal mask before initiation of chest compressions.[25] The optimal interval of ventilation before initiation of cardiac compressions is unknown. Rationally, there needs to be a balance between ensuring there is adequate ventilation in the hope of avoiding the need for compressions altogether and the risk of additional hypoxic/ischemic injury if circulation is not assisted in a timely manner. A study in a neonatal animal model of asphyxia-induced asystole found that under conditions of asystole, there was no advantage or disadvantage in delaying initiation of compressions for 1 minute rather than an initial 30 seconds of room air ventilation; however, when initiation of compressions was delayed for 90 seconds of ventilation, fewer animals were successfully resuscitated.[124] Animals exposed to 90 seconds of initial ventilation before support of the circulation with compressions required more doses of epinephrine to stabilize the heart rate and had lower blood pressures after resuscitation. Whether longer delays in initiation of compressions for bradycardia as opposed to asystole would have the same potential harm is unknown. There are no clinical data to offer guidance.

Chest Compression Technique

Compressions should be centered over the lower third of the sternum to compress most directly over the heart.[125–127] A compression depth of approximately one-third the anterior-posterior (AP) diameter of the chest should be adequate to produce a palpable pulse. Mathematical modeling based on neonatal chest CT scan dimensions suggests that a compression depth of one-third the AP diameter of the chest should be more effective than one-quarter and safer than one-half the AP chest diameter.[128,129] Although a small case series of six infants suggested that a compression depth of one-half the AP diameter of the chest resulted in higher systolic, mean, and systemic perfusion pressures, this greater depth did not result in better diastolic blood pressure (the critical determinant of coronary perfusion) than a depth of one-third the AP diameter.[130]

The two-thumb method, in which the thumbs compress the sternum while the provider's hands encircle the chest, should be used for neonatal chest compressions.[131] Compared with the previously recommended two-finger method, the two-thumb method improves the quality and consistency of compressions while decreasing compressor fatigue.[132,133] A piglet study of asphyxia-induced asystole found that over 2-minute intervals, the two-thumb method produced higher systolic blood pressures than the two-finger method, although the diastolic blood pressures were equivalent.[134] When the two techniques were compared over longer (10-minute) compression intervals using a manikin with an artificial fixed volume "arterial system," the two-thumb method produced higher mean, systolic, and diastolic blood pressures.[135] Another neonatal manikin study demonstrated that over 2-minute intervals of chest

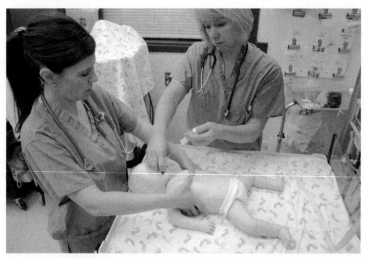

Fig. 10.5 The two-thumb compression technique can be continued from the head of the bed once the airway is secured, leaving ample access to the umbilical stump for emergency placement of an umbilical venous catheter.

compressions, the two-thumb method resulted in improved depth and consistency of compressions as well as less drift away from correct thumb/finger position.[132]

In the past, the two-finger technique was used while umbilical access was obtained so that the compressor's arms would be out of the way. Now it is recommended that once the airway is secured, which should have been completed before initiating compressions, the compressor should move to the head of the bed and continue two-thumb compressions.[12] This position allows unrestricted access to the umbilical stump for another team member to insert a catheter for emergency medication administration (Fig. 10.5).

Compression-to-Ventilation Ratio

The ratio of compressions to ventilations that would truly optimize the dual goals of perfusion and ventilation during resuscitation from asphyxial arrest is unknown.[131] A compression-to-ventilation ratio of 3:1, such that 90 compressions and 30 breaths are achieved per minute, is currently recommended to optimize ventilation.[25] During adult CPR, continuous chest compressions and infrequent, asynchronous ventilations are recommended; however, the pathophysiology of adult cardiac arrest is different. Most adults have a primary cardiac arrhythmia without respiratory failure, whereas most neonatal arrests are preceded by respiratory failure. What is known is that asphyxiated, asystolic piglets resuscitated with a combination of chest compressions and ventilations have better outcomes than those resuscitated with ventilations or compressions alone,[136,137] especially during prolonged resuscitation.[138] A physiologic mathematical modeling study suggests that higher compression-to-ventilation ratios would result in underventilation of asphyxiated infants.[139] The model predicts that three to five compressions to one ventilation should be most efficient for newborns. Later studies have compared 3:1 with 9:3 and 3:1 with 15:2 compression-to-ventilation ratios in piglet models of asystole owing to asphyxia.[140,141] Although the 15:2 ratio provided more compressions per minute without compromising $PaCO_2$ and generated statistically higher diastolic blood pressures, the diastolic blood pressure was still inadequate until epinephrine was given, and so there was no difference in time to return of spontaneous circulation. In a manikin model comparing a 3:1 versus a 15:2 ratio, providers using the 3:1 ratio achieved a greater depth of compression over 2 minutes and more consistent compression depth.[142] Thus there is no evidence from quality human, animal, manikin, or mathematical modeling studies to warrant a change from the current 3:1 compression-to-ventilation ratio.

Strategies for optimizing the quality of the compressions and ventilations with as few interruptions as possible should be considered. In an effort to avoid critical interruptions in coronary perfusion, the guidelines recommend waiting 60 seconds after starting compressions to check the heart rate response.[25] Because physical examination methods used to assess the newborn's heart rate are inaccurate and the pulse oximeter may not display a reliable signal during cardiovascular collapse, the NRP recommends using an ECG monitor to monitor the infant's heart rate if compressions are initiated.[12]

Coordination of Compressions and Ventilations

Coordination of the compressions and ventilations, with three rapid compressions followed by a short pause to interpose one ventilation so that they are not delivered simultaneously, is still recommended, but the evidence for this recommendation is weak.[18,133] Based on physiologic plausibility, there is historical concern that if compressions and ventilations were delivered at the same time, ventilation might be critically compromised. One small study using a neonatal piglet asphyxia model evaluated continuous compressions with asynchronous ventilations and found those resuscitated with this method had similar rates of return of spontaneous circulation, survival, and hemodynamic recovery compared to piglets resuscitated by the traditional 3:1 synchronized ratio.[143] A similar animal model evaluated sustained (30-second) inflations with continuous compressions and showed an improvement in the return of circulation compared with the current 3:1 synchronized ratio; however, there are currently no data from human studies using this approach.[144] Given the current lack of evidence of significant benefit, the ILCOR and NRP continue to recommend coordination of compressions and ventilations.[12,18,25]

Capnography During Cardiac Compressions

Frequent repetitive pauses in chest compressions and ventilation make it difficult to achieve and maintain adequate coronary perfusion pressure. Use of end-tidal CO_2 ($ETCO_2$) capnography during CPR may provide a continuous, noninvasive tool to eliminate frequent pauses during CPR to assess the infant's heart rate. $ETCO_2$ values reflect a balance between CO_2 production by cellular metabolism, alveolar ventilation, and pulmonary perfusion. During asystole there is no cardiac output and CO_2 is not carried to the lungs to be exhaled. During CPR, cellular metabolism and alveolar ventilation are presumed to be at a steady state (provided that PPV is given in a steady manner), so changes in $ETCO_2$ primarily reflect changes in cardiac output.[119] A piglet model of asphyxia-induced asystole has demonstrated that after PPV, $ETCO_2$ falls to near zero with loss of PBF and then increases slightly with initiation of cardiac compressions, reflecting blood being pumped through the lungs by effective CPR.[145] When circulation is restored, there is a sudden increase in $ETCO_2$ as the reestablished perfusion brings CO_2-rich blood back to the lungs. In that animal model, an $ETCO_2$ greater than 15 mm Hg correlated well with return of an audible heart rate higher than 60 beats/min. Since 2010, adult AHA guidelines have recommended continuous waveform capnography for monitoring CPR quality and detecting return of circulation by an abrupt increase in $ETCO_2$.[146] There are currently no studies in human newborns evaluating this method.

Medications During Delivery Room Resuscitation

When asphyxia is so severe that it results in asystole or agonal bradycardia, the newborn heart has become depleted of energy substrate and can no longer beat effectively.[147] Adequate perfusion of the heart with oxygenated blood must be restored or resuscitation efforts will be unsuccessful. During CPR, coronary blood flow occurs exclusively during diastole, presumably because of increased right atrial pressure during chest compressions.[148] Therefore coronary perfusion pressure is determined by the aortic diastolic blood pressure minus the right atrial diastolic blood pressure. Cardiac compressions plus adequate systemic vascular resistance must generate diastolic blood pressure adequate to achieve return of spontaneous circulation. Given the profound acidemia and resultant vasodilation induced by asphyxia, a vasopressor agent such as epinephrine is frequently required to achieve an adequate aortic diastolic pressure for sufficient coronary perfusion during CPR. A single study in a

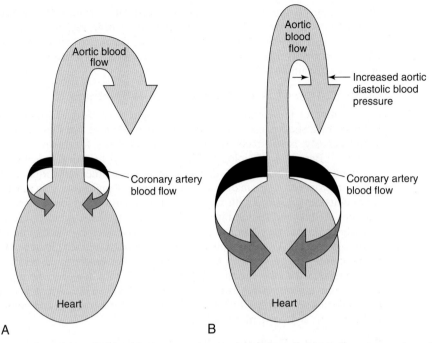

Fig. 10.6 The effect of diastolic blood pressure on coronary blood flow during cardiac compressions. A, Cardiac compressions with minimal aortic diastolic blood pressure preferentially send the majority of the cardiac output around the aortic arch to the periphery. B, Cardiac compressions with improved aortic diastolic blood pressure sends more blood into the coronary arteries to bring oxygenated blood that will help generate adenosine triphosphate to get the heart beating again. (From Wyckoff MH. Neonatal cardiopulmonary resuscitation: critical hemodynamics. *NeoReviews.* 2010;11:e123–e129.)

neonatal piglet model of asphyxial cardiac arrest suggested that vasopressin, a pulmonary vasodilator and systemic vasopressor, may improve survival but no human neonatal data are available.[149]

Epinephrine is a catecholamine that stimulates α-adrenergic receptor–mediated vasoconstriction to elevate the diastolic blood pressure and thus the coronary perfusion pressure during CPR (Fig. 10.6). Consequently, if the heart rate remains less than 60 beats/min despite 1 minute of effective PPV with coordinated chest compressions, then 0.01 to 0.03 mg/kg of epinephrine (equal to 0.1 to 0.3 mL/kg of a 0.1-mg/mL solution) should be given rapidly through a central venous catheter or intraosseous needle followed by a 1.0-mL flush with normal saline solution.[12] Data evaluating the most effective and safest dose for intravenous epinephrine during delivery room CPR are lacking and have been largely based on animal models and extrapolation from clinical trials in older children and adults. Although neonatal health care providers are trained to insert umbilical venous catheters (UVCs), other health care providers may be less comfortable with this procedure. Prehospital providers and emergency department personnel frequently insert intraosseous (IO) needles for rapid vascular access. One case series has described 27 newborns ranging from 25 to 41 weeks' gestation who were resuscitated with medications administered through an IO needle.[150] A simulation study using a neonatal manikin model demonstrated that IO needle insertion was faster than UVC placement with no difference in the participants' perceived ease of use.[151] Given the importance of administering emergency epinephrine when it is indicated during resuscitation, delivery room resuscitation personnel should have ready access to both of these devices and adequate training to reliably insert them without delay.

While securing vascular access, some providers may consider endotracheal administration of epinephrine; however, newborn transitional physiology does not favor this route for several reasons. Decreased blood flow during cardiac collapse may be insufficient to transport drugs from the alveoli to the central circulation, pulmonary vasoconstriction from acidosis could impede drug absorption, alveolar fluid may dilute the epinephrine, and right-to-left intracardiac shunts could bypass the pulmonary circulation altogether. Newborn animal and human studies indicate that endotracheal epinephrine absorption is unreliable and less effective.[152] In one cohort, 77% of newborns who did not respond to endotracheal epinephrine had return of circulation after receiving an intravenous dose.[153] If providers choose to administer one dose of endotracheal epinephrine, a higher dose (0.05 to 0.1 mg/kg = 0.5 to 1 mL/kg of a 0.1-mg/mL solution) has been recommended.[25] This higher dose should not be given intravenously.

The vast majority of asphyxiated, severely depressed newborns are not hypovolemic. Newborns may develop hypovolemic shock from acute blood caused by fetal-maternal hemorrhage, bleeding vasa previa, placental laceration, umbilical cord prolapse, or umbilical cord disruption. Volume infusion should be given only if the infant does not respond to the steps of resuscitation in the setting of acute blood loss and the infant has clinical signs of hypovolemic shock (pallor, weak pulses, poor perfusion) or the infant has signs of hypovolemic shock and there is a clinical suspicion for occult blood loss.[12] The best replacement fluid for shock associated with acute blood loss is O-negative blood, but an isotonic crystalloid such as normal saline solution is acceptable until blood is available. Emergency volume replacement during resuscitation should be administered in 10-mL/kg aliquots slowly (5–10 minutes) through a UVC or an IO needle. Additional volume may be required but caution should be used to avoid infusing excessive volume and increasing demands on the already compromised neonatal heart. In an asphyxia-induced hypotension and bradycardia model (without hypovolemia), volume infusion during resuscitation increased pulmonary edema, decreased pulmonary dynamic compliance, and did not improve blood pressure either during or after the resuscitation.[154] Thus routine volume infusions during delivery room resuscitations not complicated by hypovolemia may be detrimental, exacerbate poor cardiac output, and are not recommended.

Special Situations

Other conditions that can lead to severe respiratory depression or distress at birth and that require early resuscitation include bacterial or viral sepsis, pneumothorax, airway obstruction associated with micrognathia (Pierre Robin sequence), bilateral choanal atresia, upper airway tumors or webs, hydrops fetalis (pleural effusions, ascites, anasarca), congenital diaphragmatic hernia, massive cardiomegaly, and pulmonary hypoplasia.[12] Many of these conditions interfere with effective ventilation and oxygenation immediately after birth and require specific management interventions. These conditions are described in more detail elsewhere in this volume and therefore are not within the scope of this section on delivery room resuscitation.

The decision when to stop resuscitative efforts if there is no detectable heart rate and the infant is not responding remains controversial. Data from birth cohort studies published before the standard use of therapeutic hypothermia indicated near universal death or severe disability if the infant had no observable heart rate (Apgar score of 0) for 10 minutes. Combining multiple birth cohorts (1991–2004), Harrington et al. reported that 94% (88/94) of newborns with an absent heart rate at 10 minutes either died or survived with a severe disability.[155] Recent reports that include a series of infants enrolled in therapeutic hypothermia clinical trials, or receiving hypothermia outside a trial, have suggested that the outcome for infants with an Apgar score of 0 at 10 minutes may be improving. These studies report that 20% to 30% of infants with an Apgar score of 0 at 10 minutes who survived to be admitted to a neonatal intensive care unit and enrolled in a hypothermia trial had favorable neurodevelopmental outcomes.[156–159] Caution is required when interpreting these data because they do not describe the resuscitation procedures that were provided and are subject to significant selection bias. Infants in these reports survived the delivery room resuscitation, and frequently were transported to a neonatal intensive care unit where they qualified for enrollment in a clinical trial. These studies do not report outcomes of the infants who did not achieve return of circulation despite

10

prolonged resuscitation, were not transferred, died in the first hours of life, or did not meet enrollment criteria when they arrived at the referral center. It is likely these studies overestimate both survival and favorable outcome; however, discontinuing resuscitation at 10 minutes certainly would have led to the deaths of some infants who survived without severe disability and some who are developmentally normal. Based on the available evidence, the 2015 ILCOR science consensus reaffirmed the previous conclusion that an Apgar score of 0 at 10 minutes is a strong predictor of mortality and morbidity in late preterm and term infants and suggest that if a heart rate remains undetectable after 10 minutes of resuscitation, it may be reasonable to discontinue assisted ventilation.[18] The current European Resuscitation Council and AHA guidelines suggest that decisions to continue resuscitation beyond 10 minutes should be individualized and consider factors such as the presumed etiology of asystole, the clinical situation before birth, the infant's gestational age, whether resuscitative efforts have been optimized, the availability of advanced neonatal care, and the parents' desires.[25,52] If resuscitation is continued beyond 10 minutes, when is a reasonable time to stop? In a series of 23 newborns who received intravenous epinephrine in the delivery room (most of whom had asystole), Barber and Wyckoff reported that it took an average of 5.2 minutes (standard deviation 3.1) to administer the first dose of epinephrine and the average time to return of circulation was 11.7 minutes (standard deviation 5.8).[153] In another series of 29 term newborns who had no detectable heart rate at 10 minutes but were successfully resuscitated and transferred to an intensive care unit, the median time to achieve the first detectable heart rate was 15 minutes.[160] In another small series, all 5 surviving infants who had resuscitation continued beyond 10 minutes had return of circulation documented by 20 minutes.[157] Given the relatively low quality of evidence, the actual time required to administer intravenous epinephrine, and the difficulty of adequately counseling parents during the intense time pressure of resuscitation, some have suggested that, in the absence of a detectable heart rate, most resuscitations should continue for 20 minutes.[161]

REFERENCES

1. Harding R, Hooper SB. Regulation of lung expansion and lung growth before birth. *J Appl Physiol (Bethesda, Md: 1985)*. 1996;81(1):209–224.
2. Rudolph AM. Fetal and neonatal pulmonary circulation. *Annu Rev Plant Physiol*. 1979;41:383–395.
3. Hooper SB, Te Pas AB, Lang J, et al. Cardiovascular transition at birth: a physiological sequence. *Pediatr Res*. 2015;77(5):608–614.
4. Hooper SB, Te Pas AB, Kitchen MJ. Respiratory transition in the newborn: a three-phase process. *Arch Dis Child Fetal Neonatal Ed*. 2016;101(3):F266–F271.
5. Hooper SB, Kitchen MJ, Wallace MJ, et al. Imaging lung aeration and lung liquid clearance at birth. *FASEB*. 2007;21(12):3329–3337.
6. Siew ML, Wallace MJ, Kitchen MJ, et al. Inspiration regulates the rate and temporal pattern of lung liquid clearance and lung aeration at birth. *J Appl Physiol (Bethesda, Md: 1985)*. 2009;106(6):1888–1895.
7. Siew ML, Te Pas AB, Wallace MJ, et al. Positive end-expiratory pressure enhances development of a functional residual capacity in preterm rabbits ventilated from birth. *J Appl Physiol (Bethesda, Md: 1985)*. 2009;106(5):1487–1493.
8. Bhatt S, Alison BJ, Wallace EM, et al. Delaying cord clamping until ventilation onset improves cardiovascular function at birth in preterm lambs. *J Physiol*. 2013;591(8):2113–2126.
9. Hooper SB, Polglase GR, te Pas AB. A physiological approach to the timing of umbilical cord clamping at birth. *Arch Dis Child Fetal Neonatal Ed*. 2015;100(4):F355–F360.
10. Lang JA, Pearson JT, te Pas AB, et al. Ventilation/perfusion mismatch during lung aeration at birth. *J Appl Physiol (Bethesda, Md: 1985)*. 2014;117(5):535–543.
11. Lang JA, Pearson JT, Binder-Heschl C, et al. Increase in pulmonary blood flow at birth: role of oxygen and lung aeration. *J Physiol*. 2016;594(5):1389–1398.
12. Weiner GM, Zaichkin J, Kattwinkel J, American Academy of Pediatrics, American Heart Association. *Textbook of Neonatal Resuscitation*. 7th ed. Elk Grove Village, IL: American Academy of Pediatrics; 2016.
13. Owen LS, Weiner GM, Davis PG. Delivery room stabilization and respiratory support. In: Goldsmith JP, Karotkin EH, Keszler M, Suresh G, eds. *Assisted Ventilation of the Neonate: An Evidence-Based Approach to Newborn Respiratory Care*. 6th ed. Philadelphia, PA: Elsevier; 2017:275–290.
14. Aziz K, Chadwick M, Baker M, Andrews W. Ante- and intra-partum factors that predict increased need for neonatal resuscitation. *Resuscitation*. 2008;79(3):444–452.
15. Berazategui JP, Aguilar A, Escobedo M, et al. Risk factors for advanced resuscitation in term and near-term infants: a case-control study. *Arch Dis Child Fetal Neonatal Ed*. 2016.

16. Katheria A, Rich W, Finer N. Development of a strategic process using checklists to facilitate team preparation and improve communication during neonatal resuscitation. *Resuscitation.* 2013;84(11):1552–1557.
17. DeMauro SB, Douglas E, Karp K, et al. Improving delivery room management for very preterm infants. *Pediatrics.* 2013;132(4):e1018–e1025.
18. Perlman JM, Wyllie J, Kattwinkel J, et al. Part 7: neonatal resuscitation: 2015 International Consensus on Cardiopulmonary Resuscitation and Emergency Cardiovascular Care Science With Treatment Recommendations (Reprint). *Pediatrics.* 2015;136(suppl 2):S120–S166.
19. Trevisanuto D, Doglioni N, Cavallin F, Parotto M, Micaglio M, Zanardo V. Heat loss prevention in very preterm infants in delivery rooms: a prospective, randomized, controlled trial of polyethylene caps. *J Pediatr.* 2010;156(6):914–917, 917.e911.
20. Singh A, Duckett J, Newton T, Watkinson M. Improving neonatal unit admission temperatures in preterm babies: exothermic mattresses, polythene bags or a traditional approach? *J Perinatol.* 2010;30(1):45–49.
21. Simon P, Dannaway D, Bright B, et al. Thermal defense of extremely low gestational age newborns during resuscitation: exothermic mattresses vs polyethylene wrap. *J Perinatol.* 2011;31(1):33–37.
22. Vohra S, Roberts RS, Zhang B, Janes M, Schmidt B. Heat loss prevention (HeLP) in the delivery room: a randomized controlled trial of polyethylene occlusive skin wrapping in very preterm infants. *J Pediatr.* 2004;145(6):750–753.
23. Pillow JJ, Hillman NH, Polglase GR, et al. Oxygen, temperature and humidity of inspired gases and their influences on airway and lung tissue in near-term lambs. *Intensive Care Med.* 2009;35(12):2157–2163.
24. te Pas AB, Lopriore E, Dito I, Morley CJ, Walther FJ. Humidified and heated air during stabilization at birth improves temperature in preterm infants. *Pediatrics.* 2010;125(6):e1427–e1432.
25. Wyckoff MH, Aziz K, Escobedo MB, et al. Part 13: neonatal resuscitation: 2015 American Heart Association guidelines update for cardiopulmonary resuscitation and emergency cardiovascular care (Reprint). *Pediatrics.* 2015;136(suppl 2):S196–S218.
26. Ersdal HL, Mduma E, Svensen E, Perlman JM. Early initiation of basic resuscitation interventions including face mask ventilation may reduce birth asphyxia related mortality in low-income countries: a prospective descriptive observational study. *Resuscitation.* 2012;83(7):869–873.
27. Dawson JA, Kamlin CO, Wong C, et al. Changes in heart rate in the first minutes after birth. *Arch Dis Child Fetal Neonatal Ed.* 2010;95(3):F177–F181.
28. O'Donnell CP, Kamlin CO, Davis PG, Carlin JB, Morley CJ. Clinical assessment of infant colour at delivery. *Arch Dis Child Fetal Neonatal Ed.* 2007;92(6):F465–F467.
29. Kamlin CO, O'Donnell CP, Davis PG, Morley CJ. Oxygen saturation in healthy infants immediately after birth. *J Pediatr.* 2006;148(5):585–589.
30. Dawson JA, Kamlin CO, Vento M, et al. Defining the reference range for oxygen saturation for infants after birth. *Pediatrics.* 2010;125(6):e1340–e1347.
31. Gungor S, Kurt E, Teksoz E, Goktolga U, Ceyhan T, Baser I. Oronasopharyngeal suction versus no suction in normal and term infants delivered by elective cesarean section: a prospective randomized controlled trial. *Gynecol Obstet Invest.* 2006;61(1):9–14.
32. Katheria A, Poeltler D, Durham J, et al. Neonatal resuscitation with an intact cord: a randomized clinical trial. *J Pediatr.* 2016;178:75–80.e73.
33. McCall EM, Alderdice F, Halliday HL, Jenkins JG, Vohra S. Interventions to prevent hypothermia at birth in preterm and/or low birthweight infants. *Cochrane Database Syst Rev.* 2010;(3):CD004210.
34. Laptook AR, Salhab W, Bhaskar B, Neonatal Research Network. Admission temperature of low birth weight infants: predictors and associated morbidities. *Pediatrics.* 2007;119(3):e643–e649.
35. Russo A, McCready M, Torres L, et al. Reducing hypothermia in preterm infants following delivery. *Pediatrics.* 2014;133(4):e1055–e1062.
36. Pinheiro JM, Furdon SA, Boynton S, Dugan R, Reu-Donlon C, Jensen S. Decreasing hypothermia during delivery room stabilization of preterm neonates. *Pediatrics.* 2014;133(1):e218–e226.
37. Knobel RB, Wimmer JE Jr, Holbert D. Heat loss prevention for preterm infants in the delivery room. *J Perinatol.* 2005;25(5):304–308.
38. Meyer MP, Hou D, Ishrar NN, Dito I, te Pas AB. Initial respiratory support with cold, dry gas versus heated humidified gas and admission temperature of preterm infants. *J Pediatr.* 2015;166(2):245–250. e241.
39. Perlman JM. Hyperthermia in the delivery: potential impact on neonatal mortality and morbidity. *Clin Perinatol.* 2006;33(1):55–63, vi.
40. Kasdorf E, Perlman JM. Hyperthermia, inflammation, and perinatal brain injury. *Pediatr Neurol.* 2013;49(1):8–14.
41. Ball MK, Hillman NH, Kallapur SG, Polglase GR, Jobe AH, Pillow JJ. Body temperature effects on lung injury in ventilated preterm lambs. *Resuscitation.* 2010;81(6):749–754.
42. Carson BS, Losey RW, Bowes WA Jr, Simmons MA. Combined obstetric and pediatric approach to prevent meconium aspiration syndrome. *Am J Obstet Gynecol.* 1976;126(6):712–715.
43. Gregory GA, Gooding CA, Phibbs RH, Tooley WH. Meconium aspiration in infants—a prospective study. *J Pediatr.* 1974;85(6):848–852.
44. Ting P, Brady JP. Tracheal suction in meconium aspiration. *Am J Obstet Gynecol.* 1975;122(6): 767–771.
45. Vivian-Taylor J, Sheng J, Hadfield RM, Morris JM, Bowen JR, Roberts CL. Trends in obstetric practices and meconium aspiration syndrome: a population-based study. *BJOG.* 2011;118(13): 1601–1607.

10

46. Yoder BA, Kirsch EA, Barth WH, Gordon MC. Changing obstetric practices associated with decreasing incidence of meconium aspiration syndrome. *Obstet Gynecol*. 2002;99(5 Pt 1):731–739.

47. Dargaville PA, Copnell B, Australian and New Zealand Neonatal Network. The epidemiology of meconium aspiration syndrome: incidence, risk factors, therapies, and outcome. *Pediatrics*. 2006; 117(5):1712–1721.

48. Vain NE, Szyld EG, Prudent LM, Wiswell TE, Aguilar AM, Vivas NI. Oropharyngeal and nasopharyngeal suctioning of meconium-stained neonates before delivery of their shoulders: multicentre, randomised controlled trial. *Lancet*. 2004;364(9434):597–602.

49. Wiswell TE, Gannon CM, Jacob J, et al. Delivery room management of the apparently vigorous meconium-stained neonate: results of the multicenter, international collaborative trial. *Pediatrics*. 2000;105(1 Pt 1):1–7.

50. Chettri S, Adhisivam B, Bhat BV. Endotracheal suction for nonvigorous neonates born through meconium stained amniotic fluid: a randomized controlled trial. *J Pediatr*. 2015;166(5):1208–1213. e1201.

51. Nangia S, Sunder S, Biswas R, Saili A. Endotracheal suction in term non vigorous meconium stained neonates—a pilot study. *Resuscitation*. 2016;105:79–84.

52. Wyllie J, Bruinenberg J, Roehr CC, Rudiger M, Trevisanuto D, Urlesberger B. European Resuscitation Council Guidelines for Resuscitation 2015: section 7. Resuscitation and support of transition of babies at birth. *Resuscitation*. 2015;95:249–263.

53. Owen CJ, Wyllie JP. Determination of heart rate in the baby at birth. *Resuscitation*. 2004;60(2): 213–217.

54. Kamlin CO, O'Donnell CP, Everest NJ, Davis PG, Morley CJ. Accuracy of clinical assessment of infant heart rate in the delivery room. *Resuscitation*. 2006;71(3):319–321.

55. Phillipos E, Solevag AL, Pichler G, et al. Heart rate assessment immediately after birth. *Neonatology*. 2016;109(2):130–138.

56. McCarthy LK, Morley CJ, Davis PG, Kamlin CO, O'Donnell CP. Timing of interventions in the delivery room: does reality compare with neonatal resuscitation guidelines? *J Pediatr*. 2013; 163(6):1553–1557.e1551.

57. Bennett S, Finer NN, Rich W, Vaucher Y. A comparison of three neonatal resuscitation devices. *Resuscitation*. 2005;67(1):113–118.

58. Rafferty AR, Johnson L, Maxfield D, Dawson JA, Davis PG, Thio M. The accuracy of delivery of target pressures using self-inflating bag manometers in a benchtop study. *Acta Paediatr*. 2016;105(6):e247–e251.

59. Morley CJ, Dawson JA, Stewart MJ, Hussain F, Davis PG. The effect of a PEEP valve on a Laerdal neonatal self-inflating resuscitation bag. *J Paediatr Child Health*. 2010;46(1–2):51–56.

60. Thallinger M, Ersdal HL, Morley C, et al. Neonatal ventilation with a manikin model and two novel PEEP valves without an external gas source. *Arch Dis Child Fetal Neonatal Ed*. 2016.

61. Roehr CC, Kelm M, Fischer HS, Buhrer C, Schmalisch G, Proquitte H. Manual ventilation devices in neonatal resuscitation: tidal volume and positive pressure-provision. *Resuscitation*. 2010;81(2):202–205.

62. Dawson JA, Gerber A, Kamlin CO, Davis PG, Morley CJ. Providing PEEP during neonatal resuscitation: which device is best? *J Paediatr Child Health*. 2011;47(10):698–703.

63. Szyld E, Aguilar A, Musante GA, et al. Comparison of devices for newborn ventilation in the delivery room. *J Pediatr*. 2014;165(2):234–239. e233.

64. Dawson JA, Schmolzer GM, Kamlin CO, et al. Oxygenation with T-piece versus self-inflating bag for ventilation of extremely preterm infants at birth: a randomized controlled trial. *J Pediatr*. 2011;158(6):912–918.e911–e912.

65. Wood FE, Morley CJ. Face mask ventilation—the dos and don'ts. *Semin Fetal Neonatal Med*. 2013;18(6):344–351.

66. Schmolzer GM, Dawson JA, Kamlin CO, O'Donnell CP, Morley CJ, Davis PG. Airway obstruction and gas leak during mask ventilation of preterm infants in the delivery room. *Arch Dis Child Fetal Neonatal Ed*. 2011;96(4):F254–F257.

67. Schmolzer GM, Kamlin OC, O'Donnell CP, Dawson JA, Morley CJ, Davis PG. Assessment of tidal volume and gas leak during mask ventilation of preterm infants in the delivery room. *Arch Dis Child Fetal Neonatal Ed*. 2010;95(6):F393–F397.

68. Kattwinkel J, Stewart C, Walsh B, Gurka M, Paget-Brown A. Responding to compliance changes in a lung model during manual ventilation: perhaps volume, rather than pressure, should be displayed. *Pediatrics*. 2009;123(3):e465–e470.

69. Leone TA, Lange A, Rich W, Finer NN. Disposable colorimetric carbon dioxide detector use as an indicator of a patent airway during noninvasive mask ventilation. *Pediatrics*. 2006;118(1):e202–e204.

70. Hooper SB, Fouras A, Siew ML, et al. Expired CO_2 levels indicate degree of lung aeration at birth. *PLoS One*. 2013;8(8):e70895.

71. Kaufman J, Schmolzer GM, Kamlin CO, Davis PG. Mask ventilation of preterm infants in the delivery room. *Arch Dis Child Fetal Neonatal Ed*. 2013;98(5):F405–F410.

72. Schmolzer GM, Morley CJ, Wong C, et al. Respiratory function monitor guidance of mask ventilation in the delivery room: a feasibility study. *J Pediatr*. 2012;160(3):377–381.e372.

73. Bowman TA, Paget-Brown A, Carroll J, Gurka MJ, Kattwinkel J. Sensing and responding to compliance changes during manual ventilation using a lung model: can we teach healthcare providers to improve? *J Pediatr*. 2012;160(3):372–376. e371.

74. Cocucci C, Madorno M, Aguilar A, Acha L, Szyld E, Musante G. A metronome for pacing manual ventilation in a neonatal resuscitation simulation. *Arch Dis Child Fetal Neonatal Ed*. 2015;100(1): F47–F49.

75. Sobotka KS, Hooper SB, Allison BJ, et al. An initial sustained inflation improves the respiratory and cardiovascular transition at birth in preterm lambs. *Pediatr Res.* 2011;70(1):56–60.

76. te Pas AB, Siew M, Wallace MJ, et al. Effect of sustained inflation length on establishing functional residual capacity at birth in ventilated premature rabbits. *Pediatr Res.* 2009;66(3):295–300.

77. O'Donnell CP, Bruschettini M, Davis PG, et al. Sustained versus standard inflations during neonatal resuscitation to prevent mortality and improve respiratory outcomes. *Cochrane Database Syst Rev.* 2015;(7):CD004953.

78. Palme-Kilander C, Tunell R. Pulmonary gas exchange during facemask ventilation immediately after birth. *Arch Dis Child.* 1993;68(1 Spec No):11–16.

79. Morley C, Davis P. Continuous positive airway pressure: current controversies. *Curr Opin Pediatr.* 2004;16(2):141–145.

80. Committee on Fetus and Newborn, American Academy of Pediatrics. Respiratory support in preterm infants at birth. *Pediatrics.* 2014;133(1):171–174.

81. Schmolzer GM, Kumar M, Pichler G, Aziz K, O'Reilly M, Cheung PY. Non-invasive versus invasive respiratory support in preterm infants at birth: systematic review and meta-analysis. *BMJ.* 2013;347:f5980.

82. Morley CJ, Davis PG, Doyle LW, et al. Nasal CPAP or intubation at birth for very preterm infants. *N Engl J Med.* 2008;358(7):700–708.

83. Kamlin CO, O'Connell LA, Morley CJ, et al. A randomized trial of stylets for intubating newborn infants. *Pediatrics.* 2013;131(1):e198–e205.

84. van Os S, Cheung PY, Kushniruk K, O'Reilly M, Aziz K, Schmolzer GM. Assessment of endotracheal tube placement in newborn infants: a randomized controlled trial. *J Perinatol.* 2016;36(5):370–375.

85. Wozniak M, Arnell K, Brown M, et al. The 30 second rule: the effects of prolonged intubation attempts on oxygen saturation and heart rate in preterm infants in the delivery room. *Minerva Pediatr.* 2016.

86. Goel S, Lim SL. The intubation depth marker: the confusion of the black line. *Paediatr Anaesth.* 2003;13(7):579–583.

87. Gill I, O'Donnell CP. Vocal cord guides on neonatal endotracheal tubes. *Arch Dis Child Fetal Neonatal Ed.* 2014;99(4):F344.

88. Tochen ML. Orotracheal intubation in the newborn infant: a method for determining depth of tube insertion. *J Pediatr.* 1979;95(6):1050–1051.

89. Peterson J, Johnson N, Deakins K, Wilson-Costello D, Jelovsek JE, Chatburn R. Accuracy of the 7-8-9 Rule for endotracheal tube placement in the neonate. *J Perinatol.* 2006;26(6):333–336.

90. Amarilyo G, Mimouni FB, Oren A, Tsyrkin S, Mandel D. Orotracheal tube insertion in extremely low birth weight infants. *J Pediatr.* 2009;154(5):764–765.

91. Kempley ST, Moreiras JW, Petrone FL. Endotracheal tube length for neonatal intubation. *Resuscitation.* 2008;77(3):369–373.

92. Shukla HK, Hendricks-Munoz KD, Atakent Y, Rapaport S. Rapid estimation of insertional length of endotracheal intubation in newborn infants. *J Pediatr.* 1997;131(4):561–564.

93. Thayyil SNP, Gowers H, Sinha A. Optimal endotracheal tube tip position in extremely premature infants. *Am J Perinatol.* 2008;25(1):13–16.

94. Bismilla Z, Breakey VR, Swales J, et al. Prospective evaluation of residents on call: before and after duty-hour reduction. *Pediatrics.* 2011;127(6):1080–1087.

95. Leone TA, Rich W, Finer NN. Neonatal intubation: success of pediatric trainees. *J Pediatr.* 2005;146(5):638–641.

96. O'Donnell CP, Kamlin CO, Davis PG, Morley CJ. Endotracheal intubation attempts during neonatal resuscitation: success rates, duration, and adverse effects. *Pediatrics.* 2006;117(1):e16–e21.

97. Sauer CW, Kong JY, Vaucher YE, et al. Intubation attempts increase the risk for severe intraventricular hemorrhage in preterm infants—a retrospective cohort study. *J Pediatr.* 2016;177:108–113.

98. Trevisanuto D, Micaglio M, Ferrarese P, Zanardo V. The laryngeal mask airway: potential applications in neonates. *Arch Dis Child Fetal Neonatal Ed.* 2004;89(6):F485–F489.

99. Zanardo V, Weiner G, Micaglio M, Doglioni N, Buzzacchero R, Trevisanuto D. Delivery room resuscitation of near-term infants: role of the laryngeal mask airway. *Resuscitation.* 2010;81(3):327–330.

100. Schmolzer GM, Agarwal M, Kamlin CO, Davis PG. Supraglottic airway devices during neonatal resuscitation: an historical perspective, systematic review and meta-analysis of available clinical trials. *Resuscitation.* 2013;84(6):722–730.

101. Wanous AA, Wey A, Rudser KD, Roberts KD. Feasibility of laryngeal mask airway device placement in neonates. *Neonatology.* 2016;111(3):222–227.

102. Pinheiro JM, Santana-Rivas Q, Pezzano C. Randomized trial of laryngeal mask airway versus endotracheal intubation for surfactant delivery. *J Perinatol.* 2016;36(3):196–201.

103. Pandit JJ, MacLachlan K, Dravid RM, Popat MT. Comparison of times to achieve tracheal intubation with three techniques using the laryngeal or intubating laryngeal mask airway. *Anaesthesia.* 2002;57(2):128–132.

104. Ruetzler K, Roessler B, Potura L, et al. Performance and skill retention of intubation by paramedics using seven different airway devices—a manikin study. *Resuscitation.* 2011;82(5):593–597.

105. Reinhart DJ, Simmons G. Comparison of placement of the laryngeal mask airway with endotracheal tube by paramedics and respiratory therapists. *Ann Emerg Med.* 1994;24(2):260–263.

106. Perlman JM, Wyllie J, Kattwinkel J, et al. Neonatal resuscitation: 2010 International Consensus on Cardiopulmonary Resuscitation and Emergency Cardiovascular Care Science With Treatment Recommendations. *Pediatrics.* 2010;126(5):e1319–e1344.

10

107. Rabi Y, Yee W, Chen SY, Singhal N. Oxygen saturation trends immediately after birth. *J Pediatr*. 2006;148(5):590–594.

108. Kapadia VS, Chalak LF, DuPont TL, Rollins NK, Brion LP, Wyckoff MH. Perinatal asphyxia with hyperoxemia within the first hour of life is associated with moderate to severe hypoxic-ischemic encephalopathy. *J Pediatr*. 2013;163(4):949–954.

109. Naumburg E, Bellocco R, Cnattingius S, Jonzon A, Ekbom A. Supplementary oxygen and risk of childhood lymphatic leukaemia. *Acta Paediatr*. 2002;91(12):1328–1333.

110. Spector LG, Klebanoff MA, Feusner JH, Georgieff MK, Ross JA. Childhood cancer following neonatal oxygen supplementation. *J Pediatr*. 2005;147(1):27–31.

111. Cnattingius S, Zack MM, Ekbom A, et al. Prenatal and neonatal risk factors for childhood lymphatic leukemia. *J Natl Cancer Inst*. 1995;87(12):908–914.

112. Davis PG, Tan A, O'Donnell CP, Schulze A. Resuscitation of newborn infants with 100% oxygen or air: a systematic review and meta-analysis. *Lancet*. 2004;364(9442):1329–1333.

113. Rabi Y, Rabi D, Yee W. Room air resuscitation of the depressed newborn: a systematic review and meta-analysis. *Resuscitation*. 2007;72(3):353–363.

114. Oei JL, Vento M, Rabi Y, et al. Higher or lower oxygen for delivery room resuscitation of preterm infants below 28 completed weeks gestation: a meta-analysis. *Arch Dis Child Fetal Neonatal Ed*. 2016.

115. Sola A. Oxygen for the preterm newborn: one infant at a time. *Pediatrics*. 2008;121(6):1257.

116. Solevag AL, Dannevig I, Nakstad B, Saugstad OD. Resuscitation of severely asphyctic newborn pigs with cardiac arrest by using 21% or 100% oxygen. *Neonatology*. 2010;98(1):64–72.

117. Linner R, Werner O, Perez-de-Sa V, Cunha-Goncalves D. Circulatory recovery is as fast with air ventilation as with 100% oxygen after asphyxia-induced cardiac arrest in piglets. *Pediatr Res*. 2009;66(4):391–394.

118. Solevag AL, Schmolzer GM, O'Reilly M, et al. Myocardial perfusion and oxidative stress after 21% vs. 100% oxygen ventilation and uninterrupted chest compressions in severely asphyxiated piglets. *Resuscitation*. 2016;106:7–13.

119. Wyckoff MH. Neonatal cardiopulmonary resuscitation: critical hemodynamics. *NeoReviews*. 2010;11:e123–e129.

120. Perlman JM, Risser R. Cardiopulmonary resuscitation in the delivery room. Associated clinical events. *Arch Pediatr Adolesc Med*. 1995;149(1):20–25.

121. Wyckoff MH, Perlman JM, Laptook AR. Use of volume expansion during delivery room resuscitation in near-term and term infants. *Pediatrics*. 2005;115(4):950–955.

122. Shah PS. Extensive cardiopulmonary resuscitation for VLBW and ELBW infants: a systematic review and meta-analyses. *J Perinatol*. 2009;29(10):655–661.

123. Soraisham AS, Lodha AK, Singhal N, et al. Neonatal outcomes following extensive cardiopulmonary resuscitation in the delivery room for infants born at less than 33 weeks gestational age. *Resuscitation*. 2014;85(2):238–243.

124. Dannevig I, Solevag AL, Wyckoff M, Saugstad OD, Nakstad B. Delayed onset of cardiac compressions in cardiopulmonary resuscitation of newborn pigs with asphyctic cardiac arrest. *Neonatology*. 2011;99(2):153–162.

125. Orlowski JP. Optimum position for external cardiac compression in infants and young children. *Ann Emerg Med*. 1986;15(6):667–673.

126. Phillips GW, Zideman DA. Relation of infant heart to sternum: its significance in cardiopulmonary resuscitation. *Lancet*. 1986;1(8488):1024–1025.

127. Finholt DA, Kettrick RG, Wagner HR, Swedlow DB. The heart is under the lower third of the sternum. Implications for external cardiac massage. *Am J Dis Chil*. 1986;140(7):646–649.

128. Meyer A, Nadkarni V, Pollock A, et al. Evaluation of the neonatal resuscitation program's recommended chest compression depth using computerized tomography imaging. *Resuscitation*. 2010;81(5):544–548.

129. Braga MS, Dominguez TE, Pollock AN, et al. Estimation of optimal CPR chest compression depth in children by using computer tomography. *Pediatrics*. 2009;124(1):e69–e74.

130. Maher KO, Berg RA, Lindsey CW, Simsic J, Mahle WT. Depth of sternal compression and intra-arterial blood pressure during CPR in infants following cardiac surgery. *Resuscitation*. 2009;80(6):662–664.

131. Solevag AL, Cheung PY, O'Reilly M, Schmolzer GM. A review of approaches to optimise chest compressions in the resuscitation of asphyxiated newborns. *Arch Dis Child Fetal Neonatal Ed*. 2016;101(3):F272–F276.

132. Christman C, Hemway RJ, Wyckoff MH, Perlman JM. The two-thumb is superior to the two-finger method for administering chest compressions in a manikin model of neonatal resuscitation. *Arch Dis Child Fetal Neonatal Ed*. 2011;96(2):F99–F101.

133. Mildenhall LF, Huynh TK. Factors modulating effective chest compressions in the neonatal period. *Semin Fetal Neonatal Med*. 2013;18(6):352–356.

134. Houri PK, Frank LR, Menegazzi JJ, Taylor R. A randomized, controlled trial of two-thumb vs two-finger chest compression in a swine infant model of cardiac arrest [see comment]. *Prehosp Emerg Care*. 1997;1(2):65–67.

135. Dorfsman ML, Menegazzi JJ, Wadas RJ, Auble TE. Two-thumb vs. two-finger chest compression in an infant model of prolonged cardiopulmonary resuscitation. *Acad Emerg Med*. 2000;7(10):1077–1082.

136. Berg RA, Hilwig RW, Kern KB, Babar I, Ewy GA. Simulated mouth-to-mouth ventilation and chest compressions (bystander cardiopulmonary resuscitation) improves outcome in a swine model of prehospital pediatric asphyxial cardiac arrest. *Crit Care Med*. 1999;27(9):1893–1899.

137. Berg RA, Hilwig RW, Kern KB, Ewy GA. "Bystander" chest compressions and assisted ventilation independently improve outcome from piglet asphyxial pulseless "cardiac arrest." *Circulation.* 2000;101(14):1743–1748.

138. Dean JM, Koehler RC, Schleien CL, et al. Improved blood flow during prolonged cardiopulmonary resuscitation with 30% duty cycle in infant pigs. *Circulation.* 1991;84(2):896–904.

139. Babbs CF, Nadkarni V. Optimizing chest compression to rescue ventilation ratios during one-rescuer CPR by professionals and lay persons: children are not just little adults. *Resuscitation.* 2004;61(2):173–181.

140. Solevag AL, Dannevig I, Wyckoff M, Saugstad OD, Nakstad B. Extended series of cardiac compressions during CPR in a swine model of perinatal asphyxia. *Resuscitation.* 2010;81(11):1571–1576.

141. Solevag AL, Dannevig I, Wyckoff M, Saugstad OD, Nakstad B. Return of spontaneous circulation with a compression:ventilation ratio of 15:2 versus 3:1 in newborn pigs with cardiac arrest due to asphyxia. *Arch Dis Child Fetal Neonatal Ed.* 2011;96(6):F417–F421.

142. Hemway RJ, Christman C, Perlman J. The 3:1 is superior to a 15:2 ratio in a newborn manikin model in terms of quality of chest compressions and number of ventilations. *Arch Dis Child Fetal Neonatal Ed.* 2013;98(1):F42–F45.

143. Schmolzer GM, O'Reilly M, Labossiere J, et al. 3:1 compression to ventilation ratio versus continuous chest compression with asynchronous ventilation in a porcine model of neonatal resuscitation. *Resuscitation.* 2014;85(2):270–275.

144. Schmolzer GM, O'Reilly M, Labossiere J, et al. Cardiopulmonary resuscitation with chest compressions during sustained inflations: a new technique of neonatal resuscitation that improves recovery and survival in a neonatal porcine model. *Circulation.* 2013;128(23):2495–2503.

145. Chalak LF, Barber CA, Hynan L, Garcia D, Christie L, Wyckoff MH. End-tidal CO_2 detection of an audible heart rate during neonatal cardiopulmonary resuscitation after asystole in asphyxiated piglets. *Pediatr Res.* 2011;69(5 Pt 1):401–405.

146. Travers AH, Rea TD, Bobrow BJ, et al. Part 4: CPR overview: 2010 American Heart Association Guidelines for Cardiopulmonary Resuscitation and Emergency Cardiovascular Care. *Circulation.* 2010;122(18 suppl 3):S676–S684.

147. Kapadia V, Wyckoff MH. Chest compressions for bradycardia or asystole in neonates. *Clin Perinatol.* 2012;39(4):833–842.

148. Kern KB, Hilwig R, Ewy GA. Retrograde coronary blood flow during cardiopulmonary resuscitation in swine: intracoronary Doppler evaluation. *Am Heart J.* 1994;128(3):490–499.

149. McNamara PJ, Engelberts D, Finelli M, Adeli K, Kavanagh BP. Vasopressin improves survival compared with epinephrine in a neonatal piglet model of asphyxial cardiac arrest. *Pediatr Res.* 2014;75(6):738–748.

150. Ellemunter H, Simma B, Trawoger R, Maurer H. Intraosseous lines in preterm and full term neonates. *Arch Dis Child Fetal Neonatal Ed.* 1999;80(1):F74–F75.

151. Rajani AK, Chitkara R, Oehlert J, Halamek LP. Comparison of umbilical venous and intraosseous access during simulated neonatal resuscitation. *Pediatrics.* 2011;128(4):e954–e958.

152. Weiner GM, Niermeyer S. Medications in neonatal resuscitation: epinephrine and the search for better alternative strategies. *Clin Perinatol.* 2012;39(4):843–855.

153. Barber CA, Wyckoff MH. Use and efficacy of endotracheal versus intravenous epinephrine during neonatal cardiopulmonary resuscitation in the delivery room. *Pediatrics.* 2006;118(3):1028–1034.

154. Wyckoff M, Garcia D, Margraf L, Perlman J, Laptook A. Randomized trial of volume infusion during resuscitation of asphyxiated neonatal piglets. *Pediatr Res.* 2007;61(4):415–420.

155. Harrington DJ, Redman CW, Moulden M, Greenwood CE. The long-term outcome in surviving infants with Apgar zero at 10 minutes: a systematic review of the literature and hospital-based cohort. *Am J Obstet Gynecol.* 2007;196(5):463.e461–e465.

156. Laptook AR, Shankaran S, Ambalavanan N, et al. Outcome of term infants using apgar scores at 10 minutes following hypoxic-ischemic encephalopathy. *Pediatrics.* 2009;124(6):1619–1626.

157. Shah P, Anvekar A, McMichael J, Rao S. Outcomes of infants with Apgar score of zero at 10 min: the West Australian experience. *Arch Dis Child Fetal Neonatal Ed.* 2015;100(6):F492–F494.

158. Natarajan G, Shankaran S, Laptook AR, et al. Apgar scores at 10 min and outcomes at 6–7 years following hypoxic-ischaemic encephalopathy. *Arch Dis Child Fetal Neonatal Ed.* 2013;98(6):F473–F479.

159. Kasdorf E, Laptook A, Azzopardi D, Jacobs S, Perlman JM. Improving infant outcome with a 10 min Apgar of 0. *Arch Dis Child Fetal Neonatal Ed.* 2015;100(2):F102–F105.

160. Patel H, Beeby PJ. Resuscitation beyond 10 minutes of term babies born without signs of life. *J Paediatr Child Health.* 2004;40(3):136–138.

161. Wilkinson DJ, Stenson B. Don't stop now? How long should resuscitation continue at birth in the absence of a detectable heartbeat? *Arch Dis Child Fetal Neonatal Ed.* 2015;100(6):F476–F478.

10

CHAPTER 11

Noninvasive Ventilation of Preterm Infants: An Alternative to Mechanical Ventilation

Brett J. Manley, Bradley A. Yoder, and Peter G. Davis

11

- Continuous positive airway pressure (CPAP) is an effective respiratory support for preterm infants for a range of indications, especially when delivered via binasal prongs at set pressures equal to or greater than 25 cm H_2O.
- Extremely preterm infants may be managed with CPAP from the delivery room onward as an alternative to routine intubation.
- Nasal intermittent positive-pressure ventilation is a useful method for augmenting the benefits of CPAP, especially when synchronized with the infant's breathing.
- Noninvasive high-frequency ventilation is a promising modality that requires further study in randomized trials.
- Nasal high-flow is an alternative to CPAP as postextubation support for preterm infants and as primary support if CPAP is available as backup.

The primary concern of the clinician making choices about treatment is whether one therapy leads to better outcomes than the alternatives. This chapter draws heavily on evidence from randomized controlled trials (RCTs), and reviews found in the neonatal module of the Cochrane Library (http://www.nichd.nih.gov/cochrane/defau lt.cfm). Consistent with presentation in the library, estimates of treatment effect are expressed as relative risk (RR) or risk difference (RD) and the differences are statistically significant if the 95% confidence interval (CI) does not include 1 (for RR) or 0 (for RD). Other levels of evidence—for example, from observational studies—are presented, particularly when no RCTs exist.

We believe that before the examination of available evidence, a summary of the physiologic principles underpinning noninvasive ventilation (NIV) usefully informs clinicians and researchers. This chapter focuses on current modes of NIV in clinical use or under investigation in clinical trials: nasal continuous positive airway pressure (NCPAP), nasal intermittent positive-pressure ventilation (NIPPV), high-frequency nasal ventilation (HFNV), and nasal high-flow therapy (NHFT).

Why Do Preterm Infants Experience Respiratory Failure and How Can Noninvasive Ventilation Help?

Respiratory Distress Syndrome

Respiratory distress syndrome (RDS) is a disease of newborns, increasing in prevalence with decreasing gestational age. It is characterized by immature lung development and inadequate surfactant production. The lungs of affected infants may not expand normally immediately after birth, do not easily maintain a residual volume, and are at risk of atelectasis. Other factors also contribute to a loss of lung volume, including muscle hypotonia, a compliant chest wall, and slow clearance of fetal lung liquid.

Repeated lung expansion, followed by atelectasis during expiration, leads to shearing forces and stretch injury that damage the airway and saccular alveolar epithelium, causing leakage of protein-rich fluid from the pulmonary capillaries. This leakage in turn inhibits any endogenous surfactant present.[1] Damage to the lungs is exacerbated by mechanical ventilation (MV), high oxygen concentrations, and infection.[2]

Apnea of Prematurity

The pharyngeal airway of the preterm newborn is very compliant. The cartilaginous components are more flexible, and the fat-laden superficial fascia of the neck that stabilizes the upper airway of term infants is not well developed. The intrathoracic airways, including trachea, bronchi, and small airways, are similarly compliant and prone to collapse during expiration. The breathing patterns of very premature infants are frequently erratic and at times inadequate. The causes of apnea of prematurity include hypoxia owing to a reduced functional residual capacity, particularly in active sleep. Upper airway obstruction, alone or in combination with a central respiratory pause, accompanies most apneic events.[3]

The Role of CPAP

CPAP effectively supports the breathing of preterm infants through a number of mechanisms. It mechanically splints the upper airway, thereby minimizing obstruction and reducing apnea.[4] Distention of the airways reduces resistance to air flow and so diminishes work of breathing.[5] CPAP aids lung expansion and so reduces ventilation-perfusion mismatch and improves oxygenation. By preventing repeated alveolar collapse and reexpansion, CPAP reduces protein leak and helps conserve surfactant.

Why Might NIV Be Superior to Mechanical Ventilation via an Endotracheal Tube?

MV via an endotracheal tube (ETT) has been the mainstay of neonatal intensive care almost since its inception. Many lives have been saved by this technique but its adverse effects are well documented, as follows:
- Cardiovascular and cerebrovascular instability during intubation
- Complications of the ETT, including subglottic stenosis and tracheal lesions
- Infections, both pulmonary and systemic
- Acute and chronic lung damage, primarily related to stretch-mediated effects of nonhomogeneous tidal volume delivery at the cellular level. Studies have demonstrated a differential effect between MV and NIV on both abundance and activation of membrane-based mechanotransducer molecules.

By avoiding the local mechanical problems of an ETT and those of volutrauma, CPAP has been shown to have an advantage over MV, not just in theory but in chronic animal models as well as RCTs.[6–10]

A Brief History of Invasive and Noninvasive Neonatal Ventilation

The first form of assisted ventilation for neonates was MV provided via an ETT, which became widespread in the late 1960s and early 1970s. Gregory and associates[11] were the first to describe the use of CPAP in neonates in 1971, a therapy they developed because of the high mortality observed in infants weighing less than 1500 g, particularly those requiring assisted ventilation in the first 24 hours of life. The first series of 20 "severely ill" infants with RDS were treated with CPAP delivered predominantly via an ETT. In an attempt to avoid the complications of endotracheal intubation, other interfaces were developed, including a pressurized plastic bag[12] and a tight-fitting face mask.[13] Two infants in the initial Gregory series were managed in a pressure chamber around the infant's head.[11] In 1976, Ahlström and colleagues[14] described the use of a face chamber providing pressures up to 15 cm H_2O. Rhodes and Hall[15] conducted a controlled trial involving alternate allocation of subjects to CPAP via a tight-fitting face mask or to conventional therapy consisting of warmed humidified oxygen. A trend toward increased survival was noted in the CPAP group, which was statistically significant in the subgroup of infants weighing more than 1500 g.

The local pressure effects of these devices, combined with the problems of accessibility, particularly for suctioning and feeding, led to the development of alternative interfaces for the delivery of CPAP. Novogroder and coworkers[16] described a device composed of two ETTs inserted through the nose and then positioned under direct laryngoscopy in the posterior pharynx, joined by a Y-connector, and attached to a pressure source. Others described shorter binasal devices that were simpler to manufacture and insert.[17,18] An even simpler single nasal prong, made by cutting down an ETT, became widely used.[19] A later development in the field is that of a variable-flow device that uses jet nozzles to assist inspiratory flow while diverting flow away from the patient in expiration.[20] This design is claimed to be superior to "conventional" CPAP in reducing work of breathing.[21]

It should be noted that of all these trials, only the one conducted by Rhodes and Hall[15] used a control group. Novogroder and coworkers[16] had plans to subject their device to a randomized trial but abandoned them when "the dramatic effect of CPAP (was) observed after a brief period of treatment in all patients." It is likely that other researchers were so convinced of the virtues of endotracheal intubation that trials comparing this therapy with CPAP were considered inappropriate. In an accompanying commentary to the study by Rhodes and Hall, Chernick[22] congratulated the investigators on conducting a "daring controlled study" and suggested that although one or two such studies of CPAP would be welcome, many more "would be foolish." With some notable exceptions, it seems researchers heeded his advice. The following sections describe these exceptions.

Nasal Continuous Positive Airway Pressure

Nasal Continuous Positive Airway Pressure Devices

Several interfaces have been developed for delivering nasal CPAP (Fig. 11.1). Nasal prongs may be short, lying 1 to 2 cm inside the nose, or long, with the tip in the nasopharynx. They may be single or binasal. An important determinant of effectiveness of nasal CPAP devices is their ability to transmit the pressure to the airways. This ability depends on the resistance to flow of the device, which in turn depends on the length and diameter of the prongs. In an in vitro comparison of popular devices, short binasal prongs with the largest internal diameters had the lowest resistance.[23]

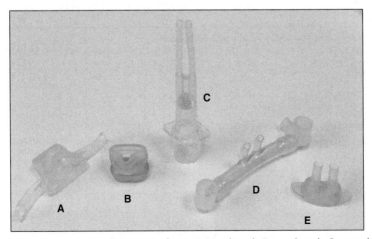

Fig. 11.1   Examples of noninvasive nasal CPAP interfaces. A, Nasal mask; B, nasal mask; C, nasopharyngeal prongs; D, short binasal prongs; and E, Infant Flow System nasal prongs. (Used with permission from Dr. Louise Owen, The Royal Women's Hospital, Melbourne, Australia.)

Since its description by Moa and coworkers[20] in 1988, the variable-flow nasal CPAP device (Aladdin nasal CPAP Infant Flow System [now called the Arabella [Hamilton Medical AG, Reno, NV], EME Infant Flow Nasal CPAP [CareFusion, San Diego, CA], or Infant Flow Driver (Electro Medical Equipment Ltd., Brighton, Sussex, UK] has become widely used around the world. In vitro studies using models of neonatal ventilation have demonstrated less pressure variation and work of breathing with the variable-flow device. Pandit and colleagues[24] measured the work of breathing in preterm infants using respiratory inductance plethysmography and esophageal pressure monitoring. They demonstrated less work of breathing with variable-flow CPAP than with constant-flow CPAP. The same group showed, in a crossover study, that the variable-flow device led to better lung recruitment than either nasal cannulae or constant-flow CPAP.[25]

An understanding of the properties of different devices is useful, but for clinicians the primary question is which device performs best at reducing the severity of the respiratory problems and intubation. Head-to-head comparisons of different devices are few. Pooled analysis of the two trials[26,27] comparing single and binasal prongs after extubation of preterm infants confirms that binasal prongs are superior at preventing extubation failure (RR 0.59, 95% CI 0.41 to 0.85) (Fig. 11.2).[28] Two trials have compared different binasal devices. Stefanescu and associates[29] compared the EME Infant Flow nasal CPAP with INCA prongs (Ackrad Laboratories Inc., Cranford, NJ) and found no difference in rates of extubation failure, death, or bronchopulmonary dysplasia (BPD). Sun and coworkers[30] reported a lower rate of reintubation using the EME Infant Flow system than with short binasal prongs.

Mazzella and associates[31] compared the Infant Flow Driver with a single long nasopharyngeal tube for the treatment of preterm infants with respiratory distress. Although infants randomly assigned to the Infant Flow Driver had lower fraction of inspired oxygen (F_{IO_2}) and respiratory rates, there were no significant differences in the need for ventilation or the duration of CPAP. The lower resistance offered by binasal prongs appears to translate to a clinical advantage for these devices over short or long single nasal prongs.

Gupta and colleagues[32] compared bubble CPAP with the Infant Flow Driver for postextubation management of preterm infants with RDS. The duration of CPAP support was halved in the bubble CPAP group. In the subgroup of infants in which ventilation was used less than 14 days, extubation failed less often in the bubble CPAP group.

COMPARISON: SHORT BINASAL PRONG VS. SINGLE PRONG (NASAL OR NASOPHARYNGEAL) NCPAP
OUTCOME: EXTUBATION FAILURE

Study	Short Binasal Prong n/N	Single Prong n/N	RR (Fixed) 95% CI	RR (Fixed) 95% CI
Endotracheal intubation within 7 days post extubation				
Davis 2001 (26)	9/41	19/46		0.53 [0.27, 1.04]
Roukema 1999 (27)	18/48	27/45		0.63 [0.40, 0.97]
Pooled analysis (95% CI)				0.59 [0.41, 0.85]

Test for heterogeneity: Chi^2 = 0.16, df = 1 (P = .69), I^2 = 0%
Test for overall effect: z = 2.80 (P = .005)

Respiratory failure within 7 days post extubation				
Davis 2001 (61)	10/41	26/46		0.43 [0.24, 0.78]
				0.43 [0.24, 0.78]

Test for overall effect: z = 2.77 (P = .006)

0.1 0.2 0.5 1   2   5 10
Favors binasal prong   Favors single prong

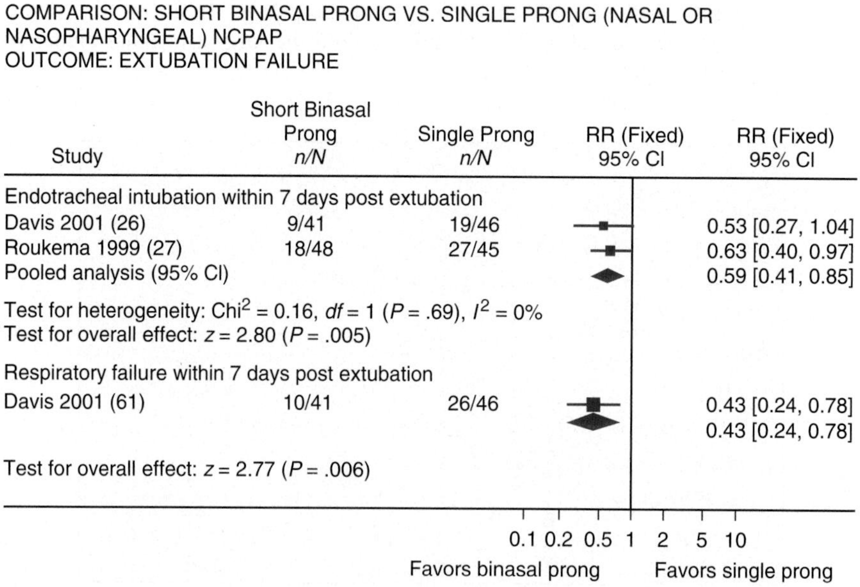

Fig. 11.2 Comparison of single-prong (nasal) and double-prong (nasopharyngeal) nasal continuous positive airway pressure (NCPAP): effect on extubation failure. See text for details. CI, Confidence interval; df, degrees of freedom; RR, relative risk.

As noted early, there are a variety of devices and interfaces through which nasal CPAP is delivered. A recent bench study by Poli and colleagues[33] suggests there may be differences in the functionality of different bubble CPAP delivery systems. Clinical trials have not been performed to compare the clinical effect, if any, of such functional differences. Over the past few years a number of centers have incorporated the "RAM" nasal cannula (Neotech, Valencia, CA) into their management scheme for delivering NIV in lieu of standard approaches to nasal CPAP. Although two small observational studies have been reported,[34,35] no randomized trials have been performed to date comparing the RAM nasal cannula to other forms of NIV, including CPAP, NIPPV, or NHFT. It is important to note that several recent bench studies suggest significant limitations in the ability of the RAM nasal cannula to provide ventilator set peak or distending pressure during CPAP or NIPPV support.[36–38] These studies show that only 60% to 70% of the set pressure is delivered to the proximal airway and that there is only minimal volume delivery as well. Clearly, RCTs are required to evaluate this nasal interface.

How Much Supporting Pressure Should Be Used?

The purpose of nasal CPAP is to deliver a pressure to the airways and lungs. If this purpose is achieved consistently, which device is used may not be important. A pressure of 5 cm H_2O is a traditional starting point. Some neonatal intensive care units (NICUs) hardly vary this pressure and claim good results.[39] There is some evidence from the Cochrane Review of postextubation nasal CPAP that pressures less than 5 cm H_2O are ineffective in this setting.[40] In their landmark publication on CPAP, Gregory and associates used pressures up to 15 mm Hg.[11] A study of infants with mild RDS showed the highest end-expiratory lung volume and tidal volume, the lowest respiratory rate, and the least thoracoabdominal asynchrony occurred at a pressure of 8 cm H_2O, which was compared with 0, 2, 4, and 6 cm H_2O.[41]

A more recent study from Buzzella and colleagues[42] suggests that CPAP pressures of 8 cm H_2O compared with 5 cm H_2O may be more effective at preventing extubation failure in extremely low-birth-weight infants. Additionally, the higher pressure seems to be well tolerated from a cardiorespiratory standpoint. Comparisons of cardiac output, cerebral circulation, and venous return suggest the higher pressure does not compromise cerebral circulation or venous return, but it may reduce pulmonary shunting across the ductus arteriosus.[43] An infant with RDS, relatively stiff lungs, a high F_{IO_2}, and a chest radiograph showing opaque lungs may need a higher pressure to support lung volume than an infant with a low F_{IO_2} treated for apneic episodes. If CPAP is to be effective, the pressure may need to be increased to the 8- to 10-cm H_2O range in infants with very low lung compliance. If an infant shows evidence of lung disease with increasing oxygen requirements and a more opaque chest radiograph, we recommend increasing the distending pressure by increments of 1 cm H_2O and observing the effect. It is important to note, however, that high distending pressures, if used in an infant with compliant lungs, can interfere with pulmonary blood flow and cause lung overdistention, leading to carbon dioxide retention.

The optimal CPAP pressure is not known and likely depends on the condition treated. Judging the distending airway pressure needed to optimize lung inflation, pulmonary, and systemic blood flow to result in the lowest needed F_{IO_2} remains an art. Future research should evaluate strategies of titrating CPAP pressures to an infant's requirements. In the absence of evidence-based guidelines, we typically use CPAP pressures in the 5- to 8-cm H_2O range, adjusting them on the basis of oxygen requirements and clinical assessment of work of breathing.

Nasal CPAP for Infants With RDS or at Risk of Developing RDS

The focus of studies on the use of nasal CPAP in infants who have, or are at risk for, RDS has changed over the decades. Questions about the topic are dealt with here in roughly historical order. From a clinical perspective, studies conducted before the availability of surfactant are of limited relevance in the modern neonatal intensive care era. In general, presurfactant trials comparing the risk and benefit of prophylactic

CPAP versus no continuous distending pressure (i.e., oxygen by hood or standard nasal cannula therapy) showed that CPAP reduced the rate of treatment failure (death or use of assisted ventilation; RR 0.70, 95% CI 0.55 to 0.88), and mortality (RR 0.52, 95% CI 0.32 to 0.87) (Fig. 11.3). However, more pneumothoraces occurred in the patients receiving continuous distending pressure (RR 2.36, 95% CI 1.25 to 5.54).

CPAP in the Surfactant Era

Surfactant is the most comprehensively evaluated treatment in neonatology. Initial randomized trials of surfactant were done nearly 30 years ago, when early CPAP was not commonly used for very preterm infants, antenatal corticosteroids were given to only 10% of eligible mothers, and neonatal mortality and morbidity rates were much higher than current rates. Surfactant therapy was provided via the ETT, and whether given prophylactically or as treatment, surfactant reduced mortality and the combined outcome of death or chronic lung disease.[44,45] Surfactant therapy appeared more beneficial when given early in the course of RDS.[46] It became common practice for all very preterm infants to be intubated in the delivery room for surfactant administration. In the past few years a number of randomized trials have evaluated "less invasive" approaches to surfactant administration in conjunction with CPAP support and are discussed in the following text. Although other methods of administration have been tried,[47] surfactant is usually given via an ETT.

Is CPAP an Alternative to Routine Intubation of Very Preterm Infants at Birth?

More than a decade ago, several groups reported their experience following policy change from early intubation to early nasal CPAP,[48,49] describing lower mortality and morbidity in the CPAP-treated group. Since then, several RCTs have compared intubation in the delivery room with early nasal CPAP. The Nasal CPAP or Intubation at Birth for Very Preterm Infants (COIN) trial[50] randomly assigned 610 breathing infants born at 25 to 29 weeks' gestation to CPAP or intubation and ventilation if they manifested signs of respiratory distress at 5 minutes after birth. Surfactant was administered to intubated infants at the discretion of the treating clinician. There were no differences in the rates of death or BPD between the groups. The benefits of CPAP included halving the intubation rate, a lower risk of the combined outcome of death or the need for oxygen therapy at 28 days, and fewer days of MV. However, the CPAP group had a higher rate of pneumothoraces (9% vs. 3% in the intubated group).

The Surfactant, Positive Pressure, and Oxygenation Randomized Trial (SUPPORT)[51] group enrolled 1316 infants between 24 and 27 weeks' gestation who

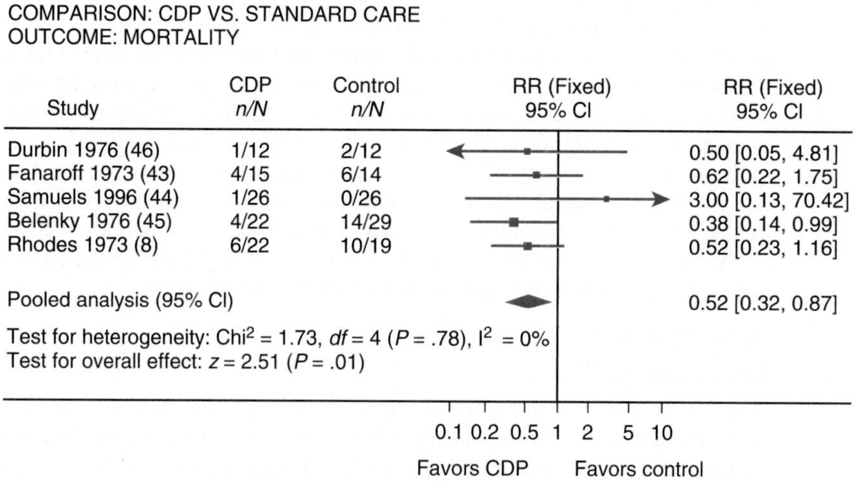

COMPARISON: CDP VS. STANDARD CARE
OUTCOME: MORTALITY

Study	CDP n/N	Control n/N	RR (Fixed) 95% CI	RR (Fixed) 95% CI
Durbin 1976 (46)	1/12	2/12		0.50 [0.05, 4.81]
Fanaroff 1973 (43)	4/15	6/14		0.62 [0.22, 1.75]
Samuels 1996 (44)	1/26	0/26		3.00 [0.13, 70.42]
Belenky 1976 (45)	4/22	14/29		0.38 [0.14, 0.99]
Rhodes 1973 (8)	6/22	10/19		0.52 [0.23, 1.16]
Pooled analysis (95% CI)				0.52 [0.32, 0.87]

Test for heterogeneity: Chi^2 = 1.73, df = 4 (P = .78), I^2 = 0%
Test for overall effect: z = 2.51 (P = .01)

0.1 0.2 0.5 1 2 5 10
Favors CDP   Favors control

Fig. 11.3 Comparison of continuous distending pressure *(CDP)* and standard care for respiratory distress syndrome: effect on rate of mortality. See text for details. *CI,* Confidence interval; *df,* degrees of freedom; *RR,* relative risk.

were randomly allocated to immediate CPAP or intubation in the delivery room. Intubated infants were also treated with surfactant within 1 hour after birth. The rates of death or BPD did not differ significantly between the groups after adjustment for gestational age, center, and familial clustering. Although 83.1% of infants in the CPAP group ultimately required intubation and MV, 34.4% were intubated in the delivery room. Overall, infants randomly assigned to CPAP were less likely to be intubated, less likely to receive postnatal corticosteroids, had fewer days of MV, and were more likely to be alive without MV by day 7.

A Vermont Oxford Network trial[52] compared three approaches to initial respiratory management in 648 very preterm infants born at 26 to 29 completed weeks' gestation: (1) prophylactic surfactant followed by a period of MV, (2) prophylactic surfactant with rapid extubation to CPAP, or (3) initial management with CPAP and selective surfactant treatment. The primary outcome was the incidence of death or BPD at 36 weeks postmenstrual age. Both prophylactic surfactant with rapid extubation to CPAP and initial management with CPAP reduced the RR of death or BPD compared with prophylactic surfactant followed by a period of MV. About half the infants managed with initial CPAP avoided MV and surfactant. Mortality and other adverse outcomes were similar between the groups.

A meta-analysis including the previous RCTs and a fourth trial[53] found a significant reduction in the combined outcome of death or BPD, at 36 weeks' corrected gestation for infants treated with early CPAP: RR 0.91 (95% CI 0.84 to 0.99), number needed to treat: 25. The trials show that nasal CPAP can be used from birth in very preterm infants and that nearly half of such infants may not need ventilation or surfactant treatment. The absence of evidence for increased risk or adverse event rates supports increasing the use of early aggressive nasal CPAP as the initial respiratory mode in an effort to prevent intubation/MV and subsequent BPD for most extremely preterm infants.

Is CPAP With Early Intubation for Surfactant and Brief Mechanical Ventilation Better Than CPAP Alone?

A systematic review has investigated whether early, brief intubation for surfactant administration followed by extubation to nasal CPAP was better than nasal CPAP and selective intubation, surfactant, and continued MV.[54] Meta-analysis of the six studies identified showed that intubation, ventilation, and early surfactant therapy followed by extubation to nasal CPAP ventilation was associated with lower incidences of later MV (typical RR 0.67, 95% CI 0.57 to 0.79), air leak syndromes (typical RR 0.52, 95% CI 0.28 to 0.96), and BPD (typical RR 0.51, 95% CI 0.26 to 0.99). The early surfactant group received about 60% more surfactant. Stratified analysis of F_{IO_2} at study entry suggested that a lower treatment threshold ($F_{IO_2} <0.45$) reduced air leaks and BPD.

Further studies have been published since this review. The Colombian Neonatal Research Network enrolled infants of 27 to 31 weeks' gestation, who were receiving oxygen and had increased work of breathing, at 15 to 60 minutes after birth.[55] The infants were treated with bubble nasal CPAP 6 cm H_2O and then were randomly allocated to either nasal CPAP plus surfactant ($n = 141$) or nasal CPAP alone ($n = 137$). The primary outcome was the need for MV started because either the F_{IO_2} was higher than 0.75 or the partial pressure of carbon dioxide (Pa_{CO_2}) was higher than 65 mm Hg. The nasal CPAP plus surfactant group received two doses of surfactant (Survanta, Abbott Nutrition, Abbott Park, IL), 2 minutes apart, and were then extubated if possible to nasal CPAP 6 cm H_2O. The need for MV was significantly lower in the nasal CPAP ventilation plus surfactant group (26% vs. 39%), although all infants who had received surfactant had been temporarily intubated and ventilated. Mortality, BPD, duration of MV, and oxygen therapy did not differ between the groups. There were fewer air leaks in the group receiving surfactant.

The CURPAP study group randomly assigned 208 infants born at 25 to 28 weeks' gestation who were not intubated within 30 minutes of birth to either (1) intubation, surfactant (Curosurf; Cornerstone Therapeutics Inc., Cary, NC) and extubation within an hour (if possible) to nasal CPAP, or (2) nasal CPAP with early selective surfactant.[56] Infants were intubated for MV when F_{IO_2} exceeded 0.4, the infant had four episodes of apnea per hour, or for Pa_{CO_2} higher than 65 mm Hg. There were no significant differences between the groups in the need for MV at 5 days of life, death, or BPD, or the rate of pneumothoraces.

All these trials show that outcomes in infants stabilized in the delivery room with either nasal CPAP or prophylactic surfactant and extubation to nasal CPAP appear to be similar to those in infants managed with surfactant followed by MV.

Less Invasive Surfactant Administration

Techniques of administering surfactant without using an ETT, less invasive surfactant administration (LISA), have recently been described. Kribs and associates[57] performed an RCT in extremely premature infants receiving nasal CPAP with ongoing signs of RDS, comparing surfactant given via an intratracheal catheter during spontaneous breathing (LISA) to conventional therapy with surfactant via ETT. Although survival without BPD was not different, the LISA group had significantly fewer rates of intubation, days of MV, and pneumothoraces. The combined outcome of survival without serious adverse event was significantly improved in the LISA group. Dargaville and colleagues[58] have also proposed a less invasive method of surfactant administration; in a feasibility study, nonsedated preterm infants undergoing nasal CPAP received surfactant via a 16-gauge vascular catheter under direct vision of the vocal cords. In all cases, surfactant was successfully administered and nasal CPAP was reestablished. A large RCT of this method is underway.[59]

LISA techniques have been further evaluated in RCTs[57,60–63] and subsequent meta-analyses.[64,65] These trials, including nearly 900 preterm infants, vary by the overall LISA approach, the mode of NIV, and study population. Additionally, none of the trials has been effectively blinded. Meta-analysis of the trials to date demonstrate a significant reduction in several important respiratory outcomes, including early CPAP failure (RR 0.67, 95% CI 0.47 to 0.93), any need for MV (RR 0.66, 95% CI 0.47 to 0.93), and death or BPD (RR 0.74, 95% CI 0.58 to 0.94).[64,65] Importantly, no increases in other common neonatal morbidities such as intraventricular hemorrhage, necrotizing enterocolitis, or retinopathy of prematurity were found with the LISA approach. Long-term neurodevelopmental follow-up studies remain to be completed.

Nasal CPAP for Postextubation Support

It is generally accepted that early extubation of preterm infants is desirable. The perceived benefits include reducing the risks of infection, local tissue damage, and BPD. On the other hand, failure of extubation and the need for reintubation is associated with instability and more local trauma. The Cochrane Review on the topic[40] identified nine randomized trials of varying methodologic quality and using different CPAP pressures and devices.[66–74] Pooled analysis showed that nasal CPAP was associated with a lower rate of respiratory failure (apnea, respiratory acidosis, or increased oxygen requirements) after extubation than management in an oxygen hood (RR 0.62, 95% CI 0.51 to 0.76). Four of the studies allowed rescue nasal CPAP for infants in whom the oxygen hood failed. Because rescue treatment with nasal CPAP was frequently successful, there was no significant difference in the rate of reintubation between the groups (RR 0.93, 95% CI 0.72 to 1.19). A study that directly compared elective with rescue nasal CPAP ventilation after extubation found no differences in reintubation rates.[75]

Therefore it can reasonably be concluded that nasal CPAP should be used when a very preterm infant is extubated to prevent the instability associated with possible subsequent respiratory failure and reintubation. However, it appears that reserving the use of nasal CPAP for preterm infants in whom respiratory failure is developing after extubation does not lead to increased reintubation.

CPAP Failure: When Should Preterm Infants Be Intubated?

There is no universally accepted definition of CPAP "failure." Polin and Sahni[76] suggested that an infant with ventilation that is not improving or inadequate oxygenation with F_{IO_2} >0.6 should be intubated and given surfactant. Others recommend intubation when the F_{IO_2} exceeds 0.35 to 0.40.[77] Studies suggest that lower gestational age (<26–27 weeks), more radiographic evidence of severe disease, and evidence of escalating F_{IO_2} are key markers for preterm infants likely to have nasal CPAP failure.[78,79] The following failure criteria were set for infants randomly allocated to nasal CPAP in the COIN trial: F_{IO_2} greater than 0.6 or pH less than 7.25 with a $Paco_2$ higher than 60 mm Hg, or more than one apneic episode per hour requiring stimulation.[50] Regardless of which threshold is applied, it is important that remediable causes of CPAP failure are sought and treated before intubation. They include airway obstruction with secretions, inappropriate (too small) prong size, and inadequate distending pressure. Treating a large mouth leak and raising the applied pressure may be useful strategies before CPAP is deemed to have failed.

Complications of Nasal CPAP

Nasal CPAP ventilation is a comparatively simple form of respiratory support, yet it is not without complications. The major problems of the early days of CPAP, intracerebellar hemorrhages[80] and hydrocephalus,[81] were solved by alterations in delivery technique. However, nasal trauma may still occur when prongs are used, ranging in severity from redness and excoriation of the nares to necrosis of the columella and nasal septum requiring surgery. Observational studies suggest that all nasal CPAP devices may cause trauma.[82] Robertson and coworkers[83] reported a complication rate of 20% in a series of very low-birth-weight infants managed with the Infant Flow Driver. To minimize the incidence of nasal trauma, we try to select a prong with a diameter that is sufficient to snugly fit the infant's nostril (avoiding excessive leak around the device), but which does not cause blanching of the nares. Positioning of binasal prongs so that there is no pressure on the columella is sometimes difficult to achieve but is critical. We have observed that supervision by skilled nurses experienced in the technique of securing nasal CPAP prongs has led to a low rate of nasal trauma.

Pneumothoraces occur in preterm infants treated with CPAP. In the COIN trial,[50] there were significantly more pneumothoraces in the CPAP group than in the ventilated group (9% vs. 3%, respectively), raising concerns in some quarters about the use of early nasal CPAP. In the previously described Colombian Neonatal Research Network study, the group managed with early surfactant therapy had fewer pneumothoraces compared with the group managed with nasal CPAP alone (2% vs. 9%).[55] Conversely, the SUPPORT trial found no difference in the rate of pneumothoraces between early CPAP and early MV.[51] An RCT of early CPAP compared with passive oxygen therapy after birth for newborn infants with respiratory distress born in Australian nontertiary centers by Buckmaster and colleagues found an almost threefold increase in pneumothorax rates in the CPAP-treated group (9% vs. 3%).[84]

Weaning CPAP

The optimal method of weaning an infant from nasal CPAP remains uncertain, and practices vary among units. An RCT comparing a strategy of weaning through reducing pressure with one of increasing time "off" nasal CPAP showed a significantly shorter duration of weaning with the "pressure" strategy.[85] A more recent trial determined that weaning directly off nasal CPAP, rather than gradual titration over increasing time intervals, resulted in discontinuing nasal CPAP earlier.[86] Recent follow-up from that study suggests that using a standardized approach to weaning from nasal CPAP in preterm infants younger than 30 weeks' gestation is associated with improved outcomes, including decreased rates of BPD.[87]

Four RCTs have assessed the role of NHFT, discussed at length later in this chapter, in weaning from nasal CPAP. Trials by Tang et al.[88] and Soonsawad et al.[89] found NHFT contributed to shorter time receiving nasal CPAP, but the overall duration of NIV was not different. In the study by Abdel-Hadys et al.,[90] the use of NHFT at 2 L/min to wean from CPAP resulted in more days on oxygen and respiratory support, with no difference in success of CPAP weaning. In contrast, Badiee[91] found NHFT at 2 L/min significantly reduced the duration of supplemental oxygen and hospital stay, without increasing successful weaning from CPAP. The use of NHFT ventilation to facilitate weaning from nasal CPAP ventilation requires further investigation.

In the absence of good evidence, our practice is to incrementally wean infants to a CPAP of 5 cm H_2O, discontinue the nasal CPAP ventilation when the infant is stable with FIO_2 less than 0.30, and recommence it if oxygen requirements or the frequency of apneas increases. We do not recommend the use of NHFT as a routine weaning method.

Nasal Intermittent Positive-Pressure Ventilation

Although nasal CPAP is an effective method of postextubation support, researchers have added positive-pressure "inflations" to a background of nasal CPAP: NIPPV. This technique was first used in the 1980s but became unpopular when it was linked to gastrointestinal perforation.[92] The availability of ventilators that "synchronized" with an infant's inspirations led to additional studies of NIPPV. The most recent systematic review identified 10 trials enrolling 1431 infants comparing extubation of infants to NIPPV or nasal CPAP.[93] Pooled analysis showed NIPPV to be associated with a significant reduction in the risk of extubation failure (typical RR 0.70, 95% CI 0.60 to 0.80), as well as the risk of needing reintubation (typical RR 0.76, 95% CI 0.65 to 0.88) (Fig. 11.4). Despite these benefits, there was not a reduction in BPD with NIPPV compared with nasal CPAP (typical RR 0.94, 95% CI 0.80 to 1.10). Reassuringly, there was no significant difference between the two approaches in the rate of abdominal distention, gastrointestinal perforation, or necrotizing enterocolitis.

Synchronized NIPPV (S-NIPPV) appears more effective in preventing intubation than nasal CPAP alone. However, most modern neonatal ventilators do not enable synchronization during NIV. Neurally adjusted ventilatory assist (NAVA), which synchronizes ventilator breaths to diaphragmatic electrical activity, has recently been applied to NIV of neonates. Preliminary studies suggest improved synchrony and lower peak inspiratory pressures compared with conventional approaches to NIPPV.[94] Large RCTs are needed to compare the safety and efficacy of NAVA-NIV to other NIV approaches for the prevention of BPD.

There is limited information to help clinicians optimize NIPPV settings. No RCTs have compared the safety or efficacy of different approaches to NIPPV settings, including the effect of rate. As many neonatal units are now using nonsynchronized NIPPV, it is important to recognize one potential adverse effect of this approach to the dynamic function of the upper airway and glottis. During normal breathing, the glottis musculature relaxes during inspiration, presumably to optimize the airway compliance and resistance to gas flow and minimize work of breathing. This neuromuscular response is unchanged when nasal CPAP is applied. However, recent studies demonstrate that nonsynchronized NIPPV (NS-NIPPV) induces a glottis constrictor response, mediated by bronchopulmonary receptors, leading to narrowing of the glottis region.[95] On the other hand, a normal glottic relaxation response was noted when NIV was applied with either NAVA or NHFV.[96,97]

NIPPV is also used in other clinical situations. A systematic review of NIPPV for treating apnea of prematurity found only two studies with a total of 54 infants.[98,99] The pooled analysis showed a modest benefit for NIPPV over nasal CPAP and no evidence

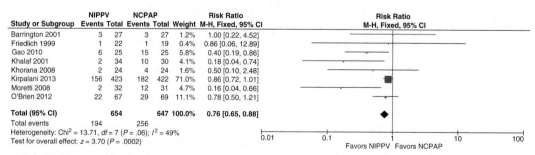

Study or Subgroup	NIPPV Events	Total	NCPAP Events	Total	Weight	Risk Ratio M-H, Fixed, 95% CI
Barrington 2001	3	27	3	27	1.2%	1.00 [0.22, 4.52]
Friedlich 1999	1	22	1	19	0.4%	0.86 [0.06, 12.89]
Gao 2010	6	25	15	25	5.8%	0.40 [0.19, 0.86]
Khalaf 2001	2	34	10	30	4.1%	0.18 [0.04, 0.74]
Khorana 2008	2	24	4	24	1.6%	0.50 [0.10, 2.48]
Kirpalani 2013	156	423	182	422	71.0%	0.86 [0.72, 1.01]
Moretti 2008	2	32	12	31	4.7%	0.16 [0.04, 0.66]
O'Brien 2012	22	67	29	69	11.1%	0.78 [0.50, 1.21]
Total (95% CI)		**654**		**647**	**100.0%**	**0.76 [0.65, 0.88]**
Total events	194		256			

Heterogeneity: Chi² = 13.71, df = 7 (P = .06); I² = 49%
Test for overall effect: z = 3.70 (P = .0002)

Favors NIPPV   Favors NCPAP

Fig. 11.4 Nasal intermittent positive pressure ventilation (*NIPPV*) versus nasal continuous positive airway pressure (*NCPAP*) for preterm neonates after extubation See text for details. *CI*, Confidence interval; *df*, degrees of freedom; *M-H*, Mantel-Haenszel (random-effects method for dichotomous data); *RR*, relative risk.

of harm.[100] It therefore seems reasonable to try NIPPV in infants experiencing troublesome apnea during treatment with nasal CPAP. Following its success in these situations, some investigators have suggested that NIPPV be used as an initial form of support for preterm infants with respiratory distress. Meneses and colleagues[101] studied NIPPV in this role: 200 preterm infants (26–34 weeks' gestation) with RDS were randomly assigned to NIPPV or nasal CPAP, with surfactant given as a rescue therapy. The rates of reintubation within the first 72 hours of life were no different between the groups (RR 0.71, 95% CI 0.48 to 1.14). Observational studies suggest that the use of NIPPV for primary treatment of RDS is worth testing in further RCTs, either alone or in conjunction with prior intubation and surfactant therapy.[102,103]

The mechanisms by which NIPPV improves clinical outcomes are uncertain. Owen[104] studied 10 premature infants receiving NS-NIPPV and found that the pressure peaks resulted in only a small increase in relative tidal volumes when delivered during spontaneous inspiration, and only occasionally led to chest inflations when delivered during apneic periods. Another study of 11 infants demonstrated that during NS-NIPPV, the delivered positive inflation pressure was variable and frequently lower than that set.[105] Chang and associates[106] compared short-term effects of NS-NIPPV and S-NIPPV with nasal CPAP. Sixteen very preterm infants, 15 ± 14 days old and undergoing treatment with the Infrasonic Infant Star Ventilator (Monet Medical, Salt Lake City, UT) were randomly allocated to nasal CPAP, NS-NIPPV at 20 or 40 inflations/min, or S-NIPPV at 20 or 40 inflations/min for 1 hour each in random order. Tidal volume, minute ventilation, and gas exchange values did not differ significantly among the groups. S-NIPPV resulted in less inspiratory effort than nasal CPAP or NS-NIPPV, but NS-NIPPV had no advantage over nasal CPAP. Active expiratory effort and expiratory duration increased during NS-NIPPV. There were no benefits for gas exchange of either form of nasal ventilation over nasal CPAP. S-NIPPV reduced breathing effort and resulted in better infant-ventilator interaction than NS-NIPPV.

NIPPV appears to be useful for augmenting nasal CPAP. Further studies of NIPPV are required to determine the optimal pressure and rate settings, the safety of the nonsynchronized mode, and the role of NIPPV as primary therapy for RDS.

Noninvasive High-Frequency Nasal Ventilation

Over the past decade, noninvasive HFNV has been increasingly studied as an approach to NIV of the neonate.[107–114] For interested readers, the clinical and pathologic effects of prolonged MV compared to early, sustained HFNV on lung injury and development in a sustainable preterm lamb model of BPD are available but are not discussed here.[8,9,115–118]

Factors Affecting Gas Exchange During HFNV

During neonatal HFNV, several factors related to tidal volume delivery and effective gas exchange need to be considered. First, as with nasal CPAP and NIPPV, satisfactory oxygenation is achieved by establishing and maintaining adequate functional residual lung volume via the mean distending pressure within the trachea and distal airway. Second, during NIV, unlike invasive MV, the mean intratracheal pressure is proportional to, but less than, the pressure set at the ventilator.[9,118] Additionally, the set peak pressure and/or amplitude setting at the ventilator is markedly attenuated (by as much as 70%) across the nasopharyngeal tube/prongs to the distal nasopharynx; pressure attenuation is greater with smaller internal diameter interfaces.[9,119,120] Third, despite this pressure attenuation, measurable small tidal volumes can be delivered at very rapid rates assisting minute ventilation.[9,119–121] Thus HFNV can maintain positive, albeit relatively low, end-expiratory pressure in the lungs to support oxygenation, while supporting ventilation by providing small tidal volumes at a high rate.

One factor influencing the effectiveness of any form of NIV is leak. Depending on the HFNV-nasal interface, leak may occur at the nares insertion site, contralateral nares, and the mouth. Shortened single nasopharyngeal tubes have been used, allowing leak from the contralateral nares, as well as short binasal CPAP prongs and masks. The least amount of leak is likely from a mask interface. The major consequence of leak is pressure reduction in the nasopharynx, trachea, and beyond.[9,121,122] However, there may be an "optimal" leak that enhances ventilation by washing out dead space.[122]

Laryngeal Effects of HFNV

During normal spontaneous breathing laryngeal muscles act in synchrony to open the upper airway during inspiration, decreasing resistance and improving the flow of gas through the glottis.[123] This normal muscle activity during inspiration is markedly altered with the application of pressure-supported NIPPV, inducing an increase in inspiratory constrictor (thryoarytenoid) muscle activity while suppressing normal inspiratory dilator (cricothyroid) muscle activity.[123] Contrary to the effect of NIPPV, the application of HFNV was shown been not to increase inspiratory constrictor muscle activity while maintaining normal dilator muscle activity.[97]

Clinical Reports on Neonatal HFNV

Use of high-frequency ventilation as an NIV technique in neonates was first published almost 20 years ago by van der Hoeven and colleagues.[107] Table 11.1 shows data from four retrospective studies ($n = 114$) and two prospective trials ($n = 79$) of HFNV in mostly preterm neonates.[107–112] There is considerable variability across studies in study population as well as in the high-frequency ventilator used and the initial settings applied. A variety of nasal interfaces have been used. Each of the published studies suggest HFNV could successfully support many (but not all) infants more effectively than conventional nasal CPAP or nasal ventilation. Significant adverse events related to HFNV have not been reported, although the majority of neonates have been supported for only relatively short periods of time.

Current Use of HFNV in the NICU

Despite the limited evidence from prospective RCTs and the lack of data identifying an optimal approach (device, interface, settings) for HFNV, the clinical use of HFNV appears to be increasing.[113,114] Fischer reported 17% (30/172) of responding NICUs in European countries (mostly Germany) use HFNV clinically in the management

Table 11.1 HIGH-FREQUENCY NASAL VENTILATION: FEATURES AND OUTCOMES FROM PUBLISHED STUDIES OF AT LEAST 10 INFANTS

Study Type	Gestation (Weeks)	Birth Weight (g)	Study Age (Days)	Device and Interface	Outcome
Retrospective					
Van der Hoeven ($n = 21$)	29 (27–32)	1010 (750–2170)	1 (0.2–20)	InfantStar NP tube (Infrasonics, Inc., San Diego, CA)	Success: 76%
Colaizy ($n = 14$)	27 (25–30)	995 (438–1371)	30 (18–147)	InfantStar NP tube (Infrasonics, Inc., San Diego, CA)	Success: 93%
Czernik ($n = 20$)	25 (23–27)	635 (382–1020)	31 (10–183)	Leoni Plus NP tube (Löwenstein Medical, Rheinland-Pfalz, Germany)	Success: 70%
Mukerji ($n = 59$)	25 (23–35)	740 (500–2860)	20 (2–147)	Drager prongs/mask (Drägerwerk, Lübeck, Germany)	Success: 58%
Prospective					
Dumas de la Roque (HFNV vs. CPAP; $n = 40$)	>37	>2000	0	Percussionaire (Percussionaire, Sandpoint, ID)	Decreased duration of distress/ F_{IO_2}
Mukerji (HFNV vs. BiPAP; $n = 39$)	26 (±2)	850 (±150)	17 (±10)	Drager binasal prongs (Drägerwerk, Lübeck, Germany)	Success: 65% vs. 35%

BiPAP, Biphasic positive airway pressure; F_{IO_2}, fraction of inspired oxygen; *HFNV*, high-frequency nasal ventilation; *NP*, nasopharyngeal.

of preterm and term neonates, most commonly for failure of nasal CPAP.[113] These investigators noted significant variation in the devices and initial support settings, but most infants were managed via short binasal prongs or a single nasopharyngeal tube. Mukerji reported a similar rate, 17% (5/28), among responding NICUs from the Canadian Neonatal Network.[114]

Device-Specific Comments Regarding HFNV

None of the human studies published to date have incorporated intermittent conventional inflations during HFNV support, in essence a combination of NIPPV with HFNV. Intermittent provision of a conventional breath during HFNV may potentially augment tidal volume delivery, improve functional resting lung volume, and improve gas exchange. Not all high-frequency ventilation devices are capable of providing conventional breaths during HFNV.

It is critical to understand that each high-frequency device may have an "optimal" approach for HFNV. Current evidence suggests HFNV may be optimized with the use of lower frequencies.[117,119] Additionally, studies suggest improved tidal volume delivery with larger nasal prong/cannula interface, with a longer inspiratory time and a higher-pressure amplitude.[120,122] However, no clinical studies (animal or human) have compared the effects of these potential modifiers on in vivo gas exchange. Given the marked loss of pressure and volume across the interface and within the respiratory passages, these differences noted in bench studies may not necessarily translate to clinical care. The routine use of HFNV cannot be recommended until the results of randomized trials are available.

Nasal High-Flow Therapy for Preterm Infants

Heated, humidified NHFT (Fig. 11.5) is an increasingly popular mode of NIV for newborn infants, particularly preterm infants. NHFT is defined as the delivery of heated, humidified, blended air and oxygen at gas flows of 1 L/min or higher through small, thin, tapered nasal cannulae.[124] In contrast to CPAP interfaces, NHFT prongs do not occlude the nares.[124] The perceived benefits of NHFT over CPAP include the simpler interface. The device is easier to apply than CPAP and more comfortable for infants[125] and is preferred by parents[126] and nurses.[127]

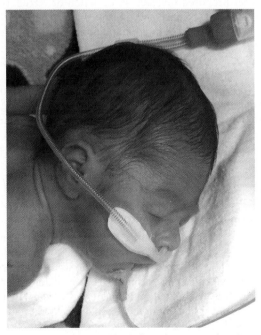

Fig. 11.5   A very preterm infant treated with nasal high-flow therapy. (Fisher & Paykel Optiflow Junior, Fisher & Paykel Healthcare, Auckland, New Zealand.)

In neonatology, NHFT use as an alternative to CPAP in developed countries has dramatically increased over the past decade. Surveys from Australia and New Zealand,[128] the United Kingdom,[129,130] and Japan[131] have reported the majority of respondent NICUs use NHFT to treat preterm infants. In 2014 in the Australian and New Zealand Neonatal Network, about 60% of very preterm infants born before 32 weeks' gestation were treated with NHFT.[132] In NICUs, NHFT is being used as an alternative to nasal CPAP for preterm infants as initial support for early respiratory distress, to treat apnea of prematurity, as postextubation support after a period of MV, to reduce nasal trauma, and as a weaning mode (previously discussed) from nasal CPAP.[128–131]

The two most widely used commercially available NHFT systems marketed for use in premature and term infants are Vapotherm Precision Flow (Vapotherm Inc., Stevensville, MD), and Optiflow Junior (Fisher & Paykel Healthcare, Auckland, NZ). These systems include a range of infant nasal prong sizes (with varying outer diameters and septum widths). The Fisher & Paykel system includes a pressure-relief valve in the circuit, whereas Vapotherm does not. Only one small trial comparing older versions of the devices has been published.[133] Hence, there is no strong evidence that one device is superior to the other.

How Does NHFT Work?

NHFT provides respiratory support through a number of mechanisms. There is probably some overlap between the mechanisms of action of NHFT and CPAP. Commercially available NHFT systems effectively deliver heated, humidified gas[134–136] with some variations between devices and between different gas flows. Nasal high flow produces a distending airway pressure, which compared with CPAP, is not set or measured when applied during routine use. In vivo and in vitro studies with different methodologies have attempted to measure the distending airway pressure produced by NHFT devices. In these studies, measured pressures were similar to, or less than, those commonly set with CPAP provided a leak in the circuit is maintained.[137–141] Measured pressures increase with increasing gas flow[135,137,138,140–145] and decreasing infant weight (higher pressures are measured in smaller infants at the same gas flow),[138,139] and pressures vary considerably between patients and with varying leak.[138,141,143,145,146]

Another proposed mechanism of action of NHFT is washout of gas from the nasopharyngeal dead space and improved gas exchange.[147,148] In vitro studies have shown that NHFT results in continuous flushing of the gas in the nasopharyngeal dead space.[149] This results in carbon dioxide clearance from the dead space, with a greater effect observed when higher gas flows were applied.[150,151] An animal study[144] showed that the effect of increasing gas flow on carbon dioxide removal and oxygenation was independent of the pressures generated, and that both ventilation and oxygenation improved in a flow-dependent manner. A high-leak interface produced better ventilation than a low-leak interface until flow rates were high. NHFT may minimize the resistance to gas flow in the nasopharynx by providing a gas flow matching or exceeding the peak inspiratory flow of the patient, thus reducing the work of breathing, similar to CPAP.[152–157]

Evidence from Randomized Trials for NHFT Use in Preterm Infants

Stabilization in the Delivery Room

There are no published randomized trials of NHFT use in the delivery room; however, Reynolds et al. recently published a single-center case series of 28 preterm infants born before 30 weeks' gestation who were stabilized with NHFT.[158] The center has extensive experience using NHFT in preterm infants. Most infants (25/28) were successfully stabilized and transferred to the NICU while receiving NHFT. Three of the four infants born at 23 or 24 weeks' gestation required intubation and ventilation in the delivery room. Overall, about half the infants who remained on NHFT went on to require surfactant treatment. RCTs are required before the use of NHFT for delivery room stabilization can be recommended.

Nasal HFT as Primary Respiratory Support After Admission to the Neonatal Unit

Nasal HFT Versus CPAP

Four published RCTs[159–162] and one unpublished[163] RCT have compared NHFT to CPAP as primary support, enrolling more 1100 preterm infants in total. These trials vary in the gestational ages and birth weights of the infants enrolled, and only the small, unpublished study by Nair[163] enrolled any extremely preterm infants. They also differ in the use of CPAP to treat infants in the NHFT group before inclusion, the NHFT and CPAP devices studied, the starting and maximal gas flows (for NHFT) and pressures (for CPAP) studied, the administration of surfactant before the primary outcome was determined, and the use of "rescue" modes of NIV once treatment failure has occurred. The study by Yoder et al.[160] included two treatment indication arms and enrolled preterm and term infants. In our pooled analysis we include only preterm infants enrolled in the primary support arm of the trial.

Pooled analyses of these studies for the outcomes of treatment failure (based on trial definitions, five studies), and intubation within 72 hours (four studies) are shown in the following text. The NHFT treatment failure rate was significantly higher than CPAP (RD 6, 95% CI 2 to 10, $P = .003$) (Fig. 11.6). This result was mainly due to the findings of the largest study by Roberts et al.,[162] which, in contrast to the other studies, found a 12% higher rate of treatment failure in the NHFT group. This may be in part due to surfactant therapy not being permitted before satisfying treatment failure criteria in that trial. However, because that study allowed rescue CPAP therapy before intubation, the overall rates of intubation within 72 hours on pooled analysis were not significantly different (RD 2, 95% CI –2 to 6, $P = .28$).

NHFT Versus NIPPV

One randomized trial compared NHFT to synchronized NIPPV as primary respiratory support. Kugelman et al.[164] randomly assigned 76 preterm infants and found no difference in the rate of treatment failure (32% vs. 34%) or intubation (29% vs. 34%) between the NHFT or NIPPV groups, respectively.

NHFT to Prevent Extubation Failure in Preterm Infants

Six published randomized trials[160,165–169] have compared NHFT with CPAP as postextubation support after a period of MV, or as support after intubation for surfactant administration and immediate extubation [INSURE] when possible). These 6 trials enrolled a total of 936 preterm infants. Although gestational age subgroup data are not available from all trials, it appears fewer than 250 extremely preterm infants born before 28 weeks' gestation were included, with the majority in two studies from Australia by Collins et al.[166] and Manley et al.[167]

Pooled analyses for the outcomes of extubation failure (based on study definitions, six studies) and reintubation within 7 days (six studies) are shown in the

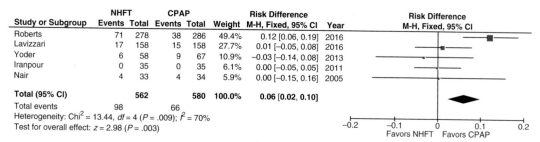

Fig. 11.6 Nasal high-flow therapy *(NHFT)* versus continuous positive airway pressure *(CPAP)* as primary support for preterm infants: treatment failure (study definition) (five studies, 1142 infants). *CI,* Confidence interval; *df,* degrees of freedom; *RR,* relative risk.

following text (Figs. 11.7 and 11.8.). Both analyses are required because the studies by Collins et al.[166] and Manley et al.[167] permitted the use of rescue CPAP/NIPPV in the NHFT group after extubation failure criteria were satisfied. There were no statistically significant differences between NHFT and CPAP on pooled analysis overall for either extubation failure (risk ratio [RR] 1.12 [0.88 to 1.43], $P = .35$) or reintubation within 7 days (RR 0.89 [0.66 to 1.19], $P = .42$).

Safety of NHFT

Adverse events, including death, BPD, and pneumothorax, were included outcomes in the Cochrane Review[170] and a systematic review by Kotecha et al.[171] No differences were demonstrated in the rates of death or BPD between NHFT and CPAP/NIPPV for any of the studied clinical indications. Trials published since these systematic reviews have similarly found no difference in rates of death or BPD.[161,162] Despite early concerns that unregulated distending pressure generation in the lung with NHFT might increase the risk of air leaks from the lung, pneumothorax rates were low in all randomized trials; there was no difference in rates of pneumothorax between NHFT and CPAP on pooled analysis[170,171] or between groups in the largest trial by Roberts et al., although fewer pneumothoraces occurred *during* NHFT treatment in that study.[162] Trials have consistently reported lower rates of nasal trauma with NHFT compared to CPAP, and this reduction is confirmed with pooled analysis in the Cochrane Review.[170] However, none of the studies included blinded assessment of this outcome, and methods of screening for and grading nasal injury varied. It should also be noted that individual studies were not powered to detect differences in the rates of most secondary outcomes.

Potential Concerns With Use of NHFT in Neonates

While the results of clinical trials are generally reassuring, there are several factors that warrant caution and further investigation. Though no differences in rates of BPD have been described with NHFT use compared to CPAP/NIPPV, the trials

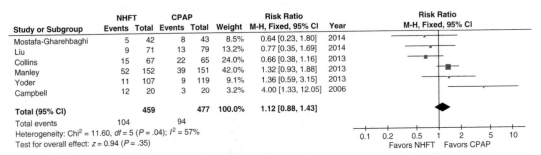

Study or Subgroup	NHFT Events	NHFT Total	CPAP Events	CPAP Total	Weight	Risk Ratio M-H, Fixed, 95% CI	Year
Mostafa-Gharehbaghi	5	42	8	43	8.5%	0.64 [0.23, 1.80]	2014
Liu	9	71	13	79	13.2%	0.77 [0.35, 1.69]	2014
Collins	15	67	22	65	24.0%	0.66 [0.38, 1.16]	2013
Manley	52	152	39	151	42.0%	1.32 [0.93, 1.88]	2013
Yoder	11	107	9	119	9.1%	1.36 [0.59, 3.15]	2013
Campbell	12	20	3	20	3.2%	4.00 [1.33, 12.05]	2006
Total (95% CI)		**459**		**477**	**100.0%**	**1.12 [0.88, 1.43]**	
Total events	104		94				

Heterogeneity: Chi^2 = 11.60, df = 5 (P = .04); I^2 = 57%
Test for overall effect: z = 0.94 (P = .35)

Fig. 11.7 Nasal high-flow therapy *(NHFT)* versus continuous positive airway pressure *(CPAP)* as postextubation or post-INSURE support: extubation failure (study definition) (six studies, 936 infants). *CI,* Confidence interval; *df,* degrees of freedom; *RR,* relative risk.

Study or Subgroup	NHFT Events	NHFT Total	CPAP Events	CPAP Total	Weight	Risk Ratio M-H, Fixed, 95% CI	Year
Liu	9	71	13	79	15.2%	0.77 [0.35, 1.69]	2014
Mostafa-Gharehbaghi	5	42	8	43	9.8%	0.64 [0.23, 1.80]	2014
Collins	7	67	8	65	10.0%	0.85 [0.33, 2.21]	2013
Yoder	11	107	12	117	14.2%	1.00 [0.46, 2.18]	2013
Manley	27	152	38	151	47.1%	0.71 [0.46, 1.09]	2013
Campbell	12	20	3	20	3.7%	4.00 [1.33, 12.05]	2006
Total (95% CI)		**459**		**475**	**100.0%**	**0.89 [0.66, 1.19]**	
Total events	71		82				

Heterogeneity: Chi^2 = 8.82, df = 5 (P = .12); I^2 = 43%
Test for overall effect: z = 0.81 (P = .42)

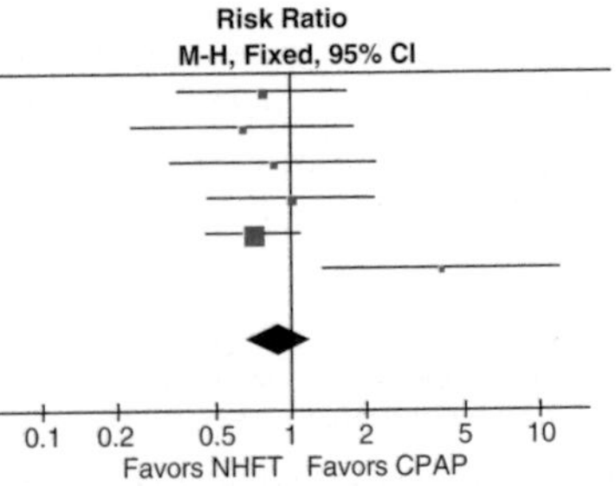

Fig. 11.8 Nasal high-flow therapy *(NHFT)* versus continuous positive airway pressure *(CPAP)* as postextubation or post-INSURE support: reintubation within 7 days (six studies, 934 infants).

have used varying definitions of BPD, or did not define it clearly, and only one[168] included BPD as part of its primary outcome. No NHFT trials have been powered sufficiently to demonstrate a difference in BPD rates, and none have reported using an oxygen reduction test or grading the severity of BPD. Four studies have reported a longer duration of weaning from respiratory support or oxygen with NHFT use compared with CPAP.[90,160,162,164] Importantly, relatively few extremely preterm infants born before 28 weeks' gestation—the population at highest risk of BPD—have been included in randomized trials, and caution is recommended when using NHFT in this population.

Should NHFT Be Used to Treat Preterm Infants?

There seems to be adequate evidence that NHFT may be used as an alternative to nasal CPAP as postextubation support in preterm infants, with caution recommended in extremely preterm infants for whom few data exist. NHFT may be a good option for stable preterm infants with (or at risk of) CPAP-related nasal trauma or other pressure injuries. The HIgh Flow Nasal Cannulae as Primary Support in the Treatment of Early Respiratory distress (HIPSTER) trial suggests that NHFT may be used as primary support in preterm infants born at 28 weeks or later of gestation who have not received surfactant, but only in care units that also have CPAP support available for those infants in whom NHFT therapy is inadequate. Until further data are available, we do not recommend the use of NHFT as primary support for extremely preterm infants or for the stabilization of newborn infants in the delivery room.

In the absence of an evidence-based NHFT weaning guideline, it is important to be diligent in weaning the gas flow as clinically indicated to avoid unnecessarily prolonging exposure to respiratory support. It is not recommended to prescribe gas flows higher than 8 L/min for preterm infants unless in a clinical trial setting. When using NHFT to treat preterm infants, care units should determine clear, objective criteria to expedite escalation of therapy when NHFT is failing.

Future Directions

Opportunities to advance knowledge in the field of NIV include studies of the following:
- Alternative techniques of surfactant administration in spontaneously breathing infants receiving NIV
- Methods available at the bedside to (1) judge optimal levels of CPAP and (2) predict which preterm infants will require intubation and surfactant
- NIPPV to determine the best settings in terms of pressures, rates, and synchronization, as well as testing its role in the initial management of RDS
- HFNV to identify optimal approach(es), including comparison of devices and settings, and to assess systemic effects as well as the effects on lung injury and developmental lung biology
- Nasal HFT to compare devices, assess efficacy and safety in extremely preterm infants, assess optimal gas flows and how best to increase and wean them, and whether NHFT may be used for stabilization of newborn infants in the delivery room

Acknowledgments

The authors thank Professor Colin Morley for his work on the previous versions of this chapter.

BJM is supported by an Australian National Health and Medical Research Council (NHMRC) Early Career Fellowship (No. 1088279). BAY is partially supported by the NICHD (No. UG1-HD0872266-01). PGD is supported by an NHMRC Practitioner Fellowship (No. 1059111).

REFERENCES

1. Ikegami M, Jacobs H, Jobe A. Surfactant function in respiratory distress syndrome. *J Pediatr.* 1983;102(3):443–447.

2. deLemos RA, Coalson JJ. The contribution of experimental models to our understanding of the pathogenesis and treatment of bronchopulmonary dysplasia. *Clin Perinatol.* 1992;19(3):521–539.

3. Di Fiore JM, Martin RJ, Gauda EB. Apnea of prematurity–perfect storm. *Respir Physiol Neurobiol.* 2013;189(2):213–222.

4. Alex CG, Aronson RM, Onal E, Lopata M. Effects of continuous positive airway pressure on upper airway and respiratory muscle activity. *J Appl Physiol (1985).* 1987;62(5):2026–2030.

5. Saunders RA, Milner AD, Hopkin IE. The effects of continuous positive airway pressure on lung mechanics and lung volumes in the neonate. *Biol Neonate.* 1976;29(3–4):178–186.

6. Thomson MA, Yoder BA, Winter VT, et al. Treatment of immature baboons for 28 days with early nasal continuous positive airway pressure. *Am J Respir Crit Care Med.* 2004;169(9):1054–1062.

7. Thomson MA, Yoder BA, Winter VT, Giavedoni L, Chang LY, Coalson JJ. Delayed extubation to nasal continuous positive airway pressure in the immature baboon model of bronchopulmonary dysplasia: lung clinical and pathological findings. *Pediatrics.* 2006;118(5):2038–2050.

8. Reyburn B, Li M, Metcalfe DB, et al. Nasal ventilation alters mesenchymal cell turnover and improves alveolarization in preterm lambs. *Am J Respir Crit Care Med.* 2008;178(4):407–418.

9. Null DM, Alvord J, Leavitt W, et al. High-frequency nasal ventilation for 21 d maintains gas exchange with lower respiratory pressures and promotes alveolarization in preterm lambs. *Pediatr Res.* 2014;75(4):507–516.

10. Subramaniam P, Ho JJ, Davis PG. Prophylactic nasal continuous positive airway pressure for preventing morbidity and mortality in very preterm infants. *Cochrane Database Syst Rev.* 2016;(6):CD001243.

11. Gregory GA, Kitterman JA, Phibbs RH, Tooley W, Hamilton WK. Treatment of the idiopathic respiratory-distress syndrome with continuous positive airway pressure. *New England Journal of Medicine.* 1971;284:1333–1340.

12. Barrie H. Simple method of applying continuous positive airway pressure in respiratory-distress syndrome. *Lancet.* 1972;1(7754):776–777.

13. Ackerman BD, Stein MP, Sommer JS, Schumacher M. Continuous positive airway pressure applied by means of a tight-fitting face-mask. *J Pediatr.* 1974;85:408–411.

14. Ahlström H, Jonson B, Svenningsen NW. Continuous positive airways pressure treatment by a face chamber in idiopathic respiratory distress syndrome. *Arch Dis Child.* 1976;51:13–21.

15. Rhodes PG, Hall RT. Continuous positive airway pressure delivered by face mask in infants with the idiopathic respiratory distress syndrome: a controlled study. *Pediatrics.* 1973;52(1):1–5.

16. Novogroder M, MacKuanying N, Eidelman AI, Gartner LM. Nasopharyngeal ventilation in respiratory distress syndrome. A simple and efficient method of delivering continuous positive airway pressure. *J Pediatr.* 1973;82(6):1059–1062.

17. Wung JT, Driscoll JM Jr, Epstein RA, Hyman AI. A new device for CPAP by nasal route. *Crit Care Med.* 1975;3(2):76–78.

18. Caliumi-Pellegrini G, Agostino R, Orzalesi M, et al. Twin nasal cannula for administration of continuous positive airway pressure to newborn infants. *Arch Dis Child.* 1974;49(3):228–230.

19. Field D, Vyas H, Milner AD, Hopkin IE. Continuous positive airway pressure via a single nasal catheter in preterm infants. *Early Hum Dev.* 1985;11(3-4):275–280.

20. Moa G, Nilsson K, Zetterstrom H, Jonsson LO. A new device for administration of nasal continuous positive airway pressure in the newborn: an experimental study. *Crit Care Med.* 1988;16(12):1238–1242.

21. Courtney SE, Aghai ZH, Saslow JG, Pyon KH, Habib RH. Changes in lung volume and work of breathing: a comparison of two variable-flow nasal continuous positive airway pressure devices in very low birth weight infants. *Pediatr Pulmonol.* 2003;36(3):248–252.

22. Chernick V. Continuous distending pressure in hyaline membrane disease: of devices, disadvantages, and a daring study. *Pediatrics.* 1973;52(1):114–115.

23. Klausner JF, Lee AY, Hutchison AA. Decreased imposed work with a new nasal continuous positive airway pressure device. *PediatrPulmonol.* 1996;22(3):188–194.

24. Pandit PB, Courtney SE, Pyon KH, Saslow JG, Habib RH. Work of breathing during constant- and variable-flow nasal continuous positive airway pressure in preterm neonates. *Pediatrics.* 2001;108(3):682–685.

25. Courtney SEM. Lung recruitment and breathing pattern during variable versus continuous flow nasal continuous positive airway pressure in premature infants: an evaluation of three devices. *Pediatrics.* 2001;107(2):304–308.

26. Davis P, Davies M, Faber B. A randomised controlled trial of two methods of delivering nasal continuous positive airway pressure after extubation to infants weighing less than 1000 g: binasal (Hudson) versus single nasal prongs. *Arch Dis Child Fetal Neonatal Ed.* 2001;85(2):F82–F85.

27. Roukema H, O'Brine K, Nesbitt Z, Zaw W. A randomized controlled trial of Infant Flow continuous positive airway pressure (CPAP) versus nasopharyngeal CPAP in the extubation of babies ≤1250 g (Abstract). *Pediatr Res.* 1999;45:318A.

28. De Paoli A, Davis P, Faber B, Morley C. Devices and pressure sources for administration of nasal continuous positive airway pressure (NCPAP) in preterm neonates. *Cochrane Database Syst Rev.* 2008;(1):CD002977.

29. Stefanescu BM, Murphy WP, Hansell BJ, Fuloria M, Morgan TM, Aschner JL. A randomized, controlled trial comparing two different continuous positive airway pressure systems for the successful extubation of extremely low birth weight infants. *Pediatrics.* 2003;112(5):1031–1038.

30. Sun SC, Tien HC. Randomized controlled trial of two methods of nasal CPAP (NCPAP): flow driver vs conventional NCPAP. *Ped Res.* 1999;45:322A.

31. Mazzella M, Bellini C, Calevo MG, et al. A randomised control study comparing the infant flow driver with nasal continuous positive airway pressure in preterm infants. *Arch Dis Child Fetal Neonatal Ed.* 2001;85(2):F86–F90.
32. Gupta S, Sinha SK, Tin W, Donn SM. A randomized controlled trial of post-extubation bubble continuous positive airway pressure versus infant flow driver continuous positive airway pressure in preterm infants with respiratory distress syndrome. *J Pediatr.* 2009;154(5):645–650.
33. Poli JA, Richardson CP, DiBlasi RM. Volume oscillations delivered to a lung model using 4 different bubble CPAP systems. *Respir Care.* 2015;60(3):371–381.
34. Paz P, Ramanathan R, Hernandez R, Biniwale M. Neonatal resuscitation using a nasal cannula: a single-center experience. *Am J Perinatol.* 2014;31(12):1031–1036.
35. Nzegwu NI, Mack T, DellaVentura R, et al. Systematic use of the RAM nasal cannula in the yale-new haven children's hospital neonatal intensive care unit: a quality improvement project. *J Matern Fetal Neonatal Med.* 2015;28(6):718–721.
36. Iyer NP, Chatburn R. Evaluation of a nasal cannula in noninvasive ventilation using a lung simulator. *Respir Care.* 2015;60(4):508–512.
37. Mukerji A, Belik J. Neonatal nasal intermittent positive pressure ventilation efficacy and lung pressure transmission. *J Perinatol.* 2015;35(9):716–719.
38. Gerdes JS, Sivieri EM, Abbasi S. Factors influencing delivered mean airway pressure during nasal CPAP with the RAM cannula. *Pediatr Pulmonol.* 2016;51(1):60–69.
39. De Klerk AM, De Klerk RK. Nasal continuous positive airway pressure and outcomes of preterm infants. *J Paediatr Child Health.* 2001;37(2):161–167.
40. Davis PG, Henderson-Smart DJ. Nasal continuous positive airways pressure immediately after extubation for preventing morbidity in preterm infants. *Cochrane Database Syst Rev.* 2003;(2):CD000143.
41. Elgellab A, Riou Y, Abbazine A, et al. Effects of nasal continuous positive airway pressure (NCPAP) on breathing pattern in spontaneously breathing premature newborn infants. *Intensive Care Med.* 2001;27(11):1782–1787.
42. Buzzella B, Claure N, D'Ugard C, Bancalari E. A randomized controlled trial of two nasal continuous positive airway pressure levels after extubation in preterm infants. *J Pediatr.* 2014;164(1):46–51.
43. Fajardo MF, Claure N, Swaminathan S, et al. Effect of positive end-expiratory pressure on ductal shunting and systemic blood flow in preterm infants with patent ductus arteriosus. *Neonatology.* 2014;105(1):9–13.
44. Soll RF. Prophylactic synthetic surfactant for preventing morbidity and mortality in preterm infants. *Cochrane Database Syst Rev.* 2000;(2):CD001079.
45. Soll RF. Prophylactic natural surfactant extract for preventing morbidity and mortality in preterm infants. *Cochrane Database Syst Rev.* 2000;(2):CD000511.
46. Yost CC, Soll RF. Early versus delayed selective surfactant treatment for neonatal respiratory distress syndrome. *Cochrane Database Syst Rev.* 2000;(2):CD001456.
47. Kattwinkel J, Robinson M, Bloom BT, Delmore P, Ferguson JE. Technique for intrapartum administration of surfactant without requirement for an endotracheal tube. *J Perinatol.* 2004;24(6):360–365.
48. Lindner W, Vossbeck S, Hummler H, Pohlandt F. Delivery room management of extremely low birth weight infants: spontaneous breathing or intubation? *Pediatrics.* 1999;103:961–967.
49. Aly H, Massaro AN, Patel K, El Mohandes AA. Is it safer to intubate premature infants in the delivery room? *Pediatrics.* 2005;115(6):1660–1665.
50. Morley CJ, Davis PG, Doyle LW, Brion LP, Hascoet JM, Carlin JB. Nasal CPAP or intubation at birth for very preterm infants. *N Engl J Med.* 2008;358(7):700–708.
51. Finer NN, Carlo WA, Walsh MC, et al. Early CPAP versus surfactant in extremely preterm infants. *N Engl J Med.* 2010;362(21):1970–1979.
52. Dunn MS, Kaempf J, de Klerk A, et al. Randomized trial comparing 3 approaches to the initial respiratory management of preterm neonates. *Pediatrics.* 2011;128(5):e1069–e1076.
53. Sandri F, Plavka R, Ancora G, et al. Prophylactic or early selective surfactant combined with nCPAP in very preterm infants. *Pediatrics.* 2010;125(6):e1402–e1409.
54. Stevens TP, Harrington EW, Blennow M, Soll RF. Early surfactant administration with brief ventilation vs. selective surfactant and continued mechanical ventilation for preterm infants with or at risk for respiratory distress syndrome. *Cochrane Database Syst Rev.* 2007;(4):CD003063.
55. Rojas MA, Lozano JM, Rojas MX, et al. Very early surfactant without mandatory ventilation in premature infants treated with early continuous positive airway pressure: a randomized, controlled trial. *Pediatrics.* 2009;123(1):137–142.
56. Sandri F, Plavka R, Ancora G, et al. Prophylactic or early selective surfactant combined with nCPAP in very preterm infants. *Pediatrics.* 2010;125(6):e1402–e1409.
57. Kribs A, Roll C, Gopel W, et al. Nonintubated surfactant application vs conventional therapy in extremely preterm infants: a randomized clinical trial. *JAMA Pediatr.* 2015;169(8):723–730.
58. Dargaville PA, Aiyappan A, Cornelius A, Williams C, De Paoli AG. Preliminary evaluation of a new technique of minimally invasive surfactant therapy. *Arch Dis Child Fetal Neonatal Ed.* 2010.
59. Dargaville PA, Kamlin CO, De Paoli AG, et al. The OPTIMIST-A trial: evaluation of minimally-invasive surfactant therapy in preterm infants 25–28 weeks gestation. *BMC Pediatr.* 2014;14:213.
60. Gopel W, Kribs A, Ziegler A, et al. Avoidance of mechanical ventilation by surfactant treatment of spontaneously breathing preterm infants (AMV): an open-label, randomised, controlled trial. *Lancet.* 2011;378(9803):1627–1634.
61. Mohammadizadeh M, Ardestani AG, Sadeghnia AR. Early administration of surfactant via a thin intratracheal catheter in preterm infants with respiratory distress syndrome: feasibility and outcome. *J Res Pharm Pract.* 2015;4(1):31–36.

11

62. Kanmaz HG, Erdeve O, Canpolat FE, Mutlu B, Dilmen U. Surfactant administration via thin catheter during spontaneous breathing: randomized controlled trial. *Pediatrics*. 2013;131(2):e502–e509.
63. Bao Y, Zhang G, Wu M, Ma L, Zhu J. A pilot study of less invasive surfactant administration in very preterm infants in a chinese tertiary center. *BMC Pediatr*. 2015;15:21.
64. Aldana-Aguirre JC, Pinto M, Featherstone RM, Kumar M. Less invasive surfactant administration versus intubation for surfactant delivery in preterm infants with respiratory distress syndrome: a systematic review and meta-analysis. *Arch Dis Child Fetal Neonatal Ed*. 2017;102(1):F17–F23.
65. Rigo V, Lefebvre C, Broux I. Surfactant instillation in spontaneously breathing preterm infants: a systematic review and meta-analysis. *Eur J Pediatr*. 2016;175(12):1933–1942.
66. Annibale DJ, Hulsey TC, Engstrom PC, Wallin LA, Ohning BL. Randomized, controlled trial of nasopharyngeal continuous positive airway pressure in the extubation of very low birth weight infants. *J Pediatr*. 1994;124:455–460.
67. Davis P, Jankov R, Doyle L, Henschke P. Randomised, controlled trial of nasal continuous positive airway pressure in the extubation of infants weighing 600 to 1250 g. *Arch Dis Child Fetal Neonatal Ed*. 1998;79(1):F54–F57.
68. Dimitriou G, Greenough A, Kavvadia V, et al. Elective use of nasal continuous positive airways pressure following extubation of preterm infants. *Eur J Pediatr*. 2000;159(6):434–439.
69. Tapia JL, Bancalari A, Gonzalez A, Mercado ME. Does continuous positive airway pressure (CPAP) during weaning from intermittent mandatory ventilation in very low birth weight infants have risks or benefits? A controlled trial. *Pediatr Pulmonol*. 1995;19(5):269–274.
70. Engelke SC, Roloff DW, Kuhns LR. Postextubation nasal continuous positive airway pressure. A prospective controlled study. *AmJ Dis Child*. 1982;136(4):359–361.
71. Higgins RD, Richter SE, Davis JM. Nasal continuous positive airway pressure facilitates extubation of very low birth weight neonates. *Pediatrics*. 1991;88(5):999–1003.
72. So BH, Tamura M, Mishina J, Watanabe T, Kamoshita S. Application of nasal continuous positive airway pressure to early extubation in very low birthweight infants. *Arch Dis Child Fetal Neonatal Ed*. 1995;72(3):F191–F193.
73. Chan V, Greenough A. Randomised trial of methods of extubation in acute and chronic respiratory distress [see comments]. *Arc Dis Child*. 1993;68:570–572.
74. Peake M, Dillon P, Shaw NJ. Randomized trial of continuous positive airways pressure to prevent reventilation in preterm infants. *Pediatr Pulmonol*. 2005;39(3):247–250.
75. Robertson NJ, Hamilton PA. Randomised trial of elective continuous positive airway pressure (CPAP) compared with rescue CPAP after extubation. *Arch Dis Child Fetal Neonatal Ed*. 1998;79(1):F58–F60.
76. Polin RA, Sahni R. Newer experience with CPAP. *Semin Neonatol*. 2002;7(5):379–389.
77. Goldbart AD, Gozal D. Non-invasive ventilation in preterm infants. *Pediatr Pulmonol Suppl*. 2004;26:158–161.
78. Ammari A, Suri M, Milisavljevic V, et al. Variables associated with the early failure of nasal CPAP in very low birth weight infants. *J Pediatr*. 2005;147(3):341–347.
79. Dargaville PA, Aiyappan A, De Paoli AG, et al. Continuous positive airway pressure failure in preterm infants: incidence, predictors and consequences. *Neonatology*. 2013;104(1):8–14.
80. Pape KE, Armstrong DL, Fitzhardinge PM. Central nervous system patholgoy associated with mask ventilation in the very low birthweight infant: a new etiology for intracerebellar hemorrhages. *Pediatrics*. 1976;58(4):473–483.
81. Vert P, Andre M, Sibout M. Continuous positive airway pressure and hydrocephalus. *Lancet*. 1973;2(7824):319.
82. Buettiker V, Hug MI, Baenziger O, Meyer C, Frey B. Advantages and disadvantages of different nasal CPAP systems in newborns. *Intensive Care Med*. 2004;30(5):926–930.
83. Robertson NJ, McCarthy LS, Hamilton PA, Moss AL. Nasal deformities resulting from flow driver continuous positive airway pressure. *Arch Dis Child Fetal Neonatal Ed*. 1996;75(3):F209–F212.
84. Buckmaster AG, Arnolda G, Wright IM, Foster JP, Henderson-Smart DJ. Continuous positive airway pressure therapy for infants with respiratory distress in non tertiary care centers: a randomized, controlled trial. *Pediatrics*. 2007;120(3):509–518.
85. Bowe L, Smith J, Clarker P, Glover K, Pasquill A, Robinson M. Nasal CPAP weaning of VLBW Infants: is decreasing CPAP pressure or increasing time off the better strategy—results of a randomised controlled trial. *Pediatric Academic Society Meeting, San Francisco (Abstract)*. 2006.
86. Todd DA, Wright A, Broom M, et al. Methods of weaning preterm babies <30 weeks gestation off CPAP: a multicentre randomised controlled trial. *Arch Dis Child Fetal Neonatal Ed*. 2012;97(4):F236–F240.
87. Heath Jeffery RC, Broom M, Shadbolt B, Todd DA. CeasIng Cpap At standarD criteriA (CICADA): implementation improves neonatal outcomes. *J Paediatr Child Health*. 2016;52(3):321–326.
88. Tang J, Reid S, Lutz T, Malcolm G, Oliver S, Osborn DA. Randomised controlled trial of weaning strategies for preterm infants on nasal continuous positive airway pressure. *BMC Pediatr*. 2015;15:147.
89. Soonsawad S, Tongsawang N, Nuntnarumit P. Heated humidified high-flow nasal cannula for weaning from continuous positive airway pressure in preterm infants: a randomized controlled trial. *Neonatology*. 2016;110(3):204–209.
90. Abdel-Hady H, Shouman B, Aly H. Early weaning from CPAP to high flow nasal cannula in preterm infants is associated with prolonged oxygen requirement: a randomized controlled trial. *Early Hum Dev*. 2011;87(3):205–208.

91. Badiee Z, Eshghi A, Mohammadizadeh M. High flow nasal cannula as a method for rapid weaning from nasal continuous positive airway pressure. *Int J Prev Med.* 2015;6:33.

92. Garland JS, Nelson DB, Rice T, Neu J. Increased risk of gastrointestinal perforations in neonates mechanically ventilated with either face mask or nasal prongs. *Pediatrics.* 1985;76(3):406–410.

93. Lemyre B, Davis PG, De Paoli AG, Kirpalani H. Nasal intermittent positive pressure ventilation (NIPPV) versus nasal continuous positive airway pressure (NCPAP) for preterm neonates after extubation. *Cochrane Database Syst Rev.* 2017;2:CD003212.

94. Lee J, Kim HS, Jung YH, et al. Non-invasive neurally adjusted ventilatory assist in preterm infants: a randomised phase II crossover trial. *Arch Dis Child Fetal Neonatal Ed.* 2015;100(6):F507–F513.

95. Roy B, Samson N, Moreau-Bussiere F, et al. Mechanisms of active laryngeal closure during non-invasive intermittent positive pressure ventilation in nonsedated lambs. *J Appl Physiol (1985).* 2008;105(5):1406–1412.

96. Hadj-Ahmed MA, Samson N, Bussieres M, Beck J, Praud JP. Absence of inspiratory laryngeal constrictor muscle activity during nasal neurally adjusted ventilatory assist in newborn lambs. *J Appl Physiol (1985).* 2012;113(1):63–70.

97. Hadj-Ahmed MA, Samson N, Nadeau C, Boudaa N, Praud JP. Laryngeal muscle activity during nasal high-frequency oscillatory ventilation in nonsedated newborn lambs. *Neonatology.* 2015;107(3):199–205.

98. Ryan CA, Finer NN, Peters KL. Nasal intermittent positive-pressure ventilation offers no advantages over nasal continuous positive airway pressure in apnea of prematurity. *Am J Dis Child.* 1989;143(10):1196–1198.

99. Lin CH, Wang ST, Lin YJ, Yeh TF. Efficacy of nasal intermittent positive pressure ventilation in treating apnea of prematurity. *Pediatr Pulmonol.* 1998;26(5):349–353.

100. Lemyre B, Davis PG, De Paoli AG. Nasal intermittent positive pressure ventilation (NIPPV) versus nasal continuous positive airway pressure (NCPAP) for apnea of prematurity. *Cochrane Database Syst Rev.* 2002;(1):CD002272.

101. Meneses J, Bhandari V, Alves JG, Herrmann D. Noninvasive ventilation for respiratory distress syndrome: a randomized controlled trial. *Pediatrics.* 2011;127(2):300–307.

102. Manzar S, Nair AK, Pai MG, et al. Use of nasal intermittent positive pressure ventilation to avoid intubation in neonates. *Saudi Med J.* 2004;25(10):1464–1467.

103. Santin R, Brodsky N, Bhandari V. A prospective observational pilot study of synchronized nasal intermittent positive pressure ventilation (SNIPPV) as a primary mode of ventilation in infants > or = 28 weeks with respiratory distress syndrome (RDS). *J Perinatol.* 2004;24(8):487–493.

104. Owen L. Effects of non-synchronised nasal intermittent positive pressure ventilation on spontaneous breathing in preterm infants. *Arch Dis Child.* 2011, in press.

105. Owen LS, Morley CJ, Davis PG. Pressure variation during ventilator generated nasal intermittent positive pressure ventilation in preterm infants. *Arch Dis Child Fetal Neonatal Ed.* 2010;95(5):F359–F364.

106. Chang HY, Claure N, D'Ugard C, Torres J, Nwajei P, Bancalari E. Effects of synchronization during nasal ventilation in clinically stable preterm infants. *Pediatr Res.* 2011;69(1):84–89.

107. van der Hoeven M, Brouwer E, Blanco CE. Nasal high frequency ventilation in neonates with moderate respiratory insufficiency. *Arch Dis Child Fetal Neonatal Ed.* 1998;79(1):F61–F63.

108. Colaizy TT, Younis UM, Bell EF, Klein JM. Nasal high-frequency ventilation for premature infants. *Acta Paediatr.* 2008;97(11):1518–1522.

109. Czernik C, Schmalisch G, Buhrer C, Proquitte H. Weaning of neonates from mechanical ventilation by use of nasopharyngeal high-frequency oscillatory ventilation: a preliminary study. *J Matern Fetal Neonatal Med.* 2012;25(4):374–378.

110. Mukerji A, Singh B, Helou SE, et al. Use of noninvasive high-frequency ventilation in the neonatal intensive care unit: a retrospective review. *Am J Perinatol.* 2015;30(2):171–176.

111. Mukerji A, Sarmiento K, Lee B, Hassall K, Shah V. Non-invasive high-frequency ventilation versus bi-phasic continuous positive airway pressure (BP-CPAP) following CPAP failure in infants <1250 g: a pilot randomized controlled trial. *J Perinatol.* 2017;37(1):49–53.

112. Dumas De La Roque E, Bertrand C, Tandonnet O, et al. Nasal high frequency percussive ventilation versus nasal continuous positive airway pressure in transient tachypnea of the newborn: a pilot randomized controlled trial (NCT00556738). *Pediatr Pulmonol.* 2011;46(3):218–223.

113. Fischer HS, Bohlin K, Buhrer C, et al. Nasal high-frequency oscillation ventilation in neonates: a survey in five European countries. *Eur J Pediatr.* 2015;174(4):465–471.

114. Mukerji A, Shah PS, Shivananda S, et al. Survey of noninvasive respiratory support practices in Canadian neonatal intensive care units. *Acta Paediatr.* 2017;106(3):387–393.

115. Albertine KH, Jones GP, Starcher BC, et al. Chronic lung injury in preterm lambs. Disordered respiratory tract development. *Am J Respir Crit Care Med.* 1999;159(3):945–958.

116. Rehan VK, Fong J, Lee R, et al. Mechanism of reduced lung injury by high-frequency nasal ventilation in a preterm lamb model of neonatal chronic lung disease. *Pediatr Res.* 2011;70(5):462–466.

117. Joss-Moore LA, Hagen-Lillevik SJ, Yost C, et al. Alveolar formation is dysregulated by restricted nutrition but not excess sedation in preterm lambs managed by noninvasive support. *Pediatr Res.* 2016;80(5):719–728.

118. Sondergaard S, Karason S, Hanson A, et al. Direct measurement of intratracheal pressure in pediatric respiratory monitoring. *Pediatr Res.* 2002;51(3):339–345.

119. De Luca D, Piastra M, Pietrini D, Conti G. Effect of amplitude and inspiratory time in a bench model of non-invasive HFOV through nasal prongs. *Pediatr Pulmonol.* 2012;47(10):1012–1018.

120. De Luca D, Carnielli VP, Conti G, Piastra M. Noninvasive high frequency oscillatory ventilation through nasal prongs: bench evaluation of efficacy and mechanics. *Intensive Care Med.* 2010;36(12):2094–2100.

121. Yoder BA, Albertine KH, Null DM Jr. High-frequency ventilation for non-invasive respiratory support of neonates. *Semin Fetal Neonatal Med.* 2016;21(3):162–173.

122. Klotz D, Schaefer C, Stavropoulou D, Fuchs H, Schumann S. Leakage in nasal high-frequency oscillatory ventilation improves carbon dioxide clearance-A bench study. *Pediatr Pulmonol.* 2017;52(3):367–372.

123. Moreau-Bussiere F, Samson N, St-Hilaire M, et al. Laryngeal response to nasal ventilation in non-sedated newborn lambs. *J Appl Physiol (1985).* 2007;102(6):2149–2157.

124. Wilkinson D, Andersen C, O'Donnell CP, De Paoli AG. High flow nasal cannula for respiratory support in preterm infants. *Cochrane Database Syst Rev.* 2011;(5):CD006405.

125. Osman M, Elsharkawy A, Abdel-Hady H. Assessment of pain during application of nasal-continuous positive airway pressure and heated, humidified high-flow nasal cannulae in preterm infants. *J Perinatol.* 2015;35(4):263–267.

126. Klingenberg C, Pettersen M, Hansen EA, et al. Patient comfort during treatment with heated humidified high flow nasal cannulae versus nasal continuous positive airway pressure: a randomised cross-over trial. *Arch Dis Child Fetal Neonatal Ed.* 2014;99(2):F134–137.

127. Roberts CT, Manley BJ, Dawson JA, Davis PG. Nursing perceptions of high-flow nasal cannulae treatment for very preterm infants. *J Paediatr Child Health.* 2014;50(10):806–810.

128. Hough JL, Shearman AD, Jardine LA, Davies MW. Humidified high flow nasal cannulae: current practice in Australasian nurseries, a survey. *J Paediatr Child Health.* 2012;48(2):106–113.

129. Ojha S, Gridley E, Dorling J. Use of heated humidified high-flow nasal cannula oxygen in neonates: a UK wide survey. *Acta Paediatr.* 2013;102(3):249–253.

130. Shetty S, Sundaresan A, Hunt K, Desai P, Greenough A. Changes in the use of humidified high flow nasal cannula oxygen. *Arch Dis Child Fetal Neonatal Ed.* 2016;101(4):F371–F372.

131. Motojima Y, Ito M, Oka S, Uchiyama A, Tamura M, Namba F. Use of high-flow nasal cannula in neonates: nationwide survey in Japan. *Pediatr Int.* 2016;58(4):308–310.

132. Chow SSW, Le Marsney R, Haslam R, Lui K. *Report of the Australian and New Zealand Neonatal Network 2014.* Sydney, 2016.

133. Miller SM, Dowd SA. High-flow nasal cannula and extubation success in the premature infant: a comparison of two modalities. *J Perinatol.* 2010;30(12):805–808.

134. Waugh JB, Granger WM. An evaluation of 2 new devices for nasal high-flow gas therapy. *Respir Care.* 2004;49(8):902–906.

135. Chang GY, Cox CA, Shaffer TH. Nasal cannula, CPAP, and high-flow nasal cannula: effect of flow on temperature, humidity, pressure, and resistance. *Biomed Instrum Technol.* 2011;45(1):69–74.

136. Roberts CT, Kortekaas R, Dawson JA, Manley BJ, Owen LS, Davis PG. The effects of non-invasive respiratory support on oropharyngeal temperature and humidity: a neonatal manikin study. *Arch Dis Child Fetal Neonatal Ed.* 2016;101(3):F248–F252.

137. Spence KL, Murphy D, Kilian C, McGonigle R, Kilani RA. High-flow nasal cannula as a device to provide continuous positive airway pressure in infants. *J Perinatol.* 2007;27(12):772–775.

138. Kubicka ZJ, Limauro J, Darnall RA. Heated, humidified high-flow nasal cannula therapy: yet another way to deliver continuous positive airway pressure? *Pediatrics.* 2008;121(1):82–88.

139. Wilkinson DJ, Andersen CC, Smith K, Holberton J. Pharyngeal pressure with high-flow nasal cannulae in premature infants. *J Perinatol.* 2008;28(1):42–47.

140. Volsko TA, Fedor K, Amadei J, Chatburn RL. High flow through a nasal cannula and CPAP effect in a simulated infant model. *Respir Care.* 2011;56(12):1893–1900.

141. Lampland AL, Plumm B, Meyers PA, Worwa CT, Mammel MC. Observational study of humidified high-flow nasal cannula compared with nasal continuous positive airway pressure. *J Pediatr.* 2009;154(2):177–182.

142. Collins CL, Barfield C, Horne RS, Davis PG. A comparison of nasal trauma in preterm infants extubated to either heated humidified high-flow nasal cannulae or nasal continuous positive airway pressure. *Eur J Pediatr.* 2014;173(2):181–186.

143. Hasan RA, Habib RH. Effects of flow rate and airleak at the nares and mouth opening on positive distending pressure delivery using commercially available high-flow nasal cannula systems: a lung model study. *Pediatr Crit Care Med.* 2011;12(1):e29–e33.

144. Frizzola M, Miller TL, Rodriguez ME, et al. High-flow nasal cannula: impact on oxygenation and ventilation in an acute lung injury model. *Pediatr Pulmonol.* 2011;46(1):67–74.

145. Iyer NP, Mhanna MJ. Association between high-flow nasal cannula and end-expiratory esophageal pressures in premature infants. *Respir Care.* 2016;61(3):285–290.

146. Sivieri EM, Gerdes JS, Abbasi S. Effect of HFNC flow rate, cannula size, and nares diameter on generated airway pressures: an in vitro study. *Pediatr Pulmonol.* 2013;48(5):506–514.

147. Dysart K, Miller TL, Wolfson MR, Shaffer TH. Research in high flow therapy: mechanisms of action. *Respir Med.* 2009;103(10):1400–1405.

148. Shaffer TH, Alapati D, Greenspan JS, Wolfson MR. Neonatal non-invasive respiratory support: physiological implications. *Pediatr Pulmonol.* 2012;47(9):837–847.

149. Spence CJT, Buchmann NA, Jermy MC. Unsteady flow in the nasal cavity with high flow therapy measured by stereoscopic PIV. *Exp Fluids.* 2011;52(3):569–579.

150. Van Hove SC, Storey J, Adams C, et al. An experimental and numerical investigation of CO_2 distribution in the upper airways during nasal high flow therapy. *Ann Biomed Eng.* 2016;44(10):3007–3019.

151. Sivieri EM, Foglia EE, Abbasi S. Carbon dioxide washout during high flow nasal cannula versus nasal CPAP support: an in vitro study. *Pediatr Pulmonol.* 2017.
152. Saslow JG, Aghai ZH, Nakhla TA, et al. Work of breathing using high-flow nasal cannula in preterm infants. *J Perinatol.* 2006;26(8):476–480.
153. de Jongh BE, Locke R, Mackley A, et al. Work of breathing indices in infants with respiratory insufficiency receiving high-flow nasal cannula and nasal continuous positive airway pressure. *J Perinatol.* 2014;34(1):27–32.
154. Shetty S, Hickey A, Rafferty GF, Peacock JL, Greenough A. Work of breathing during CPAP and heated humidified high-flow nasal cannula. *Arch Dis Child Fetal Neonatal Ed.* 2016;101(5): F404–F407.
155. Locke RG, Wolfson MR, Shaffer TH, Rubenstein SD, Greenspan JS. Inadvertent administration of positive end-distending pressure during nasal cannula flow. *Pediatrics.* 1993;91(1):135–138.
156. Boumecid H, Rakza T, Abazine A, Klosowski S, Matran R, Storme L. Influence of three nasal continuous positive airway pressure devices on breathing pattern in preterm infants. *Arch Dis Child Fetal Neonatal Ed.* 2007;92(4):F298–F300.
157. Lavizzari A, Veneroni C, Colnaghi M, et al. Respiratory mechanics during NCPAP and HHHFNC at equal distending pressures. *Arch Dis Child Fetal Neonatal Ed.* 2014;99(4):F315–F320.
158. Reynolds P, Leontiadi S, Lawson T, Otunla T, Ejiwumi O, Holland N. Stabilisation of premature infants in the delivery room with nasal high flow. *Arch Dis Child Fetal Neonatal Ed.* 2016;101(4):F284–F287.
159. Iranpour R, Sadeghnia A, Hesaraki M. High-flow nasal cannula versus nasal continuous positive airway pressure in the management of respiratory distress syndrome. *J Isfahan Med School.* 2011;29:761–771.
160. Yoder BA, Stoddard RA, Li M, King J, Dirnberger DR, Abbasi S. Heated, humidified high-flow nasal cannula versus nasal CPAP for respiratory support in neonates. *Pediatrics.* 2013;131(5):e1482–e1490.
161. Lavizzari A, Colnaghi M, Ciuffini F, et al. Heated, humidified high-flow nasal cannula vs nasal continuous positive airway pressure for respiratory distress syndrome of prematurity: a randomized clinical noninferiority trial. *JAMA Pediatr.* 2016.
162. Roberts CT, Owen LS, Manley BJ, et al. Nasal high-flow therapy for primary respiratory support in preterm infants. *N Engl J Med.* 2016;375(12):1142–1151.
163. Nair G, Karna P. Comparison of the effects of Vapotherm and nasal CPAP in respiratory distress. *Pediatric Academic Societies.* 2005;1 (Unpublished data).
164. Kugelman A, Riskin A, Said W, Shoris I, Mor F, Bader D. A randomized pilot study comparing heated humidified high-flow nasal cannulae with NIPPV for RDS. *Pediatr Pulmonol.* 2015;50(6):576–583.
165. Campbell DM, Shah PS, Shah V, Kelly EN. Nasal continuous positive airway pressure from high flow cannula versus Infant Flow for Preterm infants. *J Perinatol.* 2006;26(9):546–549.
166. Collins CL, Holberton JR, Barfield C, Davis PG. A randomized controlled trial to compare heated humidified high-flow nasal cannulae with nasal continuous positive airway pressure postextubation in premature infants. *J Pediatr.* 2013;162(5):949–954.e941.
167. Manley BJ, Owen LS, Doyle LW, et al. High-flow nasal cannulae in very preterm infants after extubation. *N Engl J Med.* 2013;369(15):1425–1433.
168. The Collaborative Group for the Multicenter Study on Heated Humidified High flow Nasal Cannula Ventilation. Efficacy and safety of heated humidified high-flow nasal cannula for prevention of extubation failure in neonates. *Chin J Pediatr.* 2014;52(4):271–276.
169. Mostafa-Gharehbaghi M, Mojabil H. Comparing the effectiveness of nasal continuous positive airway pressure (NCPAP) and high flow nasal cannula (HFNC) in prevention of post extubation assisted ventilation. *Zahedan J Res Med Sci.* 2015:29–32.
170. Wilkinson D, Andersen C, O'Donnell CP, De Paoli AG, Manley BJ. High flow nasal cannula for respiratory support in preterm infants. *Cochrane Database Syst Rev.* 2016;2:CD006405.
171. Kotecha SJ, Adappa R, Gupta N, Watkins WJ, Kotecha S, Chakraborty M. Safety and efficacy of high-flow nasal cannula therapy in preterm infants: a meta-analysis. *Pediatrics.* 2015;136(3):542–553.

11

CHAPTER 12

Newer Strategies for Surfactant Delivery

Peter A. Dargaville

- As fewer preterm infants are managed with an endotracheal tube in early life, the usual conduit for surfactant delivery is lacking. With this approach has come a dilemma regarding how and when to deliver surfactant to those showing features of surfactant-deficient respiratory distress syndrome (RDS).

- Brief intubation solely for surfactant delivery has been widely practiced but has disadvantages, not the least of which is difficulty with extubation.

- A number of less invasive approaches to delivering surfactant have been used in preterm infants with RDS, including aerosolization, pharyngeal instillation, laryngeal mask administration, and brief tracheal catheterization.

- Most experience has been gained with the approach of surfactant delivery using a thin catheter briefly inserted through the vocal cords; this method has found its way into clinical practice.

- Six randomized controlled trials of surfactant administration via a thin catheter have been reported to date, with heterogeneity with regard to the settings in which the studies were conducted and many aspects of trial design.

- Pooled data from these trials suggest that surfactant delivery via a thin catheter has advantages over delivery via an endotracheal tube, with improvement in survival free of bronchopulmonary dysplasia and reduction in the need for mechanical ventilation in the first 72 hours of life.

- The question of whether a preterm infant whose condition is stable with continuous positive airway pressure (CPAP) with early signs of RDS should receive surfactant via a thin catheter or simply continue CPAP has yet to be answered with certainty.

- Circumstantial evidence suggests that delivery of surfactant to a spontaneously breathing infant being treated with CPAP is better distributed within the lung than when an equivalent dose is given via an endotracheal tube with the aid of positive-pressure ventilation. Further laboratory and clinical studies are needed to confirm this.

- Application of surfactant therapy via a thin catheter needs to be considered as part of a less invasive approach to respiratory support in preterm infants, taking account of gestation, age, and apparent severity of RDS.

In surveying the well-chronicled history of respiratory management for the preterm infant with respiratory distress syndrome (RDS), there is the strong impression of having come full circle. The allure of continuous positive airway pressure (CPAP), announced with fanfare half a century ago as a means of overcoming the symptomatology of RDS in the pre-surfactant era,[1,2] appeared for the most part to lose favor in the 1970s. The landscape was then dominated by intubation and mechanical ventilation, only for CPAP to be gradually rediscovered[3,4] and finally reembraced as the results and meta-analyses of large clinical trials became known.[5–7] Similarly, not long after its advent into clinical practice, exogenous surfactant therapy became universal and was used early, repeatedly, and certainly to good effect, in dealing with the scourge of RDS and its complications.[8] Now, as more infants avoid intubation at the beginning of life—and thus lose the usual conduit for surfactant instillation—there is the appreciation that many infants with RDS can be successfully supported without a dose of surfactant, and the routine use of this is once indispensable drug is being questioned.[9]

In relation to the use of CPAP, the rhetoric still remains well ahead of the practice, particularly for the smallest infants who appear to have the most to gain from a lung-protective approach to respiratory support.[10–12] Well into the 21st century, the majority of infants born before 29 weeks' gestation are still intubated routinely at the beginning of life.[13–15] For many neonatologists, intubation continues to bring the certainty of the infant's lungs being ventilated even when apneic and the timely administration of a dose of surfactant, the enduring security blanket in treating RDS. The hesitation to apply CPAP more liberally from the outset is in part fueled by the appreciation that for some infants with CPAP as initial treatment, this modality fails to provide enough support, with subsequent resorting to intubation followed by a dose of surfactant given at a later than ideal time.[15–21] This pathway is known from both cohort[16–21] and population-based[15] studies to be associated with adverse outcomes, including a higher incidence of pneumothorax, bronchopulmonary dysplasia (BPD), and severe intraventricular hemorrhage (IVH). A dilemma thus exists in the management of preterm infants with RDS—should they be intubated early in life to be given a dose of surfactant or managed by CPAP to avoid the pitfalls of ventilation and the risk of ventilator-induced lung injury?[22,23]

Administration of Surfactant to Infants Treated by CPAP

A first attempt at overcoming the CPAP–surfactant dilemma was in the form of the technique of intubation, surfactant administration, and extubation (INSURE).[24] This method has been widely practiced, but its advantages over continuation of CPAP have more recently come into question. Whereas some clinical trials have found a reduced need for mechanical ventilation with INSURE,[25,26] others have not, mostly attributable to difficulty with extubation after the procedure.[7,27] This limitation, and the difficulty of the intubation itself,[28] has deterred many clinicians from using INSURE in clinical practice.

In view of the difficulties and limitations of the INSURE technique, several less invasive means of delivering surfactant to the preterm infant with RDS have been developed and pursued. These newer strategies for surfactant delivery are the subject of this chapter, which draws on the published evidence from nonrandomized and randomized studies, as well as reviews[22,23,29–36] and meta-analyses[37–45] to portray the current state of knowledge and bounds of accepted practice, and to highlight the numerous areas of uncertainty in this rapidly changing field.

Techniques of Surfactant Administration Without an Endotracheal Tube

The long-standing ingenuity of neonatologists has led to a multiplicity of methods for delivery of exogenous surfactant to the lung without using an endotracheal tube (ETT).[31,32] In some cases, these methods are far from new but have been rediscovered and reapplied as more infants avoid intubation in early life. Table 12.1 documents the full range of reported techniques, which are described in further detail in the following sections.

Table 12.1 TECHNIQUES FOR SURFACTANT DELIVERY WITHOUT INTUBATION

Technique	First Report(s)	Equipment Used
Aerosolization	Robillard et al.[46] (1964), Chu et al.[47] (1967)	Variety of aerosolization devices
Pharyngeal instillation	Ten Centre Study Group[48] (1987)	Instillation catheter
Laryngeal mask administration	Brimacombe et al.[49] (2004)	Laryngeal mask airway, size 1
Tracheal catheterization	Verder et al.[50] (1992)	Laryngoscope, variety of thin catheters, Magill forceps (some cases), other devices for directing catheter (some cases)

12

Aerosolization

Although aerosolization is currently used infrequently to deliver medications of any sort to the neonatal lung, it has the attraction of being potentially the least invasive approach to surfactant administration, involving no direct instrumentation of the airway.[32] It is little known that aerosolization was the first method of surfactant therapy in newborn infants with RDS, being first described in 1964.[46] The clinical effects in this and another pioneering clinical study[47] were modest, a testament to the difficulties in effective surfactant delivery and distribution using aerosolized surfactant, but also attributable in these early studies to the surfactant preparation used (pure dipalmitoylphosphatidylcholine with no spreading agents). Unfortunately, even with the advent of third-generation surfactant preparations with enhanced biophysical properties and the development of sophisticated nebulization devices capable of dispersion of surfactant into droplets less than 5 μm, surfactant aerosolization for infants with RDS remains in the province of research. Results of a series of observational studies[51–53] and one small clinical trial[54] have been recently reviewed.[32] Clinical benefits have been noted in some studies[51,53] but not in others.[52,54] A further clinical trial using a vibrating membrane nebulizer for surfactant aerosolization in infants between 29 and 33 weeks' gestation reported a clinical benefit in relation to need for subsequent intubation (odds ratio 0.56, 95% confidence interval 0.34–0.93).[55] However, the proportion of infants requiring intubation and surfactant therapy in the control group was considerably higher than that usually reported at this gestation.

Pharyngeal Instillation of Surfactant

Although it was established several decades ago as a method of initial surfactant delivery,[48] pharyngeal surfactant instillation shortly after birth has been largely forgotten. Kattwinkel and coworkers rediscovered the technique and applied it in preterm infants of 27 to 30 weeks' gestational age.[56] Most infants studied showed an improvement in oxygenation, indicative of surfactant delivery to the lung. Four required redosing after endotracheal intubation, and there were some reservations expressed by the authors about the applicability of the technique during cesarean delivery (especially using general anesthesia) and with breech presentation. Some enthusiasm for the method continues to the present day, with a recent report of pharyngeal surfactant administration in extremely preterm infants (<25 weeks' gestation), suggesting better transition and lesser need for intubation compared with nonrandomized controls.[57] A further randomized controlled trial (RCT) examining the efficacy of delivery room pharyngeal surfactant administration is underway in infants 28 weeks' gestation or less (the POPART [Prophylactic Oropharyngeal Surfactant For Preterm Infants: A Randomised Trial, EudraCT 2016-004198-41). For such infants, administration of surfactant with the first inflations of the lung may have a marked physiologic effect in lung fluid clearance and aeration, beyond any effect on replenishment of the surfactant pool.[58] For infants beyond 28 weeks' gestation, any form of surfactant delivery used unselectively in the delivery room is unlikely to offer an advantage over early rescue therapy in those exhibiting features of RDS not manageable by CPAP alone.[59]

Delivery of Surfactant by Laryngeal Mask Airway

The laryngeal mask airway (LMA) is designed to enclose the larynx in a cuffed seal and is increasingly promoted as a tool for facilitating neonatal resuscitation.[60,61] After initial reports of its use as a conduit for the administration of exogenous surfactant,[49,62] further studies, including a number of clinical trials, have been conducted in preterm infants.[63–67] In a group of 8 infants of 28 to 35 weeks' gestational age, Trevisanuto et al. reported the placement of an LMA without sedation, through which surfactant was administered by rapid bolus, followed by positive-pressure inflations.[63] Improvement in oxygenation was noted in all cases; two infants were subsequently intubated, including one with a pneumothorax. More recently, interest in surfactant delivery by LMA has burgeoned, with two RCTs comparing LMA administration with surfactant therapy after intubation,[65,67] and two others in which the comparator group was continuation of CPAP.[64,66] All studies concentrate on infants at 28 weeks' gestation and older, this being the lower limit of gestation at which the smallest LMA (size 1) can be reliably positioned. Surfactant delivery via LMA has been noted to be relatively easy to perform, with placement achievable in almost all cases. Two of the studies used postprocedure gastric aspiration as a way of confirming surfactant delivery to the lung, although the validity of this method has been questioned.[68] The rate of surfactant redosing has also been rather high after LMA administration (~38% in two studies combined[65,67]). A figure of ~20% might be expected in infants of 28 weeks' gestation or older, both with ETT administration or by a thin catheter.[69] Ultimately, the applicability of LMA surfactant delivery will depend on (1) the results of head-to-head comparisons with other forms of less invasive surfactant administration and (2) the willingness of clinicians to gain familiarity with LMA placement, a procedure that is otherwise uncommon in most neonatal intensive care nurseries (NICUs).

Delivery of Surfactant Via a Thin Catheter

The alternative of using a thin catheter to deliver surfactant to the trachea rather than an ETT was first reported by Verder et al., with an unstated number of preterm infants treated by this method among 34 preterm infants supported with CPAP and given surfactant therapy in a pilot study.[50] The method was rediscovered and championed by Kribs and colleagues in Cologne,[70] and enthusiasm for tracheal catheterization as a means of surfactant delivery has intensified since. Given the wide experience and clinical applicability of this technique, the remainder of this chapter focuses on this approach to surfactant delivery.

Surfactant Administration Via Brief Tracheal Catheterization

Methods of Surfactant Delivery Via a Thin Catheter

Table 12.2 shows reported techniques for surfactant delivery via thin catheter. Some techniques involve the use of instrumentation to aid passage of the catheter tip through the vocal cords (e.g. Magill forceps), yet others use no internal guide and rely on the skill of the clinician to direct the catheter into the trachea. A semirigid rather than flexible catheter has generally been used for this latter approach, with the exception of the RCT by Kanmaz et al.,[71] in which the trachea was catheterized

Table 12.2   PUBLISHED METHODS OF TRACHEAL CATHETERIZATION

Method, Reference	Catheter Type	Guidance Through Vocal Cords
Cologne method (LISA)[70]	Flexible nasogastric tube	Magill forceps
Take Care method[71]	Flexible nasogastric tube	No forceps
Hobart method[74]	Semirigid vascular catheter	No forceps
SONSURE[75]	Flexible nasogastric tube	Magill forceps
QuickSF[76]	Soft catheter	Intrapharyngeal guide

LISA, Less-invasive surfactant administration; *SONSURE*, Sonda Nasogástrica Surfactante Extubación.

with a flexible catheter without Magill forceps. Beyond these original reports, a wide range of different catheters has now been used for surfactant delivery, including umbilical, suction, and urethral catheters, inserted by both oral and nasal routes.[72,73]

Depth of Catheter Insertion

As with surfactant instillation via an ETT, the position of the catheter tip in the trachea is critically important; surfactant reflux into the pharynx or surfactant delivery preferentially into the right lung are the potential consequences of an overly shallow or deep tip position, respectively. Reported catheter insertion depth has been 1 to 2 cm beyond the vocal cords, depending on gestation. Based on information from a postmortem study of tracheal dimensions,[77] a recommended catheter tip position of 1.5 cm beyond the vocal cords at less than 27 weeks' gestation and 2 cm for more mature infants has been made.[78] Note that for many catheters (vascular catheter, feeding tube) a mark must be drawn near the tip to indicate the required depth; a wax pencil is most suitable for this purpose.[79]

Observational and Cohort Studies of Surfactant Delivery

Beyond the first descriptions of tracheal catheterization techniques, numerous single-center and multicenter experiences with this approach to surfactant delivery have now been reported. The experience of surfactant delivery via a thin catheter runs to several thousand infants, and information from these studies is used in later text sections. Readers are referred to recent reviews for discussion of individual studies.[35,36,44]

Clinical Trials of Surfactant Administration Via Tracheal Catheterization

The key features of the six clinical trials in which the efficacy of surfactant delivery via tracheal catheterization has been evaluated in preterm infants with RDS are shown in Tables 12.3 and 12.4, with commentary on each trial and an overall summation in the next sections.

Avoid Mechanical Ventilation Trial

The Avoid Mechanical Ventilation trial[80] was the first reported RCT of surfactant administration via tracheal catheterization and conducted in 12 tertiary-level NICUs in Germany. Enrolled infants ($n = 220$) were 26 to 28 weeks' gestational age with features of RDS managed by CPAP. A fraction of inspired oxygen (Fio_2) threshold of more than 0.30 in the first 12 hours of life was set for inclusion. Infants were randomly assigned to receive surfactant via a thin catheter or continue with CPAP. All infants were thereafter managed with CPAP unless intubation criteria were reached, including an Fio_2 threshold that varied from 0.30 to 0.60 between participating centers. The primary outcome for the study was the need for intubation on day 2 or 3 of life, and infants in the intervention group had a lower rate of this outcome. There was no difference in the rate of pneumothorax or other adverse events. The intervention group had a lower requirement for oxygen at 28 days, but not at 36 weeks' gestation.

Interpretation of the results of the Avoid Mechanical Ventilation trial is hampered by several limitations of design[29]: (1) only 65 of the 108 infants randomly assigned to the intervention actually received surfactant via a thin catheter, (2) both groups included infants intubated at the outset, and (3) postintervention management differed considerably among centers. Nevertheless, the finding of a reduction in the need for mechanical ventilation after surfactant administration via a thin catheter in this first clinical trial was important; it led the authors to speculate that this approach may be included in a bundle of gentler respiratory care for preterm infants in the years to come.[80]

Take Care Study

The Take Care study,[71] conducted in a single tertiary NICU in Turkey, included preterm infants ($n = 200$) younger than 32 weeks' gestation and was the first reported RCT comparing surfactant delivery via thin catheter with the INSURE approach.

Table 12.3 DESIGN FEATURES OF RANDOMIZED CONTROLLED TRIALS OF SURFACTANT DELIVERY VIA A THIN CATHETER

Trial Name, Author, (Year)	Gestation Range (Weeks)	Time of Entry	Entry Criteria	Intervention	Blinding	Surfactant Dose, Type	Control Group	Primary Outcome
AMV Göpel et al.[80] (2011)	26–28	<12 h	$FiO_2 \geq 0.30$	Cologne method	No	100 mg/kg, Curosurf/Survanta/Alveofact	Continue with CPAP	Intubation on day 2 or 3
Take Care Kanmaz et al.[71] (2013)	<32	<2 h	$FiO_2 \geq 0.40$	Take Care method	No	100 mg/kg, Curosurf	INSURE without sedation	Intubation <72 h
Mirnia et al.[81] (2013)	27–32	NS	$FiO_2 \geq 0.30$	Cologne method	No	200 mg/kg, Curosurf	INSURE without sedation	NS
Bao et al.[82] (2015)	28–32	<2 h	$FiO_2 \geq 0.30$ (28–29 weeks), ≥ 0.35 (30–32 weeks) with RDS	Hobart method	No	200 mg/kg, Curosurf	INSURE without sedation	Intubation <72 h
Mohammadizadeh et al.[83] (2015)	<35	<2 h	$FiO_2 \geq 0.30$ and/or Silverman score ≥ 5	Cologne method	No	200 mg/kg, Curosurf	INSURE without sedation	Intubation <72 h
NINSAPP Kribs et al.[79] (2015)	23–26	10–120 min	$FiO_2 \geq 0.30$ and/or Silverman score ≥ 5	Cologne method	No	Median 200 mg/kg, Curosurf	Intubation, ventilation, surfactant therapy	Survival without BPD

CPAP, Continuous positive airway pressure; *FiO_2*, fraction of inspired oxygen; *NS*, not stated; *RDS*, respiratory distress syndrome.

Table 12.4 CLINICAL DETAILS AND OUTCOMES OF RANDOMIZED CONTROLLED TRIALS OF SURFACTANT DELIVERY VIA A THIN CATHETER

Trial Name Author (Year)	Group	Total No.	Actual Gestation (Weeks)	No. at 29–32 Weeks	Fio₂ at Enrollment	Result re Primary Outcome (%)	Intubated in First 72 h (%)	Pneumothorax (%)	BPD in Survivors (%)	Death (%)	Death or BPD (%)
AMV trial Göpel et al.[80] (2011)	CPAP	112	27.5	0	0.45	46	46	7	13	5	15
	Surfactant via catheter	108	27.6	0	0.4	28[a]	28[a]	4	8	7	14
Take Care Kanmaz et al.[71] (2013)	INSURE	100	28.3	45	0.55	45	45	10	20	13	32
	Surfactant via catheter	100	28	41	0.6	30[a]	30[a]	7	10[a]	16	22
Mirnia et al.[81] (2013)	INSURE	70	29.6	44	0.42		22	6	7	16	23
	Surfactant via catheter	66	29.6	44	0.43		19	5	8	3[a]	11
Bao et al.[82] (2015)	INSURE	43	29.3	25	0.43	23	23	7	14	0	14
	Surfactant via catheter	47	29.1	25	0.43	17	17	9	13	2	15
Mohammadizadeh et al.[83] (2015)	INSURE	19	31	17	NS	16	16		21	16	37
	Surfactant via catheter	19	30	17	NS	11	11		16	5	21
NINSAPP Kribs et al.[79] (2015)	Intubated	104	25.2	0	NS	59	100	13	30	12	41
	Surfactant via catheter	107	25.3	0	NS	67	~40–50	5[a]	25	9	33
Total No.		895		258							

Control group data are shown in the shaded boxes.
BPD, Bronchopulmonary dysplasia; CPAP, Continuous positive airway pressure; Fio₂, fraction of inspired oxygen; NS, not stated.
[a]Differs from control group, P < .05.

12

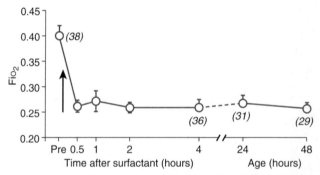

Fig. 12.1   Oxygen Requirement After Surfactant Administration Via Thin Catheter. The fraction of inspired oxygen (Fio_2) is shown for the first 4 hours after surfactant delivery and at 24 and 48 hours of life, in 38 preterm infants of median gestation of 27 weeks and birth weight of 880 g. Data are presented as the mean and standard error. The *black arrow* indicates the timing of surfactant administration, which was performed at a median age of 3.1 hours. Numbers in parentheses represent the number of data points. All postsurfactant Fio_2 values differ from those before surfactant ($P < .01$, paired *t* test). (Redrawn from Dargaville PA, Aiyappan A, De Paoli AG, et al. Minimally-invasive surfactant therapy in preterm infants on continuous positive airway pressure. *Arch Dis Child Fetal Neonatal Ed.* 2013;98:F122–F126.)

Narcotic analgesia was not used for either procedure. Inclusion in the trial required infants to demonstrate an oxygen requirement of at least 40% in the first 2 hours of life during management by CPAP. The fact that around 80% of all infants with RDS managed by CPAP achieved this Fio_2 threshold by 2 hours is somewhat surprising and is at odds with what has been observed within this gestation range in observational studies in tertiary NICUs.[20,84] This discrepancy is an issue common to several of the RCTs thus far conducted. Some important differences were noted between the groups in the Take Care study, including a lower rate of intubation before 72 hours in those receiving surfactant via a thin catheter, a shorter duration of ventilation and CPAP, as well as a reduced incidence of BPD (10% vs. 20%).

The Take Care study findings provided the first direct clinical evidence of a possible benefit in terms of surfactant distribution and tissue incorporation within the lung as a result of administration via a thin catheter in a spontaneously breathing subject. The same dose of surfactant was administered intratracheally in the two groups, which appeared to be well matched in terms of risk profile and RDS severity. Only the mode of surfactant administration differed. The INSURE group received surfactant via an ETT and in all cases positive-pressure ventilation (PPV) was applied. Infants in the intervention group were treated using a thin catheter with no PPV applied unless necessary for apnea (12% of cases). The authors speculated that the reduction in BPD rate might be due to a direct injurious effect of PPV in the INSURE group, but the intriguing possibility is also raised that surfactant is better distributed within the lung by spontaneous breathing efforts than PPV, with lasting effects on lung function and vulnerability to injury. The further evidence for this apparent benefit of spontaneous breathing, an unexpected windfall of less invasive surfactant delivery, is presented in a later section.

Bao et al.

A single-center RCT in a tertiary center in China was conducted in relatively mature infants ($n = 90$) managed by CPAP; the comparator group received surfactant via INSURE without sedation.[82] A substantial majority (~80%) of infants with RDS achieved the trial entry Fio_2 threshold of 0.30 within 2 hours of life. The trial was underpowered to detect a difference in the primary outcome, which was intubation in the first 72 hours. Oxygenation improved somewhat more rapidly after surfactant administration via a thin catheter, and fewer days of respiratory support (mechanical ventilation + CPAP) were needed by infants in this group.

Mohammadizadeh et al.

An RCT conducted in two tertiary centers in Iran enrolled infants ($n = 38$) of median gestational age 30 to 31 weeks who were managed by CPAP; the comparator group received surfactant via the INSURE procedure without sedation.[83] Two-thirds of infants achieved the entry Fio_2 threshold within 30 minutes of commencing CPAP. The study was underpowered to find any real advantage of surfactant delivery via a thin catheter; a reduction in duration of oxygen therapy in the thin catheter–treated infants was the only clinical difference noted between groups.

Mirnia et al.

An RCT was conducted in three tertiary centers in Iran, enrolling relatively mature infants with RDS ($n = 136$) managed by CPAP.[81] The report lacks detail in many aspects, including in relation to the procedures performed, the chosen primary outcome, and the determination of sample size. A significantly lower mortality rate was noted in the group receiving surfactant via a thin catheter, with no other major differences between groups.

NINSAPP Trial

In the Nonintubated Surfactant Application (NINSAPP) trial, Kribs and colleagues conducted a further RCT of the Cologne method of surfactant administration in 13 tertiary-level NICUs in Germany.[79] The study was notable for the enrollment of extremely preterm infants (<27 weeks' gestation; $n = 211$) and is the only RCT of surfactant delivery via a thin catheter to focus on this vulnerable group. Control infants received surfactant via an ETT and remained intubated and ventilated until extubation criteria were met. Enrollment was in the first 2 hours of life and could occur after 10 minutes if Fio_2 was 0.30 or higher and/or a Silverman score reached 5. Caffeine was administered before surfactant delivery in the group receiving it via a thin catheter but was delayed in the intubation group.

The primary outcome for the NINSAPP trial (survival without BPD) did not differ in incidence between the study groups, but there were some significant differences in secondary outcomes suggesting a benefit of surfactant delivery via a thin catheter. More infants survived without major complications (50% vs. 36%), the rate of severe IVH was reduced (10% vs. 22%), as were the pneumothorax rate and the overall duration of mechanical ventilation.

The intervention in the NINSAPP trial was applied as part of a less invasive bundle of respiratory management for extremely preterm infants, with avoidance of intubation in the delivery room even at 23 and 24 weeks' gestation. This is a substantial departure from what would be considered standard practice in the most immature infants. It is noteworthy that the improvement in survival free of major complications occurred despite nearly half the infants receiving surfactant via a thin catheter who progressed to intubation in the first 72 hours, and almost all infants at 23 and 24 weeks' undergoing intubation at some time. The implication is that even a few days when the extremely preterm infant is spontaneously breathing supported with CPAP (facilitated by less invasive surfactant administration) may be to their advantage in early life.

Summation of the Clinical Trials, and Findings of Meta-Analyses

The RCTs of surfactant delivery via tracheal catheterization are heterogeneous in many aspects of design, including gestation range, thresholds for study entry, surfactant administration technique, comparator group, and postintervention management. Moreover, some trials were conducted in established centers of excellence with low rates of mortality and morbidity even at extremely low gestation,[79] whereas others were conducted in NICUs in low- or middle-income countries with a developing experience of neonatal intensive care, in some cases hampered by lack of resources (e.g., nurse/patient ratio of 1:10).[83] Higher rates of mortality and morbidity are thus inevitable in studies from these centers, and these outcomes may be affected by a simple one-time intervention, such as less invasive surfactant delivery, in a way that cannot be replicated in advanced NICUs. Caution is thus required in the interpretation of the pooled findings of both the RCTs and the published meta-analyses regarding the applicability of the findings to NICUs with different resources and clinical expertise.

12

A further note of caution relates to the gestation range studies in the RCTs to date; there is an overrepresentation of infants between 26 and 28 weeks' gestation (~475 of 895), in whom the combination of effective surfactant delivery and avoidance of intubation is most likely to have sustained effects, including the possibility of an effect on BPD. Only ~250 infants have been included in RCTs beyond 28 weeks' gestation. Such infants are unlikely to receive lasting benefits on clinical outcomes from less invasive surfactant delivery in an advanced NICU setting, in which rates of BPD, other complications, and mortality should already be very low in infants starting life supported by CPAP.[84] Conversely, for infants less than 26 weeks' gestation (only ~170 randomly assigned), any advantage of surfactant via a thin catheter on lung injury may be obscured or negated by the influence of a large number of other factors that contribute to the development of BPD. The possibility that even brief avoidance of ventilation in the first days of life could have lasting effects on nonpulmonary morbidities such as intraventricular hemorrhage is raised by the result of the NINSAPP trial,[79] but this deserves further confirmation.

Meta-analyses of the RCTs[41–45]—and of the RCTs along with nonrandomized studies[40,45]—are now published. In summary, the most important findings of these studies are that surfactant administration via a thin catheter appears to have advantages over delivery via ETT, with pooled data from five studies showing a reduction in the incidence of death or BPD (risk ratio ~0.70), and the need for early mechanical ventilation (risk ratio ~0.75). A forthcoming Cochrane review will reexamine this evidence using standardized methodology.

Scientific and Practical Considerations

Effectiveness of Surfactant Delivery and Distribution

The clinical experience of surfactant therapy via a thin catheter in spontaneously breathing preterm infants supported by CPAP is of a rapid, profound, and sustained improvement in oxygenation, equivalent or better than that seen after administration via an ETT (Fig. 12.2). Several lines of inquiry have been pursued to more fully understand how spontaneous breathing and an active glottis may help to optimize the distribution of surfactant delivered into the trachea with these techniques.

Laboratory Studies of Surfactant Distribution

Exogenous surfactant distribution after administration by ETT has long been studied in animal models of lung disease, with evidence for a benefit of higher surfactant

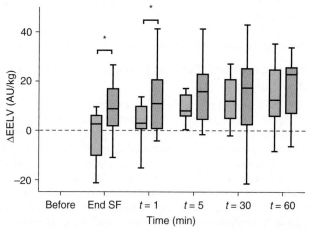

Fig. 12.2   Alteration in End-Expiratory Lung Volume (ΔEELV) After Surfactant Administration by a Thin Catheter. EELV changes in ventral (gray boxes) and dorsal (reddish boxes) lung regions are shown directly after surfactant administration (End SF) and at time points 1, 5, 30, and 60 minutes after the end of surfactant administration, relative to before surfactant. Data are from 15 preterm infants of median gestation of 29 weeks and birth weight of 1385 g. ΔEELV is measured by electrical impedance tomography and expressed as arbitrary units (AU) per kilogram of body weight. The boxes show the median and interquartile range; the whiskers show the minimum and maximum values. The asterisks indicate $P < .05$ versus before surfactant. (From van der Burg PS, de Jongh FH, Miedema M, et al. Effect of minimally invasive surfactant therapy on lung volume and ventilation in preterm infants. *J Pediatr.* 2016;170:67–72.)

concentration, larger surfactant volume, and more rapid instillation time.[85] On the other hand, given the recent emergence of less invasive approaches to surfactant therapy, the laboratory evidence is currently lagging behind clinical practice. Two published studies have examined the impact of spontaneous breathing (compared to PPV) *during*[86] or *after*[87] surfactant administration, with somewhat conflicting and inconclusive results. Niemarkt and coworkers compared the effect on surfactant distribution of spontaneous breathing or PPV during surfactant administration in preterm lambs ($n = 4$ per group).[86] Lobar distribution of surfactant was *less* even in the spontaneous breathing group, with a reduction in delivery to the right upper lobe. The small number of animals in each group limits the interpretation of this finding, which should be verified in further studies. Bohlin and coworkers[87] found spontaneous breathing *after* surfactant administration led to greater tissue incorporation of labeled exogenous surfactant and improved dynamic compliance in preterm rabbits ($n = 8$–15 per group). The conclusion drawn was that mechanical ventilation impaired or delayed tissue incorporation of surfactant, reinforcing the notion that surfactant delivery in the clinical setting should be followed by spontaneous breathing wherever possible.

The advent of surfactant administration via a thin catheter now requires some further laboratory studies to reexamine questions previously investigated in the era of surfactant delivery by PPV in intubated subjects. Factors influencing surfactant distribution, including the optimal rate of administration of surfactant, need to be reexplored. Clinical studies report a wide range of different approaches to deliver the surfactant dose, including as 3 boluses over ~30 seconds or as an infusion over 3 to 5 minutes. This latter approach requires careful appraisal; past studies of surfactant delivery by intratracheal infusion found this method to be inferior to bolus therapy in terms of surfactant distribution and postsurfactant lung function.[88,89]

Some clinical evidence regarding surfactant distribution has been gained from two studies that have examined the effect of surfactant administration on regional lung aeration measured using electrical impedance tomography in preterm infants with RDS.[90,91] Combined data from these studies, which were done several years apart in the same NICU, suggest that the aeration changes after intratracheal surfactant administration were more evenly distributed if surfactant was given via a thin catheter and under conditions of spontaneous breathing,[91] rather than via an ETT with PPV.[90] The gravity-dependent (dorsal) regions were seen to increase in aeration immediately after surfactant instillation with both delivery methods, but a delayed increase in aeration in the nondependent (ventral) lung regions was then noted preferentially in the group receiving surfactant via a thin catheter (Fig. 12.2). The authors conclude that surfactant distribution may have been optimized by spontaneous breathing, but acknowledged that the evidence is circumstantial and needs further verification by a direct comparison between methods.

Use of Premedication for Tracheal Catheterization

Minimization of Discomfort

Tracheal catheterization is currently performed under direct vision using a standard laryngoscope and in some cases instrumentation with Magill forceps, followed by insertion of a catheter through the glottis. These maneuvers, although brief, are likely to be uncomfortable and may induce apnea and/or bradycardia. For this reason, due consideration has been given to methods of maintaining comfort and enhancing tolerability during the procedure. Evidence concerning the safety and tolerability of tracheal catheterization is far from complete and at present consists of nonrandomized observational studies[92] and surveys of practice.[72,73] Premedication with narcotic or anesthetic agents appears more common in Nordic countries[73] than elsewhere.[69,71,93,94] A single-center retrospective study of discretionary use of propofol (1 mg/kg) before tracheal catheterization has suggested that this agent relieves discomfort during the procedure, but it leads to a higher need for PPV, a longer period of hypoxemia, and likely a greater chance of intubation during or after the procedure. A randomized trial of propofol therapy is now being conducted at this center.

Nonpharmacologic means of enhancing tolerance of the tracheal catheterization procedure include swaddling, tactile stimulation, and administration of 25% sucrose. The individual or combined benefit of these measures has not been formally evaluated.

Maintenance of Respiratory Effort and Avoidance of Bradycardia

It is widely accepted, although not evidence-based, that premedication with caffeine should be a prerequisite to surfactant delivery via thin catheter for infants younger than 30 weeks' gestation, with selective use of caffeine in more mature infants. Beyond this, respiratory effort during the procedure is promoted by maintenance of CPAP wherever possible, cutaneous stimulation in the event of apnea, and PPV if absolutely necessary.

Bradycardia during brief tracheal catheterization usually occurs mostly during the direct laryngoscopy, sometimes requiring easing of blade pressure on the anterior hypopharyngeal wall or even temporary cessation of laryngoscopy to resolve. Premedication with atropine in doses of 5 to 20 µg/kg has been used sporadically but is not in current favor.

Procedural Complications

Repeated Catheterization Attempts

Most studies of tracheal catheterization for surfactant delivery report high rates of catheterization of the trachea on the first attempt (first introduction of the laryngoscope), with a second or subsequent attempt required in around 20% to 30% of cases. Failure of catheterization on repeated attempts occurs with a frequency of less than 5%.

Hypoxia and Bradycardia

Not surprisingly, hypoxic and bradycardic episodes are commonly reported during tracheal catheterization for surfactant delivery, with arterial oxygen saturation less than 80% in ~40% to 60% of cases and heart rate less than 100 beats/min in 10% to 20% of cases. The need for PPV to aid recovery from these events remains relatively low and can mostly be avoided by skilled clinicians. Intubation during or after the procedure is rarely needed.

Surfactant Reflux

The appearance of some surfactant in the mouth during instillation via the catheter is noted in around one-third of reported cases. Closure of the mouth and promotion of spontaneous breathing may aid in returning the surfactant to the lung. PPV and suction are rarely needed in this circumstance.

Recommendations

Notwithstanding the gaps in the evidence, and recognizing the relatively widespread uptake of brief tracheal catheterization as an alternative to standard intubation for surfactant delivery,[72,73,79] some recommendations regarding application of this approach in a specific NICU environment are proposed in the following sections.

Selection of Infants

Gestational Age Range

Given the considerations previously mentioned, it is apparent that NICUs will need to examine their local profile of prematurity-related complications, in addition to the unit philosophy in relation to the use of CPAP from the outset, in choosing the gestation range at which to apply a less invasive approach to surfactant delivery. The thresholds at which infants receiving noninvasive support would be considered eligible are also gestation-specific and should be selected based on local experience.

Inclusion Criteria

It is clear from observational and interventional studies that not all preterm infants managed with noninvasive respiratory support will gain a benefit from surfactant delivery via a thin catheter. Particularly at more mature gestations, when surfactant deficiency is relative rather than absolute, many infants with RDS have sufficient respiratory resilience to be sustained by CPAP alone without surfactant therapy. The thresholds for treatment used in previous studies, and those proposed in the following text, aim to

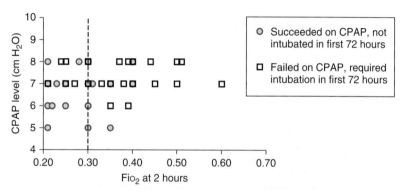

Fig. 12.3 Prediction of Continuous Positive Airway Pressure *(CPAP)* Failure in Preterm Infants Supported by CPAP. The figure shows individual data points for the highest CPAP level and appropriate fraction of inspired oxygen *(Fio₂)* in the first 2 hours in preterm infants between 25 and 28 weeks' gestation who commenced life supported by CPAP (n = 66), including those succeeding with CPAP (n = 36) and those requiring intubation at less than 72 hours (n = 30). The *dashed line* at Fio₂ of 0.30 indicates the predictive cut point. Odds ratio for CPAP failure in infants above and below this Fio₂ threshold: 5.6 (95% confidence interval 1.7–18). (Data from Dargaville PA, Aiyappan A, De Paoli AG, et al. Continuous positive airway pressure failure in preterm infants: incidence, predictors and consequences. *Neonatology.* 2013;104:8–14.)

pragmatically identify those infants with RDS of at least moderate severity, for whom surfactant therapy is likely to provide benefit and for whom CPAP failure is more likely to occur without surfactant. Previous studies of CPAP failure provide examples of how local data can help to identify a suitable threshold (Fig. 12.3). Such analysis should take into account the unit approach to CPAP (conservative vs. aggressive titration), the use (if any) of nasal high flow as primary therapy, and the uptake of adjuncts such as nasal intermittent positive-pressure ventilation. A lower Fio₂ threshold would be appropriate when high CPAP levels or nasal intermittent positive-pressure ventilation are commonly used at an early stage. Silverman scores and scoring of radiologic appearances could also contribute to the inclusion criteria if familiar to local clinicians. Similarly, a functional surfactant assay may identify infants with more serious RDS at an early stage, but such tests are not commonly used outside the province of research.

Exclusion Criteria

Some infants surpassing the treatment threshold have factors that may (1) limit the effectiveness of surfactant delivery via a thin catheter or (2) determine that surfactant alone may be insufficient to overcome the degree of respiratory compromise. Examples would be the infant with severe or very severe RDS or a comorbidity such as pneumothorax or recurrent apnea. Adoption of locally agreed-upon exclusion criteria will thus also be essential, acknowledging that surfactant therapy by standard intubation will remain the best option in some circumstances, including the lack of staff sufficiently skilled and experienced in the method of surfactant delivery via thin catheter (Box 12.1).

Future Research Directions

Longer-Term Outcomes After Surfactant Delivery Via a Thin Catheter

Although there do appear to be clinical advantages of delivering surfactant via tracheal catheterization, a comparison of longer-term outcomes is lacking, because no trial has yet reported neurodevelopmental follow-up.

Clinical Advantages of Surfactant Via a Thin Catheter Versus No Surfactant (i.e., Continuation of CPAP)

It seems clear that early surfactant delivery using a thin catheter results in fewer instances of CPAP failure, but whether this translates into further clinical benefits (e.g., reduction in BPD) has not been established. Further adequately powered studies are needed to clarify this.

> **Box 12.1   EXAMPLES OF INCLUSION AND EXCLUSION CRITERIA FOR SURFACTANT DELIVERY VIA A THIN CATHETER**
>
> Inclusion Criteria
>
> **All gestations**
> - Respiratory insufficiency thought related to RDS and managed with noninvasive respiratory support
>
> **23–25 weeks' gestation[a]**
> - CPAP level ≥6 cm H_2O
> - Any requirement for oxygen to maintain SpO_2 in the local target range
> - Age <6 h, and preferably <2 h
>
> **26–28 weeks' gestation**
> - CPAP level ≥6 cm H_2O, or nasal high flow with flow ≥7 L/min
> - FiO_2 ≥0.30 to maintain SpO_2 in the local target range.
> - Age <24 h, with an emphasis on early recognition and treatment at an age <6–12 h
>
> **Beyond 28 weeks' gestation**
> - CPAP level ≥6 cm H_2O, or HF with flow ≥7 L/min
> - FiO_2 ≥0.30 to 0.35[b] to maintain SpO_2 in the local target range
> - Age <24 h
>
> Exclusion Criteria
>
> **Absolute contraindications**
> - Severe RDS with high oxygen requirements and/or severe respiratory acidosis with prominent atelectasis radiologically, such that ongoing ventilatory support will be necessary after surfactant therapy. Suggested FiO_2 threshold at which intubation for surfactant should be considered: FiO_2>0.40-0.50 (lower gestations); FiO_2> 0.60 (more mature infants)
> - Maxillofacial, tracheal, or known pulmonary malformations
> - An alternative cause for respiratory distress (e.g., congenital pneumonia or pulmonary hypoplasia)
> - No experienced personnel available to perform the tracheal catheterization
>
> **Relative contraindications**
> - Infant <26 weeks' gestation—procedure can be technically challenging and destabilizing in inexperienced hands
> - Pneumothorax requiring drainage
> - Prominent apnea despite caffeine administration
>
> [a]Delivery room therapy controversial.
> [b]For infants >28 weeks gestation, the lower FiO_2 threshold (FiO_2 ≥ 0.30) may be preferable (1) at an age <6 h, (2) at higher CPAP levels (≥7 cm H_2O), and (3) for less mature or growth-restricted infants.
> *CPAP*, Continuous positive airway pressure; *FiO_2*, fraction of inspired oxygen; *RDS*, respiratory distress syndrome; *SpO_2*, oxygen saturation measured by pulse oximetry.

The Role of Spontaneous Breathing in Surfactant Distribution

The clinical studies showing benefits of surfactant via a thin catheter over INSURE in delivery of surfactant raise the possibility that spontaneous breathing is more effective for dispersion and distribution of surfactant from the trachea than positive-pressure ventilation. Experimental studies in which surfactant distribution has been directly measured during spontaneous breathing are few, and the results are thus far contradictory. Further laboratory and clinical studies are needed to completely understand the influence of an infant's respiratory effort on surfactant distribution.

Optimal Premedication for Infants at Different Gestation Ranges

Opinions range widely on the use of premedication for tracheal catheterization. At least one RCT examining the effect of anesthetic premedication is now being conducted, and others are needed to reach a conclusion on the risk/benefit ratio associated with the use of agents with the potential to cause respiratory depression.

Methods for Determining That the Catheter Is Correctly Positioned in the Trachea

There are no studies examining the role of carbon dioxide measurement or other means of identifying catheter tip position in confirming correct placement of the surfactant delivery catheter. Beyond its use as a training tool, videolaryngoscopy may be of benefit in confirming catheter placement and in minimizing the discomfort associated with standard laryngoscopy.

Acknowledgment

As chief investigator of the OPTIMIST-A trial (NCT02140580), the author has received support from the Royal Hobart Hospital Research Foundation, the Australian National Health and Medical Research Council (grant No. 1049114), and in-kind support from Chiesi Farmaceutici S.p.A.

REFERENCES

1. Gregory GA, Kitterman JA, Phibbs RH, Tooley WH, Hamilton WK. Treatment of the idiopathic respiratory-distress syndrome with continuous positive airway pressure. *N Engl J Med*. 1971;284: 1333–1340.
2. Tooley WH. Hyaline membrane disease. Telling it like it was. *Am Rev Resp Dis*. 1977;115:19–28.
3. Avery ME, Tooley WH, Keller JB, et al. Is chronic lung disease in low birth weight infants preventable? A survey of eight centers. *Pediatrics*. 1987;79:26–30.
4. Van Marter LJ, Allred EN, Pagano M, et al. Do clinical markers of barotrauma and oxygen toxicity explain interhospital variation in rates of chronic lung disease? The Neonatology Committee for the Developmental Network. *Pediatrics*. 2000;105:1194–1201.
5. Morley CJ, Davis PG, Doyle LW, Brion LP, Hascoet JM, Carlin JB. Nasal CPAP or intubation at birth for very preterm infants. *N Engl J Med*. 2008;358:700–708.
6. Finer NN, Carlo WA, Walsh MC, et al. Early CPAP versus surfactant in extremely preterm infants. *N Engl J Med*. 2010;362:1970–1979.
7. Dunn MS, Kaempf J, de KA, et al. Randomized trial comparing 3 approaches to the initial respiratory management of preterm neonates. *Pediatrics*. 2011;128:e1069–e1076.
8. Suresh GK, Soll RF. Overview of surfactant replacement trials. *J Perinatol*. 2005;25(suppl 2): S40–S44.
9. Jobe AH. Transition/adaptation in the delivery room and less RDS: "Don't just do something, stand there!" *J Pediatr*. 2005;147:284–286.
10. Clark RH, Slutsky AS, Gerstmann DR. Lung protective strategies of ventilation in the neonate: what are they? *Pediatrics*. 2000;105:112–114.
11. van Kaam AH, Rimensberger PC. Lung-protective ventilation strategies in neonatology: what do we know–what do we need to know? *Crit Care Med*. 2007;35:925–931.
12. Dargaville PA, Tingay DG. Lung protective ventilation in extremely preterm infants. *J Paediatr Child Health*. 2012;48:740–746.
13. Soll RF, Edwards EM, Badger GJ, et al. Obstetric and neonatal care practices for infants 501 to 1500 g from 2000 to 2009. *Pediatrics*. 2013;132:222–228.
14. Stoll BJ, Hansen NI, Bell EF, et al. Neonatal outcomes of extremely preterm infants from the NICHD Neonatal Research Network. *Pediatrics*. 2010;126:443–456.
15. Dargaville PA, Gerber A, Johansson S, et al. Incidence and outcome of CPAP failure in preterm infants. *Pediatrics*. 2016;138:e20153985.
16. Ammari A, Suri M, Milisavljevic V, et al. Variables associated with the early failure of nasal CPAP in very low birth weight infants. *J Pediatr*. 2005;147:341–347.
17. Aly H, Massaro AN, Patel K, El Mohandes AA. Is it safer to intubate premature infants in the delivery room? *Pediatrics*. 2005;115:1660–1665.
18. Fuchs H, Lindner W, Leiprecht A, Mendler MR, Hummler HD. Predictors of early nasal CPAP failure and effects of various intubation criteria on the rate of mechanical ventilation in preterm infants of <29 weeks gestational age. *Arch Dis Child Fetal Neonatal Ed*. 2011;96:F343–F347.
19. De Jaegere AP, van der Lee JH, Cante C, van Kaam AH. Early prediction of nasal continuous positive airway pressure failure in preterm infants less than 30 weeks gestation. *Acta Paediatr*. 2011;101: 374–379.
20. Dargaville PA, Aiyappan A, De Paoli AG, et al. Continuous positive airway pressure failure in preterm infants: incidence, predictors and consequences. *Neonatology*. 2013;104:8–14.
21. Tagliaferro T, Bateman D, Ruzal-Shapiro C, Polin RA. Early radiologic evidence of severe respiratory distress syndrome as a predictor of nasal continuous positive airway pressure failure in extremely low birth weight newborns. *J Perinatol*. 2014.
22. Bohlin K. RDS–CPAP or surfactant or both. *Acta Paediatr Suppl*. 2012;101:24–28.
23. Dargaville PA. CPAP, surfactant or both for the preterm infant. Resolving the dilemma. *JAMA Pediatr*. 2015;169:715–717.
24. Verder H, Robertson B, Greisen G, et al. Surfactant therapy and nasal continuous positive airway pressure for newborns with respiratory distress syndrome. Danish-Swedish Multicenter Study Group. *N Engl J Med*. 1994;331:1051–1055.
25. Escobedo MB, Gunkel JH, Kennedy KA, et al. Early surfactant for neonates with mild to moderate respiratory distress syndrome: a multicenter, randomized trial. *J Pediatr*. 2004;144:804–808.
26. Reininger A, Khalak R, Kendig JW, et al. Surfactant administration by transient intubation in infants 29 to 35 weeks' gestation with respiratory distress syndrome decreases the likelihood of later mechanical ventilation: a randomized controlled trial. *J Perinatol*. 2005;25:703–708.
27. Sandri F, Plavka R, Ancora G, et al. Prophylactic or early selective surfactant combined with nCPAP in very preterm infants. *Pediatrics*. 2010;125:e1402–e1409.

12

28. O'Donnell CP, Kamlin CO, Davis PG, Morley CJ. Endotracheal intubation attempts during neonatal resuscitation: success rates, duration, and adverse effects. *Pediatrics*. 2006;117:e16–e21.

29. Cools F. A new method of surfactant administration in preterm infants. *Lancet*. 2011;378:1607–1608.

30. Kribs A. How best to administer surfactant to VLBW infants? *Arch Dis Child Fetal Neonatal Ed*. 2011;96:F238–F240.

31. Dargaville PA. Innovation in surfactant therapy I: surfactant lavage and surfactant administration by fluid bolus using minimally invasive techniques. *Neonatology*. 2012;101:326–336.

32. Pillow JJ, Minocchieri S. Innovation in surfactant therapy II: surfactant administration by aerosolization. *Neonatology*. 2012;101:337–344.

33. Blennow M, Bohlin K. Surfactant and noninvasive ventilation. *Neonatology*. 2015;107:330–336.

34. Aguar M, Vento M, Dargaville PA. Minimally-invasive surfactant therapy—an update. *Neoreviews*. 2014;15:e275.

35. Kribs A. Minimally invasive surfactant therapy and noninvasive respiratory support. *Clin Perinatol*. 2016;43:755–771.

36. Shim GH. Update of minimally invasive surfactant therapy. *Korean J Pediatr*. 2017;60:273–281.

37. Abdel-Latif ME, Osborn DA. Nebulised surfactant in preterm infants with or at risk of respiratory distress syndrome. *Cochrane Database Syst Rev*. 2012;10:CD008310.

38. Abdel-Latif ME, Osborn DA. Pharyngeal instillation of surfactant before the first breath for prevention of morbidity and mortality in preterm infants at risk of respiratory distress syndrome. *Cochrane Database Syst Rev*. 2011;3:CD008311.

39. Abdel-Latif ME, Osborn DA. Laryngeal mask airway surfactant administration for prevention of morbidity and mortality in preterm infants with or at risk of respiratory distress syndrome. *Cochrane Database Syst Rev*. 2011:CD008309.

40. More K, Sakhuja P, Shah PS. Minimally invasive surfactant administration in preterm infants: a meta-narrative review. *JAMA Pediatr*. 2014;168:901–908.

41. Isayama T, Iwami H, McDonald S, Beyene J. Association of noninvasive ventilation strategies with mortality and bronchopulmonary dysplasia among preterm infants: a systematic review and meta-analysis. *JAMA*. 2016;316:611–624.

42. Ali E, Abdel WM, Alsalami Z, et al. New modalities to deliver surfactant in premature infants: a systematic review and meta-analysis. *J Matern Fetal Neonatal Med*. 2016;29:3519–3524.

43. Aldana-Aguirre JC, Pinto M, Featherstone RM, Kumar M. Less invasive surfactant administration versus intubation for surfactant delivery in preterm infants with respiratory distress syndrome: a systematic review and meta-analysis. *Arch Dis Child Fetal Neonatal Ed*. 2017;102:F17–F23.

44. Rigo V, Lefebvre C, Broux I. Surfactant instillation in spontaneously breathing preterm infants: a systematic review and meta-analysis. *Eur J Pediatr*. 2016;175:1933–1942.

45. Wu W, Shi Y, Li F, Wen Z, Liu H. Surfactant administration via a thin endotracheal catheter during spontaneous breathing in preterm infants. *Pediatr Pulmonol*. 2017;52:844–854.

46. Robillard E, Alarie Y, Dagenais-Perusse P, Baril E, Guilbeault A. Microaerosol administration of synthetic beta-gamma-dipalmitoyl-l-alpha-lecithin in the respiratory distress syndome: a preliminary report. *Can Med Assoc J*. 1964;90:55–57.

47. Chu J, Clements JA, Cotton EK, et al. Neonatal pulmonary ischemia. I. Clinical and physiological studies. *Pediatrics*. 1967;40(suppl 82).

48. Ten Centre Study Group. Ten centre trial of artificial surfactant (artificial lung expanding compound) in very premature babies. Ten Centre Study Group. *Br Med J*. 1987;294:991–996.

49. Brimacombe J, Gandini D, Keller C. The laryngeal mask airway for administration of surfactant in two neonates with respiratory distress syndrome. *Paediatr Anaesth*. 2004;14:188–190.

50. Verder H, Agertoft L, Albertsen P, et al. Surfactant treatment of newborn infants with respiratory distress syndrome primarily treated with nasal continuous positive air pressure. A pilot study. [Danish]. *Ugeskr Laeger*. 1992;154:2136–2139.

51. Jorch G, Hartl H, Roth B, et al. Surfactant aerosol treatment of respiratory distress syndrome in spontaneously breathing premature infants. *Pediatr Pulmonol*. 1997;24:222–224.

52. Arroe M, Pedersen-Bjergaard L, Albertsen P, Bode S, Griesen G, Jonsbo F. Inhalation of aerosolized surfactant (exosurf) to neonates treated with nasal continuous positive airway pressure. *Prenat Neonat Med*. 1998;3:346–352.

53. Finer NN, Merritt TA, Bernstein G, Job L, Mazela J, Segal R. An open label, pilot study of Aerosurf(R) combined with nCPAP to prevent RDS in preterm neonates. *J Aerosol Med Pulm Drug Deliv*. 2010;23:303–309.

54. Berggren E, Liljedahl M, Winbladh B, et al. Pilot study of nebulized surfactant therapy for neonatal respiratory distress syndrome. *Acta Paediatr*. 2000;89:460–464.

55. Minocchieri S, Berry CA, Pillow JJ. Nebulized surfactant for treatment of respiratory distress in the first hours of life: the CureNeb study [abstract]. *PAS Abstract*. 2013:3500.

56. Kattwinkel J, Robinson M, Bloom BT, Delmore P, Ferguson JE. Technique for intrapartum administration of surfactant without requirement for an endotracheal tube. *J Perinatol*. 2004;24:360–365.

57. Lamberska T, Settelmayerova E, Smisek J, Luksova M, Maloskova G, Plavka R. Oropharyngeal surfactant can improve initial stabilisation and reduce rescue intubation in infants born below 25 weeks of gestation. *Acta Paediatr*. 2017.

58. Tingay DG, Wallace MJ, Bhatia R, et al. Surfactant before the first inflation at birth improves spatial distribution of ventilation and reduces lung injury in preterm lambs. *J Appl Physiol*. 2014;116:251–258.

59. Rojas-Reyes MX, Morley CJ, Soll R. Prophylactic versus selective use of surfactant in preventing morbidity and mortality in preterm infants. *Cochrane Database Syst Rev*. 2012;3:CD000510.

60. Schmolzer GM, Agarwal M, Kamlin CO, Davis PG. Supraglottic airway devices during neonatal resuscitation: an historical perspective, systematic review and meta-analysis of available clinical trials. *Resuscitation*. 2013;84:722–730.

61. Wyckoff MH, Aziz K, Escobedo MB, et al. Part 13: Neonatal resuscitation: 2015 American Heart Association guidelines update for cardiopulmonary resuscitation and emergency cardiovascular care. *Circulation*. 2015;132:S543–S560.

62. Fraser J, Hill C, McDonald D, Jones C, Petros A. The use of the laryngeal mask airway for interhospital transport of infants with type 3 laryngotracheo-oesophageal clefts. *Intensive Care Med*. 1999;25:714–716.

63. Trevisanuto D, Grazzina N, Ferrarese P, Micaglio M, Verghese C, Zanardo V. Laryngeal mask airway used as a delivery conduit for the administration of surfactant to preterm infants with respiratory distress syndrome. *Biol Neonate*. 2005;87:217–220.

64. Attridge JT, Stewart C, Stukenborg GJ, Kattwinkel J. Administration of rescue surfactant by laryngeal mask airway: lessons from a pilot trial. *Am J Perinatol*. 2013;30:201–206.

65. Pinheiro JM, Santana-Rivas Q, Pezzano C. Randomized trial of laryngeal mask airway versus endotracheal intubation for surfactant delivery. *J Perinatol*. 2016;36:196–201.

66. Roberts KD, Brown R, Lampland AL, et al. Laryngeal mask airway for surfactant administration in neonates: a randomized, controlled trial. *J Pediatr*. 2017. [Epub ahead of print].

67. Barbosa RF, Simões e Silva AC, Silva YP. A randomized controlled trial of laryngeal mask airway for surfactant administration in neonates. *J Pediatr*. 2017;93; in press.

68. Dargaville PA. Administering surfactant without intubation - what does the laryngeal mask offer us? *J Pediatr (Rio J)*. 2017;93:313–316.

69. Dargaville PA, Aiyappan A, De Paoli AG, et al. Minimally-invasive surfactant therapy in preterm infants on continuous positive airway pressure. *Arch Dis Child Fetal Neonatal Ed*. 2013;98:F122–F126.

70. Kribs A, Pillekamp F, Hunseler C, Vierzig A, Roth B. Early administration of surfactant in spontaneous breathing with nCPAP: feasibility and outcome in extremely premature infants (postmenstrual age <=27 weeks). *Paediatr Anaesth*. 2007;17:364–369.

71. Kanmaz HG, Erdeve O, Canpolat FE, Mutlu B, Dilmen U. Surfactant administration via thin catheter during spontaneous breathing: randomized controlled trial. *Pediatrics*. 2013;131:e502–e509.

72. Klotz D, Porcaro U, Fleck T, Fuchs H. European perspective on less invasive surfactant administration-a survey. *Eur J Pediatr*. 2017;176:147–154.

73. Heiring C, Jonsson B, Andersson S, Bjorklund LJ. Survey shows large differences between the Nordic countries in the use of less invasive surfactant administration. *Acta Paediatr*. 2017;106:382–386.

74. Dargaville PA, Aiyappan A, Cornelius A, Williams C, De Paoli AG. Preliminary evaluation of a new technique of minimally invasive surfactant therapy. *Arch Dis Child Fetal Neonatal Ed*. 2011;96:F243–F248.

75. Aguar M, Cernada M, Brugada M, Gimeno A, Gutierrez A, Vento M. Minimally invasive surfactant therapy with a gastric tube is as effective as the intubation, surfactant, and extubation technique in preterm babies. *Acta Paediatr*. 2014;103:e229–e233.

76. Maiwald CA, Neuberger P, Vochem M, Poets C. QuickSF: a new technique in surfactant administration. *Neonatology*. 2017;111:211–213.

77. Embleton ND, Deshpande SA, Scott D, Wright C, Milligan DW. Foot length, an accurate predictor of nasotracheal tube length in neonates. *Arch Dis Child Fetal Neonatal Ed*. 2001;85:F60–F64.

78. Dargaville PA, Kamlin CO, De Paoli AG, et al. The OPTIMIST-A trial: evaluation of minimally-invasive surfactant therapy in preterm infants 25–28 weeks gestation. *BMC Pediatr*. 2014;14:213.

79. Kribs A, Roll C, Gopel W, et al. Nonintubated surfactant application vs conventional therapy in extremely preterm infants: a randomized clinical trial. *JAMA Pediatr*. 2015;169:723–730.

80. Göpel W, Kribs A, Ziegler A, et al. Avoidance of mechanical ventilation by surfactant treatment of spontaneously breathing preterm infants (AMV): an open-label, randomised, controlled trial. *Lancet*. 2011;378:1627–1634.

81. Mirnia K, Heidarzadeh M, Hosseini M, Balila M, Ghojazadeh M. Comparison outcome of surfactant administration via tracheal catheterization during spontaneous breathing with INSURE. *Med J Islamic World Acad Sci*. 2013;21:143–148.

82. Bao Y, Zhang G, Wu M, Ma L, Zhu J. A pilot study of less invasive surfactant administration in very preterm infants in a Chinese tertiary center. *BMC Pediatr*. 2015;15:21.

83. Mohammadizadeh M, Ardestani AG, Sadeghnia AR. Early administration of surfactant via a thin intratracheal catheter in preterm infants with respiratory distress syndrome: feasibility and outcome. *J Res Pharm Pract*. 2015;4:31–36.

84. Dargaville PA, Ali SKM, Jackson HD, Williams C, De Paoli AG. Impact of minimally invasive surfactant therapy in preterm infants at 29–32 weeks gestation. *Neonatology*. 2018;113:7–14.

85. Jobe AH. Techniques for administering surfactant. In: Robertson B, Taeusch HW, eds. *Surfactant Therapy for Lung Disease*. New York: Marcel Dekker; 1995:309–324.

86. Niemarkt HJ, Kuypers E, Jellema R, et al. Effects of less-invasive surfactant administration on oxygenation, pulmonary surfactant distribution, and lung compliance in spontaneously breathing preterm lambs. *Pediatr Res*. 2014;76:166–170.

87. Bohlin K, Bouhafs RK, Jarstrand C, Curstedt T, Blennow M, Robertson B. Spontaneous breathing or mechanical ventilation alters lung compliance and tissue association of exogenous surfactant in preterm newborn rabbits. *Pediatr Res*. 2005;57:624–630.

88. Ueda T, Ikegami M, Rider ED, Jobe AH. Distribution of surfactant and ventilation in surfactant-treated preterm lambs. *J Appl Physiol*. 1994;76:45–55.

12

89. Hentschel R, Brune T, Franke N, Harms E, Jorch G. Sequential changes in compliance and resistance after bolus administration or slow infusion of surfactant in preterm infants. *Intensive Care Med.* 2002;28:622–628.
90. Miedema M, de Jongh FH, Frerichs I, van Veenendaal MB, van Kaam AH. Changes in lung volume and ventilation during surfactant treatment in ventilated preterm infants. *Am J Respir Crit Care Med.* 2011;184:100–105.
91. van der Burg PS, de Jongh FH, Miedema M, Frerichs I, van Kaam AH. Effect of minimally invasive surfactant therapy on lung volume and ventilation in preterm infants. *J Pediatr.* 2016;170:67–72.
92. Dekker J, Lopriore E, Rijken M, Rijntjes-Jacobs E, Smits-Wintjens V, Te PA. Sedation during minimal invasive surfactant therapy in preterm infants. *Neonatology.* 2016;109:308–313.
93. Göpel W, Kribs A, Hartel C, et al. Less invasive surfactant administration is associated with improved pulmonary outcomes in spontaneously breathing preterm infants. *Acta Paediatr.* 2015;104:241–246.
94. Klebermass-Schrehof K, Wald M, Schwindt J, et al. Less invasive surfactant administration in extremely preterm infants: impact on mortality and morbidity. *Neonatology.* 2013;103:252–258.

CHAPTER 13

Respiratory Control and Apnea in Premature Infants

Vidhi P. Shah, Juliann M. Di Fiore, and Richard J. Martin

- Understanding the physiology of neonatal respiratory control has served as an effective guide to common therapeutic approaches.
- Both the acute and longer-term consequences of intermittent hypoxia secondary to apnea of prematurity are subjects of intense interest.
- Intermittent hypoxemia may contribute to an inflammatory stress response.
- Although caffeine is the mainstay of apnea therapy, there remains considerable controversy regarding optimal treatment regimens.
- Innovative newer approaches to stabilizing respiratory control may hold promise as future interventions.

There are a multitude of reasons why immaturity in respiratory control is of interest to scientists and clinicians alike. From a biologic perspective it represents a unique link between the developing respiratory and central nervous systems. The resultant apnea precipitates repetitive oxygen desaturation and, hence, preterm infants serve as a novel biologic model for studying the consequences of such episodic desaturation. From a clinical perspective the combination of immature respiratory control, an immature lung, and the resultant therapeutic ventilatory support predispose these infants to chronic respiratory morbidity. Finally, there is a need to optimize and provide safe pharmacotherapy that enhances respiratory neural output in this high-risk population of neonates. These are some of the current high-profile issues and controversies that this chapter addresses.

Biologic Challenges in Characterizing Neonatal Respiratory Control

The ability to challenge respiratory neural output with hypoxic or hypercapnic exposures is quite limited in human infants. Therefore one must rely on older studies to better understand the maturation of peripheral and central components of chemoreception. We are also very dependent on neonatal animal models, particularly data derived from rodents, although, unfortunately, such models rarely exhibit long spontaneous apnea or periodic breathing as seen in preterm infants.

Central Respiratory Control

The neural circuitry that generates respiratory rhythm and governs inspiratory and expiratory motor patterns is distributed throughout the pons and medulla. The medulla contains a specialized region known as the pre-Bötzinger complex, which contains neurons that exhibit intrinsic pacemaker activity capable of producing rhythmic respiratory motor output without sensory feedback. Although a fundamental feature of this network is that it enables breathing to occur automatically, this systematic central rhythmicity may fail in preterm infants.[1] Meanwhile, central and peripheral sensory inputs from multiple sources allow adjustments to the patterns of inspiratory and expiratory activity in response to changing metabolic conditions. For example, inhibitory sensory inputs from the upper airway may be particularly prominent in early postnatal life to serve a protective function, although this may trigger potentially clinically significant apnea.

A poorly understood concept is the relationship between periodic breathing—that is, repetitive cycles of respiratory output and pauses of approximately 5 to 10 seconds' duration, and apneic episodes typically of 10 to 20 seconds' duration that do not exhibit a cyclic pattern. Available data suggest that periodic breathing occurs predominantly in quiet sleep, whereas apnea is more common in active sleep. This would suggest a different central or peripheral biologic basis for those breathing patterns as discussed later.

Excitatory and inhibitory neurotransmitters and neuromodulators mediate the rhythmogenic synaptic communications between neurons of the medulla. Glutamate, acting on α-amino-3-hydroxy-5-methyl-4-isoxazolepropionic acid and N-methyl-D-aspartate receptors, is the major neurotransmitter mediating excitatory synaptic input to brainstem respiratory neurons. Gamma-aminobutyric acid (GABA) and glycine are the two primary inhibitory neurotransmitters in the network, mediating the waves of inhibitory postsynaptic potentials during the silent phase of respiratory neurons. Interestingly, during late embryonic and early postnatal development, GABA and glycine can mediate *excitatory* neurotransmission secondary to changes in the chloride gradient across the membrane. It is unclear how this phenomenon relates to the inhibition of respiratory output and resultant apnea seen in preterm infants.[2] Neonatal rodent data suggest that caffeine, which is a nonselective adenosine receptor inhibitor, may block excitatory A_{2A} receptors at GABAergic neurons, and so inhibit GABA output and contribute to the ability of caffeine to enhance respiratory drive.[3] Serotonin may be of particular importance in the modulation of respiratory function. Serotonergic neurons and their projections may represent the neuroanatomic substrate for the integration of cardiorespiratory responses. Defects in the medullary serotonergic system likely contribute importantly to the pathogenesis of sudden infant death syndrome.[4] For future advances in the pharmacotherapy of neonatal apnea, greater understanding of the maturation of these neurotransmitters/neuromodulators is imperative.

Central and Peripheral Chemosensitivity

Responsiveness to carbon dioxide (CO_2) is the major chemical driver of respiratory neural output. This is apparent in fetal life where breathing movements increase under hypercapnic conditions in animal models. As in later life, CO_2/hydrogen ion (H^+) responsiveness is predominantly based in the brainstem, although peripheral chemoreceptors contribute to the ventilatory response and respond more rapidly. The reduced ventilatory response to CO_2 in small preterm infants, especially those with apnea, is primarily the result of decreased central chemosensitivity; however, mechanical factors such as poor respiratory function and an unstable, compliant chest wall may contribute.[5] It is difficult to distinguish the neural from mechanical factors that contribute to respiratory failure in this population.[6]

It has been known for many years that preterm infants respond to a fall in inspired oxygen concentration with a transient increase in ventilation over approximately 1 minute, followed by a return to baseline or even depression of ventilation. The characteristic response to low oxygen in infants appears to result from initial peripheral chemoreceptor stimulation, followed by overriding depression of the respiratory center as a result of hypoxemia. Such hypoxic respiratory depression may be useful in the hypoxic intrauterine environment where respiratory activity is only intermittent and not contributing to gas exchange. The nonsustained response to low inspired oxygen concentration may, however, be a disadvantage postnatally. It may play an important role in the origin of neonatal apnea, and offers a physiologic rationale for the decrease in incidence of apnea observed when a slightly increased concentration of inspired oxygen is administered to apneic infants who have a low baseline oxygen saturation. Decreased peripheral chemoreceptor responsiveness to oxygen or central hypoxic depression of respiratory neural output may impair recovery from apnea. In contrast, excessive peripheral chemosensitivity has also been shown to compromise ventilatory stability and predispose to periodic breathing and even apnea in preterm infants.[7,8] Periodic breathing is thought to result from a combination of dominant peripheral chemosensitivity combined with a CO_2 level close to the apneic threshold, resulting in the characteristic cycles of breaths and pauses. These findings are consistent with the observed postnatal delay in onset of periodic breathing, as peripheral chemoreceptors may be silenced in the initial postnatal period.[2,9–11]

Contribution from Inflammatory Mechanisms

It is well recognized that apnea may be the first indication of neonatal sepsis. There is also considerable current biologic interest in the role of inflammation on respiratory neural output at both central and peripheral levels. Although inflammatory cytokines probably do not readily cross the blood-brain barrier, systemic infection does upregulate inflammatory cytokines at the blood-brain barrier, resulting in activation of prostaglandin signaling and resultant inhibition of respiratory neural output.[12] Chorioamnionitis is a major precipitant of preterm birth. It is possible that antenatal or postnatal exposure of the lung to a proinflammatory stimulus may activate brain circuits that destabilize respiratory neural output. In neonatal rodents there is a response of proinflammatory cytokine gene expression in the brainstem after intrapulmonary lipopolysaccharide exposure, which is partially vagally mediated.[13] This is accompanied by significant ventilatory depression to hypoxic exposure. An interesting related line of investigation is the role of intermittent hypoxia (IH) and resultant oxidant stress on inflammatory pathways that regulate respiratory neural output. Much work is needed to explore these potential interrelationships between impaired respiratory neural output and inflammation, IH, and any resultant oxidant stress as discussed later.

Clinical Challenges in Defining Neonatal Apnea

During early postnatal life apneic events are ubiquitous; they can vary widely in duration and are often accompanied by bradycardia and/or intermittent hypoxemia.[14] Accordingly, American Academy of Pediatrics guidelines have historically defined clinical apnea of prematurity as a respiratory pause of 20 seconds or shorter if accompanied by hypoxemia (<80%) and/or bradycardia (<80 beats/min).[15] It should be noted that even short respiratory pauses, approximating 10 seconds or less, may be associated with desaturation and/or bradycardia. Apnea is categorized as (1) central with loss of central respiratory drive resulting in complete cessation of flow and absence of respiratory effort; (2) obstructive with absence of flow in the presence of respiratory efforts; and (3) mixed with both central and obstructive components. Mixed apnea accounts for approximately 40% to 50% of all events in preterm infants[14,16] and is often initiated by a loss of central drive, followed by a delay in resolution owing to upper airway closure.[17] However, airway narrowing and/or collapse, as measured by cardiac signal transmission on the flow waveform, can also occur during central apnea.[18] Unfortunately, standard impedance monitoring, which reflects chest wall motion, may fail to differentiate obstructed versus unobstructed inspiratory efforts.

The true incidence of apnea during early postnatal life has been grossly underestimated because of the historical practice of using nursing documentation, shown to underreport the true frequency of clinical events by more than 50%.[19] More accurate pneumogram recordings have revealed a high incidence of cardiorespiratory events even in convalescing infants. For example, in very low-birth-weight (VLBW) neonates, 91% of pneumograms performed within 72 hours of anticipated discharge revealed apnea accompanied by a fall in heart rate or oxygen saturation.[20] This has been supported in a more recent expanded cohort of 1211 infants younger than 35 weeks' gestation showing that preterm infants continue to experience short apnea with bradycardia and/or desaturation in the week before discharge.[21] It is therefore not surprising that hospitalization is frequently prolonged owing to concern about persistent cardiorespiratory events. Neonatal intensive care unit (NICU) electronic medical record databases are beginning to incorporate automated detection of apnea/bradycardia/desaturation in contrast to manual entries by the nursing staff. Because hospital discharge is often driven by the presence (or absence) of events, it is unclear how the anticipated increased frequency of documentation with automated bedside monitoring may affect duration of hospitalization.

Association Between Apnea of Prematurity, Intermittent Hypoxemia, and Bradycardia and Neonatal Outcomes

Multiple studies in preterm infants have shown an association between apnea of prematurity and morbidity. However, more recent data in neonatal models suggest that the accompanying desaturation and/or bradycardia may be the contributing factor(s) in initiating a pathologic cascade. In preterm infants, IH is almost always preceded by a respiratory pause and often occurs rapidly (~10 seconds) after cessation of airflow.[14] Factors that can influence the initiation, duration, and severity of IH include baseline oxygen saturation,[22] oxygen uptake from the alveoli, pulmonary oxygen stores, total blood oxygen-carrying capacity, the slope of the hemoglobin oxygen dissociation curve, and metabolic oxygen consumption.[23] In extremely preterm infants, IH events are pervasive and transient during early postnatal life with a relatively low incidence during the first week of life, followed by a rapid increase during the second and third weeks and a plateau or decrease thereafter.[24] A significant challenge is that we are only beginning to understand the implications of patterns of IH events on morbidity (Fig. 13.1).

Strong evidence in both animal and infant models suggests an association between cardiorespiratory events and impaired executive function. For example, in VLBW infants delayed resolution and increased event severity during early postnatal life are risk factors for severe handicap at 13 months of age.[25] Apnea during hospitalization has also been shown as a predictor of neurodevelopmental impairment at 2 to 3 years of age[26,27] and diminished adaptive behavior at early school age (Vineland Adaptive Behavior Scale composite score).[28] Many of the infant studies relied on chart documentation of apnea, limiting the reliability of study findings, and do not address the question of whether it is the apnea or accompanying desaturation that initiates the pathologic sequelae. Unfortunately, it is very difficult to implicate causality as opposed to association when relating apnea and IH to outcome.

Long-term recordings have now allowed for more reliable and detailed analyses of oxygen saturation patterns and morbidity. For instance, continuous pulse oximetry

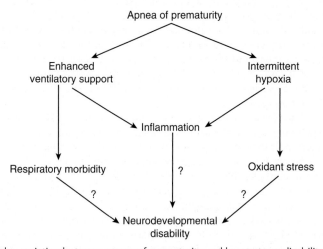

Fig. 13.1   Potential association between apnea of prematurity and longer-term disability in preterm infants.

monitoring over the first 2 months of life revealed an association between severe retinopathy of prematurity and a higher frequency of IH, of longer duration, and a distinct timing between IH events.[29] A secondary analysis of infants enrolled in the Canadian Oxygen Trial has shown an association between increased time spent less than 80% during IH events and a greater probability of death or disability, cognitive or language delay, severe retinopathy of prematurity, and motor impairment at 18 months of age[30] that was limited to IH events of 1 minute or longer in duration.

Association Between Apnea of Prematurity, Intermittent Hypoxemia, and Bradycardia and Longer-Term Outcomes

Interpretations of infant trial findings have been limited to associations between IH and morbidity in contrast to animal models that have been able to show direct causation. For example, in rodents, exposure to IH events during the first weeks of life causes impaired working memory,[31] decreased brain weight,[31] increased expression of caspase 3,[31] locomotor hyperactivity, and alterations in dopamine signaling in adulthood,[32] reinforcing long-term effects of IH exposure on brain development.

Sleep-disordered breathing is a relatively common condition in children and young adults.[33,34] Former preterm infants are especially at risk, although the mechanisms are currently unknown.[34] Early postnatal exposure to chronic intermittent exposure in rodents resulted in a blunted acute ventilatory response to hypoxia during adulthood, suggesting that early IH patterns can also have long-lasting effects on respiratory stability.[35] This may be one explanation why former preterm infants have an approximately fourfold increase in the obstructive apnea hypopnea index at 8 to 11 years of age compared with former healthy term infants.[34] A more recent trial in former preterm infants assessed the effect of early postnatal caffeine exposure on sleep architecture and breathing patterns at 5 to 12 years of age. Although there were no differences between caffeine groups, approximately 10% of the infants had obstructive sleep apnea, again suggesting former preterm birth is a risk factor for sleep-disordered breathing in later childhood.[36]

Finally, IH may be one of many factors that contribute to growth trajectory in preterm infants. Data in neonatal rats have shown that IH induces both brain[37] and body[38] growth restrictions, which were followed by catch-up growth after a few weeks of recovery. Thus the effect of IH on growth restriction may be short term and reversible. In contrast, the effect of IH on cardiovascular control may be long-lasting and dependent on the pattern of IH exposure. For example, rat pups exposed to a clustered pattern of IH exhibited lower blood pressure that was sustained after 2 months of exposure. In contrast, an equally dispersed paradigm of IH had no effect on blood pressure.[38]

In summary, the potential consequences of apnea of prematurity are most likely associated with the accompanying fall in oxygenation. Pathologic cascades may be initiated by specific high-risk patterns of IH and have both short-term and long-lasting effects, including sleep-disordered breathing, growth restriction, retinopathy of prematurity, neurodevelopmental impairment, and alterations in cardiovascular regulation. Identification of high-risk patterns may provide insight on future intervention protocols in the NICU setting.

Mechanistic Insights Into Morbidity

Little information is known regarding the mechanism underlying morbidities associated with IH, although alterations in oxidative stress, inflammatory mediators, and trophic factors may be attributed to initiating a pathophysiologic cascade. Low levels of oxygenation alter transcriptional responses that are mediated by hypoxia-inducible factors (HIFs). In animal models, IH has been shown to initiate accumulation of HIF-1α[39,40] and reactive oxygen species generation[41] during the onset of reoxygenation. At the same time, IH exposure initiates degradation of HIF-2α and downregulation of superoxide dismutase.[40] The net result is overall prooxidant signaling leading to pathophysiology. These effects are supported by data in healthy volunteers demonstrating that CIH increases oxidative stress by increasing production of reactive oxygen species without a compensatory increase in antioxidant activity.[42] Future therapeutic interventions could include inhibition of oxidative stress associated with resolution of IH.

The increase in IH events during early postnatal life in extremely preterm infants may also play a role in enhancing inflammatory cytokine levels. In animal models IH initiates an inflammatory response during early postnatal life[43] with increments in tumor necrosis factor α, interleukin (IL)-8 and IL-6 from onset of IH exposure. Correspondingly, in ELBW infants recurrent or persistent elevations of serum inflammatory proteins during the first 2 weeks of life have been associated with attention deficit behavior at 2 years of age.[44] Therefore it is reasonable to suggest that IH during early postnatal life may play a role in the inflammatory response associated with later neurodevelopmental dysfunction. This may be one possible explanation why caffeine, a known antiinflammatory, improves the rate of survival of VLBW infants without neurodevelopmental impairment (NDI) at 18 to 21 months.[45]

Controversies in Therapy

There are various pharmacologic and nonpharmacologic therapies for apnea of prematurity. Therapies are initiated depending on variations in NICU clinical practice, nursing documentation of events, clinical status, and infant respiratory requirements. Some therapies are shown to be beneficial in larger trials; however, other treatments are controversial and require further investigation.

Accepted Treatments

Caffeine

Caffeine is the most common therapy used to treat apnea and intermittent hypoxemia. Caffeine and other methylxanthines have been prescribed in preterm infants for the past 40 years[46,47] and have been shown to reduce apnea and the need for ventilation.[48] In a recent study Rhein et al. demonstrated that caffeine therapy, administered to infants of 25 to 32 weeks' gestation, decreased the number of intermittent hypoxemic events and time with hypoxemia at 35 and 36 weeks' postmenstrual age.[49]

The largest trial of caffeine (Caffeine for Apnea of Prematurity Trial) randomly assigned 2006 infants with birth weights between 500 and 1250 g to caffeine or placebo in the first 10 days of life. Although apnea of prematurity was not measured in this clinical trial, caffeine administration was associated with a reduction in the duration of positive-pressure support, oxygen supplementation, and the incidence of bronchopulmonary dysplasia.[50] Caffeine also significantly improved survival without neurodevelopmental disability at 18 to 21 months, although the two treatment groups were no longer statistically different at 5 years of age.[45,51]

There are various pharmacologic effects of caffeine in apnea of prematurity. Most importantly, it stimulates the respiratory center in the brainstem and increases sensitivity to CO_2.[52] Mechanisms of action include blockade of adenosine A_1 and A_{2A} receptor subtypes resulting in excitation of respiration neural output.[53,54] Caffeine has also been shown to enhance peripheral chemoreceptor activation.[55] A loading dose of caffeine showed a rapid (within 5 min) and prolonged (2-hour) increase in diaphragmatic activity that was associated with an increase in tidal volume.[56] Lastly, caffeine may have antiinflammatory properties in the lung. For example, rat pups exposed prenatally to lipopolysaccharide had improved lung resistance and cytokine profiles after caffeine treatment.[57]

Optimal strategies of caffeine therapy have yet to be determined (Box 13.1). For example, common practice entails a caffeine citrate loading dose of 20 mg/kg followed by 5 to 10 mg/kg per day[45,50,51] with potential side effects including tachycardia, dysrhythmia, feeding intolerance, gastroesophageal reflux disease, jitteriness,

---

Box 13.1   CAFFEINE THERAPY CONTROVERSIES

Prophylactic versus therapeutic: Optimal onset of therapy?
Optimal maintenance dosing: Upper limit?
Role for additional loading dose?
Optimal duration of therapy: When to stop?
Mechanism of action: Optimizing respiratory control versus antiinflammatory?

---

irritability, or rarely observed seizures.[52] However, higher doses of 80 mg/kg have been associated with an increased incidence of cerebellar hemorrhage and should most likely be avoided.[58]

There have been no randomized control trials to address the optimal time to start or stop treatment with caffeine. The ideal time to start caffeine treatment has been examined by a few retrospective cohort studies. Early caffeine administration during the first 2 to 3 days of life was associated with reduction of bronchopulmonary dysplasia,[49,59,60] patent ductus arteriosus requiring treatment,[59–61] and duration of positive-pressure ventilation.[60] American Academy of Pediatrics guidelines suggest discontinuing caffeine when cardiorespiratory events are insignificant for 5 to 7 days or 33 to 34 weeks' postmenstrual age, whichever comes first.[53] However, it is important to realize that preterm infants born at very young gestational ages may continue to have apnea and intermittent hypoxemia events even beyond 33 to 34 weeks' postmenstrual age.[53]

Noninvasive Ventilation

Nasal continuous positive airway pressure (CPAP) is safe and effective and has a prominent role in treatment for apnea of prematurity. CPAP is a noninvasive form of applying constant distending pressure level during inhalation and exhalation. It supports infants who are spontaneously breathing but who have airway instability, pulmonary edema, and atelectasis.[62] CPAP enhances functional residual capacity, reduces work of breathing, and decreases mixed and obstructive apnea.[63–65]

There is considerable controversy regarding the best mode of CPAP delivery. This is further complicated by the various low- and high-flow cannulas that are widely used for CPAP delivery despite limited comparative studies. Refinement of techniques to both deliver CPAP and provide effective synchronized noninvasive ventilation may be the answer.

Oxygen Administration

As discussed earlier, centrally mediated hypoxic depression is prominent in early postnatal life. It follows that avoidance of hypoxemia should benefit apnea; additionally, hypoxia increases the pauses associated with periodic breathing. Earlier studies found that increases in the fraction of inspired oxygen (F_{IO_2}) decreased apnea of prematurity and periodic breathing.[66,67] More recent data demonstrated that targeting a lower baseline oxygen saturation (85%–89%) compared with higher oxygen saturation (91%–95%) was associated with an increased rate of intermittent hypoxemic events in preterm infants.[22] Because major complications of oxygen toxicity include retinopathy of prematurity and lung damage with resultant bronchopulmonary dysplasia, it is important to balance the level of supplemental oxygen with potential risks associated with oxygen.

Positioning

Earlier studies have demonstrated that prone positioning may stabilize the chest wall, improve oxygenation, and decrease apnea. Of course, this approach cannot occur close to discharge when prone positioning should be avoided. Excessive neck flexion clearly needs to be avoided to prevent upper airway obstruction. It is possible that there may be a modest benefit from a head elevated at a 15-degree tilt position.[68]

Controversial Approaches

Kangaroo Care

Multiple studies encompassing various age groups of premature infants have compared the effects of kangaroo care on decreasing apnea of prematurity and intermittent desaturation episodes. In one study, skin-to-skin care increased bradycardia and desaturation episodes.[69] However, in a separate study, no significant effects were found.[70] Therefore, although the use of skin-to-skin contact has benefits in newborn care, including bonding between mother and infant and improved breastfeeding, there is currently no known benefit for kangaroo care for the treatment of apnea of prematurity.

Blood Transfusions

There have been conflicting views regarding blood transfusions to reduce the incidence of apnea of prematurity. Zagol et al. found an association between blood transfusions and a decreased number of apnea/bradycardia/desaturation events in addition to a reduction of apneas at higher hematocrits.[71] In a separate randomized controlled trial, the frequency of apneas was twice as high in the restrictive-transfusion versus liberal-transfusion group.[72] For intubated infants, the hematocrit for which transfusion was indicated was less than 46% for the liberal-transfusion group, and less than 34% for the restricted-transfusion group. The threshold level was set at lower hematocrits in infants receiving noninvasive ventilation or breathing room air. In contrast, other studies have shown no significant difference in frequency of apnea,[73,74] bradycardia,[73] or hypoxemia.[73] Abu Jawdeh et al. showed that improvement in intermittent hypoxemic events occurs only after the first week of life, which may explain some of the discrepancy between studies.[75] Although the results among studies are conflicting, they do suggest that severe anemia may contribute to worsening of apnea of prematurity and an increase in hematocrit may protect against the desaturation that accompanies apnea. Additionally, it should be noted that blood transfusions have been associated with potentially more complications, including increased respiratory support after transfusions, necrotizing enterocolitis, and bronchopulmonary dysplasia.[74]

Mechanosensory Stimulation

Kinesthetic stimulation using oscillating mattresses for prevention of apnea has been proposed as a treatment for apnea of prematurity. In a meta-analysis that included 154 infants there was no clear evidence of effect of this therapy on apnea or bradycardia.[76] By contrast, in a more recent small-scale study of 10 preterm infants, stochastic (random) stimulation reduced desaturation episodes.[77] There may be a future for such novel modes of kinesthetic or related stimulation to improve respiratory drive.

Carbon Dioxide Therapy

As discussed earlier, neonates are vulnerable to apneic episodes owing to minor oscillations in breathing, which may bring eupneic partial pressure of carbon dioxide (P_{CO_2}) below the apneic threshold.[78] In a randomized, double-blinded, controlled trial including 87 premature infants (27–32 weeks' gestational age), very low supplemental CO_2 treatment decreased apnea time from baseline. However, theophylline was twice as effective as CO_2 treatment.[79] Hence, CO_2 therapy for apnea of prematurity cannot be routinely recommended, complicated in part by the fact that many preterm infants may already have baseline hypercapnia.

Doxapram

Doxapram stimulates peripheral and central chemoreceptors, which results in augmentation of breathing. Significant reductions in apnea have been shown with increasing dose of doxapram. However, higher doses have been accompanied by elevations in blood pressure,[80] and prolonged use in the neonatal period has been associated with an adverse Mental Developmental Index in infants with birth weights less than 1250 g.[81] In the Caffeine for Apnea of Prematurity Trial, infants in the placebo group were more likely to develop cerebral palsy than those in the caffeine group; however, in the placebo group infants were three times more likely to receive doxapram.[45] Because of the possibility of long-term adverse effects of doxapram, this therapy has limited appeal.

Discharge Practice

There is virtually no evidence for practice regarding discharge decisions for infants who have apnea of prematurity. It is known that infants born at a younger gestational age have delayed resolution of apnea and bradycardia events. In a retrospective cohort study that included 1400 infants at 34 weeks' gestation or earlier, a 5- to 7-day apnea/bradycardia-free interval had a success rate between 94% and 96% of predicting no events after discharge. Success rates were dependent on the gestational age and postmenstrual age of the infant.[82] In most NICU settings, an apnea event-free period before discharge of 5 to 7 days is commonly used.[53] Often this is based on nursing observation and monitor alarm thresholds for recording of apnea and bradycardia events. Preterm infants have clinically undetected apnea events that may not be apparent unless continuous electronic recording is investigated. However, there is no evidence that they predict acute life-threatening events.[20] At this time, routine home monitoring for resolved apnea of prematurity is not recommended,[53] although this is an option for selected infants who are sent home while using oxygen or have certain congenital disorders requiring frequent monitoring.

REFERENCES

1. Stryker CC, Dylag A, Martin RJ. Apnea and control of breathing. In: Jobe AH, Whitsett JA, Abman SH, eds. *Fetal and Neonatal Lung Development: Clinical Correlates and Technologies for the Future.* New York: Cambridge University Press; 2016:chap 12.
2. Gauda EB, Martin RJ. Control of breathing. In: Gleason C, ed. *Avery's Diseases of the Newborn.* 9th ed. Philaldelphia: Elsevier; 2016:chap 43.
3. Mayer CA, Haxhiu MA, Martin RJ, et al. Adenosine A_{2A} receptors mediate GABAergic inhibition of respiration in immature rats. *J Appl Physiol.* 2006;100:91–97.
4. Kinney HC, Broadbelt KG, Haynes RL, et al. The serotonergic anatomy of the developing human medulla oblongata: implications for pediatric disorders of homeostasis. *J Chem Neuroanat.* 2011;41:182–199.
5. Gerhardt T, Bancalari E. Apnea of prematurity. I. Lung function and regulation of breathing. *Pediatrics.* 1984;74:58–62.
6. Martin RJ. Pathophysiology of apnea of prematurity. In: Polin RA, Abman SH, Rowitch DH, Benitz WE, Fox WW, eds. *Fetal & Neonatal Physiology.* 5th ed. Philadelphia: Elsevier; 2016:chap 157.
7. Cardot V, Chardon K, Tourneux P, et al. Ventilatory response to a hyperoxic test is related to the frequency of short apneic episodes in late preterm neonates. *Pediatr Res.* 2007;62:591–596.
8. Nock ML, Di Fiore JM, Arko MK, et al. Relationship of the ventilatory response to hypoxia with neonatal apnea in preterm infants. *J Pediatr.* 2004;144:291–295.
9. Patel M, Mohr M, Lake D, et al. Clinical associations with immature breathing in preterm infants: part 2—periodic breathing. *Pediatr Res.* 2016;80:28–34.
10. Khan A, Qurashi M, Kwiatkowski K, et al. Measurement of the CO_2 apneic threshold in newborn infants: possible relevance for periodic breathing and apnea. *J Appl Physiol.* 2005;98:1171–1176.
11. Al-Matary A, Kutbi I, Qurashi M, et al. Increased peripheral chemoreceptor activity may be critical in destabilizing breathing in neonates. *Semin Perinatol.* 2004;28:264–272.
12. Hofstetter AO, Saha S, Silijehav V, et al. The induced prostaglandin E2 pathway is a key regulator of the respiratory response to infection and hypoxia in neonates. *Proc Natl Acad Sci U S A.* 2007;104:9894–9899.
13. Balan KV, Kc P, Hoxha Z, et al. Vagal afferents modulate cytokine-mediated respiratory control at the neonatal medulla oblongata. *Respir Physiol Neurobiol.* 2011;178:458–464.
14. Di Fiore JM, Arko MK, Miller MJ, et al. Cardiorespiratory events in preterm infants referred for apnea monitoring studies. *Pediatrics.* 2001;108:1304–1308.
15. Finer NN, Higgins R, Kattwinkel J, Martin RJ. Summary proceedings from the apnea-of-prematurity group. *Pediatrics.* 2006;117:S47–S51.
16. Barrington KJ, Finer NN. Periodic breathing and apnea in preterm infants. *Pediatr Res.* 1990;27:118–121.
17. Gauda EB, Miller MJ, Carlo WA, Di Fiore JM, Johnsen DC, Martin RJ. Genioglossus response to airway occlusion in apneic versus nonapneic infants. *Pediatr Res.* 1987;22:683–687.
18. Lemke RP, Idiong N, Al-Saedi S, Kwiatkowski K, Cates DB, Rigatto H. Evidence of a critical period of airway instability during central apneas in preterm infants. *Am J Respir Crit Care Med.* 1998;157:470–474.
19. Brockmann PE, Wiechers C, Pantalitschka T, Diebold J, Vagedes J, Poets CF. Under-recognition of alarms in a neonatal intensive care unit. *Arch Dis Child Fetal Neonatal Ed.* 2013;98:F524–F527.

20. Barrington KJ, Finer N, Li D. Predischarge respiratory recordings in very low birth weight newborn infants. *J Pediatr.* 1996;129:934–940.
21. Fairchild K, Mohr M, Paget-Brown A, et al. Clinical associations of immature breathing in preterm infants: part 1—central apnea. *Pediatr Res* 2016;80:21–27.
22. Di Fiore JM, Walsh M, Wrage L, et al. Low oxygen saturation target range is associated with increased incidence of intermittent hypoxemia. *J Pediatr.* 2012;161:1047–1052.
23. Sands SA, Edwards BA, Kelly VJ, et al. Mechanism underlying accelerated arterial oxygen desaturation during recurrent apnea. *Am J Respir Crit Care Med.* 2010;182:961–969.
24. Di Fiore JM, Bloom JN, Orge F, et al. A higher incidence of intermittent hypoxemic episodes is associated with severe retinopathy of prematurity. *J Pediatr.* 2010;157:69–73.
25. Pillekamp F, Hermann C, Keller T, von Gontard A, Kribs A, Roth B. Factors influencing apnea and bradycardia of prematurity—implications for neurodevelopment. *Neonatology.* 2007;91:155–161.
26. Janvier A, Khairy M, Kokkotis A, Cormier C, Messmer D, Barrington KJ. Apnea is associated with neurodevelopmental impairment in very low birth weight infants. *J Perinatol.* 2004;24:763–768.
27. Cheung PY, Barrington KJ, Finer NN, Robertson CM. Early childhood neurodevelopment in very low birth weight infants with predischarge apnea. *Pediatr Pulmonol.* 1999;27:14–20.
28. Taylor HG, Klein N, Schatschneider C, Hack M. Predictors of early school age outcomes in very low birth weight children. *J Dev Behav Pediatr.* 1998;19:235–243.
29. Di Fiore JM, Kaffashi F, Loparo K, et al. The relationship between patterns of intermittent hypoxia and retinopathy of prematurity in preterm infants. *Pediatr Res.* 2012;72:606–612.
30. Poets CF, Roberts RS, Schmidt B, et al. Association between intermittent hypoxemia or bradycardia and late death or disability in extremely preterm infants. *JAMA.* 2015;314:595–603.
31. Ratner V, Kishkurno SV, Slinko SK, et al. The contribution of intermittent hypoxemia to late neurological handicap in mice with hyperoxia-induced lung injury. *Neonatology.* 2007;92:50–58.
32. Decker MJ, Jones KA, Solomon IG, Keating GL, Rye DB. Reduced extracellular dopamine and increased responsiveness to novelty: neurochemical and behavioral sequelae of intermittent hypoxia. *Sleep.* 2005;28:169–176.
33. Paavonen EJ, Strang-Karlsson S, Raikkonen K, et al. Very low birth weight increases risk for sleep-disordered breathing in young adulthood: the Helsinki study of very low birth weight adults. *Pediatrics.* 2007;120:778–784.
34. Rosen CL, Larkin EK, Kirchner HL, et al. Prevalence and risk factors for sleep-disordered breathing in 8- to 11-year-old children: association with race and prematurity. *J Pediatr.* 2003;142:383–389.
35. Reeves SR, Gozal D. Respiratory and metabolic responses to early postnatal chronic intermittent hypoxia and sustained hypoxia in the developing rat. *Pediatr Res.* 2006;60:680–686.
36. Marcus CL, Meltzer LJ, Roberts RS, et al. Long-term effects of caffeine therapy for apnea of prematurity on sleep at school age. *Am J Respir Crit Care Med.* 2014;190:791–799.
37. Kanaan A, Farahani R, Douglas RM, Lamanna JC, Haddad GG. Effect of chronic continuous or intermittent hypoxia and reoxygenation on cerebral capillary density and myelination. *Am J Physiol Regul Integr Comp Physiol.* 2006;290:R1105–R1114.
38. Pozo ME, Cave A, Köroğlu OA, et al. Effect of postnatal intermittent hypoxia on growth and cardiovascular regulation of rat pups. *Neonatology.* 2012;102:107–113.
39. Yuan G, Nanduri J, Khan S, Semenza GL, Prabhakar NR. Induction of HIF-1α expression by intermittent hypoxia: involvement of NADPH oxidase, Ca^{2+} signaling, prolyl hydroxylases, and mTOR. *J Cell Physiol.* 2008;217:674–685.
40. Nanduri J, Wang N, Yuan G, et al. Intermittent hypoxia degrades HIF-2α via calpains resulting in oxidative stress: implications for recurrent apnea-induced morbidities. *Proc Natl Acad Sci U S A.* 2009;106:1199–1204.
41. Fabian RH, Perez-Polo JR, Kent TA. Extracellular superoxide concentration increases following cerebral hypoxia but does not affect cerebral blood flow. *Int J Dev Neurosci.* 2004;22:225–230.
42. Pialoux V, Hanly PJ, Foster GE, et al. Effects of exposure to intermittent hypoxia on oxidative stress and acute hypoxic ventilatory response in humans. *Am J Respir Crit Care Med.* 2009;180:1002–1009.
43. Li S, Qian XH, Zhou W, et al. Time-dependent inflammatory factor production and NFκB activation in a rodent model of intermittent hypoxia. *Swiss Med Wkly.* 2011;141:w13309.
44. O'Shea TM, Joseph RM, Kuban KC, et al. Elevated blood levels of inflammation-related proteins are associated with an attention problem at age 24 mo in extremely preterm infants. *Pediatr Res.* 2014;75:781–787.
45. Schmidt B, Roberts RS, Davis P, et al. Long-term effects of caffeine therapy for apnea of prematurity. *N Engl J Med.* 2007;357:1893–1902.
46. Kuzemko JA, Paala J. Apnoeic attacks in the newborn treated with aminophylline. *Arch Dis Child.* 1973;48:404–406.
47. Aranda JV, Gorman W, Bergsteinsson H, Gunn T. Efficacy of caffeine in treatment of apnea in the low-birth-weight infant. *J Pediatr.* 1977;90:467–472.
48. Henderson-Smart DJ, Steer P. Methylxanthine treatment for apnea in preterm infants. *Cochrane Database Syst Rev.* 2000;(2).
49. Rhein LM, Dobson NR, Darnall RA, et al. Effects of caffeine on intermittent hypoxia in infants born prematurely. *JAMA Pediatr.* 2014;4799:1–8.
50. Schmidt B, Roberts RS, Davis P, et al. Caffeine therapy for apnea of prematurity. *NEJM.* 2006;354:2112–2121.
51. Schmidt B, Anderson PJ, Doyle LW, et al. Survival without disability to age 5 years after neonatal caffeine therapy for apnea of prematurity. *JAMA.* 2012;307:275–282.

52. Abdel-Hady H, Nasef N, Shabaan AE, Nour I. Caffeine therapy in preterm infants. *World J Clin Pediatr.* 2015;4:81–93.
53. Eichenwald EC. Apnea of prematurity. *Pediatrics.* 2016;137:e20153757.
54. Wilson CG, Martin RJ, Jaber M, et al. Adenosine A2A receptors interact with GABAergic pathways to modulate respiration in neonatal piglets. *Respir Physiol Neurobiol.* 2004;141:201–211.
55. Chardon K, Bach V, Telliez F, et al. Effect of caffeine on peripheral chemoreceptor activity in premature neonates: interaction with sleep stages. *J Appl Physiol.* 2004;96:2161–2166.
56. Kraaijenga JV, Hutten GJ, De Jongh FH, Van Kaam AH. The effect of caffeine on diaphragmatic activity and tidal volume in preterm infants. *J Pediatr.* 2015;167:70–75.
57. Köroğlu ÖA, MacFarlane PM, Balan KV, Zenebe WJ, Martin RJ, Kc P. Anti-inflammatory effect of caffeine is associated with improved lung function after lipopolysaccharide-induced amnionitis. *Neonatology.* 2014;106:235–240.
58. McPherson C, Neil JJ, Tjoeng TH, Pineda R, Inder TE. A pilot randomized trial of high-dose caffeine therapy in preterm infants. *Pediatr Res.* 2015;78:198–204.
59. Lodha A, Seshia M, McMillan DD, et al. Association of early caffeine administration and neonatal outcomes in very preterm neonates. *JAMA Pediatr.* 2015;169:33–38.
60. Dobson NR, Patel RM, Smith PB, et al. Trends in caffeine use and association between clinical outcomes and timing of therapy in very low birth weight infants. *J Pediatr.* 2014;164:992–998.
61. Patel RM, Leong T, Carlton DP, Vyas-Read S. Early caffeine therapy and clinical outcomes in extremely preterm infants. *J Perinatol.* 2013;33:134–140.
62. Diblasi RM. Nasal continuous positive airway pressure [CPAP] for the respiratory care of the newborn infant. *Respir Care.* 2009;54:1209–1235.
63. Pantalitschka T, Sievers J, Urschitz MS, Herberts T, Reher C, Poets CF. Randomised crossover trial of four nasal respiratory support systems for apnoea of prematurity in very low birthweight infants. *Arch Dis Child Fetal Neonatal Ed.* 2009;94:F245–F248.
64. Millar D, Kirpalani H. Benefits of non invasive ventilation. *Indian Pediatrics.* 2004;41:1008–1017.
65. Zhao J, Gonzalez F, Mu D. Apnea of prematurity: from cause to treatment. *Euro J Pediatr.* 2011;170:1097–1105.
66. Weintraub Z, Alvaro R, Kwiatkowski K, Cates D, Rigatto H. Effects of inhaled oxygen (up to 40%) on periodic breathing and apnea in preterm infants. *J Appl Physiol.* 1992;72:116–120.
67. Simakajornboon N, Beckerman RC, Mack C, Sharon D, Gozal D. Effect of supplemental oxygen on sleep architecture and cardiorespiratory events in preterm infants. *Pediatrics.* 2002;110:884–888.
68. Di Fiore JM, Poets CF, Gauda E, Martin RJ, MacFarlane P. Cardiorespiratory events in preterm infants: etiology and monitoring technologies. *J Perinatol.* 2015;36:1–8.
69. Bohnhorst B, Gill D, Dördelmann M, Peter CS, Poets CF. Bradycardia and desaturation during skin-to-skin care: no relationship to hyperthermia. *J Pediatr.* 2004;145:499–502.
70. Heimann K, Vaessen P, Peschgens T, Stanzel S, Wenzl TG, Orlikowsky T. Impact of skin to skin care, prone and supine positioning on cardiorespiratory parameters and thermoregulation in premature infants. *Neonatology.* 2010;97:311–317.
71. Zagol K, Lake DE, Vergales B, et al. Anemia, apnea of prematurity, and blood transfusions. *J Pediatr.* 2012;161:417–421.
72. Bell EF. Randomized trial of liberal versus restrictive guidelines for red blood cell transfusion in preterm infants. *Pediatrics.* 2005;115:1685–1691.
73. Poets CF, Pauls U, Bohnhorst B. Effect of blood transfusion on apnoea, bradycardia and hypoxaemia in preterm infants. *Eur J Pediatr.* 1997;156:311–316.
74. Valieva OA, Strandjord TP, Mayock DE, Sandra E. Effects of transfusions in extremely low birth weight infants: a retrospective study. *J Pediatr.* 2009;155:331–337.
75. Abu Jawdeh EG, Martin RJ, Dick TE, Walsh MC, Di Fiore JM. The effect of red blood cell transfusion on intermittent hypoxemia in ELBW infants. *J Perinatol.* 2014;34:921–925.
76. Osborn DA, Henderson-Smart DJ. Kinesthetic stimulation versus theophylline for apnea in preterm infants. *Cochrane Database Syst Rev.* 2000;2.
77. Bloch-Salisbury E, Indic P, Bednarek F, Paydarfar D. Stabilizing immature breathing patterns of preterm infants using stochastic mechanosensory stimulation. *J Appl Physiol.* 2009;107:1017–1027.
78. Khan A, Qurashi M, Kwiatkowski K, Cates D, Rigatto H. Measurement of the CO_2 apneic threshold in newborn infants: possible relevance for periodic breathing and apnea. *J Appl Physiol.* 2005;98:1171–1176.
79. Alvaro RE, Khalil M, Qurashi M, et al. CO_2 inhalation as a treatment for apnea of prematurity: a randomized double-blind controlled trial. *J Pediatrs.* 2012;160:252–257.
80. Barrington KJ, Finer NN, Torok-Both G, Jamali F, Coutts RT. Dose-response relationship of doxapram in the therapy for refractory idiopathic apnea of prematurity. *Pediatrics.* 1987;80:22–27.
81. Sreenan C, Etches PC, Demianczuk N, Robertson CMT. Isolated mental developmental delay in very low birth weight infants: association with prolonged doxapram therapy for apnea. *J Pediatr.* 2001;139:832–837.
82. Lorch SA, Srinivasan L, Escobar GJ. Epidemiology of apnea and bradycardia resolution in premature infants. *Pediatrics.* 2011;128:e366–e373.

13

CHAPTER 14

Oxygenation Instability in the Premature Infant

Nelson Claure, Richard J. Martin, Juliann M. Di Fiore, and
Eduardo Bancalari

14

- Premature infants present with frequent episodes of spontaneous intermittent hypoxemia. These episodes are more prevalent in infants who require prolonged mechanical ventilation.

- A common mechanism triggering intermittent hypoxemia is contractions of the abdominal muscles that splint the respiratory system, resulting in decreased lung volume, impaired lung mechanics, and hypoventilation.

- Episodes of intermittent hypoxemia are often followed by hyperoxemia induced by excessive oxygen supplementation used to prevent or correct the episodes.

- Because of the frequency and severity of intermittent hypoxemia, it can have detrimental effects on long-term outcome.

- The mechanisms and consequences of intermittent hypoxemia need to be further investigated to identify effective therapeutic and preventive strategies.

As a consequence of their respiratory instability, premature infants experience frequent fluctuations in oxygenation and intermittent hypoxemia (IH) episodes. These episodes can be induced, but most are spontaneous and their severity and duration can be influenced by staff responsiveness. Premature infants who show fluctuations in arterial oxygen saturation as measured by pulse oximetry (Spo_2) require frequent adjustment to the fraction of inspired oxygen (Fio_2). However, maintenance of Spo_2 within the prescribed range is not always achieved, and infants can spend considerable time with Spo_2 below or above this range.

This chapter describes the mechanisms leading to fluctuations in oxygenation, discusses the management strategies used to prevent or attenuate these fluctuations, and provides an overview of the possible long-term consequences of oxygenation instability in the premature infant.

Mechanisms of Oxygenation Instability in Ventilated Infants

Most preterm infants receiving mechanical ventilation present with respiratory instability that make them susceptible to IH. These episodes of IH can complicate the respiratory management and prolong the need for respiratory support and oxygen supplementation, both of which may be associated with long-term sequelae. The mechanisms leading to IH, their clinical management, and possible consequences are discussed in the following sections.

Episodic hypoxemia in neonates has been traditionally attributed to hypoventilation owing to central or obstructive apnea, but these mechanisms mainly apply to spontaneously breathing infants. Most extremely premature infants present with

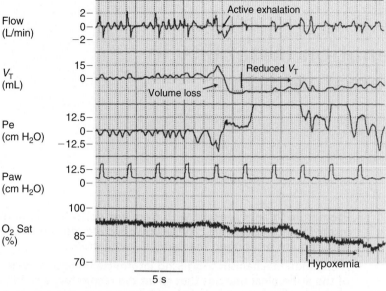

Fig. 14.1 Mechanism triggering an episode of hypoxemia in a ventilated infant. Recordings of flow, tidal volume (V_T), esophageal pressure (Pe), airway pressure (Paw), and oxygen (O_2) saturation (Spo_2) illustrate the mechanism triggering hypoxemia. At first, an active exhalation produces an increase in intrathoracic pressure and a loss in end-expiratory lung volume that is followed by a period of reduced V_T despite continuous cycling of the ventilator. This results in a decline in Spo_2 and hypoxemia. (From Bolivar JM, Gerhardt T, Gonzalez A, et al. Mechanisms for episodes of hypoxemia in preterm infants undergoing mechanical ventilation. *J Pediatr.* 1995:127:767–773.)

an increasing frequency of IH after the first weeks after birth while they still require mechanical ventilation and supplemental oxygen. The occurrence of spontaneous IH in mechanically ventilated infants is often perplexing because they occur despite continued cycling of the ventilator and patency of the airway. These episodes of hypoxemia are characterized by a rapid decline in Spo_2 that become more frequent with advancing postnatal age.[1–3]

One of the most common mechanisms leading to spontaneous IH in mechanically ventilated preterm infants are forced exhalations secondary to contractions of the abdominal musculature that impinge on the respiratory system and impair respiratory mechanics. The resultant decrease in lung volume and hypoventilation cause hypoxemia that becomes more severe and persistent with successive abdominal contractions.[4–6] This is illustrated in Fig. 14.1.

Electromyographic measurements show that these forced exhalations are caused by contractions of the abdominal muscles that produce a marked increase in abdominal and intrathoracic pressure, some in excess of 25 cm H_2O.[6] As shown in Fig. 14.2, repeated contractions of the abdominal muscles can prolong the episodes and increase their severity. It is important to note that in ventilated infants, the endotracheal tube bypasses the glottis and eliminates the protective upper airway's function to preserve lung volume during the rise in intrathoracic pressure.

The factors that elicit these forced exhalations leading to loss in lung volume and hypoventilation with hypoxemia have not been clearly defined. However, behavioral disturbances appear to trigger IH. Increased body activity, agitation, squirming, and tachycardia are frequently present moments before the onset of the episodes.[5] Intermittent hypoxia is observed more frequently during awake or indeterminate sleep states than during quiet or active sleep.[7] These observations are important because indeterminate sleep is the most common sleep state in preterm infants. The prone position has also been associated with fewer and shorter IH episodes compared with the supine position.[8,9]

The combination of increased activity leading to ventilation changes and poor lung function owing to the underlying lung disease may aggravate the frequency and severity of IH. In addition, the low functional residual capacity and decreased lung

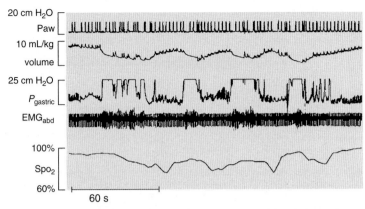

Fig. 14.2 Episode of hypoxemia associated with multiple contractions of the abdominal muscles. The recording shows repeated contractions of the abdominal muscles detected by abdominal electromyography (*EMG*$_{abd}$) producing increases in gastric pressure (*P*$_{gastric}$). Each contraction is associated with a decline in end-expiratory lung volume and an acute reduction in tidal volume despite continuous cycling of the ventilator followed by a progressive decline in oxygen saturation (*Spo*$_2$). *Paw*, Airway pressure; *s*, seconds. (From Esquer C, Claure N, D'Ugard C, et al. Role of abdominal muscles activity on duration and severity of hypoxemia episodes in mechanically ventilated preterm infants. *Neonatology.* 2007;92:182–186.)

compliance characteristic of these infants, combined with bypassing of the glottis by the endotracheal tube, may increase the likelihood of reaching closing volume in some areas of the lung with even small decreases in lung volume.

The decline in Spo$_2$ during these episodes of hypoxemia is more abrupt than what is expected from a decline in ventilation alone and often persists after ventilation has been reestablished.[5] This observation suggests that the initial loss in lung volume and hypoventilation may produce ventilation-perfusion inequalities and some degree of intrapulmonary shunting, thereby causing a rapid decline in Spo$_2$. The onset of hypoxemia can also provoke an increase in pulmonary vascular resistance and induce right-to-left shunting through extrapulmonary channels. These circulatory changes can explain why episodes of IH are observed more frequently in infants with chronic lung disease and increased pulmonary vascular reactivity. In many of these infants, normoxemia is restored only after the fraction of inspired oxygen (F$_{IO_2}$) is increased, which may restore oxygenation not only by increasing the alveolar-capillary oxygen gradient but also by attenuating the hypoxia-induced pulmonary vasoconstriction.

Oxygenation Instability in Spontaneously Breathing Infants After Mechanical Ventilation

Episodes of hypoxemia are frequently observed in premature infants after extubation while the infants are receiving noninvasive respiratory support or breathing spontaneously. IH during this period have been mainly attributed to central or mixed apnea. However, a study showed that most IH in spontaneously breathing preterm infants after a prolonged course of ventilation may also be caused by episodes of forced exhalation, which induce a decline in lung volume and hypoventilation[10] similar to the IH observed in intubated infants (Fig. 14.3). In this study almost all infants were receiving caffeine. Hence, it is possible that use of stimulants after extubation may have decreased the proportion of IH caused by central apnea during the postextubation period. It is also possible that preterm infants after prolonged mechanical ventilation may be more susceptible to lung volume instability because the prolonged presence of the endotracheal tube may impair the upper airway's ability to preserve lung volume. The extent to which this contributes to extubation failure remains to be determined. (Oxygenation instability in spontaneously breathing infants resulting from central and obstructive apnea is discussed in Chapter 13.)

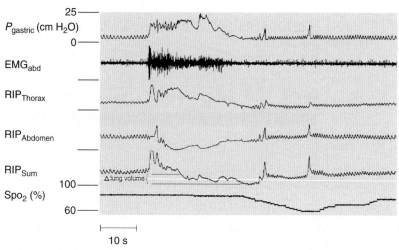

Fig. 14.3 Mechanism triggering an episode of hypoxemia in a preterm infant after extubation. The recording from an infant breathing spontaneously shows a contraction of the abdominal muscles (recorded by abdominal electromyography [EMG_{abd}]) that produced an increase in gastric pressure ($P_{gastric}$). This was associated with a decline in the abdominal volume (measured by respiratory inductance plethysmography [$RIP_{Abdomen}$]) that coincided with an initial increase in thoracic volume (RIP_{Thorax}). After these events, a decrease in end-expiratory lung volume was noticed in the sum signal of the thoracic and abdominal RIP bands (RIP_{Sum}) and a brief absence of spontaneous breathing. This was followed by a decline in oxygen saturation (Spo_2) that persisted for some time despite resumption of spontaneous breathing. s, seconds. (From Esquer C, Claure N, D'Ugard C, et al. Mechanisms of hypoxemia episodes in spontaneously breathing preterm infants after mechanical ventilation. *Neonatology*. 2008;94:100–104.)

Management of Oxygenation Instability

Ventilatory Strategies

To reduce the frequency, severity, or duration of IH, clinicians often resort to higher levels of mechanical respiratory support. However, this may be of limited efficacy and can lead to unwanted consequences. A high positive end-expiratory pressure (PEEP) may increase lung volume and increase basal oxygenation levels, but this maneuver may be only partially effective in preventing IH caused by active exhalations. This is because the rise in intrathoracic pressure during forceful contraction of the abdominal muscles exceeds the level of positive end-expiratory pressure considerably. Higher peak inspiratory pressure (PIP) or ventilator frequency can be effective in attenuating IH, but this strategy provides excessive support during periods when the infant is not presenting with episodic hypoxemia. Improving infant-ventilator interaction by using synchronized ventilation has been shown to reduce IH in preterm infants.[11]

Volume-targeted ventilation (VTV) automatically adjusts the ventilator PIP to maintain a set tidal volume (V_T). The efficacy of VTV in attenuating the decrease in V_T and minute ventilation that precedes each episode of hypoxemia was evaluated in preterm infants with frequent IH. In these studies, VTV attenuated the decrease in ventilation and the severity and duration of the episodes of IH compared with conventional pressure-controlled (PC) ventilation but failed to prevent them.[12-14] However, this required setting a target V_T that was larger than the V_T delivered during PC ventilation, possibly exposing the infants to excessive V_T and PIP during periods when ventilation was stable. In a recent study matching the target V_T during VTV to that during PC ventilation, VTV reduced the duration of episodes of IH and the F_{IO_2} provided by the caregivers in response to these episodes. The limited effectiveness of VTV is likely because infants continue to increase intrathoracic pressure and reduce their lung volume despite the continuous cycling of the ventilator. Fig. 14.4 shows VTV adjustments in PIP during an episode of hypoxemia.

Automatic increases in ventilator frequency when minute ventilation or Spo_2 declines are effective in reducing the duration but not the frequency of IH.[15,16] The parallel increase in ventilator frequency and PIP, to maintain minute ventilation and V_T, respectively, was more effective in reducing the duration and severity of IH in an animal model.[17] This approach has not been evaluated in infants.

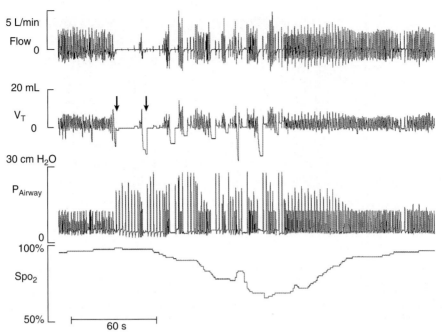

Fig. 14.4 Recordings of flow, tidal volume (V_T), airway pressure (P_{Airway}), and oxygen saturation (Spo_2) during volume guarantee ventilation. Active exhalations that decrease lung volume are marked by *arrows*. A period of reduced V_T precedes the decline in Spo_2. Active exhalations continue to occur during the episode. Peak inspiratory pressure is automatically increased in response to the decline in V_T. Resumption of spontaneous breathing and cessation of active exhalations lead to reestablishment of V_T and resolution of the hypoxemia episode. (From Jain D, Claure N, D'Ugard C, et al. Volume guarantee ventilation: effect on preterm infants with frequent hypoxemia episodes. *Neonatology.* 2016;110:129–134.)

Supplemental Oxygen

The goal of oxygen supplementation in preterm infants is to maintain adequate oxygenation while minimizing hyperoxemia and oxygen exposure. However, this is complicated by fluctuations in oxygenation. Fio_2 is adjusted to maintain Spo_2 within a target range and avoid exposure to high and low Spo_2, but this is only partially achieved during routine care. Data from 14 centers showed that in preterm infants receiving supplemental oxygen the Spo_2 was within the target range only 48% of the time.[18,19] These data showed preterm infants spend 16% of the time below the target range (0%–47% between centers).[18] This is mainly due to IH episodes that are predominantly spontaneous but with a duration and severity that can be influenced by staff responsiveness. In these infants Spo_2 was above the target for 36% of the time (5%–90% between centers); which is almost always induced by provision of an Fio_2 that exceeds that required to maintain Spo_2 within target. This is frequently done in an attempt to avert IH, whereas in other cases the staff increases Fio_2 in response to a hypoxemia alarm but often Fio_2 is not promptly returned to baseline after the episode resolves.[20] As shown in Fig. 14.5, high basal levels of Spo_2 can attenuate the frequency or severity of IH, but this increases the exposure to high Fio_2 and hyperoxemia.

Many factors contribute to the premature infant's oxygenation instability. Fluctuations in Spo_2 increase with postnatal age and with progressing chronic lung disease.[1-3] In preterm infants the stability of oxygenation is also influenced by the target range of Spo_2. A relatively small change in the target range from 90% to 95% to 88% to 94% doubled the proportion of time with Spo_2 less than 80% (from 1.9% to 4.0%).[21] This was also observed in a study where targeting Spo_2 between 87% to 91% compared with 94% to 96% increased the proportion of time with Spo_2 less than 85% (from 1% to 17%).[22] These findings are in

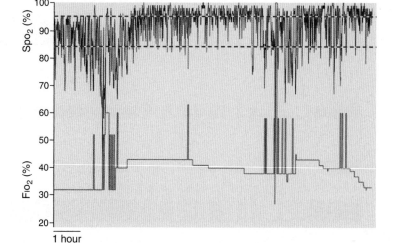

Fig. 14.5 Changes in baseline fraction of inspired oxygen *(FIO₂)* in a ventilated infant with frequent episodes of hypoxemia. The recording from an infant with frequent episodes of hypoxemia shows the response of the caregiver, who first increased FIO₂ transiently when oxygen saturation *(SpO₂)* decreased *(lower dashed red line)*. Subsequently, the persistent increase in the baseline FIO₂ reduced the severity of the fluctuations but also led to hyperoxemia *(upper dashed red line)*. Late, the severity of the IH episodes increased despite the higher baseline FIO₂.

agreement with data from the SUPPORT trial, which showed the frequency of IH was higher among infants assigned to the 85% to 89% compared with the 91% to 95% target range.[23]

Limited staff availability can further compromise SpO₂ targeting during routine clinical care.[19,24] The proportion of time with SpO₂ within the target range declined with a lower nurse-to-patient ratio (38% with 1:1 to 15% with 1:3 or lower nurse-to-patient ratio). This was mainly due to an increased time spent with SpO₂ greater than 97% (from 8% to 37%).[24] Gaps between unit policies and clinical practice can also contribute to the poor maintenance of SpO₂ ranges in the neonatal intensive care unit.[25,26] Education of the clinical staff increases the proportion of time with SpO₂ within the target range (from 20% to 40%).[26] This mainly resulted from a reduced proportion of time with SpO₂ above range (from 78% to 37%), but the unintended effect of this approach was an increased proportion of time with SpO₂ less than 85% (from 1% to 13%).

Studies have evaluated the use of systems that automatically adjust FIO₂ in preterm infants with oxygenation instability.[27–33] Although automatic FIO₂ control is more effective than the clinical staff or a fully dedicated nurse in maintaining SpO₂ within the target range, it did not abolish IH. The reason is that these systems are designed to respond to IH episodes and attenuate their severity and duration but not prevent their occurrence. Automatic FIO₂ control was more effective in reducing the most severe and prolonged episodes, but in some of these studies the frequency of brief episodes of hypoxemia was higher during automatic compared with manual FIO₂ control. This is likely due to the maintenance of high basal SpO₂ levels during routine care in an attempt to prevent IH.

Reducing Environmental Disturbances

None of the strategies mentioned previously has been shown effective in totally preventing spontaneous IH in premature infants. The reason may be that the primary trigger of these episodes in the intubated infant is more related to factors that affect the infant's behavior. Observations of less hypoxemia during the night and during periods of sleep suggest the potential benefits of strategies to reduce behavioral disturbances, facilitate sleep, and promote spontaneous respiratory stability in preterm infants who exhibit frequent IH.

Consequences of Oxygenation Instability

The short- and long-term consequences of episodic hypoxemia in the preterm infant are often subject of controversy (see also Chapter 13). Concerns regarding the deleterious effects of IH are confounded by the fact that IH is more frequently observed in infants with a more complicated respiratory course who also present with other morbidities that are independently associated with poor outcome.

Some data show that IH episodes are associated with changes in brain oxygenation.[34-39] Frequent episodes of severe hypoxemia or bradycardia may affect brain tissue oxygenation and possibly induce reoxygenation injury and oxidative damage, effects similar to those observed in animal studies of intermittent hypoxia.[40,41]

Experimental animal data have shown that exposure to intermittent hypoxia during the early postnatal period can alter the maturation of the respiratory control system,[42-44] possibly mediated by attenuated peripheral chemosensitivity, leading to more respiratory instability and apnea.[44] Early postnatal exposure to intermittent hypoxia can alter the mechanism of autoresuscitation,[44,45] which may explain the ineffective autoresuscitation described in premature infants with BPD.[46]

Although the long-term neurologic effects of IH in the preterm infant have not been clearly established, motor delays and lower mental development quotients have been reported in infants with persistent and frequent apnea and IH.[47-51] Episodes of IH caused by active exhalation produced by contraction of the abdominal muscles in premature infants during the postextubation period are often more severe than episodes associated with apnea.[10,17] Hence, they may have more striking effects on the central nervous system.

IH is common in preterm infants with underlying lung and central nervous system diseases; therefore, it is difficult to determine a causal relation between IH and brain injury. Nonetheless, a recent post hoc analysis of the Canadian Oxygen Trial revealed a strong association between prolonged episodes of IH with neurodevelopmental impairment at 18 months corrected age.[52] This was particularly evident for those episodes lasting 60 seconds or longer.

In animal models of retinopathy of prematurity, fluctuations in oxygenation have been linked to abnormal retinal vasculature development, and more so when fluctuations involved swings into hyperoxia and hypoxia.[52-60] Infants with severe retinopathy of prematurity have more IH, especially beyond postnatal week 4 and with episodes whose durations exceed 60 seconds.[61]

Persistence of IH over long periods may also have deleterious effects on lung development and function with increased airway and vasculature reactivity.[62-64] These effects may be compounded by the increased exposure to supplemental oxygen used to treat or prevent them. In animal models, intermittent hyperoxia-hypoxia led to abnormal development of alveoli and lung vasculature.[65]

Summary

Oxygenation instability is very common in the premature infant. This instability is manifested as episodic hypoxemia and is quite prevalent in the premature infant who remains ventilated beyond the first week or two after birth. These episodes increase in frequency with postnatal age, especially in infants with chronic lung disease. Because of their potential consequences, episodes of IH should neither be considered benign, nor a manifestation of immaturity or transient respiratory instability that resolves over time. Although the evidence is not conclusive, their detrimental effects on the infant's neurologic outcome may be significant.

Episodic hypoxemia needs to be carefully investigated to better understand its mechanisms and identify strategies to ameliorate its frequency and severity. Further investigation is needed to define the impact of IH on the preterm infant's developing central nervous system and other organ systems. Infants with IH need to be monitored closely to ensure prompt intervention and avoid prolonged episodes. An effort to avoid specific conditions leading to severe hypoxemia and hypoventilation is important.

REFERENCES

1. Garg M, Kurzner SI, Bautista DB, Keens TG. Clinically unsuspected hypoxia during sleep and feeding in infants with bronchopulmonary dysplasia. *Pediatrics*. 1988;81:635–642.
2. Durand M, McEvoy C, MacDonald K. Spontaneous desaturations in intubated very low birth weight infants with acute and chronic lung disease. *Pediatr Pulmonol*. 1992;13:136–142.
3. Di Fiore JM, Bloom JN, Orge F, et al. A higher incidence of intermittent hypoxemic episodes is associated with severe retinopathy of prematurity. *J Pediatr*. 2010;157:69–73.
4. Bolivar JM, Gerhardt T, Gonzalez A, et al. Mechanisms for episodes of hypoxemia in preterm infants undergoing mechanical ventilation. *J Pediatr*. 1995;127:767–773.
5. Dimaguila MA, Di Fiore JM, Martin RJ, Miller MJ. Characteristics of hypoxemic episodes in very low birth weight infants on ventilatory support. *J Pediatr*. 1997;130:577–583.
6. Esquer C, Claure N, D'Ugard C, et al. Role of abdominal muscles activity on duration and severity of hypoxemia episodes in mechanically ventilated preterm infants. *Neonatology*. 2007;92:182–186.
7. Lehtonen L, Johnson MW, Bakdash T, et al. Relation of sleep state to hypoxemic episodes in ventilated extremely-low-birth-weight infants. *J Pediatr*. 2002;141:363–368.
8. McEvoy C, Mendoza ME, Bowling S, et al. Prone positioning decreases episodes of hypoxemia in extremely low birth weight infants (1000 grams or less) with chronic lung disease. *J Pediatr*. 1997;130:305–309.
9. Chang YJ, Anderson GC, Dowling D, Lin CH. Decreased activity and oxygen desaturation in prone ventilated preterm infants during the first postnatal week. *Heart Lung*. 2002;31:34–42.
10. Esquer C, Claure N, D'Ugard C, et al. Mechanisms of hypoxemia episodes in spontaneously breathing preterm infants after mechanical ventilation. *Neonatology*. 2008;94:100–104.
11. Firme SR, McEvoy CT, Alconcel C, et al. Episodes of hypoxemia during synchronized intermittent mandatory ventilation in ventilator-dependent very low birth weight infants. *Pediatr Pulmonol*. 2005;40:9–14.
12. Polimeni V, Claure N, D'Ugard C, Bancalari E. Effects of volume-targeted synchronized intermittent mandatory ventilation on spontaneous episodes of hypoxemia in preterm infants. *Biol Neonate*. 2006;89:50–55.
13. Hummler HD, Engelmann A, Pohlandt F, Franz AR. Volume-controlled intermittent mandatory ventilation in preterm infants with hypoxemic episodes. *Intensive Care Med*. 2006;32:577–584.
14. Jain D, Claure N, D'Ugard C, Bello J, Bancalari E. Volume guarantee ventilation: effect on preterm infants with frequent hypoxemia episodes. *Neonatology*. 2016;110:129–134.
15. Claure N, Gerhardt T, Hummler H, et al. Computer controlled minute ventilation in preterm infants undergoing mechanical ventilation. *J Pediatr*. 1997;131:910–913.
16. Herber-Jonat S, Rieger-Fackeldey E, Hummler H, Schulze A. Adaptive mechanical backup ventilation for preterm infants on respiratory assist modes—a pilot study. *Int Care Med*. 2006;32:302–308.
17. Claure N, Suguihara C, Peng J, et al. Targeted minute ventilation and tidal volume in an animal model of acute changes in lung mechanics and episodes of hypoxemia. *Neonatology*. 2009;95:132–140.
18. Hagadorn JI, Furey AM, Nghiem TH, et al. Achieved versus intended pulse oximeter saturation in infants born less than 28 weeks' gestation: the AVIOx study. *Pediatrics*. 2006;118:1574–1582.
19. Lim K, Wheeler KI, Gale TJ, et al. Oxygen saturation targeting in preterm infants receiving continuous positive airway pressure. *J Pediatr*. 2014;164:730–736.
20. van Zanten HA, Tan RN, Thio M, et al. The risk for hyperoxaemia after apnoea, bradycardia and hypoxaemia in preterm infants. *Arch Dis Child Fetal Neonatal Ed*. 2014;99:F269–F273.
21. Laptook AR, Salhab W, Allen J, Saha S, Walsh M. Pulse oximetry in very low birth weight infants: can oxygen saturation be maintained in the desired range? *J Perinatol*. 2006;26:337–341.
22. McEvoy C, Durand M, Hewlett V. Episodes of spontaneous desaturations in infants with chronic lung disease at two different levels of oxygenation. *Pediatr Pulmonol*. 1993;15:140–144.
23. Di Fiore JM, Walsh M, Wrage L, et al. Low oxygen saturation target range is associated with increased incidence of intermittent hypoxemia. *J Pediatr*. 2012;161:1047–1052.
24. Sink DW, Hope SA, Hagadorn JI. Nurse:patient ratio and achievement of oxygen saturation goals in premature infants. *Arch Dis Child Fetal Neonatal Ed*. 2011;96:F93–F98.
25. Nghiem TH, Hagadorn JI, Terrin N, Syke S, MacKinnon B, Cole CH. Nurse opinions and pulse oximeter saturation target limits for preterm infants. *Pediatrics*. 2008;121:e1039–e1046.
26. Ford SP, Leick-Rude MK, Meinert KA, et al. Overcoming barriers to oxygen saturation targeting. *Pediatrics*. 2006;118:S177–S186.
27. Claure N, Gerhardt T, Everett R, et al. Closed-loop controlled inspired oxygen concentration for mechanically ventilated very low birth weight infants with frequent episodes of hypoxemia. *Pediatrics*. 2001;107:1120–1124.
28. Urschitz MS, Horn W, Seyfang A, et al. Automatic control of the inspired oxygen fraction in preterm infants: a randomized crossover trial. *Am J Respir Crit Care Med*. 2004;170:1095–1100.
29. Claure N, D'Ugard C, Bancalari E. Automated adjustment of inspired oxygen in preterm infants with frequent fluctuations in oxygenation: a pilot clinical trial. *J Pediatr*. 2009;155:640–645.
30. Claure N, Bancalari E, D'Ugard C, et al. Multicenter crossover study of automated adjustment of inspired oxygen in mechanically ventilated preterm infants. *Pediatrics*. 2011;127:e76–e83.
31. Waitz M, Schmid MB, Fuchs H, Mendler MR, Dreyhaupt J, Hummler HD. Effects of automated adjustment of the inspired oxygen on fluctuations of arterial and regional cerebral tissue oxygenation in preterm infants with frequent desaturations. *J Pediatr*. 2015;166:240–244.
32. Zapata J, Gómez JJ, Araque Campo R, Matiz Rubio A, Sola A. A randomised controlled trial of an automated oxygen delivery algorithm for preterm neonates receiving supplemental oxygen without mechanical ventilation. *Acta Paediatr*. 2014;103(9):928–933.

33. van Kaam AH, Hummler HD, Wilinska M, et al. Automated versus manual oxygen control with different saturation targets and modes of respiratory support in preterm infants. *J Pediatr.* 2015;167:545–550. e1–2.

34. Livera LN, Spencer SA, Thorniley MS, et al. Effects of hypoxaemia and bradycardia on neonatal haemodynamics. *Arch Dis Childhood.* 1991;66:376–380.

35. Claure N, Sanchez V, D'Ugard C, Bancalari E. Changes in cerebral oxygenation during spontaneous episodes of hypoxemia in mechanically ventilated preterm infants. *Pediatric Academic Societies, E-PAS.* 2003:2529.

36. Esquer C, Claure N, Capasso C, et al. Effect of spontaneous episodes of hypoxemia on brain oxygenation and brain-stem function in preterm infants. *Pediatric Academic Societies, E-PAS.* 2005:2625.

37. Dominguez S, Claure N, D'Ugard C, Bancalari E. Effects of spontaneous episodes of hypoxemia on hemodynamics and cerebral oxygenation in preterm infants. *Pediatric Academic Societies, E-PAS.* 2011:3833.328.

38. Schmid MB, Hopfner RJ, Lenhof S, Hummler HD, Fuchs H. Cerebral desaturations in preterm infants: a crossover trial on influence of oxygen saturation target range. *Arch Dis Child Fetal Neonatal Ed.* 2013;98:F392–F398.

39. Schmid MB, Hopfner RJ, Lenhof S, Hummler HD, Fuchs H. Cerebral oxygenation during intermittent hypoxemia and bradycardia in preterm infants. *Neonatology.* 2015;107:137–146.

40. Ratner V, Kishkurno SV, Slinko SK, et al. The contribution of intermittent hypoxemia to late neurological handicap in mice with hyperoxia-induced lung injury. *Neonatology.* 2007;92:50–58.

41. Row BW, Liu R, Xu W, et al. Intermittent hypoxia is associated with oxidative stress and spatial learning deficits in the rat. *Am J Resp Crit Care Med.* 2003;167:1548–1553.

42. Gozal D, Reeves SR, Row BW, Neville JJ, Guo SZ, Lipton AJ. Respiratory effects of gestational intermittent hypoxia in the developing rat. *Am J Respir Crit Care Med.* 2003;167:1540–1547.

43. Reeves SR, Mitchell GS, Gozal D. Early postnatal chronic intermittent hypoxia modifies hypoxic respiratory responses and long-term phrenic facilitation in adult rats. *Am J Physiol Regul Integr Comp Physiol.* 2006;290:R1664–R1671.

44. Julien C, Bairam A, Joseph V. Chronic intermittent hypoxia reduces ventilatory long-term facilitation and enhances apnea frequency in newborn rats. *Am J Physiol Regul Integr Comp Physiol.* 2008;294:R1356–R1366.

45. Gozal D, Gozal E, Reeves SR, Lipton AJ. Gasping and autoresuscitation in the developing rat: effect of antecedent intermittent hypoxia. *J Appl Physiol (1985).* 2002;92:1141–1144.

46. Garg M, Kurzner SI, Bautista D, Keens TG. Hypoxic arousal responses in infants with bronchopulmonary dysplasia. *Pediatrics.* 1988;82:59–63.

47. Koons AH, Mojica N, Jadeja N, et al. Neurodevelopmental outcome of infants with apnea of infancy. *Am J Perinatol.* 1993;10:208–211.

48. Levitt GA, Mushin A, Bellman S, Harvey DR. Outcome of preterm infants who suffered neonatal apnoeic attacks. *Early Hum Dev.* 1998;16:235–243.

49. Cheung P, Barrington KJ, Finer NN, Robertson CMT. Early childhood neurodevelopment in very low birth weight infants with predischarge apnea. *Pediatr Pulmonol.* 1999;27:14–20.

50. Pillenkamp F, Hermann C, Keller T, et al. Factors influencing apnea and bradycardia of prematurity-Implications for neurodevelopment. *Neonatology.* 2007;91:155–161.

51. Janvier A, Khairy M, Kokkotis A, et al. Apnea is associated with neurodevelopmental impairment in very low birth weight infants. *J Perinatol.* 2004;24:763–768.

52. Poets CF, Roberts RS, Schmidt B, et al. Association between intermittent hypoxemia or bradycardia and late death or disability in extremely preterm infants. *JAMA.* 2015;314:595–603.

53. Penn JS, Henry MM, Tolman BL. Exposure to alternating hypoxia and hyperoxia causes severe proliferative retinopathy in the newborn rat. *Pediatr Res.* 1994;36:724–731.

54. Saito Y, Omoto T, Cho Y, et al. The progression of retinopathy of prematurity and fluctuation in blood gas tension. *Graefes Arch Clin Exp Ophthalmol.* 1993;231:151–156.

55. Reynaud X, Dorey CK. Extraretinal neovascularization induced by hypoxic episodes in the neonatal rat. *Invest Ophthalmol Vis Sci.* 1994;35:3169–3177.

56. Phelps DL, Rosenbaum A. Effects of marginal hypoxia on recovery from oxygen-induced retinopathy in the kitten model. *Pediatrics.* 1984;73:1–6.

57. Cunningham S, McColm JR, Wade J, et al. A novel model of retinopathy of prematurity simulating preterm oxygen variability in the neonatal rat. *Invest Ophthalmol Vis Sci.* 2000;41:4275–4280.

58. Coleman RJ, Beharry KD, Brock RS, et al. Effects of brief, clustered versus dispersed hypoxic episodes on systemic and ocular growth factors in a rat model of oxygen-induced retinopathy. *Pediatr Res.* 2008;64:50–55.

59. McColm JR, Cunningham S, Wade J, et al. Hypoxic oxygen fluctuations produce less severe retinopathy than hyperoxic fluctuations in a rat model of retinopathy of prematurity. *Pediatric Res.* 2004;55:107–113.

60. McColm JR, Greisen P, Hartnett ME. VEGF isoforms and their expression after a single episode of hypoxia or repeated fluctuations between hyperoxia and hypoxia: relevance to clinical ROP. *Mol Vis.* 2004;10:512–520.

61. Di Fiore JM, Kaffashi F, Loparo K, et al. The relationship between patterns of intermittent hypoxia and retinopathy of prematurity in preterm infants. *Pediatr Res.* 2012;72:606–612.

62. Tay-Uyboco JS, Kwiatkowski K, Cates DB, et al. Hypoxic airway constriction in infants of very low birth weight recovering from moderate to severe bronchopulmonary dysplasia. *J Pediatr.* 1989;115:456–459.

14

63. Unger M, Atkins M, Briscoe WA, King TK. Potentiation of pulmonary vasoconstrictor response with repeated intermittent hypoxia. *J Appl Physiol*. 1977;43:662–667.
64. Custer JR, Hales CA. Influence of alveolar oxygen on pulmonary vasoconstriction in newborn lambs versus sheep. *Am Rev Respir Dis*. 1985;132:326–331.
65. Ratner V, Slinko S, Utkina-Sosunova I, et al. Hypoxic stress exacerbates hyperoxia-induced lung injury in a neonatal mouse model of bronchopulmonary dysplasia. *Neonatology*. 2009;95:299–305.

B

CHAPTER 15

Optimal Oxygenation in Extremely Preterm Infants

Waldemar A. Carlo and Lisa M. Askie

- Targeting appropriate oxygenation in newborn infants can improve outcomes.
- Evidence from randomized controlled trials and the corresponding meta-analyses indicate that air vs 100% oxygen for resuscitation of term infants increased survival in the neonates resuscitated with room air.
- Evidence from randomized controlled trials and the corresponding meta-analyses indicate that there is a lower risk of mortality and necrotizing enterocolitis with targeting SpO_2 ranges of 91% to 95% compared to 85% to 89% without adverse effects on blindness or neurodevelopment in extremely preterm infants.
- Many updated guidelines now recommend room air for resuscitation for term infants and targeting SpO_2 levels similar to the range of SpO_2 found to reduce mortality in these trials (91% to 95%) in extremely preterm infants.

Background

There is now an emerging body of information that suggests that some of the complications associated with extreme immaturity are potentiated by an excess of free radicals in infants who are intrinsically deficient in antioxidants, such as superoxide dismutase, catalase, and glutathione peroxidase. During hypoxia, metabolic alterations prime hypoxic cells to produce free oxygen radicals when subsequently exposed to oxygen. Such reperfusion injury, in addition to increasing the production of free oxygen radicals, is associated with other metabolic changes that may produce long-lasting harmful effects. Low plasma antioxidant activity at birth in premature infants may be an independent risk factor for mortality.[1] Pulmonary oxygen toxicity, through the generation of reactive oxygen/nitrogen species in excess of antioxidant defenses, may be a contributor to the development of bronchopulmonary dysplasia (BPD).[2–4] Immaturity is a factor explaining free radical–mediated pulmonary protein oxidation in premature newborns, and oxidation of proteins is related to the development of chronic lung disease.[5] It has been reported that oxygen toxicity can also increase the risk of retinopathy of prematurity (ROP), mortality, periventricular leukomalacia, and cerebral palsy.[6] However, oxygen restriction was also associated with an increased risk of death[7–9] and cerebral palsy.[10,11]

A meta-analysis of air versus 100% oxygen for newborn resuscitation that included four randomized trials revealed a decreased rate of death in the group resuscitated with room air (relative risk [RR] 0.71 [95% confidence interval (CI) 0.54–0.94], risk difference [RD] −0.05 [95% CI −0.08 to −0.01]).[12] However, longer durations of differential oxygen exposures had not been tested in randomized controlled trials in infants before the recent oxygen saturation (SpO_2) targeting trials.

For long-term use in infants, the American Academy of Pediatrics (AAP) recommended targeting oxygen saturation (SpO_2) between 85% and 95% or partial pressure of arterial oxygen of 50 to 80 mm Hg based on opinion as data were very limited. Before the recent Spo$_2$ targeting trials, there had been limited data from observational studies that suggested that targeting oxygen saturations below 90% may improve outcomes.

Observational Studies of Oxygenation Targeting

Tin et al. reviewed outcomes for infants admitted to neonatal intensive care units (NICUs) in northern England from 1990 to 1994 with policies to maintain either lower (70%–90%) or higher Spo$_2$ ranges (88%–98%).[13] They reported that infants managed with lower Spo$_2$ targets (70%–90%) developed ROP less often (6.2% vs. 27.2%), underwent a shorter duration of ventilation (14 days vs. 31), were less likely to be receiving oxygen at 36 weeks (18% vs. 46%), and were less likely to have a weight below the third centile at discharge (17% vs. 45%) than infants managed in NICUs with the higher Spo$_2$ targets (88%–98%). Very importantly, mortality and cerebral palsy did not differ by Spo$_2$ target groups. On follow-up at 10 years of age, fewer children cared for in NICUs with the lower Spo$_2$ targets had cognitive disability compared with those treated in NICUs with higher Spo$_2$ targets (23% vs. 35%).[14] In addition, the mean intelligence quotient (IQ) of children was 8 points higher in those managed in the lower Spo$_2$ target NICUs. There were also more children with very low scores on the Vineland Adaptive Behavior Scales in the higher compared with the lower Spo$_2$ target group (34% vs. 20%). At 10 years, there were 5 blind children among 64 survivors in the higher Spo$_2$ target group versus none of 60 in the lower Spo$_2$ target group. These results provided reassurance that restrictive oxygen therapy in infants of less than 28 weeks' gestation was safe and effective in improving outcomes and that lower Spo$_2$ targeting may reduce adverse outcomes such as neurodevelopmental impairment and blindness.

Another observational study designed as a before-and-after study reported ROP and mortality outcomes in infants managed in the same unit when Spo$_2$ targets were decreased to 83% to 93%.[15] In this study, it was found that the incidence of ROP stages 3 to 4 decreased consistently in a 5-year period from 12.5% to 2.5%, and the need for laser treatment decreased from 4.5% to 0% following the institution of a detailed oxygen management policy that included strict guidelines for increasing and weaning the fraction of inspired oxygen and the monitoring of Spo$_2$. Annual survival rates showed a trend toward improvement for all infants, especially for those with birth weights of 500 to 749 g.

A prospective, multicountry observational study by Hagadorn et al. was designed to measure achieved Spo$_2$ levels in extremely preterm infants.[16] The participating NICUs reported their targeted Spo$_2$ ranges and continuous recordings of Spo$_2$ were collected. This study showed that target saturations differed markedly by center in a range from 83% to 98% and that targeted Spo$_2$ was typically achieved less than 50% of the time.

Using transcutaneous oxygen monitoring, Bancalari and collaborators were able to show that infants who received continuous monitoring had a similar incidence of ROP compared to infants who were monitored by intermittent sampling. However, for the subgroup of infants with birth weights below 1100 g, there was a decreased incidence of ROP using transcutaneous arterial oxygen targets of 50 to 80 mm Hg compared with infants managed with intermittent blood gas sampling.[17]

Two randomized controlled trials of oxygen saturation targeting have been conducted during the postneonatal period to test oxygen saturation targets above 95%. The Supplemental Therapeutic Oxygen for Prethreshold Retinopathy of Prematurity (STOP-ROP) trial included 649 infants who were born at a mean of 25 weeks and were 35 weeks at enrollment.[18] Targeting oxygen saturations above 95% slightly reduced the number of infants who went on to have severe disease requiring retinal surgery. However, targeting oxygen saturations above 95% increased the proportion of infants who required prolonged oxygen supplementation and diuretics. The Benefits of Oxygen Saturation Targeting (BOOST) trial was a double-blind, randomized controlled trial that compared an oxygen saturation target of 91% to 94% versus a target of 95% to 98% in 358 infants less than 30 weeks at birth who required oxygen at 32 weeks postmenstrual age.[19] Oxygen growth and development, which were the main outcomes, were not improved with the higher oxygen saturation targeting. Furthermore, and consistent with the STOP-ROP trial results, targeting higher oxygen saturations increased the use of postnatal steroids and diuretics and resulted in more readmissions and more pulmonary-related deaths. Given this evidence, there have not been more trials testing oxygen saturation targets above 95%.

Data from several observational studies indicated wide ranges of practices and suggested the safety and benefits of targeting transcutaneous oxygen of 50 to 80 mm Hg or SpO_2 below 90%. Many experts in the field recommended that randomized clinical trials were needed to test different oxygenation targets.[20–23] As continuous SpO_2 measurements had become the standard of care, it made more sense to test continuous SpO_2 targets rather than continuous transcutaneous partial pressure of oxygen targets or intermittent blood gas targets. One of the giants in neonatology, Dr. Bill Silverman, wrote in 2004 "Recent observations have suggested that oxygen-saturation targets used for many decades in the treatment of extremely low gestational age neonates (<28 weeks) have been too high." Silverman added "I am encouraged to learn that these disturbing findings have now inspired efforts to organize an international RCT in the hope of finding an optimum range of oxygenation to minimize the risks of four competing outcomes: mortality, retinopathy, cerebral palsy, and chronic lung disease."[22] Indeed, five randomized controlled trials were soon initiated in the United States, Canada (whose studies included many other countries), the United Kingdom, Australia, and New Zealand.

The Support Trial

The first trial of SpO_2 targeting starting soon after birth—the Surfactant, Positive Pressure, and Pulse Oximetry Trial (SUPPORT)—was conducted in the Eunice Kennedy Shriver National Institute of Child Health and Human Development Neonatal Research Network clinical centers. SUPPORT was designed to compare the effects of a lower SpO_2 target (85%–89%) and a higher SpO_2 target (91%–95%). Infants of 24 to 27 weeks' gestation were enrolled prenatally or by 2 hours after birth. Blinding was maintained with the use of electronically altered pulse oximeters (Masimo Radical Co-Oximeter, Irvine, CA) that displayed saturation levels of 88% to 92% as the target range for both groups, with a maximum variation of 3%. Targeting of arterial oxygen saturation was continued until 36 weeks of postmenstrual age or until the infant was breathing ambient air and had not received ventilator support or continuous positive airway pressure for more than 72 hours. The main outcome measures were severe ROP or death (short term) and neurodevelopmental impairment or death at 24 months corrected age (longer term). A total of 1316 infants were enrolled. The primary outcome did not differ between the lower and higher SpO_2 intervention groups (28.3% and 32.1%, respectively; RR with lower SpO_2 target group 0.90, 95% CI 0.76–1.06, $P = .21$), but unexpectedly there was a lower mortality rate in the infants in the higher SpO_2 target group (16.2% vs. 19.9%, $P = .04$). Severe ROP occurred less often in the 85% to 89% SpO_2 target group (8.6% vs. 17.9%, $P < .001$). There were no significant differences in the rate of BPD, neurodevelopmental impairment, blindness, other ophthalmologic outcomes, patent ductus arteriosus, intracranial hemorrhage, or other major outcome measures.

Other Randomized Controlled Trials

There was an international effort to conduct other randomized controlled trials similar to the SUPPORT trial. A collaboration to conduct an individual participant data prospective meta-analysis—the Neonatal Oxygen Prospective Meta-Analysis (NeOProM) Collaboration—was established and the protocol for this collaboration was published.[24] This collaboration resulted in four other funded grant applications that led to completion of the BOOST UK and BOOST Australian trials,[25] the Canadian Oxygen Trial (COT),[26] and the New Zealand BOOST trial.[27] These four trials were very similar to SUPPORT because the protocols were shared prospectively. The similar design optimized the planned individual participant data meta-analysis.

The four trials were conducted as planned, but the BOOST UK and BOOST Australia trials stopped enrollment early because of an unexpected higher mortality rate in the higher Spo_2 target groups. For brevity, the results of these trials are presented together with the SUPPORT results as a Cochrane meta-analysis has just been published.[28]

Meta-Analyses of the Oxygen Saturation Targeting Trials

The Cochrane meta-analysis assessed the effects of targeting lower versus higher arterial oxygen saturations on important long- and short-term outcomes in extremely preterm infants (Table 15.1).[28] A standard Cochrane Neonatal search of the major literature data bases yielded the 5 trials mentioned previously, which enrolled a total of 4965 infants. There were no other randomized controlled trials that met inclusion criteria. No other randomized controlled trials have been conducted with differential Spo_2 targeting for extended periods starting soon after birth in neonates. Extremely preterm infants less than 28 weeks' gestation were enrolled in all five trials. The trials were well conducted. All five trials used masking of the randomization, intervention, and outcome assessment. There was a high rate of follow-up and data reporting; thus the risk of bias was low. The lower and higher Spo_2 target group treatments achieved different cumulative oxygen saturation levels, although achieved Spo_2 levels were higher than targeted for both groups (see later). The quality of the evidence was rated as high for the outcomes of death, disability, and necrotizing enterocolitis. The quality of the evidence was rated as moderate for the outcomes of ROP receiving treatment and blindness because of moderate heterogeneity of the results for ROP receiving treatment and because of the low frequency of the events for blindness, respectively. Thus the quality of this meta-analysis indicates that the major results are reliable and lead to confidence that the true effect lies close to that of the estimates of the effects.

Death or major disability to 18 to 24 months corrected age did not differ between the lower Spo_2 (85%–89%) vs. the higher Spo_2 (91%–95%) oxygen saturation target groups (RR 1.04 [95% CI 0.98–1.10], RD 0.02 [95% CI −0.01 to −0.05]; 4754 infants). The lower Spo_2 target group had a higher rate of death at 18 to 24 months corrected age (RR 1.16 [95% CI 1.03–1.31], RD 0.03 [95% CI 0.01–0.05]; 4873 infants), a higher rate of necrotizing enterocolitis (RR 1.24 [95% CI 1.05–1.47], RD 0.02 [95% CI 0.01–0.04]; 4929 infants), and a lower rate of ROP receiving treatment (RR 0.72 [95% CI 0.61–0.85], RD −0.04 [95% CI −0.06 to −0.02]; 4089 infants) compared with the higher Spo_2 target group. Major disability, blindness, severe hearing loss, and cerebral palsy did not differ between the two Spo_2 target groups. Other major outcomes, including patent ductus arteriosus receiving treatment or weight at discharge, did not differ between the treatment groups. Because of a calibration issue detected after completion of SUPPORT, the original Spo_2 monitors were replaced with new monitors with revised software during recruitment to the COT and BOOST trials. A difference in mortality was reported in the SUPPORT group with the original oximeter calibration software. However, the subgroup analysis by type of oximeter calibration software (original vs. revised) showed a significantly larger treatment effect (interaction $P = .03$) favoring the higher saturation target group for infants assigned to revised algorithm oximeters (RR 1.38 [95% CI 1.13–1.68], RD 0.06 [95% CI 0.01–0.10]; 3 trials, 1716

Table 15.1 MAJOR OUTCOMES IN THE LOWER VERSUS THE HIGHER OXYGEN SATURATION TRIALS

	RR (CI)	RD (CI)	NNTB/NNTH
Death or major disability	1.04 (0.98, 1.10)	0.02 (−0.01, 0.05)	—
Death by 18–24 months	1.16 (1.03, 1.31)	0.03 (0.01, 0.05)	33 (100, 20)
Necrotizing enterocolitis	1.24 (1.05, 1.47)	0.02 (0.01, 0.05)	50 (100, 20)
Retinopathy of prematurity treatment	0.72 (0.61, 0.85)	−0.04 (−0.06, −0.02)	25 (16, 50)

CI, Confidence interval; *NNTB*, number need to benefit; *NNTH*, number needed to harm; *RD*, risk difference; *RR*, relative risk.
From Askie LM, Darlow BA, Davis PG, et al. Effects of targeting lower versus higher arterial oxygen saturations on death or disability in preterm infants. *Cochrane Database Syst Rev.* 2017;11(4):CD011190.

infants). Other subgroup analyses based on gestational age, gender, and multiples versus singletons did not show any differences in outcomes between the treatment groups.

The Cochrane systematic review is the most comprehensive review published at present. The NeOProM study, which has been completed and presented at international meetings, has not been published yet. The Cochrane systematic review is the only review to use unpublished data from the individual trials to derive aligned definitions for outcome measures. Some of the authors of the Cochrane meta-analysis participated in the trials but an author independent of the trials assisted with data checking and interpretation.

Subgroup Analyses

It was reported that a subgroup analysis by birth weight of infants enrolled in the SUPPORT study revealed a higher mortality rate in the small-for-gestational age infants.[29] However, in the abstract presentation of the NeOProM Collaboration at the Pediatric Academic Societies in May 2017, it was reported that there were no differences in mortality by birth weight percentile using various intrauterine growth curves. Further subgroup analysis will be published by the NeOProM investigators.

Achieved Oxygen Saturations in the Randomized Controlled Trials

As expected, achieved SpO_2 levels differed from the target SpO_2 ranges in the five trials. In the higher SpO_2 saturation target group, infants achieved actual oxygen saturations that approximated the target SpO_2 levels of 91% to 95% (Fig. 15.1). However, in the lower oxygen saturation target group (that aimed for an SpO_2 range of 85%–89%), infants recorded oxygen saturations that were substantially higher than the target. Thus the increased mortality and increased necrotizing enterocolitis in the lower

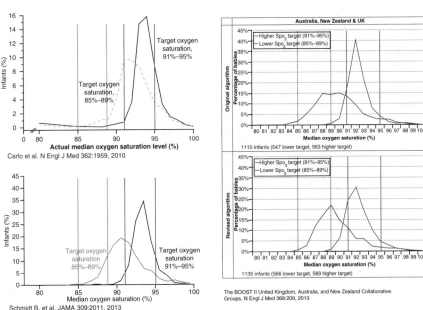

Fig. 15.1 Median achieved oxygen saturation *(SpO₂)* levels in the SUPPORT, COT, and BOOST II trials. Achieved SpO_2 levels differed from the target SpO_2 ranges in the trials. There were differences in achieved SpO_2 levels by trial. However, in all trials the higher oxygen saturation target group infants achieved oxygen saturations that approximated the target oxygen saturations. In contrast, in the lower oxygen saturation target group, infants achieved oxygen saturations that were substantially higher than the target oxygen saturations and approximated the wide range of 85% to 95%.

oxygen saturation target group occurred despite a smaller than expected difference in oxygen saturations between the treatment groups. Furthermore, the achieved oxygen saturations in the lower oxygen saturation target group mimicked the previous recommended oxygen saturations of 85% to 95% (see Fig. 15.1) Thus after a thorough analysis of achieved oxygen saturations in these trials, there is evidence that the lower oxygen saturation group achieved oxygen saturations similar to the oxygen saturations previously recommended. Targeting and achieving oxygen saturations higher than previously recommended decreased death and necrotizing enterocolitis without an increase in adverse neurologic outcomes or blindness despite the increase in treatment for ROP. This high-level evidence from the five oxygen saturation targeting trials indicates that target saturations should be 91% to 95% rather than 85% to 95% as previously recommended, 85% to 89% as tested in these trials, or other intermediate targets such as 88% to 92%, which is within the levels of SpO_2 achieved in the lower oxygen saturation target group in these trials.

Guidelines for Practice

Since publication of the SpO_2 target trials, guidance from the AAP[30] and other groups has changed. The AAP guidelines now state that target SpO_2 of 90% to 95% may be safer than 85% to 89%. The previous recommended target range of 85% to 95% is no longer recommended. Guidelines by professional societies and others in many countries have been updated accordingly. Clinical practice is changing in many countries.

Conclusions

In summary, five similarly designed and well-conducted randomized controlled trials of SpO_2 targeting have been completed. A total of 4965 infants have been enrolled, and the survivors have been followed up to at least 18 to 24 months corrected postmenstrual age. The meta-analysis of these trials shows an increased risk of mortality and necrotizing enterocolitis with targeting SpO_2 ranges of 85% to 89%. There was a decreased risk of treatment for ROP in the lower SpO_2 targeting group but no reduction in blindness. Differential SpO_2 targeting in the range tested did not affect neurodevelopment. Individual trials have not reported differences in the rates of patent ductus arteriosus or BPD. Many updated guidelines now recommend targeting SpO_2 levels similar to the range of SpO_2 found to reduce mortality in these trials (91%–95%) despite the increased risk of retinopathy particularly as blindness was not affected.

REFERENCES

1. Silvers KM, Gibson AT, Russell JM, Powers HJ. Antioxidant activity, packed cell transfusions, and outcome in premature infants. *Arch Dis Child*. 1998;78:F214–F219.
2. Saugstad OD. Bronchopulmonary dysplasia and oxidative stress: are we closer to an understanding of the pathogenesis of BPD? *Acta Paediatr*. 1997;86:1277–1282.
3. Davis JM. Role of oxidant injury in the pathogenesis of neonatal lung disease. *Acta Paediatr*. 2002:9123–9125.
4. Luo XP, Jankov RP, Ning Q, Liao LJ, Tanswell AK. Oxygen-mediated parenchymal and vascular lung injury. *Acta Pharmacol Sin*. 2002:2322–2328.
5. Varsila E, Pesonen E, Andersson S. Early protein oxidation in the neonatal lung is related to development of chronic lung disease. *Acta Paediatr*. 1995;84:1296–1299.
6. Carlo WA, Finer NN, Walsh MC. Target ranges of oxygen saturation in extremely preterm infants. *N Engl J Med*. 2010;362:1959–1969.
7. Avery ME. Recent increase in mortality from hyaline membrane disease. *J Pediatr*. 1960;57:553–559.
8. Cross KW. Cost of preventing retrolental fibroplasia? *Lancet*. 1973;2:954–960.
9. Bolton DP, Cross KW. Further observations on cost of preventing retrolental fibroplasia. *Lancet*. 1974;1:445–448.
10. Usher RH. Clinical investigation of the respiratory distress syndrome of prematurity. Interim report. *N Y State J Medicine*. 1961;61:1677–1696.
11. McDonald AD. Oxygen treatment of premature babies and cerebral palsy. *Dev Med Child Neurol*. 1964;6:313–314.
12. Tan A, Schulze A, O'Donnell CP, Davis PG. Air versus oxygen for resuscitation of infants at birth. *Cochrane Database Syst Rev*. 2005:CD002273.

13. Tin W, Milligan DW, Pennefather P, Hey E. Pulse oximetry, severe retinopathy, and outcome at one year in babies of less than 28 weeks gestation. *Arch Dis Child Fetal Neonatal Ed.* 2001;84: F106–F110.
14. Bradley S, Anderson K, Tin W, et al. Early oxygen exposure and outcome at 10 years in babies of less than 28 weeks. *Pediatr Res.* 2004;55:A373.
15. Chow LC, Wright KW, Sola A. Can changes in clinical practice decrease the incidence of severe retinopathy of prematurity in very low birth weight infants? *Pediatrics.* 2003;111:339–345.
16. Hagadorn JI, Furey AM, Nghiem TH, et al. AVIOx Study Group. Achieved versus intended pulse oximeter saturation in infants born less than 28 weeks' gestation: the AVIOx study. *Pediatrics.* 2006;118:1574–1582.
17. Bancalari E, Flynn J, Goldberg RN, et al. Influence of transcutaneous oxygen monitoring on the incidence of retinopathy of prematurity. *Pediatrics.* 1987;79:663–669.
18. The STOP-ROP Multicenter Study Group. Supplemental therapeutic oxygen for prethershold retinopathy of prematurity (STOP-ROP), a randomized, controlled trial. I. primary outcomes. *Pediatrics.* 2000;105:295–310.
19. Askie LM, Henderson-Smart DJ, Irwig L, et al. Oxygen-saturation targets and outcomes in extremely preterm infants. *N Engl J Med.* 2003;349:953–961.
20. Poets CF. When do infants need additional inspired oxygen? A review of the current literature. *Pediatr Pulmonol.* 1998;26:424–428.
21. Cole CH, Wright KW, Tarnow-Mordi W, Phelps DL. Resolving our uncertainty about oxygen. *Pediatrics.* 2003;112:1415–1419.
22. Silverman WA. A cautionary tale about supplemental oxygen: the albatross of neonatal medicine. *Pediatrics.* 2004;113:394–396.
23. Higgins RD, Raju TN, Perlman J, et al. Hypothermia and perinatal asphyxia: executive summary of the National Institute of Child Health and Human Development workshop. *J Pediatr.* 2006;148:170–175.
24. Askie LM, Brocklehurst P, Darlow BA, Finer N, Schmidt B, Tarnow-Mordi W; NeOProM Collaborative Group. NeOProM: neonatal oxygenation prospective meta-analysis collaboration study protocol. *BMC Pediatr.* 2011;11:6.
25. Stenson B, Brocklehurst P, Tarnow-Mordi W, UK BOOST II trial, Australian BOOST II trial, New Zealand BOOST II trial. Increased 36-week survival with high oxygen saturation target in extremely preterm infants. *N Engl J Med.* 2011;364:1680–1682.
26. Schmidt B, Whyte RK, Asztalos EV, et al. Effects of targeting higher vs lower arterial oxygen saturations on death or disability in extremely preterm infants: a randomized clinical trial. *JAMA.* 2013;309:2111–2120.
27. Darlow BA, Marschner SL, Donoghoe M, et al. Benefits of oxygen saturation targeting-New Zealand (BOOST-NZ) collaborative group. *J Pediatr.* 2014;165:30–35.
28. Askie LM, Darlow BA, Davis PG, et al. Effects of targeting lower versus higher arterial oxygen saturations on death or disability in preterm infants. *Cochrane Database Syst Rev.* 2017;11(4): CD011190.
29. Walsh MC, Di Fiore JM, Martin RJ, Gantz M, Carlo WA, Finer N. Association of oxygen target and growth status with increased mortality in small for gestational age infants: further analysis of the surfactant, positive pressure and pulse oximetry randomized trial. *JAMA Pediatric.* 2016;170:292–294.
30. Cummings JJ, Polin RA, AAP Committee on Fetus and Newborn. Oxygen targeting in extremely low birth weight infants. *Pediatrics.* 2016;138:e20161576.

15

CHAPTER 16

Patient-Ventilator Interaction

Nelson Claure, Martin Keszler, and Eduardo Bancalari

- Important interactions between the infant and the ventilator occur routinely during invasive and noninvasive mechanical ventilation. Some of these interactions can have significant effects on ventilation and gas exchange and may prolong the need for respiratory support.
- Asynchrony between the ventilator and the infant's breathing effort, excessive peak inflation pressure, or inspiratory time that is too long can affect the infant's respiratory rhythm and lead to agitation.
- Ventilator waveforms and monitored parameters should be used to determine the adequacy of ventilator settings and detect any adverse condition such as autotriggering.
- The interaction between the infant and new modes of ventilation that become available should be carefully examined before they are widely used.

Mechanical ventilation is an important tool in the management of premature infants with respiratory failure but is associated with an increased risk of acute and chronic lung injury and other associated morbidities. Despite continued efforts to reduce its use, a large proportion of preterm infants eventually require intubation and mechanical ventilation.

The earlier association between mechanical ventilation and the risk for lung injury was primarily believed to be due to aggressive use of the ventilator, which produced injurious lung expansion and chronic lung damage.[1] In part because of the limitations in the older ventilators, clinicians for years elected to impose a respiratory pattern on their patients to take over their ventilation completely. To achieve this, neonates with respiratory failure were sedated, paralyzed, or underwent hyperventilation to suppress their spontaneous respiratory drive. These approaches were associated with many problems that led to prolonged ventilator dependence and higher rates of complications. The likelihood of hyperventilation or hypoventilation is higher during controlled ventilation because the settings are not always adjusted to match the infant's metabolic demands and changing respiratory mechanics. Moreover, neonates who do not exercise the respiratory muscles for long periods are less likely to be weaned successfully from mechanical ventilation.

Neonatal ventilatory support has evolved from controlled ventilation to assisted ventilation with the evolution of various modes of synchronized ventilation. These gentler strategies have been developed to take maximal advantage of the patient's own respiratory effort and ameliorate ventilator-associated lung injury. These strategies involve careful management to minimize ventilator support to avoid volume injury and shorten the duration of mechanical ventilation. As a result, the ventilatory support provided to premature infants has changed from a strategy to fully control ventilation, targeting normal blood gas values, to a less aggressive approach in which the ventilator is used to supplement the infant's spontaneous respiratory effort. During the course of

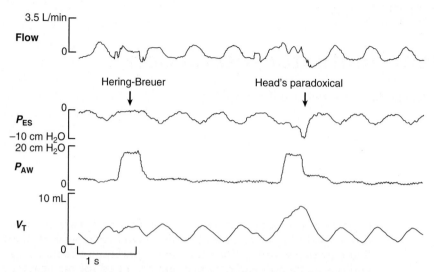

Fig. 16.1 Activation of Hering-Breuer and Head's paradoxical reflexes. Recordings of flow, esophageal pressure (P_{ES}), airway pressure (P_{AW}), and tidal volume (V_T) show the activation of the Hering-Breuer inhibitory reflex by a ventilator cycle that delays the initiation of the next spontaneous inspiration. The following ventilator cycle elicits an increase in inspiratory effort (greater negative deflection in P_{ES}) within the same spontaneous inspiration that results in a greater V_T in a pattern characteristic of the Head's paradoxical reflex.

the mechanical ventilatory support, there is continuous interaction between infant and the ventilator. Some of these interactions can have negative effects on the infant's spontaneous breathing effort and affect adversely ventilation and gas exchange, whereas other interactions can be beneficial. This chapter describes these interactions, their effects, and discusses alternatives to enhance positive interactions.

Patient-Ventilator Interaction During Conventional Mechanical Ventilation

The interaction between the patient and the ventilator can be extremely complex because it is influenced by many factors, including the patient's respiratory drive, various respiratory reflexes, the mechanical characteristics of the respiratory system, and the timing, flow, and pressure characteristics of the ventilator inflations. Respiratory reflexes influence the infant's spontaneous respiratory rhythm. Activation of the Hering-Breuer vagal inhibitory reflex by lung inflation can shorten neural inspiration, whereas its activation by lung inflation during neural expiration will delay the onset of the next spontaneous inspiration. Also active in the newborn, Head's paradoxical reflex can be activated by a rapid lung inflation and elicit a greater inspiratory effort. This could result in a greater transpulmonary pressure, larger tidal volume (V_T), and risk of alveolar overdistention. These interactions are illustrated in Fig. 16.1.

Infant-Ventilator Asynchrony

Asynchrony between the infant and the ventilator occurs frequently during intermittent mandatory ventilation (IMV) because mechanical inflations are delivered at fixed intervals and duration, which do not coincide with the infant's spontaneous inspiration. The ventilator positive pressure cycles can interact with the infant's spontaneous breathing and reflex activity. The effects vary depending on the timing and volume of the spontaneous inspiration or positive-pressure inflation.[2–4]

Inspiratory asynchrony occurs when the ventilator inflation is delivered toward the end of the spontaneous inspiration and extends beyond the end of inspiration. Fig. 16.2 shows an example of asynchrony during the spontaneous inspiratory phase. The resulting inspiratory hold can affect the spontaneous respiratory rate, and the

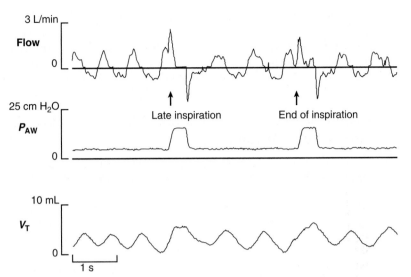

Fig. 16.2 Infant-ventilator inspiratory asynchrony. Tracings of flow, airway pressure (P_{AW}), and tidal volume (V_T) show intermittent mandatory ventilation cycles delivered toward the second half or at the end of the infant's spontaneous inspiratory phase. These asynchronous cycles produce a volume plateau or a larger V_T that delays the onset of the next spontaneous inspiration.

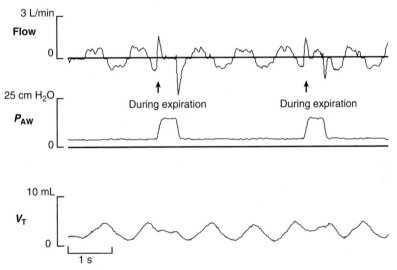

Fig. 16.3 Infant-ventilator expiratory asynchrony. Tracings of flow, airway pressure (P_{AW}), and tidal volume (V_T) show intermittent mandatory ventilation cycles delivered during the spontaneous expiratory phase. These asynchronous cycles prolong the expiration and affect the spontaneous breathing frequency by delaying the next spontaneous inspiration.

additional lung inflation on top of the spontaneous breath may cause volutrauma. Expiratory asynchrony occurs when the ventilator inflation is delivered during exhalation and prolongs the spontaneous expiratory phase, in turn affecting the spontaneous breathing frequency, as shown in Fig. 16.3. This type of asynchrony can also elicit active exhalation against an elevated pressure at the airway, producing a rise in intrathoracic and probably also intracranial pressure.

Asynchrony between the infant's spontaneous breathing and the ventilator inflations can have multiple effects, including poor gas exchange, air leaks, and increased risk of intraventricular hemorrhage (IVH).[5–8]

Asynchrony was common in earlier generations of neonatal ventilators. Monitoring was limited to visual assessment of chest expansion and breathing rate, with limited ability to determine asynchrony or the adequacy of V_T. Manipulation of the ventilator inspiratory and expiratory time has been suggested as a strategy to decrease asynchrony by adapting to the infant's breathing pattern.[9,10] This, however, requires frequent adjustment of these settings because of the variability of the infant's breathing. Use of high ventilator rates has also been suggested as a way to prevent asynchrony.[11] However, this may not be the most adequate approach for premature infants because of the risk of hypocapnia and its association with IVH and periventricular leukomalacia.

Patient-Ventilator Interaction During Synchronized Mechanical Ventilation

Because of the serious drawbacks of controlled ventilation, there has been an almost complete shift toward the use of assisted (i.e., synchronized) ventilation modes. The patient's spontaneous respiratory drive is not inhibited, so infants are more likely to be weaned sooner from mechanical ventilation because their respiratory muscles remain fit and can cope with the increased work of breathing during the weaning process. Because the ventilator is used only to supplement the infant's respiratory effort, lower peak inflation pressure (PIP) is needed to maintain adequate minute ventilation. The likelihood of hyperventilation is also reduced by allowing the infant to determine the total minute ventilation.

Ventilators used to provide assisted ventilation must respond on a timely basis to the demands of even the smallest infants. Incorporation of sensors and microprocessors for monitoring and control of different functions has made possible the development of ventilators capable of synchronizing the ventilator positive pressure cycle with the infant's spontaneous inspiration (i.e., patient-triggered ventilation).

The use of synchronized ventilation to assist the infant's spontaneous breathing while avoiding the effects of asynchrony can lead to a gentler ventilatory strategy and preservation of the infant's breathing rhythm. During synchronized ventilation, cycling of the ventilator shortly after the onset of the spontaneous inspiration achieves a larger transpulmonary pressure because of the sum of the positive-pressure cycle to the negative pressure generated by the diaphragm. This produces a larger V_T than that generated by the infant or the ventilator alone, as illustrated in Fig. 16.4. The positive interaction between the infant and the ventilator during inflation explains the better gas exchange and ventilation with more consistent V_T and lower breathing effort during synchronized than during conventional ventilation.[12–22] One of the most

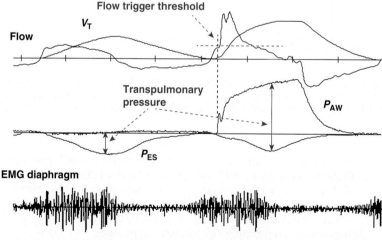

Fig. 16.4 Spontaneous inspiratory effort and synchronization of ventilator cycle. Tracings of flow, tidal volume (V_T), airway pressure (P_{AW}), esophageal pressure (P_{ES}), and electrical activity of the diaphragm obtained from a preterm infant show how the contraction of the diaphragm (measured by electromyography [EMG]) generates the negative pressure responsible for the inspiratory flow. Timely triggering of the ventilator cycle shortly after the onset of the inspiratory flow increases the transpulmonary pressure, and a larger V_T is achieved than in the preceding, nonassisted spontaneous inspiration.

consistent and important advantages of patient-triggered ventilation is that the preservation of spontaneous respiration facilitates weaning from the ventilator and shortens the duration of mechanical ventilation.[23] This explains the improved respiratory outcome with synchronized ventilation, which was more striking among the smaller infants at higher risk for bronchopulmonary dysplasia.[24,25] Synchronous ventilation has also been shown to reduce the stress response and fluctuations in blood pressure and oxygenation in preterm infants.[18,21,26,27]

Methods of Synchronization

Synchronization of the ventilator cycle with spontaneous inspiration is achieved by using different methods to detect inspiratory activity. Their efficacy and reliability vary, and these performance characteristics significantly influence the interaction between the ventilator and the infant's spontaneous inspiratory effort.

Mainstream (proximal) or internal flow sensors are used in neonatal ventilators to detect the inspiratory flow generated by the infant's spontaneous inspiratory effort. The ventilator cycle starts when the inspiratory flow exceeds a set threshold (see Fig. 16.4). Flow triggering has been shown to be more sensitive and specific than other methods; the ability to use low flow thresholds for triggering make this method appealing for use in sicker and more immature infants.[28-30] Flow triggering is limited by the presence of gas leaks around the endotracheal tube. Leaking gas travels through the flow sensor in the same direction as the inspiratory flow and may produce autocycling if this exceeds the trigger threshold. This is less of a problem with some modern ventilators designed specifically for neonatal use, which have effective compensation for even moderately large endotracheal tube leaks.

Although mainstream flow sensors are usually small, they increase the instrumental dead space and may affect carbon dioxide (CO_2) elimination, particularly in smaller infants.[31-33] This effect, however, is relatively small and is outweighed by the advantages of flow triggering.

Outward motion of the abdomen during inspiration can be detected by a pressure capsule applied on the abdominal surface. The use of this capsule for ventilator triggering is relatively simple but requires individualized sensitivity adjustment to avoid autocycling during patient activity. This capsule has been used effectively to synchronize the ventilator during invasive and noninvasive respiratory support in the past but is no longer available in the United States.[24,34-38]

The transmission of the negative pressure changes produced by spontaneous inspiration to the airway can also be used for triggering. However, because of their respiratory disease and relatively weak respiratory pump, preterm infants do not consistently produce the pressure changes at the airway required for triggering, which can lead to lack of or delayed triggering with these systems.[30,39,40] Using the electrical activity of the diaphragm (EA_{DIA}) is an attractive way of triggering ventilator inflations because it eliminates the trigger delay occasioned by pneumatic coupling. Onset of inflation is triggered by an increase in the electrical potential generated by diaphragmatic muscle contraction, as sensed by a special feeding catheter with an array of miniature electrodes. Inflation is terminated when EA_{DIA} declines below a fixed threshold, resulting in optimal synchrony for both initiation and termination of ventilator inflation. EA_{DIA} is unaffected by leakage, making it uniquely suited for synchronization during noninvasive positive-pressure ventilation. Cost and availability (it is currently only available from one manufacturer) are limiting factors for more widespread use of this promising triggering modality.[41-43]

Modalities of Synchronized Ventilation

Synchronized IMV

Synchronized IMV (SIMV) is similar to conventional IMV but with synchronous delivery of ventilator cycles. In both IMV and SIMV, the number of ventilator cycles delivered every minute is set by the clinician but the interval between cycles

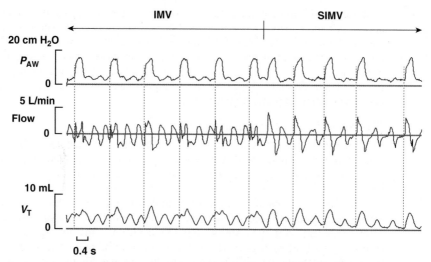

Fig. 16.5   Transition to synchronized intermittent mandatory ventilation *(IMV)*. Tracings of airway pressure *(P*$_{AW}$*)*, flow, and tidal volume *(V*$_T$*)* during transition from IMV to synchronized IMV *(SIMV)* show how IMV cycles delivered at fixed intervals occur during different phases of the spontaneous breath. In contrast, synchronous ventilator cycles during SIMV achieve a more consistent V_T and do not disturb the respiratory rhythm of the infant. Note that the interval between ventilator cycles is variable during SIMV to accommodate the infant's spontaneous breathing.

(expiratory duration, Te), which is constant in IMV, is variable in SIMV. Fig. 16.4 illustrates how synchrony is achieved during SIMV, and Fig. 16.5 shows a more regular ventilatory pattern during SIM compared with IMV. The disadvantage of SIMV in small preterm infants with narrow endotracheal tubes and insufficient muscle strength is that these immature infants often do not achieve adequate V_T with spontaneous breaths that are in excess of the supported rate. These small breaths largely rebreathe dead-space gas and contribute little to alveolar minute ventilation, which often necessitates a larger V_T for the low rate of SIMV inflations.

Assist/Control Ventilation

In assist/control (A/C) ventilation, every spontaneous inspiratory effort is assisted with a mechanical inflation. These synchronous inflations reduce the work of breathing and improve V_T, as illustrated in Fig. 16.6. Because all breaths are supported and easily clear dead space, the V_T needed with A/C is substantially lower than with SIMV.[21] Most preterm infants have an inconsistent respiratory drive. Hence, in A/C ventilation, a backup IMV rate is necessary to prevent hypoventilation during episodes of apnea. Backup ventilator cycles delivered during apnea may not always prevent hypoventilation if the rate is insufficient; optimally the backup rate is set only 10 cycles below the infant's spontaneous effort to avoid large fluctuations in minute ventilation. On the other hand, a backup rate too near the infant's breathing frequency or above it may lead to ventilator takeover if it provides all the required minute ventilation. In some neonatal ventilators, the duration of inspiration (Ti) in A/C ventilation is set by the operator, and in others, the ventilator cycle can be automatically terminated in synchrony with the declining inspiratory flow at the end of inspiration. This latter arrangement is also known as *flow cycling*. This allows the preterm infant to increase breathing frequency without shortening Te and affecting V_T, unlike A/C ventilation with a set Ti.[40] In most ventilators, the mode of A/C with flow cycling is referred to as pressure support ventilation (see the next section).

Pressure-Support Ventilation

Pressure-support ventilation (PSV) is a flow-cycled modality in which, as in A/C ventilation, every breath is assisted and the positive pressure is automatically terminated when the patient ends inspiration. This modality gives the infant complete

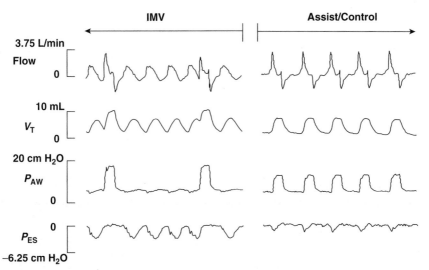

Fig. 16.6 Transition to synchronized assist/control ventilation. Tracings of flow, tidal volume (V_T), airway pressure (P_{AW}), and esophageal pressure (P_{ES}) during transition from intermittent mandatory ventilation (IMV) to assist/control ventilation show how the delivery of synchronous positive-pressure cycles reduces the inspiratory effort and avoids the disturbances to the infant's breathing rate observed when IMV cycles are delivered during exhalation.

control of the frequency and Ti. The synchronous support pressure is aimed at compensating for the loads induced by reduced lung compliance and increased airway and endotracheal tube resistance.[17,44]

A consistent respiratory drive is needed to ensure maintenance of ventilation in PSV, but if apnea occurs, a backup IMV rate prevents hypoventilation. In many ventilators PSV can be combined with SIMV and thus the spontaneous breaths are pressure-supported, eliminating some of the problems of SIMV. Because the aim of PSV is mainly to boost the V_T of spontaneous breaths, the pressure-supported breaths are usually assisted with lower pressures and result in smaller V_Ts than breaths assisted with SIMV. However, the level of pressure support should be sufficient to achieve a physiologic V_T, of at least 3.5 to 4 mL/kg or it will not be effective due to a continued high dead space-to-V_T ratio of the spontaneous breaths.

The addition of PSV to SIMV in preterm infants is aimed at boosting the spontaneous breaths and thus reducing the reliance on the larger SIMV inflations. PSV used with SIMV has been shown to reduce breathing effort and increase V_T in proportion to the support pressure used.[45–47] The combined use of SIMV and PSV was found to accelerate weaning in preterm infants compared with SIMV alone, preferentially in infants weighing more than 700 g at birth.[48] This advantage is likely due to these infants' more consistent respiratory drive, which ensures effective triggering of the ventilator.

Infant-Ventilator Maladaptation

Although synchronized ventilation can unload the respiratory pump by sharing the respiratory workload, the opposite occurs when there is maladaptation between the patient and the ventilator and the infant "fights" the ventilator. This lack of adaptation can be due to inadequate function of the synchronization mechanism, which leads to delayed triggering or trigger failure, autocycling, end-inspiratory asynchrony, or flow starvation. These problems may vary among ventilators according to their triggering methods and other characteristics, but there is also great variability during routine clinical practice, depending on the infant population, the underlying lung disease, and the ventilator settings.

Long Inspiratory Time and End-Inspiratory Asynchrony

End-inspiratory asynchrony occurs when the Ti of the ventilator cycle exceeds the patient's neural inspiration or when there is delayed triggering and the mechanical

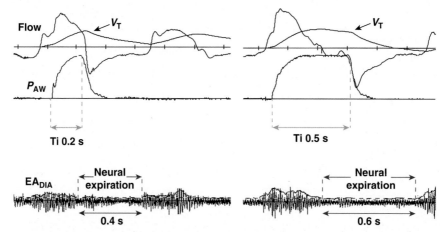

Fig. 16.7 Effect of excessive inspiratory time. Tracings of flow, tidal volume (V_T), airway pressure (P_{AW}), and electromyographic activity of the diaphragm (EA_{DIA}) show the effects of a ventilator cycle with a prolonged inspiratory time *(Ti)* on the neural respiratory activity in a preterm infant. The prolonged volume plateau extends beyond the inspiratory activity and prolongs the neural expiratory phase, delaying the start of the following spontaneous inspiration.

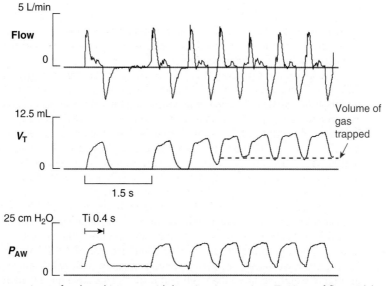

Fig. 16.8 Gas trapping at fast breathing rate with long inspiratory time. Tracings of flow, tidal volume (V_T), and airway pressure (P_{AW}) during assist/control ventilation with a constant inspiratory time *(Ti)* that exceeds the duration required to complete inspiration. Note the prolonged periods near zero flow and volume plateau. An increase in the spontaneous frequency produces an inverse inspiration-to-expiration ratio that results in gas trapping because of insufficient time to complete exhalation.

cycle starts late during spontaneous inspiration. Continuation of the mechanical inflation into neural expiration results in a prolonged inspiratory plateau similar to an inspiratory hold and decreases the time for unopposed exhalation. In some cases, this can elicit active exhalation efforts against the positive pressure. The long Ti can produce a prolonged volume plateau that keeps the lung distended, delays the initiation of the next spontaneous inspiration, and affects the infant's breathing rhythm[49,50] (illustrated in Fig. 16.7). This effect is mediated by the Hering-Breuer inhibitory reflex.

In A/C ventilation, an excessive Ti may also result in an inverse inspiration-to-expiration ratio, insufficient expiratory time, and gas trapping, if the spontaneous breathing frequency increases (Fig. 16.8). This can limit breathing frequency and disrupt the neural breathing pattern.[40,49,50] To prevent this situation, in addition to

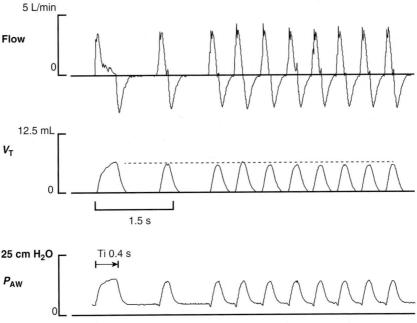

Fig. 16.9 Fast breathing rate with flow-cycling. Tracings of flow, tidal volume (V_T), and airway pressure (P_{AW}) during assist/control ventilation with flow-cycling. The shorter inspiratory time (Ti) during flow cycling permits a higher spontaneous breathing frequency with a resulting V_T that is comparable to that achieved with the longer Ti of the first breath.

avoiding a Ti that is too long, mechanical inflations can be terminated automatically based on the decline of the inspiratory flow below a set threshold, known as termination criteria. Fig. 16.9 shows an example of automatic termination of Ti (flow cycling as used in PSV). In ventilators not specifically designed for newborn infants, this automatic termination of ventilator inflations may not work properly when a large gas leak around the endotracheal tube is present, because the leak can maintain the measured inspiratory flow above the breath termination criteria. Manual adjustment of the termination criteria is possible to deal with this issue, but because the leak is often variable, this is difficult. Setting the termination criteria too high (e.g., 30% or 40% of peak flow) would lead to premature breath termination when the leak decreases. Specialized neonatal ventilators have effective leak compensation that eliminates this problem. On the other hand, a set Ti that is shorter that the infant's spontaneous inspiration can result in inadequate transpulmonary pressure and insufficient V_T. Flow cycling largely eliminates this problem by automatically adjusting the Ti in response to changing lung mechanics and spontaneous inspiratory time of the infant.

Trigger Delay

Delayed triggering of the inflation relative to the onset of the spontaneous inspiration can lead to increased work of breathing.[51] The delay can result in prolonged inspiratory hold similar to the IMV cycles that occur late in inspiration. In A/C ventilation the effects may be similar to those of long Ti described previously. Delayed triggering is usually due to a relatively insufficient trigger sensitivity setting with flow triggering. In modern neonatal ventilators with effective leak compensation that minimizes the risk of autotriggering, sensitivity should be always be set at the most sensitive level to minimize trigger delay. Long trigger delay was a common problem when pressure triggers were used in the past, but virtually all modern ventilators now use flow or diaphragmatic trigger. However, not all ventilators used in the neonatal intensive care unit (NICU) are designed for newborns. Universal ventilators are primarily designed for adults with cuffed endotracheal tubes and may not have effective leak compensation, thus requiring trigger sensitivity adjustment that may lead to inspiratory asynchrony.

Trigger Failure

Trigger failure occurs because of trigger sensitivity that is too low—for instance, an excessive flow trigger threshold that exceeds the inspiratory flow produced by the infant's spontaneous inspiratory effort. As a result, the infant will be supported only by the IMV or AC ventilation backup rate in a nonsynchronized mode. Trigger failure should be rare with appropriate settings on neonatal ventilators but remains a problem when leak compensation is lacking, a situation similar to long trigger delay.

Autotriggering

Autotriggering is one of the most common problems with patient-triggered ventilation. It occurs when the ventilator inflations are triggered by artifact, rather than in response to the patient's inspiratory effort. The most common causes of autotriggering are gas leaks around the endotracheal tube and water condensation in the ventilator circuit, both of which produce changes in gas flow or oscillations in pressure that are detected by the flow sensor as the onset of the infant's spontaneous inspiration.[52] Leaks around the endotracheal tube are common among infants who remain ventilated for long periods because the immature tissues of the larynx and trachea stretch over time with positive-pressure ventilation (acquired tracheomegaly). Less frequently, infants may actually outgrow the tube size. Small leaks can be compensated for by an increase in the flow trigger threshold. Newer specialty neonatal ventilators have automatic leak compensation systems capable of compensating for leaks of up to 60%. However, when the leaks are too large or variable, leak compensation becomes less effective and sometimes the endotracheal tube needs to be replaced with a larger one to reduce the leak and avoid autotriggering. A former 600-g infant who is 3 weeks old but still only weighs 750 g may need a 3.0-mm endotracheal tube to eliminate a large leak; the guidelines for endotracheal tube size based on birth weight apply only for the initial intubation and should not prevent the use of appropriate size tube when a large leak is present.

Autotrigger may also occur due to water condensation in the unheated expiratory limb of the circuit and generate oscillations that trigger the ventilator at a very rapid rate. This problem is not solved by leak compensation. Water traps located at the lowest point in the circuit can be helpful, but even more effective is the use of modern semipermeable expiratory circuits that allow the water to move out of the circuit, virtually eliminating autotriggering caused by condensation.

The consequences of autotriggering are more serious in A/C ventilation or PSV because none of the currently available neonatal ventilators offers the option to limit the frequency. In these modalities, autotriggering at a high ventilator rate can induce hyperventilation, hypocapnia, and gas trapping. If the autotriggering persists, it is likely to blunt the spontaneous respiratory drive through hyperventilation. In contrast, the effects of autotriggering in SIMV are limited because the ventilator rate is set by the clinician, and therefore the ventilator behaves as if it were in the IMV mode instead of SIMV. A high rate alarm should always be set at an appropriate value when using A/C or PSV to alert the caregivers to the possibility of autotriggering.

Excessive or Insufficient Circuit Flow

Flow starvation occurs when the flow through the ventilator circuit is lower than the peak inspiratory flow generated by the patient's own inspiratory effort. In older patients, flow starvation produces a sensation of air hunger and anxiety. In infants it can be a cause of agitation and maladaptation to the ventilator, because there is not enough fresh gas for the infant's spontaneous inspiration between or during ventilator cycles. Some ventilator modes have the capacity to automatically increase the flow to match the patient demand (demand flow), but if this feature is not available, it is critical that the ventilator flow be adjusted to meet the demands of the patient. Flow starvation can be recognized when the patient struggles during inspiration and by a characteristic appearance of the pressure waveform. When the circulating flow in the ventilator circuit is insufficient, the ventilator does not consistently reach the peak pressures set by the operator. Although uncommon in small infants, because their flow requirements are relatively low and seldom exceed the available flow, it is important to recognize this condition because the infant may be receiving less ventilatory support than intended, which is commonly associated with agitation.

At the other extreme, excessive circuit flows can modify the pressure profile of the ventilator cycle, resulting in a rapid increase to the PIP. Ventilators differ in how inspiratory flow is regulated. In older devices there is a fixed inspiratory flow rate adjustable by the user. More recently the rate of inspiration is controlled by adjusting the "rise time" or slope of the rate of pressure increase. Rapid inspiratory flow results in fast lung inflation rates that are not observed during normal spontaneous breathing and may be injurious to the airways. Damage from excessively high inspiratory flow, referred to as rheotrauma, is not well documented but may be a legitimate concern. Optimal inspiratory flow rate/rise time are currently unknown.

Excessive Peak Inflation Pressure

Ventilator cycles triggered by the onset of the infant's inspiration generally deliver a greater V_T than that produced by the spontaneous effort alone. Although it does not occur in a consistent manner, the larger lung inflation produced by triggered ventilator cycles with high PIP can inhibit the infant's neural inspiration through activation of the stretch inhibitory reflex, as illustrated in Fig. 16.10. The conditions that can lead to inhibition of the neural inspiratory activity by lung inflation in preterm infants have not been clearly defined. In addition to the magnitude of the inflation, the sensitivity of the infant's respiratory center to stretch receptor activity is likely modulated by the chemical respiratory drive and possibly by the rate of lung inflation.

Although the possible impact of inhibition of the infant's inspiratory effort on his ability to maintain a consistent breathing rhythm is unknown, the occurrence of such inhibition in a persistent manner over time may have unwanted consequences. On the other hand, it is possible that inhibition of spontaneous inspiration when V_T is excessive is a protective mechanism. Hence, an inconsistent or decreased sensitivity to stretch receptor activity may increase the infant's risk for lung injury when PIP is excessive during synchronized ventilation.

All modern ventilators now incorporate some means of monitoring V_T; therefore excessively high PIP and V_T are largely preventable with close monitoring even when using pressure-controlled modes of ventilation. The problem can also be avoided by the use of volume-targeted ventilation.

Excessive Positive End-Expiratory Pressure

The beneficial effect of positive end-expiratory pressure (PEEP) on oxygenation was demonstrated long ago[53] and is due to resolution of areas of atelectasis and decreased pulmonary shunting. The use of adequate PEEP to maintain alveolar recruitment

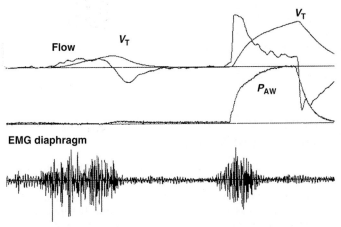

Fig. 16.10 Inhibition of spontaneous inspiration by large tidal volume. Recordings of flow, tidal volume (V_T), airway pressure (P_{AW}), and electromyographic activity (*EMG*) of the diaphragm during spontaneous intermittent mandatory ventilation show inhibition of the infant's inspiration by a synchronous ventilator cycle that produces a V_T that is considerably greater than the V_T produced by the preceding spontaneous inspiration.

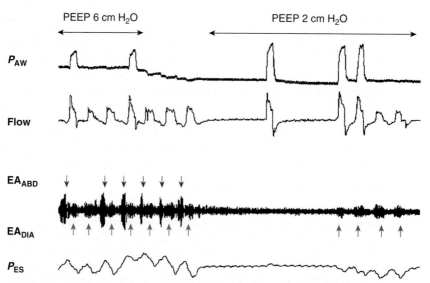

Fig. 16.11 Abdominal muscle activity with high PEEP. Tracings of airway pressure (P_{AW}), flow, electrical activity of the abdominal (EA_{ABD}, *red arrows*), and diaphragmatic (EA_{DIA}, *gray arrows*) muscles, and esophageal pressure (P_{ES}) during a decrease in positive end-expiratory pressure *(PEEP)* from 6 cm H_2O to 2 cm H_2O in a preterm infant. Contractions of the abdominal muscles during every expiration accelerate the expiratory flow rate at high PEEP but disappear when PEEP is reduced.

and functional residual capacity at end-exhalation is a crucial component of lung-protective ventilation strategies because it ensures even distribution of V_T into an open lung. However, excessive levels of PEEP can produce a rise in CO_2 owing to greater anatomic dead space resulting from distention of airways, increased alveolar dead space owing to incomplete exhalation (gas trapping), and decreased ventilation owing to overdistention of the lung, thus leading to reduced lung compliance.[54–57] The reduction in compliance is caused by a rise in lung volume to the flatter portion of the pressure-volume relationship. It is important to note that, because of alveolar recruitment, an increase in PEEP achieves a greater gain in lung volume than the gain in V_T achieved by an increase in PIP of the same magnitude.[58]

In small preterm infants, increasing PEEP does not produce a compensatory increase in diaphragmatic activity to keep ventilation unchanged.[57] The reason may be activation of inhibitory stretch receptors at higher lung volumes.[59] The inability to maintain ventilation at rising PEEP levels may also be affected by decreased contractility and tension generation when the diaphragm is displaced downward at higher lung volumes.[60] On the other hand, PEEP levels that produce excessive lung volumes can elicit activation of expiratory muscles to actively exhale against the pressure generated by the ventilator,[61] as illustrated in Fig. 16.11.

Although the optimal PEEP level in preterm infants is difficult to determine, it is clear that both insufficient and excessive PEEP can lead to negative infant-ventilator interactions.

Patient-Ventilator Interaction During Volume Targeted Ventilation

Automatic adjustment of inflation pressure in response to changing lung mechanics and alterations in patient respiratory effort is an example of a closed-loop system that maintains a relatively stable V_T during pressure-controlled ventilation. Volume guarantee (VG) has for the most part become the industry standard for volume-targeted ventilation (VTV) and some version of the algorithm is now available in most ventilators used in the NICU. The benefits and operating characteristics are described in Chapter 19; here we focus on the patient-ventilator interactions during VTV. The key concept to understanding this interaction is the recognition of

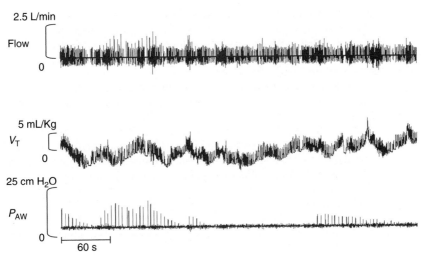

Fig. 16.12 Automatic adjustments in peak pressure during volume-targeted ventilation with a target tidal volume (V_T) that is too low. Tracings of flow, V_T, and airway pressure (P_{AW}) show a declining peak pressure as the infant maintained V_T above the target V_T. This resulted in periods when the infant was left receiving only positive end-expiratory pressure.

the fact that the V_T reaching the patient's lungs results from the combination of the positive pressure generated by the ventilator and the negative inspiratory pressure generated by the infant. With pressure-controlled ventilation, the ventilator component of the transpulmonary pressure is fixed, while the immature infant's inspiratory effort is sporadic and highly variable from breath to breath. This results in large fluctuations in transpulmonary pressure and consequently the delivered V_T. With VTV, the ventilator compares the exhaled V_T with the target V_T and adjusts the inflation pressure to attempt to maintain the target V_T. Thus the ventilator component of the transpulmonary pressure is also variable—in general in inverse proportion to the infant's effort—attempting to maintain a stable transpulmonary pressure and thus V_T. Because the breath-to-breath change in the ventilator pressure is limited to avoid overshoot, the V_T fluctuates to some extent, but less so than without this adaptive mechanism.[62] Appropriate choice of V_T is critical to the success of VTV. In general, a higher target V_T will result in a decrease in inspiratory effort,[63,64] but an excessively high V_T target will overventilate and suppress the infant's respiratory drive. On the other hand, a target V_T that is too low will provide inadequate support. This is because by design, if the measured V_T is above the target, the PIP will be decreased for the next inflation. As long as the infant continues to generate a V_T above the target value, the PIP will continue to decrease until the infant is essentially on endotracheal continuous positive airway pressure with no positive pressure generated by the ventilator (Fig. 16.12). This will eventually lead to fatigue, lung derecruitment and prolongation of respiratory support. Thus it is critical that the patient's response to the initial settings be evaluated at the bedside by careful observation of the above-described patient-ventilator interactions.

Patient-Ventilator Interaction During Neurally Adjusted Ventilatory Assist

The most recent innovation in patient-ventilator interaction is the advent of neurally adjusted ventilatory assist (NAVA). NAVA uses the EADi not only to trigger onset of inflation but also to modulate inflation pressure in proportion to the infant's diaphragmatic activity and to cycle into expiration when diaphragmatic activity wanes. The patient effectively determines the rate, volume, and inspiratory time of each inflation. This is an example of very sophisticated patient-ventilator interaction that has gained increased acceptance in the NICU, despite a lack of long-term studies that demonstrate the safety and efficacy of this approach. In short-term studies NAVA has been shown to provide ventilation comparable to SIMV with lower EA_{DIA}.[41,42] A higher NAVA gain setting can lead to a reduction in EA_{DIA}, reflecting a decreased inspiratory effort.[43] Data on the most appropriate NAVA gain or the rationale and approach to set this parameter in premature infants have not been clearly described.

Although it is theoretically very attractive, use of NAVA assumes a mature respiratory control center, which is clearly not a valid assumption in very premature infants. The concern here is that the positive feedback principle of NAVA could accentuate the periodic breathing seen in preterm infants and lead to fluctuations in the arterial partial pressure of CO_2 ($Paco_2$) and intermittently to excessively large inflations leading to volutrauma. Although the proponents of NAVA argue that excessively large inflations should not occur because of the stretch inhibitory Hering-Breuer reflex, it is equally likely that large inflations could trigger the Head paradoxical reflex, leading to an even larger inflation. There are no data on the stability of V_T during NAVA or the number of excessively large inflations, nor are there long-term studies evaluating the effect of NAVA on lung injury and risk of chronic lung disease.

NAVA assumes the respiratory control center is functioning normally and it provides proportional assist to enable the patient to do what he or she is attempting to do: a strong inspiratory effort, such as may occur when the infant is disturbed, generates higher inflation pressure, while during hypoventilation little support is provided. A backup ventilator rate needs to be set appropriately to deal with periods of apnea, but the backup will not kick in when the infant merely hypoventilates because of shallow breathing. Fig. 16.13 illustrates the need for a backup ventilator rate to avoid hypoventilation during apnea. To reduce the risk of excessive or prolonged lung inflation during NAVA it is necessary to ensure limits to peak pressure and inspiratory duration are set adequately. Fig. 16.14 provides an example of a large and prolonged increase in ventilator pressure during NAVA.

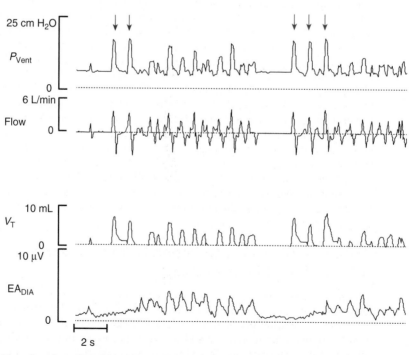

Fig. 16.13 Neurally adjusted ventilatory assist (NAVA) during variable spontaneous respiratory drive. Recordings of ventilator pressure (P_{Vent}), flow, tidal volume (V_T), and diaphragmatic electrical activity (EA_{DIA}) from a premature infant on NAVA show P_{Vent} is proportional to EA_{DIA}, while during periods of apnea the infant receives backup pressure-controlled breaths (*red arrows*) to prevent hypoventilation.

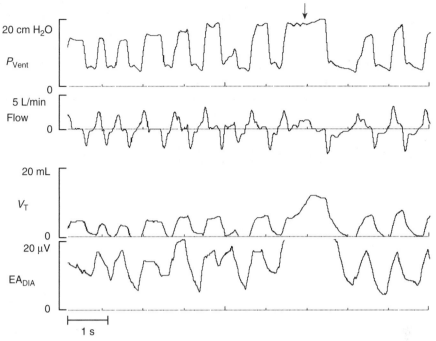

Fig. 16.14 Neurally adjusted ventilatory assist (NAVA) and increased diaphragmatic activity. Recordings of ventilator pressure (P_{Vent}), flow, tidal volume (V_T), and diaphragmatic electrical activity (EA_{DIA}) from a premature infant receiving NAVA show increased P_{Vent} during a large and prolonged contraction of the diaphragm, resulting in a considerably larger V_T *(red arrow)*.

NAVA and VG take a diametrically opposite approach. VG was specifically developed for preterm infants with immature respiratory control. With VG, when there is a decline in inspiratory effort, more pressure is generated by the ventilator to maintain a stable V_T. This is in contrast to NAVA with which a decline in breathing effort will result in lower ventilator pressure. This explains the findings of studies in which EA_{DIA} was shown to be higher during NAVA compared with VG.[65]

Patient-Ventilator Interaction During Noninvasive Ventilation

Noninvasive ventilation (NIV) was one of the earliest forms of support used in neonates, and it is again used increasingly to reduce the need for intubation or facilitate weaning from invasive ventilatory support in preterm neonates. NIV is commonly provided with the same ventilators used for conventional mechanical ventilation. In contrast to invasive ventilation, in which the endotracheal tube bypasses the infant's upper airway and ensures the transmission of the positive pressure to the infant's airways, pressure transmission during NIV depends on the patency and resistance of the upper airway and on the large leaks present in an open system. The complexity of the mechanisms that determine upper airway patency and modulate its resistance makes it difficult to predict the degree of transmission of the positive pressure applied on the nose to the infant's distal airways.[66–71]

Sufficient transmission of the positive pressure during apnea is particularly important, because nasal ventilation is often used in infants with immature respiratory control. The efficacy of nasal ventilation during apnea is not consistent, and it is inadequate if the infant's upper airway is not patent. In contrast, when the airway is patent the positive-pressure cycles produce lung inflation, as shown Fig. 16.15, but this is actually uncommon, because during apnea the upper airway is usually closed, which reduces the effectiveness of noninvasive IMV. A study demonstrated

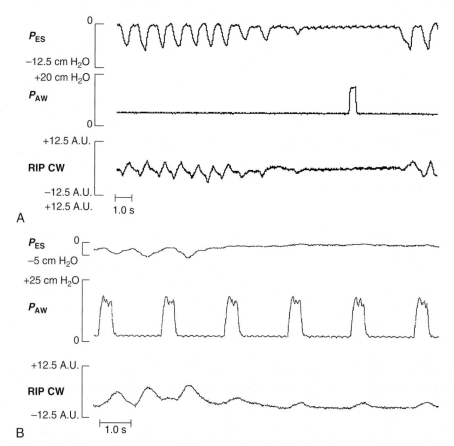

Fig. 16.15 Transmission of nasal positive-pressure cycles during apnea. A, Tracings of esophageal pressure (P_{ES}), airway pressure (P_{AW}), and chest wall expansion measured by respiratory inductance plethysmography (*RIP CW*) shows in a single nasal positive-pressure cycle delivered during a brief apneic pause that does not produce transmission of the pressure and expansion of the chest. In contrast, B shows small expansion of the chest during positive-pressure cycles. In these recordings pressure transmission may have been influenced by patency of the upper airway patency or gas leakage. *A.U.,* Arbitrary units.

that only 3% of ventilator inflations were accompanied by a measureable V_T with nonsynchronized NIV.[72] Thus synchronization during NIV appears to be important. Unfortunately, the Graseby capsule used for synchronization of NIV in many countries is no longer available in the United States.

Adequate transmission of the positive pressure during nasal synchronized ventilation can increase V_T,[73] but this process appears to be more effective in infants with greater ventilatory demands who cannot achieve sufficient ventilation.[74] Another important benefit of synchronized delivery of the positive-pressure cycle is that of unloading the respiratory pump, which is primarily reflected in a lesser inspiratory effort than with continuous positive airway pressure alone.[34,73,74] In stable preterm infants, the reduction in breathing effort appears to be mediated by inhibitory reflexes rather than by decreased central drive, as illustrated by a significant attenuation in inspiratory effort during synchronous nasal IMV cycles (Fig. 16.16). In contrast, nonsynchronized ventilator cycles during nasal IMV do not increase ventilation or reduce breathing effort; instead, they appear to negatively affect the infant's respiratory rhythm, as is observed with invasive IMV (Fig. 16.17).[34]

Noninvasive NAVA can overcome the problems of nonsynchronized nasal IMV and appears to be quite effective.[75] Its true potential needs to be evaluated in well-controlled clinical trials, which have not been conducted as of this writing.

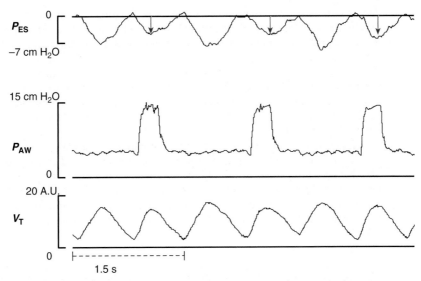

Fig. 16.16 Inspiratory effort during nasal synchronized ventilation. Tracings of esophageal pressure (P_{ES}), airway pressure (P_{AW}), and tidal volume (V_T) during synchronized nasal intermittent mandatory ventilation illustrate the reduction in the infant's spontaneous inspiratory effort with each synchronized cycle of the ventilator. *Red arrows* mark the smaller negative deflections in P_{ES} during inspiration. *A.U.,* Arbitrary units. (From Chang HY, Claure N, D'Ugard C, et al. Effects of synchronization during nasal ventilation in clinically stable preterm infants. *Pediatr Res.* 2011;69:84–89.)

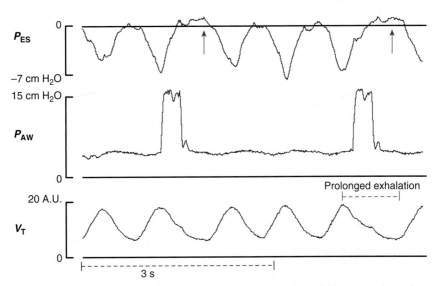

Fig. 16.17 Prolonged exhalation and active expiratory activity during asynchronous nasal ventilation. Tracings of esophageal pressure (P_{ES}), airway pressure (P_{AW}), and tidal volume (V_T) during nonsynchronized nasal intermittent mandatory ventilation (SIMV) show prolongation of the exhalation and active expiratory effort *(red arrows)* with asynchronous ventilator cycles delivered toward the end of the infant's inspiration or during exhalation. *A.U.,* Arbitrary units. (From Chang HY, Claure N, D'Ugard C, et al. Effects of synchronization during nasal ventilation in clinically stable preterm infants. *Pediatr Res.* 2011;69:84–89.)

Summary

Important interactions between the infant and the ventilator occur routinely during invasive and noninvasive ventilatory support. Some of these interactions can have significant effects on ventilation and gas exchange, but the extent to which the interactions affect long-term respiratory or neurologic outcome is unknown. Nonetheless, they may play an important indirect role by prolonging respiratory support and disturbing the development of a stable and consistent respiratory rhythm in the preterm infant. Sophisticated microprocessor-controlled ventilators specifically designed for newborn infants can eliminate most instances of asynchrony when used optimally. When other devices are used, careful attention to optimizing ventilator settings using ventilator-generated waveforms to identify and correct instances of asynchrony can minimize the adverse effects of poor synchronization. The interaction between the infant and new modes of ventilation that become available should be examined before they are widely used.

Equally important is understanding that patient agitation is an important clinical sign of suboptimal ventilator support. It is often believed that gas exchange is poor because the patient is fighting the ventilator. More often, the patient is fighting the ventilator because the settings are suboptimal, leading to poor gas exchange. Therefore, rather than prescribing sedation or paralysis, the clinician must go to the bedside and carefully evaluate patient-ventilator interactions to identify the cause of agitation.

REFERENCES

1. Northway WH Jr, Rosan RC, Porter DY. Pulmonary disease following respirator therapy of hyaline-membrane disease. Bronchopulmonary dysplasia. *N Engl J Med.* 1967;276(7):357–368.
2. Greenough A, Morley C, Davis J. Interaction of spontaneous respiration with artificial ventilation in preterm babies. *J Pediatr.* 1983;103(5):769–773.
3. Greenough A, Morley CJ, Davis JA. Respiratory reflexes in ventilated premature babies. *Early Hum Dev.* 1983;8(1):65–75.
4. Greenough A, Morley CJ, Davis JA. Provoked augmented inspirations in ventilated premature babies. *Early Hum Dev.* 1984;9(2):111–117.
5. Greenough A, Morley CJ. Pneumothorax in infants who fight ventilators. *Lancet.* 1984;1(8378):689.
6. Stark AR, Bascom R, Frantz ID 3rd. Muscle relaxation in mechanically ventilated infants. *J Pediatr.* 1979;94(3):439–443.
7. Perlman JM, McMenamin JB, Volpe JJ. Fluctuating cerebral blood-flow velocity in respiratory-distress syndrome. Relation to the development of intraventricular hemorrhage. *N Engl J Med.* 1983;309(4):204–209.
8. Perlman JM, Goodman S, Kreusser KL, Volpe JJ. Reduction in intraventricular hemorrhage by elimination of fluctuating cerebral blood-flow velocity in preterm infants with respiratory distress syndrome. *N Engl J Med.* 1985;312(21):1353–1357.
9. Field D, Milner AD, Hopkin IE. Manipulation of ventilator settings to prevent active expiration against positive pressure inflation. *Arch Dis Child.* 1985;60(11):1036–1040.
10. South M, Morley CJ. Synchronous mechanical ventilation of the neonate. *Arch Dis Child.* 1986;61(12):1190–1195.
11. Greenough A, Morley CJ, Pool J. Fighting the ventilator—are fast rates an effective alternative to paralysis? *Early Hum Dev.* 1986;13(2):189–194.
12. Mehta A, Callan K, Wright BM, Stacey TE. Patient-triggered ventilation in the newborn. *Lancet.* 328(8497):17–19.
13. Greenough A, Hird MF, Chan V. Airway pressure triggered ventilation for preterm neonates. *J Perinat Med.* 1991;19(6):471–476.
14. Greenough A, Pool J. Neonatal patient triggered ventilation. *Arch Dis Child.* 1988;63(4):394–397.
15. Hird MF, Greenough A. Patient triggered ventilation using a flow triggered system. *Arch Dis Child.* 1991;66(10 Spec No):1140–1142.
16. Hird MF, Greenough A. Patient triggered ventilation in chronically ventilator-dependent infants. *Eur J Pediatr.* 1991;150(10):732–734.
17. Brochard L, Rua F, Lorino H, Lemaire F, Harf A. Inspiratory pressure support compensates for the additional work of breathing caused by the endotracheal tube. *Anesthesiology.* 1991;75(5):739–745.
18. Amitay M, Etches PC, Finer NN, Maidens JM. Synchronous mechanical ventilation of the neonate with respiratory disease. *Crit Care Med.* 1993;21(1):118–124.
19. Bernstein G, Heldt GP, Mannino FL. Increased and more consistent tidal volumes during synchronized intermittent mandatory ventilation in newborn infants. *Am J Respir Crit Care Med.* 1994;150(5 Pt 1):1444–1448.
20. Cleary JP, Bernstein G, Mannino FL, Heldt GP. Improved oxygenation during synchronized intermittent mandatory ventilation in neonates with respiratory distress syndrome: a randomized, crossover study. *J Pediatr.* 1995;126(3):407–411.
21. Hummler H, Gerhardt T, Gonzalez A, Claure N, Everett R, Bancalari E. Influence of different methods of synchronized mechanical ventilation on ventilation, gas exchange, patient effort, and blood pressure fluctuations in premature neonates. *Pediatr Pulmonol.* 1996;22(5):305–313.
22. Jarreau PH, Moriette G, Mussat P, et al. Patient-triggered ventilation decreases the work of breathing in neonates. *Am J Respir Crit Care Med.* 1996;153(3):1176–1181.
23. Greenough A. Update on patient-triggered ventilation. *Clin Perinatol.* 2001;28(3):533–546.

24. Bernstein G, Mannino FL, Heldt GP, et al. Randomized multicenter trial comparing synchronized and conventional intermittent mandatory ventilation in neonates. *J Pediatr*. 1996;128(4):453–463.

25. Claure N, Bancalari E. New modes of mechanical ventilation in the preterm newborn: evidence of benefit. *Arch Dis Child Fetal Neonatal Ed*. 2007;92(6):F508–F512.

26. Quinn MW, de Boer RC, Ansari N, Baumer JH. Stress response and mode of ventilation in preterm infants. *Arch Dis Child Fetal Neonatal Ed*. 1998;78(3):F195–F198.

27. Firme SR, McEvoy CT, Alconcel C, Tanner J, Durand M. Episodes of hypoxemia during synchronized intermittent mandatory ventilation in ventilator-dependent very low birth weight infants. *Pediatr Pulmonol*. 2005;40(1):9–14.

28. John J, Bjorklund LJ, Svenningsen NW, Jonson B. Airway and body surface sensors for triggering in neonatal ventilation. *Acta Paediatr*. 1994;83(9):903–909.

29. Hummler HD, Gerhardt T, Gonzalez A, et al. Patient-triggered ventilation in neonates: comparison of a flow- and an impedance-triggered system. *Am J Respir Crit Care Med*. 1996;154(4 Pt 1):1049–1054.

30. Dimitriou G, Greenough A, Cherian S. Comparison of airway pressure and airflow triggering systems using a single type of neonatal ventilator. *Acta Paediatr*. 2001;90(4):445–447.

31. Figueras J, Rodriguez-Miguelez JM, Botet F, Thio M, Jimenez R. Changes in TcPCO$_2$ regarding pulmonary mechanics due to pneumotachometer dead space in ventilated newborns. *J Perinat Med*. 1997;25(4):333–339.

32. Claure N, D'Ugard C, Bancalari E. Elimination of ventilator dead space during synchronized ventilation in premature infants. *J Pediatr*. 2003;143(3):315–320.

33. Estay A, Claure N, D'Ugard C, Organero R, Bancalari E. Effects of instrumental dead space reduction during weaning from synchronized ventilation in preterm infants. *J Perinatol*. 2010;30(7):479–483.

34. Chang HY, Claure N, D'Ugard C, Torres J, Nwajei P, Bancalari E. Effects of synchronization during nasal ventilation in clinically stable preterm infants. *Pediatr Res*. 2011;69(1):84–89.

35. Kiciman NM, Andreasson B, Bernstein G, et al. Thoracoabdominal motion in newborns during ventilation delivered by endotracheal tube or nasal prongs. *Pediatr Pulmonol*. 1998;25(3):175–181.

36. Friedlich P, Lecart C, Posen R, Ramicone E, Chan L, Ramanathan R. A randomized trial of nasopharyngeal-synchronized intermittent mandatory ventilation versus nasopharyngeal continuous positive airway pressure in very low birth weight infants after extubation. *J Perinatol*. 1999;19(6 Pt 1):413–418.

37. Barrington KJ, Bull D, Finer NN. Randomized trial of nasal synchronized intermittent mandatory ventilation compared with continuous positive airway pressure after extubation of very low birth weight infants. *Pediatrics*. 2001;107(4):638–641.

38. Khalaf MN, Brodsky N, Hurley J, Bhandari V. A prospective randomized, controlled trial comparing synchronized nasal intermittent positive pressure ventilation versus nasal continuous positive airway pressure as modes of extubation. *Pediatrics*. 2001;108(1):13–17.

39. Laubscher B, Greenough A, Kavadia V. Comparison of body surface and airway triggered ventilation in extremely premature infants. *Acta Paediatr*. 1997;86(1):102–104.

40. Dimitriou G, Greenough A, Laubscher B, Yamaguchi N. Comparison of airway pressure-triggered and airflow-triggered ventilation in very immature infants. *Acta Paediatr*. 1998;87(12):1256–1260.

41. Stein H, Alosh H, Ethington P, White DB. Prospective crossover comparison between NAVA and pressure control ventilation in premature neonates less than 1500 grams. *J Perinatol*. 2013;33(6):452–456.

42. Lee J, Kim HS, Jung YH, et al. Non-invasive neurally adjusted ventilatory assist in preterm infants: a randomised phase II crossover trial. *Arch Dis Child Fetal Neonatal Ed*. 2015;100(6):F507–F513.

43. Firestone KS, Fisher S, Reddy S, White DB, Stein HM. Effect of changing NAVA levels on peak inspiratory pressures and electrical activity of the diaphragm in premature neonates. *J Perinatol*. 2015;35(8):612–616.

44. Brochard L, Harf A, Lorino H, Lemaire F. Inspiratory pressure support prevents diaphragmatic fatigue during weaning from mechanical ventilation. *Am Rev Respir Dis*. 1989;139(2):513–521.

45. Osorio W, Claure N, D'Ugard C, Athavale K, Bancalari E. Effects of pressure support during an acute reduction of synchronized intermittent mandatory ventilation in preterm infants. *J Perinatol*. 2005;25(6):412–416.

46. Gupta S, Sinha SK, Donn SM. The effect of two levels of pressure support ventilation on tidal volume delivery and minute ventilation in preterm infants. *Arch Dis Child Fetal Neonatal Ed*. 2009;94(2):F80–F83.

47. Patel DS, Rafferty GF, Lee S, Hannam S, Greenough A. Work of breathing during SIMV with and without pressure support. *Arch Dis Child*. 2009;94(6):434–436.

48. Reyes ZC, Claure N, Tauscher MK, D'Ugard C, Vanbuskirk S, Bancalari E. Randomized, controlled trial comparing synchronized intermittent mandatory ventilation and synchronized intermittent mandatory ventilation plus pressure support in preterm infants. *Pediatrics*. 2006;118(4):1409–1417.

49. Beck J, Tucci M, Emeriaud G, Lacroix J, Sinderby C. Prolonged neural expiratory time induced by mechanical ventilation in infants. *Pediatr Res*. 2004;55(5):747–754.

50. Upton CJ, Milner AD, Stokes GM. The effect of changes in inspiratory time on neonatal triggered ventilation. *Eur J Pediatr*. 1990;149(9):648–650.

51. De Luca D, Conti G, Piastra M, Paolillo PM. Flow-cycled versus time-cycled sIPPV in preterm babies with RDS: a breath-to-breath randomised cross-over trial. *Arch Dis Child Fetal Neonatal Ed*. 2009;94(6):F397–F401.

52. Bernstein G, Knodel E, Heldt GP. Airway leak size in neonates and autocycling of three flow-triggered ventilators. *Crit Care Med*. 1995;23(10):1739–1744.

16

53. DeLemos RA, McLaughlin GW, Robison EJ, Schulz J, Kirby RR. Continuous positive airway pressure as an adjunct to mechanical ventilation in the newborn with respiratory distress syndrome. *Anesth Analg*. 1973;52(3):328–332.

54. Dinger J, Topfer A, Schaller P, Schwarze R. Effect of positive end expiratory pressure on functional residual capacity and compliance in surfactant-treated preterm infants. *J Perinat Med*. 2001;29(2):137–143.

55. Dimitriou G, Greenough A, Laubscher B. Appropriate positive end expiratory pressure level in surfactant-treated preterm infants. *Eur J Pediatr*. 1999;158(11):888–891.

56. Consolo LC, Palhares DB, Consolo LZ. Assessment of pulmonary function of preterm newborn infants with respiratory distress syndrome at different positive end expiratory pressure levels. *J Pediatr*. 2002;78(5):403–408.

57. Alegria X, Claure N, Wada Y, Esquer C, D'Ugard C, Bancalari E. Acute effects of PEEP on tidal volume and respiratory center output during synchronized ventilation in preterm infants. *Pediatr Pulmonol*. 2006;41(8):759–764.

58. Bartholomew KM, Brownlee KG, Snowden S, Dear PR. To PEEP or not to PEEP? *Arch Dis Child Fetal Neonatal Ed*. 1994;70(3):F209–F212.

59. Hassan A, Gossage J, Ingram D, Lee S, Milner AD. Volume of activation of the Hering-Breuer inflation reflex in the newborn infant. *J Appl Physiol (1985)*. 2001;90(3):763–769.

60. Smith J, Bellemare F. Effect of lung volume on in vivo contraction characteristics of human diaphragm. *J Appl Physiol (1985)*. 1987;62(5):1893–1900.

61. South M, Morley CJ, Hughes G. Expiratory muscle activity in preterm babies. *Arch Dis Child*. 1987;62(8):825–829.

62. Keszler M, Abubakar K. Volume guarantee: stability of tidal volume and incidence of hypocarbia. *Pediatr Pulmonol*. 2004;38(3):240–245.

63. Patel DS, Rafferty GF, Lee S, Hannam S, Greenough A. Work of breathing and volume targeted ventilation in respiratory distress. *Arch Dis Child Fetal Neonatal Ed*. 2010;95(6):F443–F446.

64. Patel DS, Sharma A, Prendergast M, Rafferty GF, Greenough A. Work of breathing and different levels of volume-targeted ventilation. *Pediatrics*. 2009;123(4):e679–e684.

65. Longhini F, Ferrero F, De Luca D, et al. Neurally adjusted ventilatory assist in preterm neonates with acute respiratory failure. *Neonatology*. 2015;107(1):60–67.

66. Carlo WA, Martin RJ, Bruce EN, Strohl KP, Fanaroff AA. Alae nasi activation (nasal flaring) decreases nasal resistance in preterm infants. *Pediatrics*. 1983;72(3):338–343.

67. Carlo WA, Kosch PC, Bruce EN, Strohl KP, Martin RJ. Control of laryngeal muscle activity in preterm infants. *Pediatr Res*. 1987;22(1):87–91.

68. Eichenwald EC, Howell RG 3rd, Kosch PC, Ungarelli RA, Lindsey J, Stark R. Developmental changes in sequential activation of laryngeal abductor muscle and diaphragm in infants. *J Appl Physiol (1985)*. 1992;73(4):1425–1431.

69. Carlo WA, Miller MJ, Martin RJ. Differential response of respiratory muscles to airway occlusion in infants. *J Appl Physiol (1985)*. 1985;59(3):847–852.

70. Duara S, Silva Neto G, Claure N, Gerhardt T, Bancalari E. Effect of maturation on the extrathoracic airway stability of infants. *J Appl Physiol*. 1992;73(6):2368–2372.

71. Duara S, Silva Neto G, Claure N. Role of respiratory muscles in upper airway narrowing induced by inspiratory loading in preterm infants. *J Appl Physiol*. 1994;77(1):30–36.

72. Owen LS, Morley CJ, Dawson JA, Davis PG. Effects of non-synchronised nasal intermittent positive pressure ventilation on spontaneous breathing in preterm infants. *Arch Dis Child Fetal Neonatal Ed*. 2011;96(6):F422–F428.

73. Aghai ZH, Saslow JG, Nakhla T, et al. Synchronized nasal intermittent positive pressure ventilation (SNIPPV) decreases work of breathing (WOB) in premature infants with respiratory distress syndrome (RDS) compared to nasal continuous positive airway pressure (NCPAP). *Pediatr Pulmonol*. 2006;41(9):875–881.

74. Ali N, Claure N, Alegria X, D'Ugard C, Organero R, Bancalari E. Effects of non-invasive pressure support ventilation (NI-PSV) on ventilation and respiratory effort in very low birth weight infants. *Pediatr Pulmonol*. 2007;42(8):704–710.

75. Beck J, Reilly M, Grasselli G, et al. Patient-ventilator interaction during neurally adjusted ventilatory assist in low birth weight infants. *Pediatr Res*. 2009;65(6):663–668.

CHAPTER 17

Pulmonary-Cardiovascular Interaction

Shahab Noori and Martin Kluckow

- The respiratory and cardiac systems are integrally related both anatomically and functionally and as a result there are significant interactions, particularly in the newborn period.

- Inappropriately high airway pressure during mechanical ventilation leads to adverse hemodynamic effects, including a reduction in left and right ventricular output, a decrease in venous return, and an increase in pulmonary vascular resistance. Inappropriately low airway pressure can also have detrimental effects by decreasing lung volume and consequently increasing pulmonary vascular resistance.

- Positive end-expiratory pressure and mean arterial pressure in the range commonly used in clinical practice in settings of lung diseases with low compliance and in the absence of low lung volume or hyperexpansion have mild effects on hemodynamics.

- In addition to the direct effects of ventilator settings on the cardiovascular system, the chosen treatment strategy and aims, such as a particular blood gas goal, can have a significant effect on the cardiovascular system. Although the impact of acidosis on the cardiovascular system is not well studied, there is accumulating evidence that excessive hypercapnia, especially in the first few postnatal days, attenuates cerebral blood flow autoregulation and likely contributes to reperfusion injury in preterm infants.

The cardiorespiratory system consists of two organ systems—the heart and cardiovascular system and the lungs and pulmonary vasculature—that are designed to work together to deliver an adequate supply of oxygen to the tissues to meet the demands of oxygen consumption. There are complex anatomic and physiologic relationships between these two organ systems. An understanding as to how they interact both normally and in the presence of pathologic conditions or interventions, such as the provision of positive pressure, is essential for any clinician working with sick children and infants. Changes in intrathoracic pressure affect both organ systems and within the cardiovascular system there are different effects on the left- and right-sided structures. A delicate balance needs to be maintained between the distending airway pressure needed to optimize lung volume—and thus oxygenation—while also avoiding excessive pressure that would compromise global cardiac function that is necessary for adequate systemic blood flow, which is essential for normal oxygen delivery. Both optimal oxygenation and normal cardiac output are required to deliver adequate oxygen to the tissues. Reduced tissue oxygenation often has a multifactorial causation; however, many of the issues are related to what is happening at the level of the cardiorespiratory interaction.

The initial cardiorespiratory interaction is during birth at the time of the circulatory transition and umbilical cord clamping. A normal relationship between the spontaneously breathing infant with normal lungs and cardiovascular system should ensue, in which case there is a balance between the closely associated lungs and heart. If there is a pathologic condition, particularly respiratory distress, then the interventions required to support the respiratory system such as positive-pressure ventilation may adversely affect the function of the heart. Similarly, abnormalities of cardiac function such as ventricular failure can result in lung congestion and the need for respiratory support. Finally, changes in the pulmonary vasculature, particularly in the neonatal transition where failure of the normal fall in pulmonary vascular resistance (PVR) can impair cardiac function. The predominant influence on the cardiorespiratory interaction is mean airway pressure (MAP), which most directly affects the intrathoracic pressure. The effect of inspiration/expiration in addition to MAP is minimal. Adjunctive respiratory therapies such as inhaled nitric oxide may also rapidly change the balance between cardiac and respiratory systems.

Cardiorespiratory Interactions at Birth

In utero the fetus has fluid-filled lungs with a very low pulmonary blood flow (PBF; about 10% of postnatal flow[1]) and minimal tidal volume changes, such that any pressure exerted on the heart physically and via venous return is steady and unchanging. The interposition of the placenta and the unique fetal shunts—the ductus venosus, foramen ovale (FO), and patent ductus arteriosus (PDA)—into the fetoplacental circulation results in a fetal circulation quite different from that of the postnatal infant just minutes after birth. Instead of being two parallel circulations, there is admixture of blood at several levels. Oxygenated blood returning from the placenta via the umbilical vein passes through the ductus venosus and into the inferior vena cava (IVC). Blood then streams into the right atrium, where owing to the anatomy of the right atrium and FO, the oxygenated blood is directed preferentially across the FO into the left atrium, thus improving the oxygenation level of blood passing from the left atrium into the left ventricle and subsequently toward the systemic circulation. The presence of the PDA and fetal conditions (hypoxemia, vasoconstricting factors) that cause increased PVR result in preferential blood flow from the right ventricle via the right-to-left shunting PDA into the systemic circulation.[2] The significantly reduced blood flow to the pulmonary circulation means that the normal main source of preload to the left atrium (when there is no placental flow)—the pulmonary venous return—is significantly limited in utero.[3] Blood passing from the right ventricle via the PDA and from the left ventricle into the aorta travels down the descending aorta and deoxygenated blood is then sent to the placenta via iliac and eventually umbilical arteries to complete the fetoplacental circulation. The main flow to the left atrium is provided by the placental return and some flow from lower body via the IVC; this is an important consideration when the timing of umbilical cord clamping in the newborn transition is considered. Interruption of the placental blood flow return before establishment of the PBF through the lungs puts the transitioning newborn at risk of a loss of preload to the systemic ventricle with a subsequent fall in systemic cardiac output.[4]

The events of the perinatal cardiopulmonary transition constitute the first, and possibly most crucial, cardiorespiratory interaction and there is potential for significant complications. Such complications range from premature interruption of the placental blood flow, resulting in an acute drop in cardiac output,[4] to failure to properly transition, leading to the syndrome of persistent pulmonary hypertension of the newborn (PPHN; Table 17.1). Keeping the cardiorespiratory events of the transition

Table 17.1   CLINICAL RELEVANCE OF CARDIORESPIRATORY INTERACTION AT BIRTH

Event	Intervention	Impact
Inspiration	Stimulation or PPV	Fluid absorption ↑ Pulmonary blood flow Reversal of PDA shunt
Lung aeration before cord clamping	Stimulation, CPAP/PPV[a]	Placental transfusion
Establishing FRC	CPAP/PPV	Improved oxygenation, ↓ Risk of PPHN
Avoidance of hyperoxia	Avoidance of hyperoxia	Improved response to iNO in case of PPHN

[a]Excessively high CPAP and PPV can also negatively affect venous return and cardiovascular function (see text).
CPAP, Continuous positive airway pressure; *FRC,* functional residual capacity; *iNO,* inhaled nitric oxide; *PDA,* patent ductus arteriosus; *PPHN,* persistent pulmonary hypertension of the newborn; *PPV,* positive-pressure ventilation.

in sequence has become an important aspect of management at birth. The key initial event is inflation of the lungs (usually by crying but also by use of positive-pressure devices), resulting in a rapid increase in PBF and reversal of the ductal shunt to become left to right.[5] Additionally, the lung liquid must be rapidly absorbed; the most recent animal imaging data suggest that this occurs via transepithelial gradients developed during inspiration.[6,7] With the increased PBF, adequate left atrial filling is established and the umbilical cord can now be cut without acutely reducing the left atrial return. In this sequence, oxygenation is provided by the lungs before the placental "lung" is removed by cord clamping. Failure to allow the natural sequence of events to unfold may result in significant hemodynamic instability, at least in animal models.[8] The first response to clamping the umbilical cord and separating from the low-resistance placenta before lung aeration is a rapid increase in arterial pressure and blood flow and a rapid reduction in cardiac output from lack of LA filling, followed by a surge in blood pressure and blood flow as PBF is established. These hemodynamic changes are much less marked if the PBF is established by lung aeration before cord clamping (termed physiologically based cord clamping).[9] Delaying cord clamping increases the likelihood that the newborn will establish breathing/lung inflation before the umbilical cord is clamped.[10,11] The benefits of a delay in cord clamp time have generally been ascribed to the receipt of a placental transfusion.[11] The magnitude of the transfusion is dependent on a number of factors, including gravity, time, flow/patency of the umbilical vessels, and spontaneous breathing efforts. Respiratory efforts result in significant fluctuations in umbilical cord blood flow[12] and can potentially enhance the placental transfusion received as well as stabilize the hemodynamics of the transition as discussed previously. The consequences of an increased understanding of the cardiorespiratory interactions at birth are that there may be physiologic advantages to providing positive pressure and initial resuscitative measures while the infant is still attached to the umbilical cord. Equipment and techniques to allow this to happen are currently in development.[10,13]

Umbilical cord milking is another alternative for provision of a placental transfusion to the newborn. Less is known about the physiology of this technique and the cardiorespiratory effects on placental transfusion. Because transfusion occurs over a shorter period, there is less opportunity for the effect of the respiratory system on the volume of transfusion and subsequent cardiac flow on effects.[14] The cardiovascular benefits still seem to be present, including higher mean blood pressure and less inotrope use.[15]

After inflation of the lungs and the commencement of spontaneous negative-pressure breathing, there are further cardiorespiratory interactions with venous blood return to the heart enhanced by the negative-pressure generated during normal inspiration. This can be seen on blood flow traces showing a respiratory pattern, more so in adults.[16] If an infant requires positive-pressure support—either by continuous positive airway pressure (CPAP) or mechanical ventilation—some degree of impact on the cardiovascular system is inevitable. Mechanical ventilation raises intrathoracic pressure and reduces venous return and preload to the right heart, thus also impairing right ventricular (RV) performance, especially if the distending pressure is excessive relative to the compliance of the lungs. Mechanical ventilation also significantly affects PVR and RV afterload. The left ventricle, in contrast, receives venous return from within the thorax so it is less affected by changes in intrathoracic pressure. Cardiac output from the left ventricle is dependent on blood flow from the right ventricle, so changes in RV output will also affect left ventricular (LV) output. Increased pressure in the right ventricle can cause a conformational change in the heart with displacement of the interventricular septum that decreases LV preload and compliance. Although LV contractility is not affected by positive-pressure ventilation, the LV output can be significantly affected by changes in the LV myocardial wall tension (the difference between LV systolic pressure and mean intrathoracic pressure).[17,18] There is also a potentially positive effect of mechanical ventilation and raised intrathoracic pressure on the LV with lower LV afterload owing to a decreased transmyocardial pressure gradient in the setting of higher intrathoracic pressure (Fig. 17.1).[19]

After birth the neonate is exposed to higher oxygen tension compared with fetal life. Routine use of oxygen supplement can deleteriously affect the cardiovascular

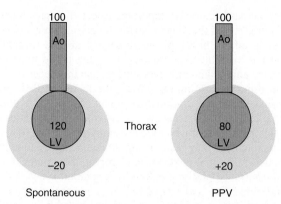

Fig. 17.1   Effects of intrathoracic pressure on left ventricular (*LV*) afterload. This is a schematic drawing of an example of the difference in intrathoracic and left ventricular pressure in spontaneously breathing versus positive-pressure ventilation (*PPV*) in an adult. On the left side, the left ventricle of a spontaneously breathing patient needs to generate a transmural pressure of 120 mm Hg in response to a systemic systolic pressure of 100 mm Hg and a mean intrathoracic pressure of –20 mm Hg. When this patient is mechanically ventilated with a mean intrathoracic pressure of +20 mm Hg, the left ventricle has to generate a pressure of only 80 mm Hg to result in the same systemic systolic pressure of 100 mm Hg. Thus an augmentation of mean intrathoracic pressure reduces left ventricular afterload and potentially improves overall left ventricular function. *Ao,* Aorta. (From Cheifetz IM. Cardiorespiratory interactions: the relationship between mechanical ventilation and hemodynamics. *Respir Care.* 2014;59:1937–1945.)

transition. Indeed, animal models have shown a reduction in response to inhaled nitric oxide in sheep with PPHN exposed to a high fraction of inspired oxygen.[20]

Each of the elements of cardiovascular function can be affected by the respiratory system—the preload via changes in intrathoracic pressure and PBF, the contractility by direct impingement on ventricles within a confined space, and the afterload by changes in the PVR (both overinflation and underinflation increase PVR)[21]—that also translates to inadequate filling of the left atrium in the setting of reduced PBF.[22,23]

The Physiology of Cardiovascular and Respiratory Interaction

During normal phasic spontaneous breathing with negative intrathoracic pressure, the passive systemic venous return can easily fill the right atrium, which is at low pressure, with the additional augmenting effect of inspiration. The end-diastolic volumes of both ventricles change in different directions: enhanced venous return into the RV from outside the thorax increases RV filling, which makes the LV stiffer and harder to fill.[24] When positive pressure is applied, the opposite happens: impaired RV filling and easier LV filling. The end result of these changes is fluctuations in the systemic arterial pressure. In a ventilated adult, ventilator-induced changes in preload can result in a variable stroke volume and subsequently variation in the pulse pressure. The rise in arterial pressure during a positive-pressure breath is counterintuitive as the expectation would be reduction in venous return and subsequently the pulse pressure should decrease. Factors that may account for this include an increase in pulmonary venous return from squeezing of capillaries, decreased LV afterload, mechanical assistance of LV contraction by compression, and adrenergic stimulation with increased inotropy.[25] The degree of pulse pressure variation can be used to predict responsiveness to a volume bolus during supportive hemodynamic management.[26] Interestingly, the effect of mechanical ventilation on the right ventricle is opposite: impaired venous return and cardiac output, which in turn reduces the venous return to the left atrium that will result in a fall in LV output as well. Pulse pressure variation is also seen in neonates in association with cardiopulmonary interactions, but it is probably not as variable and thus not likely to be as predictive of fluid responsiveness.[27] This may be due to the greater compliance of the newborn chest wall compared with that of the adult, which may decrease the transmission of positive pressure to the pleural space and mediastinum.

Table 17.2 IMPACT OF LUNG DISEASE AND VENTILATOR SUPPORT ON COMPONENTS OF CARDIAC OUTPUT

Component	Respiratory Alteration	Resultant Effect
Preload	High mean airway pressure	↓ RV preload
	High pulmonary vascular resistance	↓ LV preload
Contractility	High pulmonary vascular resistance	↓ RV contractility
	Acidosis secondary to permissive hypercapnia	↓ Contractility[a]
Afterload	High pulmonary vascular resistance	↑ RV afterload
	Positive intrathoracic pressure	↓ LV afterload

[a]This has been demonstrated in adults.
LV, Left ventricular; *RV,* right ventricular.

Preload

Preload is an important driver of adequate cardiac contractility and subsequently cardiac output and the newborn heart are particularly sensitive to changes in preload. Worsening respiratory disease can affect both right and left sides of the heart (Table 17.2). Higher MAP impairs systemic venous return to the right atrium, necessitating higher central venous pressure (CVP) to counteract the increased intrathoracic pressure, particularly in the setting of positive-pressure ventilation. If the reduced systemic venous return is not balanced by increased CVP, the preload to the right ventricle is reduced and thus right ventricular output (RVO) will fall. A reduction in RVO results in reduced PBF, which apart from the effect on oxygenation, will also have an impact on the preload and filling to the left atrium and, subsequently, the systemic cardiac output. The reduction in PBF can be exacerbated by the state of recruitment of the lungs. Underrecruited lungs result in collapse in the supporting tissues around blood vessels in the lung, thus increasing PVR. If the lungs are overinflated, the increased pressure from the air-filled structures in the lung causes compression of pulmonary vasculature and results in impaired PBF and reduced return to the left atrium (Fig. 17.2). If there is increased pulmonary vasoconstriction (such as in PPHN), this will also impair blood flow through the lungs. An index of severity of raised PVR can be obtained by assessing the pulmonary venous return, in which case the pulmonary venous velocity is reduced.[28] Direct impingement of the heart, either by excessive MAP with overdistended lungs or by dilation of either ventricle, can cause septal bowing and reduction of ventricular cavity, typically of the LV by the RV with PPHN.[29]

At low MAPs, the negative influence on cardiac output is mediated primarily through reduced systemic venous return, whereas at higher MAPs direct effects on PVR and myocardial function become important.[22] In the sickest infants, all of these factors are likely to be important. MAP is often very high, hypoxia and acidosis are common, and pulmonary artery pressure is high as suggested by the commonly observed low ductal blood flow velocity. Both ventricles also show the ability to substantially increase output when the preload is increased by a ductal or atrial shunt, confirming a degree of myocardial reserve. The effect of positive-pressure ventilation in reducing systemic venous return and cardiac output may be as important in preterm infants as it has been recognized to be in adults. There are few studies on the effect of ventilation on cardiac output in the preterm infant. Hausdorf and Hellwege[30] demonstrated a 25% to 30% reduction in ventricular stroke and cardiac output, with no effect on blood pressure, by increasing positive end-expiratory pressure (PEEP) from 0 to 8 cm H$_2$O in a group of preterm infants. This is clinically important because an aggressive effort to improve arterial oxygenation may reduce perfusion and thus compromise tissue oxygen delivery. Trang et al.[31] suggested that this occurs at PEEP levels above 6 cm H$_2$O in preterm infants. However, the absolute level of PEEP or MAP is not as important as the appropriateness of those pressures for the compliance of the lungs; the more compliant the lungs are, the greater the transmission of distending airway pressure to the mediastinum and thus the greater the impairment of cardiac output.

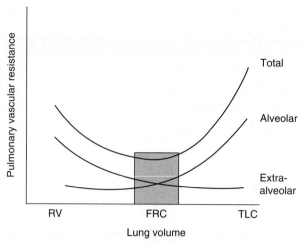

Fig. 17.2 Schematic representation of the relationship between lung volume and pulmonary vascular resistance. As lung volume increases from residual volume *(RV)* to total lung capacity *(TLC)*, the alveolar vessels become increasingly compressed by the distending alveoli; thus their resistance increases, whereas the resistance of the extraalveolar vessels (which become less tortuous as lung volume increases) falls. The combined effect of increasing lung volume on the pulmonary vasculature produces the typical U-shaped curve as shown, with its nadir, or optimum, at around normal functional residual capacity *(FRC)*. (From Shekerdemian L, Bohn D. Cardiovascular effects of mechanical ventilation. *Arch Dis Child.* 1999;80:475–480.)

Interventions to counteract the deleterious effects of respiratory diseases and ventilator support on the preload primarily involve judicious use of ventilation settings to avoid excessive MAP and addressing the underlying pathophysiology of the lung disease—for example, reducing PVR. However, there is some evidence from adults[23] and one study in the preterm newborn[32] to suggest that volume expansion can correct some of the preload deficit that results from positive-pressure ventilation and improve cardiac output in the short term.

Contractility

Mechanical ventilation does not appear to directly affect myocardial contractility. However, through a decrease in LV afterload it may enhance LV contractility. On the other hand, as discussed earlier, inappropriately high or low lung volume can increase PVR and therefore through an increase in RV afterload can impair RV contractility. In addition, ventilator strategies aimed at permissive hypercapnia with resulting acidosis can decrease myocardial contractility, at least in adults (see the "Effect of Acidosis and Permissive Hypercapnia" section). In the term infant, poor cardiac output is most often the result of an asphyxial insult or sepsis. Poor cardiac output in the preterm infant has been seen primarily as a consequence of an immature myocardium,[33] especially in the first few postnatal days of the very premature infant.[34] LV ejection fraction, admittedly a broad measure of myocardial function in the preterm infant,[35] was not significantly associated with either ventricular output. The predominantly left-to-right pattern of ductal shunting reduces RV output, and atrial shunting reduces LV output (LVO) by shunting blood from the systemic back to the pulmonary circulation. This effect is apparent even in the first postnatal days.

Afterload

Afterload also potentially has a large effect on cardiac output in the transitioning newborn. The afterload to which the right ventricle is exposed is determined primarily by what is happening in the lungs, both in terms of aeration and in terms of the pulmonary vascular pressure. Optimization of lung recruitment and addressing raised PVR are both important strategies to improve RV function. Judicious management of the shunting through the PDA may also be important with strategies to allow the PDA to remain open and promote a right-to-left shunt, sometimes reducing afterload on the RV and allowing improved forward flow out of the ventricle. Although as discussed earlier, positive-pressure ventilation can enhance LV contractility by reducing the LV afterload (wall stress), systemic vascular resistance (SVR) plays a more important role in changes in LV afterload than mechanical ventilation.

The newborn myocardium and cardiac function are more vulnerable to both preload and afterload changes than in older infants and adults and this is even more so in preterm infants. They have a simpler structure with fewer mitochondria, and differences in the myofibrils themselves result in less reserve and ability to compensate for changes in blood volume and peripheral resistance.[34,36]

Effect of the Respiratory System on the Cardiovascular System

Mechanical Ventilation

In a normal spontaneously breathing infant during inspiration, the negative intrathoracic pressure increases the transmural pressure in the right atrium (RA) and RV, thereby increasing the venous return. During expiration the opposite effects occur; however, owing to the presence of valves in the venous system, these effects are relatively small. On the other hand, when a patient is receiving positive-pressure respiratory support, during inspiration the pleural pressure increases and therefore venous return to the RA is impeded while the improvement in venous return occurs during the expiratory phase.

The effect of phases of respiration during mechanical ventilation on the left and RV filling is different. During expiration, both phases of ventricular filling (early passive and atrial) increase on the right side and decrease on the left side.[37] The increase in LV filling during inspiration may be related to the increase in intraalveolar/interalveolar pressure improving drainage to the left atrium (LA) and improved LV distensibility owing to lower RV volume.

Effects of PEEP, CPAP, and MAP

The effects of PEEP, CPAP and MAP on venous return, PVR, and cardiac function for the most part depend on the lung compliance and lung volume. Both extremes of lung volume can increase PVR (see Fig. 17.2).[38] This increase in RV afterload can impair RV function and through ventricular interdependence also adversely affect LV function.

In an experiment on premature lambs with normal lungs ventilated with a tidal volume of 5 mL/kg and receiving PEEP of 4 cm H_2O, PEEP was changed randomly to 0, 8, and 12 cm H_2O.[39] Increasing PEEP from 4 to 8 H_2O and from 4 to 12 H_2O decreased PBF by 20.5% and 41%, respectively, and caused corresponding changes in PVR; reducing PEEP from 4 to 0 H_2O did not affect PBF. Interestingly, despite decreasing PBF, increasing PEEP from 4 to 8 H_2O and then 12 cm H_2O improved oxygenation, presumably as the result of improvement in lung recruitment and ventilation-perfusion matching. Higher PVR and lower PBF with an increase in PEEP have also been shown in a swine model with normal pulmonary function test results.[40] Again, it needs to be emphasized that these animals had normal lung compliance and therefore any PEEP above 4 cm H_2O would be excessive.

Although the effects of increase in PEEP/MAP in human neonates are similar to those of animal models, they are less prominent. When the PEEP increased from 0 to 4 cm H_2O and 8 cm H_2O in preterm infants after the acute phase of respiratory distress syndrome (RDS), both left and right cardiac output decreased.[30] In a more recent and larger study, preterm and term infants supported by mechanical ventilation with a baseline PEEP of 5 cm H_2O were exposed to a brief period of higher PEEP of 8 cm H_2O.[41] The researchers found a statistically nonsignificant 5% decrease in RVO and no effect on systemic circulation as evidenced by unchanged superior vena cava (SVC) flow for the infants as a group. However, the effect on SVC flow was variable; a third of the subjects showed a significant (about 25%) increase and another third demonstrated a significant decrease in SVC flow. These divergent effects are probably explained by differences in the underlying lung pathology; those with more compliant lungs had a decrease in flow with higher PEEP, while those with more atelectatic lungs showed improved flow with higher PEEP. In this study, no change in ductal diameter or in percentage of right-to-left shunt was noted. Another study assessed the effect of change in PEEP from a baseline of 5 cm H_2O to 2 and 8 cm H_2O on ductal shunting and systemic flow in ventilated extremely preterm infants with a PDA.[42] Reduction of PEEP to 2 cm H_2O had no significant effect. There was no change in SVC flow or cerebral regional oxygen saturation, but there was a mild reduction in LVO with a resultant decrease in the LVO-to-SVC ratio when PEEP was increased to 8 cm H_2O. This is suggestive of a mild reduction in left-to-right ductal shunting. However, the low LVO could also reflect a reduction in venous return. Interestingly, a recent study found no difference in LVO, RVO, or SVC flow with CPAP of 4, 6, and 8 cm H_2O in stable preterm infants with minimal lung disease.[43] This lack of any hemodynamic effect may be attributed to ineffective pressure transmission via a noninvasive nasal interface. Studies of preterm infants being weaned from CPAP have shown variable results; some reported no effect, whereas others demonstrated lower RVO and SVC flow during CPAP treatment.[44,45]

A study of the impact of lung recruitment with high-frequency oscillation on pulmonary, systemic, and ductal blood flow in preterm infants with RDS demonstrates interesting findings.[46] Before giving surfactant, the MAP was increased stepwise until the fraction of inspired oxygen (F_{IO_2}) was less than 0.25 or no further improvement in oxygenation was noted; this was termed the opening pressure. Then the MAP was decreased until deterioration in oxygenation was noted; this was termed the closing pressure. Then lungs were recruited again and MAP was kept at 2 cm H_2O above the closing pressure; this was termed the optimal pressure. Despite very high MAP at the optimal pressure (20 cm H_2O), the hemodynamic effects were small. The RVO decreased by 17%, but no changes in SVC flow, ductal diameter, or flow pattern were noted.

Based on the available literature, the impact of PEEP or CPAP of up to 8 cm H_2O on ductal diameter and flow, systemic flow and PBF in preterm infants appear to be negligible or minimal. This is in contrast to animal studies, which have demonstrated a significant reduction in venous return and PBF and an increase in PVR. Although this may be the result of interspecies differences, the main reason for the discrepancy is likely the difference in lung compliance. Animal studies in general evaluated the impact of PEEP in models with normal lung compliance, whereas in human studies subjects had lung disease with presumably variable decrease in compliance. Indeed, as noted earlier, even a very high MAP appears to have little effect on the hemodynamics in subjects with poor lung compliance.[47] Therefore the positive airway pressure more readily affects intrapleural pressure and overdistends the alveoli if it is inappropriately high for the degree of reduced compliance. As such, inappropriately high PEEP and MAP can result in increased PVR and reduction in PBF, leading to hypoxemia and decreased systemic blood flow.

Effect of Tidal Volume

Little is known about the effect of different tidal volumes on hemodynamics. In a pediatric swine model with normal lung function, increasing tidal volume (up to 25 mL/kg) resulted in progressive and exponential increase in PVR and reduction in RVO and these effects were more pronounced with higher PEEP.[40] These deleterious effects appear to be the result of decreased preload (impaired venous return) and lung overdistention with physical compression of the microvasculature. Clearly, a grossly excessive tidal volume of this degree has deleterious effects. In addition, as discussed earlier, normal lung compliance in these animal models limits the applicability of the findings to human subjects with lung disease.

Effect of Acidosis and Permissive Hypercapnia

Permissive hypercapnia is a common lung-protective strategy used in the care of neonates with lung disease.[48] Acceptance of higher carbon dioxide (CO_2) levels than normal allows for use of lower ventilator settings and smaller tidal volumes with a resultant decrease in volutrauma and lung injury.[49] Because the renal compensatory metabolic alkalosis takes several days to take hold and may be further delayed in extremely premature infants owing to renal tubular immaturity, permissive hypercapnia leads to acidosis, especially in the first few postnatal days. Little is known about the impact of acidosis on cardiovascular function and cerebral hemodynamics in neonates.

The ionic channels in the myocyte are pH sensitive. Some promote and others reduce the influx of calcium, with the net effect of an increase in intracellular calcium with an acidic pH.[50] However, owing to the inhibition of myofibrillar responsiveness in acidic pH, myocardial contractility decreases despite an increase in intracellular calcium. In adult humans, acidosis and permissive hypercapnia affect the heart and vascular system, leading to a decrease in myocardial contractility and a drop in SVR. Despite the decrease in contractility, cardiac output increases, most likely secondary to low afterload. Most of the effects of hypercapnia on the cardiovascular system appear to be mediated via altering pH as the above-mentioned effects tend to attenuate or completely disappear with administration of a base or with passage of time as compensatory metabolic alkalosis sets in.[51,52] Interestingly, animal studies suggest that the myocardial and vascular responses to acidosis are developmentally regulated and differ in newborn versus adult subjects. Newborn animals exhibit a more tolerant myocardium but greater vasodilation in response to acidosis.[53–55] Little is known about the effects of acidosis in human neonates. A recent prospective cross-sectional study evaluated the effect of pH and CO_2 on cardiovascular function in hemodynamically stable preterm infants.[56] The pH ranged from 7.02 to 7.46 and CO_2 from 28 to 76 mm Hg and base excess from −13 to +6 mEq/L. They found no relationship between various indices of myocardial contractility and pH in the first 2 weeks after birth. There was no relationship between either LVO or SVR with pH (or CO_2) during the transitional period (first 3 days). However, a weak but significant negative correlation between LVO and pH and positive correlation between SVR and pH were noted after the transitional period (postnatal day 4–14). CO_2 had a positive and negative correlation with LVO and SVR, respectively, during the post-transitional period. The observed association remained significant even after adjusting for the effect of base deficit. This lack of reduction in contractility in contrast to the findings in adults may be due to higher intracellular buffer in neonates compared to that of the mature myocardium.[57] As for the effect of pH and CO_2 on cardiac output and SVR, there appears to be a postnatal maturational process in the cardiovascular response with the pattern becoming similar to that seen in adults only after the first 3 postnatal days.[56] Attempts at normalizing pH in the case of metabolic acidosis by giving sodium bicarbonate yields minimal hemodynamic effects. When sodium bicarbonate was given to ventilated preterm infants with metabolic acidosis, despite an increase in pH from mean 7.24 to 7.30, the increase in cardiac output was transient and likely was reflective of volume administration.[58] Similarly, correction of metabolic acidosis with sodium bicarbonate had no effect on cerebral, renal, and splanchnic regional tissue oxygenation in very low-birth-weight neonates.[59]

Effect of the Cardiovascular System on the Respiratory System

The impact of impaired cardiovascular system function on the respiratory system is primarily through alteration in normal pulmonary flow. In the case of myocardial dysfunction—for example, in the setting of perinatal asphyxia—the RVO can be low owing to poor contractility. In addition, the concomitant pulmonary hypertension that is common in this setting could lead to a severely compromised PBF and hypoxemic respiratory failure.

Excessive pulmonary flow in the setting of intracardiac shunt or PDA results in pulmonary edema and decreases lung compliance, necessitating an escalation in ventilator support. The impact of PDA on lung function and development of BPD are discussed in detail in Chapter 7.

Impaired LV diastolic function increases left atrial pressure and can result in pulmonary venous congestion and pulmonary edema. Unfortunately, owing to difficulty in noninvasive assessment of diastolic function, this problem is often unrecognized.

The close relationship between the cardiovascular and respiratory systems both functionally and anatomically means that these systems interact and influence each other significantly. In the neonate there are several specific conditions that result in important interactions that can be clinically relevant.

Pulmonary Hypertension

The syndrome of PPHN, presenting clinically as an infant with hypoxic respiratory failure disproportionate to the degree of lung abnormality, is associated with significant interaction between the lungs and cardiovascular system. It is important to understand that this PPHN is a clinical syndrome, not a single entity of raised pulmonary pressures. The syndrome of PPHN can arise from a variety of clinical conditions, the end result of which is dependent on the relative effect of each of the components. The effect of each component on the respiratory system is also variable. The underlying components of PPHN include lung pathology and ventilation-perfusion mismatch (meconium aspiration, pneumonia); the effect of asphyxia on myocardial function' the patency of the ductus arteriosus; the relative pressures across the PDA resulting in left-to-right, right-to-left, or bidirectional shunt; the PVR; and the SVR. Each of these components has some influence on the respiratory system, some more directly than others. The effect of air space abnormality, which can result in ventilation-perfusion mismatch, is clear and can result in reduced gas exchange with poor oxygenation and CO_2 retention, both of which in turn may result in increased PVR. Increased PVR can both change the direction of shunting across the PDA depending on the SVR and blood pressure, as well as reduce the PBF. PBF is reduced as the result of poor RV function, increased afterload from both PVR, and lung air space changes, which directly impinge on the patency of pulmonary blood vessels. The iatrogenic effect of mechanical ventilation or increased distending pressure also contributes to this impingement on the pulmonary blood vessels. The effect of reduced PBF owing to multiple underlying causes cascades on to the systemic side of the heart with reduced filling of the left atrium and subsequently decreased LV output. The reduced LV output may be exacerbated by asphyxial myocardial injury, with up to 70% of asphyxiated infants demonstrating evidence of abnormal cardiac function when cardiac output is measured.[60,61] The reduction in systemic blood flow may then in turn result in reduced systemic blood flow and blood pressure, which results in more right-to-left shunting through the PDA. Finally, the ventricular interdependence of the right and left ventricles, which share a septum and fibers and are constrained by the pericardium, can result in further reductions in the LV output owing to decreased cavity size and preload from septal bowing away from the right ventricle in the setting of high pulmonary vascular pressures (Fig. 17.3).[62]

Patent Ductus Arteriosus

The relationship between the PDA and the lung is extensively reviewed in Chapter 7. The effect of a PDA on the lung occurs at multiple levels and at differing time points. The initial effect occurs with increasing left-to-right shunt through a PDA that has failed to constrict fully, usually in the setting of a premature infant. Failure of full constriction in the first few hours in the setting of an infant who has rapidly improving lung compliance results in an increasing left-to-right shunt through the PDA. The resultant increased PBF has several effects. The first is the physical effect of stiffer lungs, which are more difficult for the infant to inflate or require higher positive pressure if receiving respiratory support. Premature infants may develop CO_2 retention or have increasing apnea and need for respiratory support. Second, the increased blood flow through lung blood vessels and capillaries results in fluid leakage into the interstitial tissues, predisposing infants to lung damage and the need for increased respiratory support. Finally, acute increases in PBF can lead to more significant complications, including pulmonary hemorrhage (actually hemorrhagic pulmonary edema)[63] that can cause acute pulmonary injury and clinical deterioration, with a need for high ventilator pressures and eventually long-term pulmonary damage.

The association between PDA and BPD is clear but a causal relationship has not been established. Reduction in the incidence of BPD has not been demonstrated in clinical trials of early treatment to close the PDA. These trials, however, are problematic in that there were large variations in patient clinical features and a high incidence of open-label treatment confounding the results.[64]

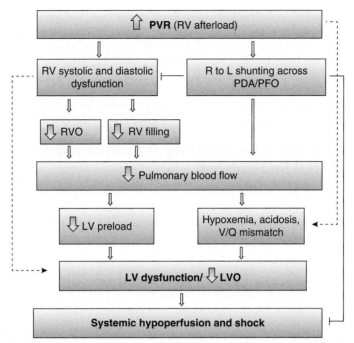

Fig. 17.3 Circulatory changes in neonates with pulmonary hypertension showing the multiple underlying pathophysiologies and the interactions between them, which can lead to a vicious cycle of hypoxemia, ventilation-perfusion *(V/Q)* mismatch and cardiac dysfunction. *LV,* Left ventricular; *LVO,* left ventricular output; *PDA,* patent ductus arteriosus; *PFO,* patent foramen ovale; *PVR,* pulmonary vascular resistance; *R to L,* right to left; *RV,* right ventricular; *RVO,* right ventricular output. (From McNamara P, Weisz D, Giesinger RE, Jain A. Hemodynamics. In MacDonald MG, Seshia MK, eds. *Avery's Neonatology: Pathophysiology & Management of the Newborn.* 7th ed. Philadelphia: Wolters Kluwer; 2016, pp 457–486.)

Asphyxia

Infants who have evidence of asphyxia at birth with low Apgar scores, acidosis, and neonatal encephalopathy frequently have associated cardiorespiratory dysfunction. The appearance of an asphyxiated infant—pale and tachycardic with impaired perfusion—suggests cardiovascular compromise and, indeed, transient myocardial ischemia is commonly associated with asphyxia.[65,66] The common association with myocardial impairment results in respiratory impairment from reduced cardiac output with venous congestion and subsequent respiratory distress.

Congenital Diaphragmatic Hernia

Infants with congenital diaphragmatic hernia have a variable degree of lung hypoplasia and pulmonary vasculature changes, which result in raised pulmonary pressures; thus congenital diaphragmatic hernia is one of the causal factors in the syndrome of PPHN. Several factors accentuate the cardiorespiratory interaction. These include displacement of the heart owing to herniated organs, pulmonary hypertension secondary to pulmonary hypoplasia and hypoxia, and the need for positive-pressure ventilation. Systemic hypotension is commonly seen in this patient population as the result of decreased venous return, hypoxia, acidosis, and LV dysfunction secondary to abnormal ventricular septal motion. This in turn can exacerbate right-to-left shunting at the PDA level. In addition, there is usually a variable degree of LV hypoplasia and dysfunction,[67,68] which appears to limit the effectiveness of pulmonary vasodilator therapy.[69]

Congenital Heart Disease

Congenital heart disease in infants represents another potential area where the cardiovascular system interacts with the respiratory system. The physiologic effects of positive-pressure ventilation on the systemic and pulmonary circulations should be carefully considered. Ductal-dependent cyanotic heart disease presents acutely at the time of ductal closure or earlier if there are signs of desaturation. Disordered blood flow and hypoxia often result in raised pulmonary pressures. Infants with congenital heart disease that is associated with increased PBF, including severe left heart abnormalities such as hypoplastic left heart syndrome and univentricular physiology, may have pulmonary overcirculation with increased risk of pulmonary edema. Systemic output may also be reduced owing to preferential flow into the pulmonary circulation.

Interaction During Early Transition and Potential Clinical Implications

The role of left-to-right PDA shunting in the pathogenesis of BPD and pulmonary hemorrhage is discussed elsewhere (see Chapter 7). In this section, we review the cardiovascular and cerebral hemodynamic effects of surfactant administration and CO_2 alteration in preterm infants.

Surfactant

Surfactant administration for RDS can be associated with significant changes in hemodynamics. Although surfactant may have vasodilatory properties, most of the hemodynamic changes are likely to be due to mechanical effects of the instillation process and rapid improvement in lung compliance and functional residual capacity. As a result, studies have shown variable effects of surfactant on indices of cerebral blood flow (CBF); some show reduction, and others report no change or an increase.[70–74] Some changes have been attributed to redistribution of blood flow and an increase in CO_2.[70,72,73]

The reported effects of surfactant on systemic and PBF are also variable. Animal studies have shown an increase in PBF. Human data on the subject are scarce. In preterm neonates in the delivery room, surfactant administration resulted in an increase in RVO but no change in SVC flow.[75] It is intriguing that despite an increase in ductal diameter in the presence of a complete left-to-right shunt, an increase in fractional shortening, and an increase in the left atrium-to-aortic root ratio, the LVO decreased in this study. In more mature preterm infants, rescue surfactant several hours after birth resulted in an increase in SVC flow and RVO but only in those who were considered surfactant-responders (defined as an FIO_2 of 0.21 by 3 hours following surfactant administration).[76] Interestingly, no change in PDA or PFO flow was noted in this study.

The effect of surfactant on the PDA is of particular interest as the improvement in lung compliance and reduction in PVR can significantly increase left-to-right ductal shunting and theoretically predispose to pulmonary hemorrhage. While animal studies have shown a significant increase in left-to-right ductal shunting after surfactant administration,[77] this has not been demonstrated in humans.[73,75,76] Although there are differences between experimental models and clinical settings, the lack of effect in humans could also be due to difficulty in assessing ductal flow using Doppler techniques.

Carbon Dioxide, Cerebral Blood Flow, and Brain Injury

As mentioned earlier, CO_2 values above the normal level are common in preterm infants. Accepting higher CO_2 allows for use of lower ventilator settings and weaning from respiratory support, although this has not been shown to affect development of BPD.[78,79] However, changes in CO_2 significantly alter cerebral hemodynamics with hypocapnia reducing and hypercapnia increasing CBF. These changes in CBF could have a significant impact on outcome.

There is a strong association between high CO_2 levels and the occurrence of periventricular/intraventricular hemorrhage (P/IVH).[80,81] A higher CO_2 level has been shown to be an independent predictor of severe P/IVH or death,[82] and maximum CO_2 in the first 3 days is a dose-dependent predictor of severe P/IVH.[83] It is postulated that a high CO_2 level potentiates the reperfusion phase of the ischemia-reperfusion injury that precedes the occurrence of P/IVH.[84] Interestingly, the effect of CO_2 on CBF is blunted on the first day. However, by the second postnatal day the cerebral vasculature becomes very reactive to high CO_2 levels.[85,86] A recent study showed a breakpoint between middle cerebral artery mean flow velocity (a surrogate for CBF) and CO_2 at about 52 mm Hg with no relationship below and a strong linear relationship above this threshold.[86] Furthermore, a high CO_2 level not only increases CBF but also, through attenuation of CBF autoregulation, makes the brain more vulnerable to blood pressure swings.[86,87] Both these mechanisms could enhance reperfusion injury.[88] Therefore permissive hypercapnia above the low 50s (mm Hg) in the first few days may put vulnerable, extremely premature infants at a higher risk for developing P/IVH. Interestingly, neurodevelopmental follow-up results of a randomized control trial of mild versus high permissive hypercapnia in intubated extremely low-birth-weight (ELBW) infants was not different between the groups.[89] A low CO_2 level, on the other hand, decreases CBF and has been associated with periventricular leukomalacia.[90,91] Unlike permissive hypercapnia, hypocapnia does not confer any benefits in preterm infants and therefore should be avoided.

Interaction After Transition and Potential Clinical Implications

Although inappropriate ventilator support and excessive MAP can have similar deleterious effects on cardiovascular function as described earlier, the clinical implications are often less apparent after the transitional period as the preterm infant becomes less vulnerable. In recent years, pulmonary hypertension and RV failure in the setting of BPD have increasingly been recognized. Pathophysiology of the pulmonary hypertension associated with BPD is unclear. It is likely related to lung injury, inflammation, and arrest of pulmonary development associated with BPD, although evidence of pulmonary hypertension has also been reported in preterm infants with seemingly mild or no BPD.[92] The reported prevalence of pulmonary hypertension is variable and depends on the studied population and the definition of pulmonary hypertension on echocardiography. Estimating pressure gradient using tricuspid regurgitation (TR) jet is the most reliable measure of estimating pulmonary pressure using echocardiography. Unfortunately, a TR jet may not be present in up to 25% of cases despite the presence of pulmonary hypertension.[93] Furthermore, estimating pulmonary pressure by assessment of the PDA shunt is often not feasible in patients with BPD, as the ductus is rarely patent. In such cases, qualitative and less reliable markers of pulmonary hypertension, such as interventricular septal flattening, RV dilatation, and hypertrophy, can be used. It is important to note that even when the TR jet is present, echocardiography may not accurately estimate the severity of pulmonary hypertension.[94] Using the TR jet, the prevalence of pulmonary hypertension after the first month of life was reported to be about 12% among ELBW infants in a prospective observational study.[95] When qualitative indices of pulmonary hypertension were used, the prevalence was about 18%.[95] In retrospective studies using both quantitative and qualitative echocardiographic indices of pulmonary hypertension, the prevalence 4 weeks after birth was about 8% in all ELBW infants[96] and about 15% in ELBW infants with BPD.[97] A recent prospective study of preterm infants with a birth weight ranging between 500 and 1250 g using both quantitative and qualitative echocardiographic indices of pulmonary hypertension reported a 42% incidence in pulmonary hypertension at 7 days after birth.[92] Interestingly, early pulmonary hypertension was a risk factor for increased severity of BPD and pulmonary hypertension at 36 weeks postmenstrual age.[92] This suggests that pulmonary vascular disease, independent of BPD, contributes to the development of pulmonary hypertension. Other risk factors for developing pulmonary hypertension in patients with BPD include extreme prematurity, low birth weight, small-for-gestational age, oligohydramnios, prolonged ventilator support, and PDA ligation.[92,95–99] It is important to screen high-risk preterm infants with BPD because pulmonary hypertension increases the risk of mortality and poor neurodevelopmental outcome in this population.[92,95,97,100]

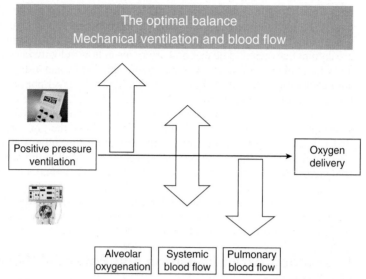

Fig. 17.4 Oxygen delivery to the tissues is determined both by the alveolar ventilation and oxygenation (mainly respiratory contribution) and by the blood flow to those tissues. There is an optimal balance between the use of positive-pressure ventilation to improve alveolar ventilation and the effects that higher mean airway pressure have on systemic, and particularly pulmonary, blood flow. Understanding this balance, particularly the effect of positive pressure on both the respiratory and cardiovascular system, is crucial to good neonatal care. (From de Waal, K. Personal communication, 2015.)

Conclusions

Understanding the interaction between the respiratory and cardiovascular systems is important in the management of neonates in the intensive care unit. The impact of respiration on circulatory function and vice versa is most evident at birth and during the early transition. During this period, unsuccessful transition of one system can significantly alter the normal sequence of events in the other system with potential for catastrophic complications. After the transitional period (first few postnatal days), although the impact of appropriate ventilator settings for the disease condition on cardiovascular system is small, excessive and inappropriately low ventilator support can severely impair the cardiovascular function and compromise both systemic and PBF. There is an optimal balance between the use of positive-pressure ventilation to improve alveolar ventilation and the effects of higher MAP on systemic blood flow and, particularly, PBF. As both alveolar oxygenation and systemic blood flow are required for oxygen delivery, this balance must be carefully considered (Fig. 17.4). Finally, we must appreciate that very little is known regarding the effects of different modes of ventilation and common ventilator strategies, such as permissive hypercapnia, on hemodynamics.

REFERENCES

1. Rasanen J, Wood DC, Weiner S, Ludomirski A, Huhta JC. Role of the pulmonary circulation in the distribution of human fetal cardiac output during the second half of pregnancy. *Circulation.* 1996;94(5):1068–1073.
2. Gao Y, Raj JU. Regulation of the pulmonary circulation in the fetus and newborn. *Physiol Rev.* 2010;90(4):1291–1335.
3. Rudolph AM. Fetal and neonatal pulmonary circulation. *Annu Rev Physiol.* 1979;41:383–395.
4. Bhatt S, Polglase GR, Wallace EM, Te Pas AB, Hooper SB. Ventilation before umbilical cord clamping improves the physiological transition at birth. *Front Pediatr.* 2014;2:113.
5. Crossley KJ, Allison BJ, Polglase GR, Morley CJ, Davis PG, Hooper SB. Dynamic changes in the direction of blood flow through the ductus arteriosus at birth. *J Physiol.* 2009;587(Pt 19):4695–4704.
6. te Pas AB, Davis PG, Hooper SB, Morley CJ. From liquid to air: breathing after birth. *J Pediatr.* 2008;152(5):607–611.
7. Hooper SB, Kitchen MJ, Wallace MJ, et al. Imaging lung aeration and lung liquid clearance at birth. *FASEB J.* 2007;21:3329–3337.

8. Bhatt S, Alison BJ, Wallace EM, et al. Delaying cord clamping until ventilation onset improves cardiovascular function at birth in preterm lambs. *J Physiol*. 2013;591(Pt 8):2113–2126.
9. Hooper SB, Binder-Heschl C, Polglase GR, et al. The timing of umbilical cord clamping at birth: physiological considerations. *Matern Health Neonatol Perinatol*. 2016;2:4.
10. Katheria A, Poeltler D, Durham J, et al. Neonatal resuscitation with an intact cord: a randomized clinical trial. *J Pediatr*. 2016;178:75–80.e73.
11. Katheria AC, Lakshminrusimha S, Rabe H, McAdams R, Mercer JS. Placental transfusion: a review. *J Perinatol*. 2016.
12. Boere I, Roest AA, Wallace E, et al. Umbilical blood flow patterns directly after birth before delayed cord clamping. *Arch Dis Child Fetal Neonatal Ed*. 2014.
13. Hutchon D. Evolution of neonatal resuscitation with intact placental circulation. *Clinical Practice*. 2014;10(2):58–61.
14. Katheria AC, Truong G, Cousins L, Oshiro B, Finer NN. Umbilical cord milking versus delayed cord clamping in preterm infants. *Pediatrics*. 2015;136(1):61–69.
15. Katheria A, Blank D, Rich W, Finer N. Umbilical cord milking improves transition in premature infants at birth. *PLoS One*. 2014;9(4):e94085.
16. Feihl F, Broccard AF. Interactions between respiration and systemic hemodynamics. Part II: practical implications in critical care. *Intensive Care Med*. 2009;35(2):198–205.
17. Pinsky MR, Summer WR. Cardiac augmentation by phasic high intrathoracic pressure support in man. *Chest*. 1983;84(4):370–375.
18. Pinsky MR, Summer WR, Wise RA, Permutt S, Bromberger-Barnea B. Augmentation of cardiac function by elevation of intrathoracic pressure. *J Appl Physiol Respir Environ Exerc Physiol*. 1983;54(4):950–955.
19. Cheifetz IM. Cardiorespiratory interactions: the relationship between mechanical ventilation and hemodynamics. *Respir Care*. 2014;59(12):1937–1945.
20. Lakshminrusimha S, Swartz DD, Gugino SF, et al. Oxygen concentration and pulmonary hemodynamics in newborn lambs with pulmonary hypertension. *Pediatr Res*. 2009;66(5):539–544.
21. Benumof JL. Mechanism of decreased blood flow to atelectatic lung. *J Appl Physiol Respir Environ Exerc Physiol*. 1979;46(6):1047–1048.
22. Biondi JW, Schulman DS, Soufer R, et al. The effect of incremental positive end-expiratory pressure on right ventricular hemodynamics and ejection fraction. *Anesth Analg*. 1988;67:144–151.
23. Dhainaut JF, Devaux JY, Monsallier JF, Brunet F, Villemant D, Huyghebaert MF. Mechanisms of decreased left ventricular preload during continuous positive pressure ventilation in ARDS. *Chest*. 1986;90:74–80.
24. Kim BH, Ishida Y, Tsuneoka Y, et al. Effects of spontaneous respiration on right and left ventricular function: evaluation by respiratory and ECG gated radionuclide ventriculography. *J Nucl Med*. 1987;28(2):173–177.
25. Jardin F, Farcot JC, Gueret P, Prost JF, Ozier Y, Bourdarias JP. Cyclic changes in arterial pulse during respiratory support. *Circulation*. 1983;68(2):266–274.
26. Marik PE, Cavallazzi R, Vasu T, Hirani A. Dynamic changes in arterial waveform derived variables and fluid responsiveness in mechanically ventilated patients: a systematic review of the literature. *Crit Care Med*. 2009;37(9):2642–2647.
27. Heskamp L, Lansdorp B, Hopman J, Lemson J, de Boode WP. Ventilator-induced pulse pressure variation in neonates. *Physiol Rep*. 2016;4(4).
28. Jain A, McNamara PJ. Persistent pulmonary hypertension of the newborn: Advances in diagnosis and treatment. *Semin Fetal Neonatal Med*. 2015;20(4):262–271.
29. Jain A, Mohamed A, El-Khuffash A, et al. A comprehensive echocardiographic protocol for assessing neonatal right ventricular dimensions and function in the transitional period: normative data and z scores. *J Am Soc Echocardiogr*. 2014;27(12):1293–1304.
30. Hausdorf G, Hellwege HH. Influence of positive end-expiratory pressure on cardiac performance in premature infants: a Doppler-echocardiographic study. *Crit Care Med*. 1987;15:661–664.
31. Trang TT, Tibballs J, Mercier JC, Beaufils F. Optimization of oxygen transport in mechanically ventilated newborns using oximetry and pulsed Doppler-derived cardiac output. *Crit Care Med*. 1988;16:1094–1097.
32. Maayan C, Eyal F, Mandelberg A, Sapoznikov D, Lewis BS. Effect of mechanical ventilation and volume loading on left ventricular performance in premature infants with respiratory distress syndrome. *Crit Care Med*. 1986;14(10):858–860.
33. Gill AB, Weindling AM. Echocardiographic assessment of cardiac function in shocked very low birthweight infants. *Arch Dis Child*. 1993;68:17–21.
34. Takahashi Y, Harada K, Kishkurno S, Arai, Ishida A, Takada G. Postnatal left ventricular contractility in very low birth weight infants. *Pediatr Cardiol*. 1997;18(2):112–117.
35. Lee LA, Kimball TR, Daniels SR, Khoury P, Meyer RA. Left ventricular mechanics in the preterm infant and their effect on the measurement of cardiac performance. *J Pediatr*. 1992;120(1):114–119.
36. Teitel DF. Physiologic development of the cardiovascular system in the fetus. In: Polin RA, Fox WW, eds. *Fetal and Neonatal Physiology*. 2nd ed. Philadelphia: WB Saunders Company; 1998:827–836.
37. Maroto E, Fouron JC, Teyssier G, Bard H, van Doesburg NH, Cartwright D. Effect of intermittent positive pressure ventilation on diastolic ventricular filling patterns in premature infants. *J Am Coll Cardiol*. 1990;16(1):171–174.
38. Shekerdemian L, Bohn D. Cardiovascular effects of mechanical ventilation. *Arch Dis Child*. 1999;80(5):475–480.
39. Polglase GR, Morley CJ, Crossley KJ, et al. Positive end-expiratory pressure differentially alters pulmonary hemodynamics and oxygenation in ventilated, very premature lambs. *J Appl Physiol*. 2005;99(4):1453–1461.

17

40. Cheifetz IM, Craig DM, Quick G, et al. Increasing tidal volumes and pulmonary overdistention adversely affect pulmonary vascular mechanics and cardiac output in a pediatric swine model. *Crit Care Med*. 1998;26(4):710–716.

41. de Waal KA, Evans N, Osborn DA, Kluckow M. Cardiorespiratory effects of changes in end expiratory pressure in ventilated newborns. *Arch Dis Child Fetal Neonatal Ed*. 2007;92(6):F444–F448.

42. Fajardo MF, Claure N, Swaminathan S, et al. Effect of positive end-expiratory pressure on ductal shunting and systemic blood flow in preterm infants with patent ductus arteriosus. *Neonatology*. 2014;105(1):9–13.

43. Beker F, Rogerson SR, Hooper SB, Wong C, Davis PG. The effects of nasal continuous positive airway pressure on cardiac function in premature infants with minimal lung disease: a crossover randomized trial. *J Pediatr*. 2014;164(4):726–729.

44. Moritz B, Fritz M, Mann C, Simma B. Nasal continuous positive airway pressure (n-CPAP) does not change cardiac output in preterm infants. *Am J Perinatol*. 2008;25(2):105–109.

45. Abdel-Hady H, Matter M, Hammad A, El-Refaay A, Aly H. Hemodynamic changes during weaning from nasal continuous positive airway pressure. *Pediatrics*. 2008;122(5):e1086–e1090.

46. de Waal K, Evans N, van der Lee J, van Kaam A. Effect of lung recruitment on pulmonary, systemic, and ductal blood flow in preterm infants. *J Pediatr*. 2009;154(5):651–655.

47. de Waal KA, Evans N, van der Lee J, van KA. Effect of lung recruitment on pulmonary, systemic, and ductal blood flow in preterm infants. *J Pediatr*. 2009;154(5):651–655.

48. van Kaam AH, De Jaegere AP, Rimensberger PC, Neovent Study Group. Incidence of hypo- and hyper-capnia in a cross-sectional European cohort of ventilated newborn infants. *Arch Dis Child Fetal Neonatal Ed*. 2013;98(4):F323–F326.

49. Miller JD, Carlo WA. Safety and effectiveness of permissive hypercapnia in the preterm infant. *Curr Opin Pediatr*. 2007;19(2):142–144.

50. Orchard CH, Kentish JC. Effects of changes of pH on the contractile function of cardiac muscle. *Am J Physiol Cell Physiol*. 1990;258(6 Pt 1):C967–C981.

51. Weber T, Tschernich H, Sitzwohl C, et al. Tromethamine buffer modifies the depressant effect of permissive hypercapnia on myocardial contractility in patients with acute respiratory distress syndrome. *Am J Respir Crit Care Med*. 2000;162(4 Pt 1):1361–1365.

52. Carvalho CR, Barbas CS, Medeiros DM, et al. Temporal hemodynamic effects of permissive hypercapnia associated with ideal PEEP in ARDS. *Am J Respir Crit Care Med*. 1997;156(5):1458–1466.

53. Nakanishi T, Gu H, Momma K. Developmental changes in the effect of acidosis on contraction, intracellular pH, and calcium in the rabbit mesenteric small artery. *Pediatr Res*. 1997;42(6):750–757.

54. Nakanishi T, Seguchi M, Tsuchiya T, Yasukouchi S, Takao A. Effect of acidosis on intracellular pH and calcium concentration in the newborn and adult rabbit myocardium. *Circ Res*. 1990;67(1):111–123.

55. Nakanishi T, Gu H, Momma K. Effect of acidosis on contraction, intracellular pH, and calcium in the newborn and adult rabbit aorta. *Heart Vessels*. 1997;12(5):207–215.

56. Noori S, Wu TW, Seri I. pH effects on cardiac function and systemic vascular resistance in preterm infants. *J Pediatr*. 2013;162(5):958–963.e951.

57. Nakanishi T, Okuda H, Nakazawa M, Takao A. Effect of acidosis on contractile function in the newborn rabbit heart. *Pediatr Res*. 1985;19(5):482–488.

58. Fanconi S, Burger R, Ghelfi D, Uehlinger J, Arbenz U. Hemodynamic effects of sodium bicarbonate in critically ill neonates [see comments]. *Intensive Care Med*. 1993;19(2):65–69.

59. Mintzer JP, Parvez B, Alpan G, LaGamma EF. Effects of sodium bicarbonate correction of metabolic acidosis on regional tissue oxygenation in very low birth weight neonates. *J Perinatol*. 2015;35(8):601–606.

60. Sehgal A, Wong F, Menahem S. Speckle tracking derived strain in infants with severe perinatal asphyxia: a comparative case control study. *Cardiovasc Ultrasound*. 2013;11:34.

61. Giesinger RE, Bailey LJ, Deshpande P, McNamara PJ. Hypoxic-ischemic encephalopathy and therapeutic hypothermia: the hemodynamic perspective. *J Pediatr*. 2017;180:22–30.e22.

62. McNamara P, Weisz D, Giesinger RE, Jain A. Hemodynamics. In: MacDonald MG, Seshia MK, eds. *Avery's Neonatology: Pathophysiology & Management of the Newborn*. 7th ed. Philadelphia: Wolters Kluwer; 2016.

63. Kluckow M, Evans N. Ductal shunting, high pulmonary blood flow, and pulmonary hemorrhage. *J Pediatr*. 2000;137(1):68–72.

64. Zonnenberg I, de Waal K. The definition of a haemodynamic significant duct in randomized controlled trials: a systematic literature review. *Acta Paediatr*. 2012;101(3):247–251.

65. Shah P, Riphagen S, Beyene J, Perlman M. Multiorgan dysfunction in infants with post-asphyxial hypoxic-ischaemic encephalopathy. *Arch Dis Child Fetal Neonatal Ed*. 2004;89(2):F152–F155.

66. Tapia-Rombo CA, Carpio-Hernandez JC, Salazar-Acuna AH, et al. Detection of transitory myocardial ischemia secondary to perinatal asphyxia. *Arch Med Res*. 2000;31(4):377–383.

67. Schwartz SM, Vermilion RP, Hirschl RB. Evaluation of left ventricular mass in children with left-sided congenital diaphragmatic hernia. *J Pediatr*. 1994;125(3):447–451.

68. Byrne FA, Keller RL, Meadows J, et al. Severe left diaphragmatic hernia limits size of fetal left heart more than right diaphragmatic hernia. *Ultrasound Obstet Gynecol*. 2015.

69. Kinsella JP, Ivy DD, Abman SH. Pulmonary vasodilator therapy in congenital diaphragmatic hernia: acute, late, and chronic pulmonary hypertension. *Semin Perinatol*. 2005;29(2):123–128.

70. Schipper JA, Mohammad GI, van Straaten HL, Koppe JG. The impact of surfactant replacement therapy on cerebral and systemic circulation and lung function. *Eur J Pediatr*. 1997;156(3):224–227.

71. Nuntnarumit P, Bada HS, Yang W, Korones SB. Cerebral blood flow velocity changes after bovine natural surfactant instillation. *J Perinatol.* 2000;20(4):240–243.

72. Kaiser JR, Gauss CH, Williams DK. Surfactant administration acutely affects cerebral and systemic hemodynamics and gas exchange in very-low-birth-weight infants. *J Pediatr.* 2004;144(6):809–814.

73. Saliba E, Nashashibi M, Vaillant MC, Nasr C, Laugier J. Instillation rate effects of exosurf on cerebral and cardiovascular haemodynamics in preterm neonates. *Arch Dis Child Fetal Neonatal Ed.* 1994;71(3):F174–F178.

74. Roll C, Knief J, Horsch S, Hanssler L. Effect of surfactant administration on cerebral haemodynamics and oxygenation in premature infants—a near infrared spectroscopy study. *Neuropediatrics.* 2000;31(1):16–23.

75. Sehgal A, Mak W, Dunn M, et al. Haemodynamic changes after delivery room surfactant administration to very low birth weight infants. *Arch Dis Child Fetal Neonatal Ed.* 2010;95(5):F345–F351.

76. Katheria AC, Leone TA. Changes in hemodynamics after rescue surfactant administration. *J Perinatol.* 2013;33(7):525–528.

77. Clyman RI, Jobe A, Heymann M, et al. Increased shunt through the patent ductus arteriosus after surfactant replacement therapy. *J Pediatr.* 1982;100(1):101–107.

78. Carlo WA, Stark AR, Wright LL, et al. Minimal ventilation to prevent bronchopulmonary dysplasia in extremely-low-birth-weight infants. *J Pediatr.* 2002;141(3):370–374.

79. Thome UH, Genzel-Boroviczeny O, Bohnhorst B, et al. Permissive hypercapnia in extremely low birthweight infants (PHELBI): a randomised controlled multicentre trial. *Lancet Respir Med.* 2015;3(7):534–543.

80. Fabres J, Carlo WA, Phillips V, Howard G, Ambalavanan N. Both extremes of arterial carbon dioxide pressure and the magnitude of fluctuations in arterial carbon dioxide pressure are associated with severe intraventricular hemorrhage in preterm infants. *Pediatrics.* 2007;119(2):299–305.

81. McKee LA, Fabres J, Howard G, Peralta-Carcelen M, Carlo WA, Ambalavanan N. PaCO$_2$ and neurodevelopment in extremely low birth weight infants. *J Pediatr.* 2009;155(2):217–221.e211.

82. Ambalavanan N, Carlo WA, Wrage LA, et al. PaCO$_2$ in surfactant, positive pressure, and oxygenation randomised trial (SUPPORT). *Arch Dis Child Fetal Neonatal Ed.* 2015;100(2):F145–F149.

83. Kaiser JR, Gauss CH, Pont MM, Williams DK. Hypercapnia during the first 3 days of life is associated with severe intraventricular hemorrhage in very low birth weight infants. *J Perinatol.* 2006;26(5):279–285.

84. Noori S, McCoy M, Anderson MP, Ramji F, Seri I. Changes in cardiac function and cerebral blood flow in relation to peri/intraventricular hemorrhage in extremely preterm infants. *J Pediatr.* 2014;164(2):264–270.e261–e263.

85. Pryds O, Greisen G, Lou H, Friis HB. Heterogeneity of cerebral vasoreactivity in preterm infants supported by mechanical ventilation. *J Pediatr.* 1989;115(4):638–645.

86. Noori S, Anderson M, Soleymani S, Seri I. Effect of carbon dioxide on cerebral blood flow velocity in preterm infants during postnatal transition. *Acta Paediatr.* 2014;103(8):e334–e339.

87. Kaiser JR, Gauss CH, Williams DK. The effects of hypercapnia on cerebral autoregulation in ventilated very low birth weight infants. *Pediatr Res.* 2005;58(5):931–935.

88. Noori S, Seri I. Hemodynamic antecedents of peri/intraventricular hemorrhage in very preterm neonates. *Semin Fetal Neonatal Med.* 2015;20(4):232–237.

89. Thome UH, Genzel-Boroviczeny O, Bohnhorst B, et al. Neurodevelopmental outcomes of extremely low birthweight infants randomised to different PCO$_2$ targets: the PHELBI follow-up study. *Arch Dis Child Fetal Neonatal Ed.* 2017.

90. Wiswell TE, Graziani LJ, Kornhauser MS, et al. Effects of hypocarbia on the development of cystic periventricular leukomalacia in premature infants treated with high-frequency jet ventilation. *Pediatrics.* 1996;98(5):918–924.

91. Shankaran S, Langer JC, Kazzi SN, et al. Cumulative index of exposure to hypocarbia and hyperoxia as risk factors for periventricular leukomalacia in low birth weight infants. *Pediatrics.* 2006;118(4):1654–1659.

92. Mourani PM, Sontag MK, Younoszai A, et al. Early pulmonary vascular disease in preterm infants at risk for bronchopulmonary dysplasia. *Am J Respir Crit Care Med.* 2015;191(1):87–95.

93. Abman SH, Hansmann G, Archer SL, et al. Pediatric pulmonary hypertension: guidelines from the American Heart Association and American Thoracic Society. *Circulation.* 2015;132(21):2037–2099.

94. Mourani PM, Sontag MK, Younoszai A, Ivy DD, Abman SH. Clinical utility of echocardiography for the diagnosis and management of pulmonary vascular disease in young children with chronic lung disease. *Pediatrics.* 2008;121(2):317–325.

95. Bhat R, Salas AA, Foster C, Carlo WA, Ambalavanan N. Prospective analysis of pulmonary hypertension in extremely low birth weight infants. *Pediatrics.* 2012;129(3):e682–e689.

96. Collaco JM, Dadlani GH, Nies MK, Leshko J, Everett AD, McGrath-Morrow SA. Risk factors and clinical outcomes in preterm infants with pulmonary hypertension. *PLoS One.* 2016;11(10):e0163904.

97. Slaughter JL, Pakrashi T, Jones DE, South AP, Shah TA. Echocardiographic detection of pulmonary hypertension in extremely low birth weight infants with bronchopulmonary dysplasia requiring prolonged positive pressure ventilation. *J Perinatol.* 2011;31(10):635–640.

98. Kim D-H, Kim H-S, Choi CW, Kim E-K, Kim BI, Choi J-H. Risk factors for pulmonary artery hypertension in preterm infants with moderate or severe bronchopulmonary dysplasia. *Neonatology.* 2012;101(1):40–46.

99. Check J, Gotteiner N, Liu X, et al. Fetal growth restriction and pulmonary hypertension in premature infants with bronchopulmonary dysplasia. *J Perinatol.* 2013;33(7):553–557.

100. Nakanishi H, Uchiyama A, Kusuda S. Impact of pulmonary hypertension on neurodevelopmental outcome in preterm infants with bronchopulmonary dysplasia: a cohort study. *J Perinatol.* 2016;36(10):890–896.

17

CHAPTER 18

Ventilator Strategies to Reduce Lung Injury and Duration of Mechanical Ventilation

Martin Keszler and Nelson Claure

- The immature lungs of extremely preterm infants are susceptible to damage from a variety of factors that are potentially modifiable by the use of lung-protective strategies of respiratory support.

- Avoidance of mechanical ventilation, optimal delivery room stabilization, and early use of noninvasive respiratory support are important elements in minimizing lung injury.

- When mechanical ventilation is needed, it should be used with care and attention to the individual patient's specific pathophysiology and with a goal of extubation at the earliest opportunity.

- Recruitment and maintenance of optimal lung volume is a key element in any lung-protective ventilation strategy, including both conventional and high-frequency ventilation.

- Volume-targeted ventilation maintains more stable tidal volume and minute ventilation, shortens the duration of mechanical ventilation, and is associated with a decrease in both lung and brain injury.

Despite appropriate emphasis on noninvasive respiratory support when feasible, mechanical ventilation (MV) remains a mainstay of therapy in extremely preterm infants.[1–3] Although it is undoubtedly lifesaving, invasive MV has many untoward effects on the brain and the lungs, especially in the most immature infants.[1] The endotracheal tube (ETT) acts as a foreign body, quickly becoming colonized and acting as a portal of entry for pathogens, increasing the risk of ventilator-associated pneumonia and late-onset sepsis.[4] For these reasons, avoidance of MV in favor of noninvasive respiratory support is considered one of the most important steps in preventing neonatal morbidity. When MV is required, the goal is to wean the patient from invasive ventilation as soon as feasible to minimize ventilator-associated lung injury (VALI). Although VALI is a key element in the pathogenesis of bronchopulmonary dysplasia (BPD), many other factors play an important role in its pathogenesis, including the intrauterine environment (inflammation and infection), postnatal infection, oxidative stress, antenatal and postnatal nutritional deprivation, presence of patent ductus arteriosus, and excessive fluid administration.

Ventilator-Associated Lung Injury

Many terms have been used to describe the mechanism of injury in VALI. *Barotrauma* refers to damage caused by inflation pressure. The conviction that pressure is the major determinant of lung injury has caused clinicians to focus on limiting inflation pressure, often to the point of precluding adequate ventilation. However, there is convincing evidence that high inflation pressure by itself, without correspondingly high tidal volume (V_T), does not result in lung injury. Rather, injury related to high inflation pressure is mediated through tissue stretch resulting from excessive

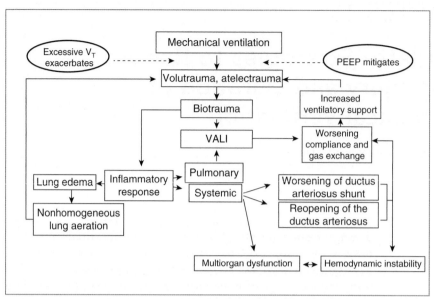

Fig. 18.1 The cycle of ventilator-associated lung injury *(VALI)* is complex and multifactorial. The initiating event is biophysical injury from excessive tissue stretching, which in turn leads to biotrauma and initiates the cascade of lung injury and repair. Both systemic and pulmonary inflammatory responses become operative and lead to secondary adverse effects that in turn worsen pulmonary status, leading to a need for escalating ventilatory settings, which in turn cause more injury. V_T, Tidal volume.

V_T or from regional overdistention when ventilating lungs with extensive atelectasis. Dreyfuss and colleagues demonstrated more than 20 years ago that severe acute lung injury occurred in small animals ventilated with large V_T, regardless of whether that volume was generated by positive or negative pressure.[5] In contrast, animals exposed to the same high inflation pressure but with an elastic bandage over the chest and abdomen to limit the delivered V_T showed substantially less acute lung injury. Similarly, Hernandez et al. demonstrated that animals exposed to pressure as high as 45 cm H_2O did not show evidence of acute lung injury when their chest and abdomen were enclosed in a plaster cast.[6] *Volutrauma* refers to injury caused by overdistention and excessive stretching of tissues, which leads to disruption of alveolar and small airway epithelium, resulting in acute edema, an outpouring of protein-rich exudate, and release of proteases, cytokines, and chemokines. This in turn leads to activation of macrophages and invasion of activated neutrophils. Collectively, this latter process is referred to as *biotrauma*. Another important concept is that of *atelectrauma*, or lung damage caused by tidal ventilation in the presence of atelectasis.[7] Atelectrauma causes lung injury via several different mechanisms. The portion of the lungs that remains atelectatic experiences increased surfactant turnover and has high critical opening pressure. There are shear forces at the boundary between the aerated and atelectatic parts of the lung, leading to structural tissue damage. Ventilation of injured lungs using inadequate end-expiratory pressure results in repeated alveolar collapse and expansion with each inflation, a process that leads to lung injury quite rapidly. Perhaps most importantly, when a portion of the lungs is atelectatic, the gas entering the lungs will preferentially distend the aerated portion of the lung, which is more compliant than the atelectatic lung with its high critical opening pressure. This fact is evident from Laplace's law and corroborated by experimental evidence, showing that the most injured portion of the lung was the aerated nondependent lung.[8] This maldistribution of V_T leads to overdistention of that portion of the lungs and regional volutrauma. Thus VALI is initiated by some form of biophysical injury, which in turn triggers a release of mediators and activated leukocytes, leading to biotrauma and initiating the complex cascade of lung injury and eventual repair. A schematic representation of the cycle of VALI is illustrated in Fig. 18.1.

How Can VALI Be Reduced?

As is evident from the prior discussion, the process of lung damage from MV is multifactorial and cannot be linked to any single variable. Consequently, any approach to reducing lung injury must be comprehensive and begin with the initial stabilization of the infant in the delivery room. Because some degree of impairment of normal pulmonary development (i.e., arrest of alveolarization) is probably inevitable when an extremely preterm fetus is suddenly thrust into what by fetal standards is a very hyperoxic environment and must initiate air breathing with incompletely developed lungs, it is unlikely that improved respiratory support and avoidance of MV can completely prevent impairment of lung structure and function. However, optimal respiratory and general supportive care can minimize the superimposition of VALI on this developmental arrest and together with optimal nutrition can facilitate lung growth and repair.

Delivery Room Stabilization

The time immediately after birth when air breathing is initiated in a structurally immature surfactant deficient lung is recognized as a critical time during which the process of lung injury and subsequent repair may be triggered in a matter of minutes. Moments after birth, the newborn must rapidly clear lung fluid from the airways and terminal air spaces, aerate the lungs, and sustain a functional residual capacity, thus facilitating a dramatic increase in pulmonary blood flow. Vigorous full-term infants are able to achieve this critical transition quickly and effectively,[9] but this is much more problematic in very preterm infants who often fail to generate sufficient critical opening pressure to achieve adequate lung inflation because of their limited muscle strength, excessively compliant chest wall, limited surfactant pool, and incomplete lung development. The excessively compliant chest wall of the preterm infant fails to sustain the lung aeration that may have been achieved spontaneously or with positive-pressure ventilation. For the same reasons, these infants may be unable to generate sufficient negative intrathoracic pressure to effectively move lung fluid from the air spaces to the interstitium, lymphatics, and veins. Subsequent tidal breathing, both spontaneous and that generated by positive-pressure ventilation, occurs in lungs that are still partially fluid-filled and incompletely expanded. This situation leads to maldistribution of V_T to a fraction of the preterm lung, a phenomenon that can generate excessive tissue stretching even when the V_T is in an appropriate range that is generally considered safe.

The use of positive end-expiratory pressure (PEEP) and/or continuous positive airway pressure (CPAP) during the initial stabilization of preterm infants compensates for the excessively compliant chest wall and surfactant deficiency by stabilizing alveoli during the expiratory phase and has been shown to help establish functional residual capacity.[10] Both Neonatal Resuscitation Program (NRP) and International Liaison Committee on Resuscitation (ILCOR) guidelines give a qualified endorsement to the use of PEEP/CPAP but cite a lack of high-quality randomized controlled trials (RCTs) to make a stronger recommendation.[11,12] However, the physiologic rationale and experimental evidence from preclinical studies is so persuasive that this practice has become the de facto standard of care in much of the developed world and thus a RCT would be very difficult to undertake at this point. However, provision of end-expiratory pressure alone may not sufficiently address the inadequate muscle strength of the preterm infant or help clear lung fluid sufficiently rapidly to avoid regional volutrauma and atelectrauma, which can occur in minutes. Owing to the much greater viscosity of liquid compared with air, resistance to moving liquid through small airways is much greater than that for air, making the time constants required to move fluid through the airways much longer. These considerations support the concept that a prolonged (aka "sustained") inflation applied soon after birth should be more effective in clearing lung fluid in the first minutes of life than the typical short inflations used during positive-pressure ventilation. Theoretically, rapid and effective lung recruitment that results in even distribution of V_T immediately after birth should reduce VALI. Some evidence supports the theoretical advantages of sustained inflation in extremely preterm infants,[10,13] but there is also potential for harm if excessive pressure is applied to relatively compliant lungs, resulting in

18

lung overdistention.[14] At present, the evidence that this intervention can reduce VALI remains inconclusive.[15–17] Clear evidence regarding the optimal way to deliver a sustained ventilation is also lacking. Therefore routine use of the procedure cannot be recommended pending the outcome of an ongoing controlled clinical trial.[18]

Noninvasive Respiratory Support

Avoiding MV is widely believed to reduce iatrogenic lung injury largely based on early cohort comparisons of CPAP versus MV, which suggested a dramatic reduction in the incidence of BPD.[19] However, a series of more recent randomized trials showed a much smaller impact of noninvasive respiratory support. A meta-analysis of four recent trials that enrolled nearly 2800 preterm infants[20–23] showed that BPD rates alone were not significantly different between infants randomly assigned to MV and those assigned to nasal CPAP (32.4% vs. 34.0%).[24] However, the more important combined outcome of death or BPD (death and BPD are competing outcomes) showed a nearly 10% reduction (relative risk [RR] 0.91, 95% confidence interval [CI] 0.84–0.99) with a number needed to treat of 25. There was also a significant decrease in the duration of MV and a trend toward shorter duration of supplemental oxygen with early CPAP in two of the trials.[20,21]

Nasal intermittent positive-pressure ventilation (NIPPV), if delivered effectively, may augment an immature infant's inadequate respiratory effort without the complications associated with endotracheal intubation.[25] This approach benefits from avoiding the use of an ETT, thus reducing the incidence of VALI and ventilator-associated pneumonia, and avoiding the contribution of postnatal inflammatory response to the development of BPD.[26] A meta-analysis of several small single-center studies concluded that NIPPV was superior to CPAP in preventing extubation failure, especially when NIPPV was synchronized with the infant's respiratory effort.[27] However, a more recent large multinational randomized trial in extremely low-birth-weight infants failed to substantiate any benefits, showing no reduction in BPD, mortality, or the combined outcome.[28] Lack of synchronization might be responsible for lack of benefit in some of these studies. Current evidence suggests that unsynchronized NIPPV rarely generates a measurable V_T,[29] likely because the vocal cords are closed except during active inspiratory effort. The cyclic inflation, however, does result in a higher mean airway pressure and it is likely that this higher distending pressure accounts for some of the observed benefits of NIPPV. The benefit of a higher continuous distending pressure may be more evident in infants with residual lung disease who require higher oxygen supplementation. This was evidenced in a small clinical trial during the extubation phase where a CPAP of 8 cm H_2O was more effective in reducing extubation failure than 5 cm H_2O.[30] Nasal high-frequency oscillatory ventilation (HVOF) has also been explored by several groups, but as of this writing, the suggestion of efficacy is based only on case reports and small series.[31–33] Noninvasive neurally adjusted ventilatory assist uses the electrical activity of the diaphragm to trigger ventilator inflations and is thus not affected by leakage of a noninvasive interface; it may thus be the best tool to deliver noninvasive ventilation in small preterm infants.[34] However, definitive studies are still lacking.

Mechanical Ventilation Strategies

The goal of MV is to maintain acceptable gas exchange with a minimum of adverse effects and to wean the patient from invasive support as expeditiously as possible. There are many choices of devices and modes of ventilation with limited high-quality data to guide the clinician's choice. Because of the wide range of clinical conditions, weights, and gestational ages of neonatal patients, there are no simple rules regarding indications for intubation and initiation of MV. "Standard" indications for intubation and initial ventilator settings often recommended in texts on this subject have limited utility. Instead, the choice of modalities of support and ventilation strategies should be guided by the specific underlying pathophysiologic considerations. Ventilators are nothing but tools in our hands that we need to use thoughtfully to optimize outcomes.

Basic Modes of Synchronized Ventilation

Despite the relative paucity of high-quality evidence, the question is no longer whether to use synchronized versus unsynchronized ventilation, but rather which modality of synchronization is optimal. Synchronization of ventilator inflations with the infant's spontaneous breaths allows the clinician to avoid or minimize sedation/muscle relaxation and to maximize the patient's own spontaneous respiratory effort. Encouraging spontaneous breathing during MV has clear advantages, but it makes managing MV more challenging for the clinician. The optimal use of assisted ventilation requires a clear understanding of the complex interaction between the awake, spontaneously breathing infant and the various modalities of synchronized ventilation discussed in depth in Chapter 16. A key ingredient is an appreciation of the additive nature of the patient's inspiratory effort and the positive pressure generated by the ventilator. The magnitude of the V_T is determined by the transpulmonary pressure, the sum of the negative inspiratory effort of the infant, and the positive inflation pressure from the ventilator. Because the spontaneous effort is often sporadic and highly variable in a preterm infant, the resulting transpulmonary pressure and V_T typically fluctuate substantially.

In the following text, we briefly review the common modes of synchronized ventilation, the important advantages of volume-targeted ventilation and the importance of the optimizing lung inflation.

Synchronized Intermittent Mandatory Ventilation

Synchronized intermittent mandatory ventilation (SIMV) is a basic synchronized mode that provides a user-selected number of inflations in synchrony with the infant's breathing. If no spontaneous effort is detected during a trigger window, a mandatory inflation is delivered. Spontaneous breaths in excess of the set ventilator rate receive no support. In small preterm infants, this results in uneven V_Ts and high work of breathing because of the high airway resistance of the narrow ETT, hindered by the limited muscle strength and mechanical disadvantage of the infant's excessively compliant chest wall. SIMV thus is not the optimal mode in this population. SIMV allows the operator to set the ventilator rate as well as inflation pressure and PEEP. Weaning is accomplished by gradual lowering of both rate and inflation pressure.

Assist/Control

In neonatal applications, assist control (A/C) is a time-cycled, pressure-controlled mode that supports every spontaneous breath, thus resulting in more uniform V_T and lower work of breathing than SIMV. The goal is for the infant and the ventilator to work together with every breath, resulting in lower ventilator pressure. A backup ventilator rate provides a minimum rate in case of apnea and should be set just below the infant's spontaneous rate, usually at 40 inflations/min. A backup rate that is too low will result in excessive fluctuations in minute ventilation and oxygen saturations during periods of apnea. Because the infant controls the ventilator rate, gradual withdrawal of support is accomplished by lowering the peak inflation pressure, reducing the support given to each breath and thus encouraging the infant to gradually take over the work of breathing. Depending on the device used, some vigilance may be necessary to avoid autotriggering. Because ventilators do not commonly have a user-set upper limit to the cycling frequency, there is a risk of hyperventilation owing to autotriggering. This is seldom a problem when specialty neonatal ventilators with effective leak compensation are used, but even with those devices, water condensation in the expiratory limb can cause autotriggering.

Pressure-Support Ventilation

Pressure-support ventilation (PSV) functions differently in adult and neonatal ventilators, a situation that frequently causes confusion. In specialty neonatal ventilators, PSV is a pressure-controlled mode that supports every spontaneous breath just like A/C but is flow-cycled. Flow cycling means that inflation is terminated when inspiratory flow declines to a preset threshold (usually 5%–20% of peak flow), eliminating inspiratory hold (prolonged inflation time) and thus providing more complete synchrony. Avoidance of prolonged inflation time likely results in less fluctuation in intrathoracic and intracranial pressure that is a consequence of infants exhaling during inspiratory hold. Additionally, PSV automatically adjusts inspiratory time (T_I) in response to the changing lung mechanics of the patient. Changing from time-cycled A/C to PSV often results in a shorter T_I and therefore lower mean airway pressure (P_{AW}). Adjustment to PEEP may be needed to maintain P_{AW} and avoid atelectasis. A substantial leak around the ETT may affect flow cycling. To prevent excessive inspiratory duration during PSV the time limit should be set appropriately. Similar to A/C, the risk of autotriggering is also present during PSV, especially when universal ventilators not specifically designed for neonates with uncuffed ETTs are used.

Similar to A/C, a backup rate will maintain a minimum inflation rate. In most devices PSV can also be used to support spontaneous breathing between low-rate SIMV to overcome the problems associated with inadequate spontaneous respiratory effort and high ETT resistance, or in a fully spontaneous mode (CPAP + PSV). When used with SIMV or with CPAP, PSV does not provide a backup mandatory rate, so a reliable spontaneous respiratory effort is required. Weaning from PSV when it is used as a primary mode is accomplished in the same way as for A/C. When used in conjunction with SIMV, both the SIMV inflation rate and peak inflation pressure (PIP) should be lowered, leaving the infant increasingly breathing spontaneously with only a modest level of PSV, at which point extubation should be attempted.

Choice of Assisted Ventilation Modes

To date, only three small randomized trials compared A/C and SIMV. These trials did not show clear advantages of one mode over the other with regard to weaning and duration of MV, though a recent meta-analysis by Greenough et al. found a strong trend favoring A/C with a shorter duration of weaning (mean difference −42.4 hours, 95% CI −94.35 to 9.60).[35–37] In the absence of large randomized trials to provide the necessary evidence base and establish the superiority of one mode or the other, the choice between A/C and SIMV—the two most widely used modalities of synchronized ventilation—remains a matter of training, personal preference, or habit. Valid physiologic considerations and short-term studies indicate that modes that support every spontaneous breath are preferable in small preterm infants breathing through narrow ETTs. Documented benefits of A/C over SIMV include smaller and less variable V_T, less tachypnea, more rapid weaning from MV, and smaller fluctuations in blood pressure.[35,38,39] Despite indications that SIMV does not provide optimal support in extremely low-gestational-age newborns, many clinicians continue to use it both in the acute phase of illness and during weaning from MV,[40] based on the common assumption that both rate and pressure must be weaned before extubation.[35,36] Preference for the lower inflation rate of SIMV appears to be based on the superficially plausible assumption that a smaller number of inflations is inherently less damaging. This concept ignores the fact that the slower ventilator rate is accomplished at the expense of a larger V_T,[38] a variable that is clearly more injurious than ventilator rate (e.g., consider high-frequency ventilation) and is contradicted by available evidence from both preclinical and clinical studies.[41,42] Many clinicians also mistakenly believe that assisting every breath prevents respiratory muscle training. This concern reflects a failure to understand that the infant contributes an increasing amount of inspiratory effort to the transpulmonary pressure during weaning, progressively taking over a greater proportion of the work of breathing as the ventilator inflation pressure is decreased, resulting in effective training of the respiratory muscles. As weaning progresses, the inflation pressure is decreased to the point where it only overcomes the added resistance of the ETT and circuit, at which point the infant can be extubated.

Volume-Targeted Ventilation

Pressure-controlled ventilation became the standard approach to MV in newborns because early attempts at volume-controlled ventilation using equipment available at the time in infants with uncuffed ETTs were disappointing. Pressure-controlled ventilation remains the dominant mode of ventilation in the neonatal intensive care unit

Table 18.1   MAJOR OUTCOMES OF VOLUME-TARGETED VERSUS PRESSURE-LIMITED VENTILATION[a]

Outcome	No. of Studies	No. of Subjects	Relative Risk (95% CI) or Mean Difference (95% CI)
Mortality	11	767	0.73 (0.51–1.05)
Any IVH	11	759	0.65 (0.42–0.99)[b]
Grade 3–4 IVH	11	707	0.55 (0.39–0.79)[b]
BPD at 36 weeks	9	596	0.61 (0.46–0.82)[b]
Cystic PVL	7	531	0.33 (0.15–0.72)[b]
Pneumothorax	8	595	0.46 (0.25–0.86)[b]
Failure of assigned mode	4	405	0.64 (0.43–0.94)[b]
Any hypocapnia	2	58	0.56 (0.33–0.96)[b]
Duration of supplemental oxygen (days)	2	133	−1.68 (−2.5 to −0.88)[b]

[a]The table summarizes the major outcomes assessed in the meta-analysis of 11 randomized clinical trials.
[b]p<0.05.
BPD, Bronchopulmonary dysplasia; *IVH,* intraventricular hemorrhage; *PVL,* periventricular leukomalacia.
From Peng W, Zhu H, Shi H, et al. Volume-targeted ventilation is more suitable than pressure-limited ventilation for preterm infants: a systematic review and meta-analysis. *Arch Dis Child Fetal Neonatal Ed.* 2014;99:F158–165.

because of its simplicity, ability to ventilate despite a large ETT leak, and improved intrapulmonary gas distribution owing to a decelerating gas flow pattern.[43,44] The fear of pressure as the major culprit in lung injury is deeply ingrained and many clinicians continue to believe that directly controlling PIP is important, despite unequivocal evidence that volume, not pressure, is the key element in VALI.[45,46] The danger of using pressure control is that V_T is not directly controlled and changes when lung compliance is altered. Consequently, minute ventilation may change substantially without any adjustment of ventilator settings with lung volume recruitment or surfactant administration, resulting in hyperventilation and volutrauma. V_T may become insufficient with decreased lung compliance, increased airway resistance, or absence of the patient's spontaneous respiratory effort and lead to hypercapnia, tachypnea, increased work of breathing and oxygen consumption, agitation, fatigue, atelectasis/atelectrauma, and acidosis. Rapid, shallow breathing leads to inefficient gas exchange owing to increased dead space/V_T ratio. It is therefore evident that relatively tight control of V_T is highly desirable and for this reason, volume-controlled ventilation remains the standard of care in adult and pediatric ventilation.

There are many ways to regulate V_T delivery during MV. Modern ventilators now make it possible to use volume-controlled ventilation in newborns by allowing for measurement of exhaled V_T at the airway opening, so that manual adjustment of set V_T at the ventilator end of the patient circuit can be made to achieve a desired exhaled V_T.[47] More convenient are volume-targeted modes that are modifications of pressure-controlled ventilation that automatically adjust inflation pressure and/or time to achieve a target V_T.[48] It is likely that the key benefit of volume-targeted ventilation (VTV) rests in the ability to regulate V_T, regardless of how that goal is achieved. With V_T as the primary control variable, inflation pressure is automatically reduced as lung compliance and patient inspiratory effort improve, resulting in real-time weaning of pressure. Although volume targeting can also be achieved by close monitoring of V_T and manual changes of PIP, VTV results in more timely adjustments. Volume guarantee (VG) is the most extensively studied form of VTV and the basic control algorithm is increasingly being adopted by ventilator manufacturers. Benefits documented in two recent meta-analyses that encompassed several different modalities of VTV include significant decrease in the rate of BPD, pneumothorax, severe intraventricular hemorrhage, and periventricular leukomalacia, as well as less hypocapnia and shorter duration of MV (Table 18.1).[49,50]

Importance of the Open Lung Strategy

Ensuring that gas entering the lungs is evenly distributed into an "open lung"—thus avoiding atelectrauma—is a key element of any lung-protective ventilation strategy.[51] Adequate PEEP is widely recognized as a means of mitigating lung injury.[51,52]

Unfortunately, the impassioned plea of Burkhard Lachmann 25 years ago to "*open the lung and keep it open!*"[53] has been ignored by many practitioners during conventional MV despite a sound physiologic basis and strong experimental evidence in its favor. In practical terms, the open lung is achieved by applying adequate PEEP.[54] One of the most important obstacles to optimizing the manner in which conventional MV is practiced is the persistence of "PEEP-o-phobia," the fear of using adequate levels of end-expiratory pressure. This may be in part due to the fact that the open lung strategy has not been extensively evaluated in the clinical setting.[52] It is important to understand that there is no single optimal PEEP level. The level of end-expiratory pressure must be tailored to the degree of lung injury (i.e., lung compliance). For infants with healthy lungs and thus normal lung compliance, PEEP of 3 cm H_2O may be appropriate; PEEP of 6 cm H_2O may well lead to overexpansion of normal lungs with circulatory impairment and elevated cerebral venous pressure. On the other hand, atelectatic, poorly compliant lungs may transiently require PEEP levels as high as 8 to 10 cm H_2O or more to achieve adequate alveolar recruitment and optimize the ventilation/perfusion ratio. Because infants with healthy lungs seldom undergo ventilation, PEEP of less than 5 cm H_2O should be seldom used. Interventions that result in interruption of PEEP should be kept to a minimum (e.g., avoidance of routine suctioning, unnecessary disconnection of the patient circuit) to avoid loss of lung volume recruitment. Maintenance of sufficient lung volume may be particularly important during the critical postextubation period in infants with significant lung disease.[30]

High-Frequency Ventilation

In contrast to conventional ventilation, the importance of optimizing lung volume has been recognized since its early days by users of high-frequency ventilation (HFV), where the optimal lung volume strategy has become standard practice and is widely understood to be critical to its success.[55,56] HFV includes several modes of ventilation, including high-frequency oscillatory ventilation (HFOV), high-frequency jet ventilation (HFJV), and high-frequency percussive ventilation (HFPV) that have been used in neonatology since the 1980s. The benefit of HFV is believed to be a function of reduced pressure and volume swings transmitted to the periphery of the lungs. A number of early animal studies demonstrated the short-term benefits of HFOV with an optimal lung volume strategy.[57] Yoder et al. compared the effect of more prolonged HFOV and low V_T positive-pressure ventilation using the immature baboon model for BPD, demonstrating that prolonged use of HFOV significantly improved early lung function with sustained improvement in pulmonary mechanics up to day 28 of life and less pulmonary inflammation in the recovery phase of their respiratory distress syndrome.[58] Clinical results with HFV have been less consistent with several RCTs of various modes of HFV showing improved outcomes, including reduction in BPD and/or duration of MV,[59–63] whereas other trials showed no improvement.[64–69] Interpretation of RCTs of HFV is made more challenging because most trials were performed many years ago in patient populations that differ markedly from infants being treated today and compared HFV with less sophisticated (more injurious) modes of conventional ventilation than those in use today.[52] Importantly, HFV trials that showed benefit were exclusively those that used the optimal lung volume strategy. In those "successful" HFV studies were two important differences between study and control groups: high frequency versus low frequency and open lung approach versus low distending pressure. The latter may be the more important difference; HFOV used without the open lung strategy was relatively ineffective in reducing lung injury.[70] At the same time, several preclinical studies demonstrated that conventional ventilation, when used with the open lung strategy, can achieve similar degrees of lung protection as HFOV, suggesting that optimizing lung volume, rather than frequency, is the key factor.[71–73] However, clinical application of the open lung strategy with conventional ventilation may be more difficult and the approach has not been adequately evaluated in clinical trials.[74]

With the inclusion of more recent clinical trials that reflect advances in conventional ventilation strategies, the lung-protective effect of HFOV is less clear than earlier studies suggested.[75] Individual patient data meta-analysis from several RCTs failed to demonstrate superiority of HFOV over conventional ventilation and did not suggest that any particular subgroup of preterm infants might uniquely benefit from HFOV.[76] Nonetheless, there may be more subtle benefits of lung-protective HFOV strategies as suggested by the long-term pulmonary follow-up from the United Kingdom Oscillation Study (UKOS), which demonstrated less severe long-term pulmonary function abnormalities in the HFOV group despite no difference in the primary outcome of BPD at 36 weeks.[76]

Evidence-Based Approach to Mechanical Ventilation

Based on the concepts outlined earlier, certain general guidelines for a lung-protective approach to MV can be formulated. The overarching goal is to minimize adverse effects on the infant's lungs, hemodynamics, and brain while supporting adequate gas exchange. Because prolonged duration of ventilation is associated with an increased likelihood of chronic lung disease, late-onset sepsis, and neurodevelopmental impairment, successful extubation at the earliest possible time is an important goal. Ventilation settings must be individualized to address each patient's specific condition but must include the dual objectives of optimizing lung volume/preventing atelectasis and avoiding excessively large V_T. The open lung strategy improves lung compliance, minimizes oxygen requirement, avoids surfactant inactivation, and achieves even V_T distribution. Prevention of excessive V_T delivery minimizes volutrauma and hypocapnia, the two most important and potentially preventable elements of lung and brain injury. Modern neonatal ventilators give clinicians access to effective volume-targeted modes, but not all neonatal intensive care units in the United States have invested in ventilators specifically designed for newborns, relying instead on so-called universal ventilators, which may not provide optimal volume-targeted modes for the smallest infants. Effective use of VTV requires practitioners to abandon their deeply ingrained "barophobia" and embrace instead the importance of consistent V_T delivery. Equally important is familiarity with the appropriate V_T targets, which are a function of patient size, postnatal age, and nature of their lung disease.[48]

When relatively high pressures are needed to achieve adequate support, HFV may be a better option. The encouraging results of long-term pulmonary outcome from the UKOS study, coupled with the recent availability (at least outside the United States) of HFOV devices capable of measuring and regulating V_T (HFOV + VG),[77,78] will likely lead to resurgence of enthusiasm for early use of HFOV as a lung-protective prevention strategy.

Mild permissive hypercapnia and the lowest fraction of inspired oxygen (F_{IO_2}) consistent with adequate oxygenation are generally considered appropriate, but partial pressure of carbon dioxide (P_{CO_2}) higher than 60 mm Hg should be avoided in the first 72 hours of life because of the increased risk of intraventricular hemorrhage.[79–81] There is no evidence to support the routine use of sedation; therefore infants should be allowed to breathe spontaneously. Routine suctioning should be avoided as it leads to derecruitment, transient hypoxemia, and perturbation of cerebral hemodynamics.[82] However, when secretions are detected by auscultation or by perturbation of the flow waveform, rapid gentle suctioning without instillation of normal saline solution should be performed.

In the absence of clear evidence from RCTs, the choice of SIMV or A/C remains a matter of personal preference and practice style. There is little difference between the two in the acute phase of respiratory failure when the set rate is relatively high with both modes, but the difference becomes more pronounced during weaning, especially in the smallest infants, owing to high ETT resistance. Prolonged ventilation with low-rate SIMV should be avoided in these infants as it imposes an undesirably high work of breathing. SIMV also results in larger V_T compared with A/C, because small preterm infants typically do not generate adequate spontaneous V_T and thus have a high dead space/V_T ratio. To a significant degree, this problem may be overcome by adding PSV to the spontaneous breaths during SIMV.[83] While this approach is effective, it adds complexity and does not appear to have any advantage over A/C or PSV used alone, as long as atelectasis is avoided by using adequate level of PEEP. Additionally, it is important to recognize that volume targeting will only be applied to the SIMV inflations when using SIMV with PSV and VG.

Some degree of arrest of normal lung development is probably inevitable in the most immature infants even with optimized respiratory support and therefore "new BPD" is probably unavoidable at the lowest gestational ages. Suboptimal respiratory support is likely to exacerbate that process and add an element of added lung injury, leading to the superimposition of "old BPD." The wide variation in the risk-adjusted incidence of BPD among the academic medical centers of the National Institute of Child Health and Human Development Neonatal Research Network suggests that MV and other clinical practices constitute potentially modifiable risk factors.[84] The concepts outlined in this chapter are based on the best available evidence and physiologic rationale and may provide an opportunity to minimize adverse respiratory outcomes in extremely immature infants requiring respiratory support.

Conflict of Interest Statement

Dr. Keszler has received honoraria for lectures and research grant support from Dräger Medical. Dr. Keszler also chairs the Data Safety Monitoring Board of a clinical trial supported by Medipost America and serves on a Data Safety Monitoring Board for a clinical trial sponsored by Chiesi USA Inc. None of the companies had any input into the content of this chapter.

REFERENCES

1. Walsh MC, Morris BH, Wrage LA, et al. Extremely low birthweight neonates with protracted ventilation: mortality and 18-month neurodevelopmental outcomes. *J Pediatr*. 2005;146(6):798–804.
2. SUPPORT Study Group of the Eunice Kennedy Shriver NICHD Neonatal Research Network, Finer NN, Carlo WA, et al. Early CPAP versus surfactant in extremely preterm infants. *N Engl J Med*. 2010;362(21):1970–1979.
3. Morley CJ, Davis PG, Doyle LW, Brion LP, Hascoet JM, Carlin JB. Nasal CPAP or intubation at birth for very preterm infants. *N Engl J Med*. 2008;358(7):700–708.
4. Garland JS. Strategies to prevent ventilator-associated pneumonia in neonates. *Clin Perinatol*. 2010;37(3):629–643.
5. Dreyfuss D, Soler P, Basset G, Saumon G. High inflation pressure pulmonary edema. Respective effects of high airway pressure, high tidal volume, and positive end-expiratory pressure. *Am Rev Respir Dis*. 1988;137(5):1159–1164.
6. Hernandez LA, Peevy KJ, Moise AA, Parker JC. Chest wall restriction limits high airway pressure-induced lung injury in young rabbits. *J Appl Physiol*. 1989;66(5):2364–2368.
7. Mols G, Priebe HJ, Guttmann J. Alveolar recruitment in acute lung injury. *Br J Anaesth*. 2006;96(2):156–166.
8. Tsuchida S, Engelberts D, Peltekova V, et al. Atelectasis causes alveolar injury in nonatelectatic lung regions. *Am J Respir Crit Care Med*. 2006;174(3):279–289.
9. Mortola JP, Fisher JT, Smith JB, Fox GS, Weeks D, Willis D. Onset of respiration in infants delivered by cesarean section. *J Appl Physiol Respir Environ Exerc Physiol*. 1982;52(3):716.
10. te Pas AB, Siew M, Wallace MJ, et al. Establishing functional residual capacity at birth: the effect of sustained inflation and positive end-expiratory pressure in a preterm rabbit model. *Pediatr Res*. 2009;65(5):537–541.
11. Wyckoff MH, Aziz K, Escobedo MB, et al. Part 13: Neonatal Resuscitation: 2015 American Heart Association guidelines update for cardiopulmonary resuscitation and emergency cardiovascular care (Reprint). *Pediatrics*. 2015;136(suppl 2):S196–S218.
12. Perlman JM, Wyllie J, Kattwinkel J, et al. Part 7: Neonatal Resuscitation: 2015 International Consensus on Cardiopulmonary Resuscitation and Emergency Cardiovascular Care Science With Treatment Recommendations. *Circulation*. 2015;132(16 suppl 1):S204–S241.
13. Schmolzer GM, O'Reilly M, Labossiere J, et al. Cardiopulmonary resuscitation with chest compressions during sustained inflations: a new technique of neonatal resuscitation that improves recovery and survival in a neonatal porcine model. *Circulation*. 2013;128(23):2495–2503.
14. Bjorklund LJ, Ingimarsson J, Curstedt T, et al. Manual ventilation with a few large breaths at birth compromises the therapeutic effect of subsequent surfactant replacement in immature lambs. *Pediatr Res*. 1997;42(3):348–355.
15. Hillman NH, Kemp MW, Miura Y, Kallapur SG, Jobe AH. Sustained inflation at birth did not alter lung injury from mechanical ventilation in surfactant-treated fetal lambs. *PLoS One*. 2014;9(11):e113473.
16. Hillman NH, Kemp MW, Noble PB, Kallapur SG, Jobe AH. Sustained inflation at birth did not protect preterm fetal sheep from lung injury. *Am J Physiol Lung Cell Mol Physiol*. 2013;305(6):L446–L453.

17. Wyckoff MH. Improving neonatal cardiopulmonary resuscitation hemodynamics: are sustained inflations during compressions the answer? *Circulation*. 2013;128(23):2468–2469.
18. Foglia EE, Owen LS, Thio M, et al. Sustained Aeration of Infant Lungs (SAIL) trial: study protocol for a randomized controlled trial. *Trials*. 2015;16:95.
19. Ammari A, Suri M, Milisavljevic V, et al. Variables associated with the early failure of nasal CPAP in very low birth weight infants. *J Pediatr*. 2005;147(3):341–347.
20. Morley CJ, Davis PG, Doyle LW, Brion LP, Hascoet JM, Carlin JB. Nasal CPAP or intubation at birth for very preterm infants. *N Engl J Med*. 2008;358(7):700–708.
21. NICHD Neonatal Research Network, Support Study Group of the Eunice Kennedy Shriver. Early CPAP versus surfactant in extremely preterm infants. *N Engl J Med*. 2010;362:1970–1979.
22. Sandri F, Plavka R, Ancora G, et al. Prophylactic or early selective surfactant combined with nCPAP in very preterm infants. *Pediatrics*. 2010;125(6):e1402–e1409.
23. Dunn MS, Kaempf J, de Klerk A, et al. Randomized trial comparing 3 approaches to the initial respiratory management of preterm neonates. *Pediatrics*. 2011;128(5):e1069–e1076.
24. Schmolzer GM, Kumar M, Pichler G, Aziz K, O'Reilly M, Cheung PY. Non-invasive versus invasive respiratory support in preterm infants at birth: systematic review and meta-analysis. *BMJ*. 2013;347. f5980.
25. Moretti C, Gizzi C, Papoff P, et al. Comparing the effects of nasal synchronized intermittent positive pressure ventilation (nSIPPV) and nasal continuous positive airway pressure (nCPAP) after extubation in very low birth weight infants. *Early Hum Dev*. 1999;56(2–3):167–177.
26. Davis PG, Morley CJ, Owen LS. Non-invasive respiratory support of preterm neonates with respiratory distress: continuous positive airway pressure and nasal intermittent positive pressure ventilation. *Semin Fetal Neonatal Med*. 2009;14(1):14–20.
27. Meneses J, Bhandari V, Alves JG. Nasal intermittent positive-pressure ventilation vs nasal continuous positive airway pressure for preterm infants with respiratory distress syndrome: a systematic review and meta-analysis. *Arch Pediatr Adolesc Med*. 2012;166(4):372–376.
28. Kirpalani H, Millar D, Lemyre B, Yoder BA, Chiu A, Roberts RS. A trial comparing noninvasive ventilation strategies in preterm infants. *N Engl J Med*. 2013;369(7):611–620.
29. Owen LS, Morley CJ, Dawson JA, Davis PG. Effects of non-synchronised nasal intermittent positive pressure ventilation on spontaneous breathing in preterm infants. *Arch Dis Child Fetal Neonatal Ed*. 2011;96(6):F422–F428.
30. Buzzella B, Claure N, D'Ugard C, Bancalari E. A randomized controlled trial of two nasal continuous positive airway pressure levels after extubation in preterm infants. *J Pediatr*. 2014;164(1):46–51.
31. van der Hoeven M, Brouwer E, Blanco CE. Nasal high frequency ventilation in neonates with moderate respiratory insufficiency. *Arch Dis Child Fetal Neonatal Ed*. 1998;79(1):F61–F63.
32. Mukerji A, Singh B, Helou SE, et al. Use of noninvasive high-frequency ventilation in the neonatal intensive care unit: a retrospective review. *Am J Perinatol*. 2015;30(2):171–176.
33. De Luca D, Dell'Orto V. Non-invasive high-frequency oscillatory ventilation in neonates: review of physiology, biology and clinical data. *Arch Dis Child Fetal Neonatal Ed*. 2016.
34. Gibu C, Cheng P, Ward RJ, Castro B, Heldt GP. Feasibility and physiological effects of non-invasive neurally-adjusted ventilatory assist (NIV-NAVA) in preterm infants. *Pediatr Res*. 2017.
35. Chan V, Greenough A. Comparison of weaning by patient triggered ventilation or synchronous intermittent mandatory ventilation in preterm infants. *Acta Paediatr*. 1994;83(3):335–337.
36. Dimitriou G, Greenough A, Griffin F, Chan V. Synchronous intermittent mandatory ventilation modes compared with patient triggered ventilation during weaning. *Arch Dis Child Fetal Neonatal Ed*. 1995;72(3):F188–F190.
37. Greenough A, Rossor TE, Sundaresan A, Murthy V, Milner AD. Synchronized mechanical ventilation for respiratory support in newborn infants. *Cochrane Database Syst Rev*. 2016;9:CD000456.
38. Hummler H, Gerhardt T, Gonzalez A, Claure N, Everett R, Bancalari E. Influence of different methods of synchronized mechanical ventilation on ventilation, gas exchange, patient effort, and blood pressure fluctuations in premature neonates. *Pediatr Pulmonol*. 1996;22(5):305–313.
39. Mrozek JD, Bendel-Stenzel EM, Meyers PA, Bing DR, Connett JE, Mammel MC. Randomized controlled trial of volume-targeted synchronized ventilation and conventional intermittent mandatory ventilation following initial exogenous surfactant therapy. *Pediatr Pulmonol*. 2000;29(1):11–18.
40. Sharma A, Greenough A. Survey of neonatal respiratory support strategies. *Acta Paediatr*. 2007; 96(8):1115–1117.
41. Albertine KH, Jones GP, Starcher BC, et al. Chronic lung injury in preterm lambs. Disordered respiratory tract development. *Am J Respir Crit Care Med*. 1999;159(3):945–958.
42. Multicentre randomised controlled trial of high against low frequency positive pressure ventilation. Oxford Region Controlled Trial of Artificial Ventilation OCTAVE Study Group. *Arch Dis Child*. 1991;66(7 Spec No):770–775.
43. Dani C, Bresci C, Lista G, et al. Neonatal respiratory support strategies in the intensive care unit: an Italian survey. *Eur J Pediatr*. 2013;172(3):331–336.
44. van Kaam AH, Rimensberger PC, Borensztajn D, De Jaegere AP. Ventilation practices in the neonatal intensive care unit: a cross-sectional study. *J Pediatr*. 2010;157(5):767–771.e763.
45. Dreyfuss D, Saumon G. Ventilator-induced lung injury: lessons from experimental studies. *Am J Respir Crit Care Med*. 1998;157(1):294–323.
46. Dreyfuss D, Saumon G. Role of tidal volume, FRC, and end-inspiratory volume in the development of pulmonary edema following mechanical ventilation. *Am Rev Respir Dis*. 1993;148(5): 1194–1203.

18

47. Singh J, Sinha SK, Clarke P, Byrne S, Donn SM. Mechanical ventilation of very low birth weight infants: is volume or pressure a better target variable? *J Pediatr*. 2006;149(3):308–313.
48. Keszler M. Update on mechanical ventilatory strategies. *Neo Reviews*. 2013;14(5):e237–e251.
49. Wheeler K, Klingenberg C, McCallion N, Morley CJ, Davis PG. Volume-targeted versus pressure-limited ventilation in the neonate. *Cochrane Database Syst Rev*. 2010;(11):CD003666.
50. Peng W, Zhu H, Shi H, Liu E. Volume-targeted ventilation is more suitable than pressure-limited ventilation for preterm infants: a systematic review and meta-analysis. *Arch Dis Child Fetal Neonatal Ed*. 2014;99(2):F158–F165.
51. Rimensberger PC, Cox PN, Frndova H, Bryan AC. The open lung during small tidal volume ventilation: concepts of recruitment and "optimal" positive end-expiratory pressure. *Crit Care Med*. 1999;27(9):1946–1952.
52. van Kaam AH, Rimensberger PC. Lung-protective ventilation strategies in neonatology: what do we know—what do we need to know? *Crit Care Med*. 2007;35(3):925–931.
53. Lachmann B. Open up the lung and keep the lung open. *Intensive Care Med*. 1992;18(6):319–321.
54. Castoldi F, Daniele I, Fontana P, Cavigioli F, Lupo E, Lista G. Lung recruitment maneuver during volume guarantee ventilation of preterm infants with acute respiratory distress syndrome. *Am J Perinatol*. 2011;28(7):521–528.
55. Bryan AC. The oscillations of HFO. *Am J Respir Crit Care Med*. 2001;163(4):816–817.
56. Froese AB. Role of lung volume in lung injury: HFO in the atelectasis-prone lung. *Acta Anaesthesiol Scand Suppl*. 1989;90:126–130.
57. Keszler M, Durand DJ. Neonatal high-frequency ventilation. Past, present, and future. *Clin Perinatol*. 2001;28(3):579–607.
58. Yoder BA, Siler-Khodr T, Winter VT, Coalson JJ. High-frequency oscillatory ventilation: effects on lung function, mechanics, and airway cytokines in the immature baboon model for neonatal chronic lung disease. *Am J Respir Crit Care Med*. 2000;162(5):1867–1876.
59. Clark RH, Gerstmann DR, Null DM Jr, deLemos RA. Prospective randomized comparison of high-frequency oscillatory and conventional ventilation in respiratory distress syndrome. *Pediatrics*. 1992;89(1):5–12.
60. Gerstmann DR, Minton SD, Stoddard RA, et al. The Provo multicenter early high-frequency oscillatory ventilation trial: improved pulmonary and clinical outcome in respiratory distress syndrome. *Pediatrics*. 1996;98(6 Pt 1):1044–1057.
61. Keszler M, Modanlou HD, Brudno DS, et al. Multicenter controlled clinical trial of high-frequency jet ventilation in preterm infants with uncomplicated respiratory distress syndrome. *Pediatrics*. 1997;100(4):593–599.
62. Plavka R, Kopecky P, Sebron V, Svihovec P, Zlatohlavkova B, Janus V. A prospective randomized comparison of conventional mechanical ventilation and very early high frequency oscillatory ventilation in extremely premature newborns with respiratory distress syndrome. *Intensive Care Med*. 1999;25(1):68–75.
63. Courtney SE, Durand DJ, Asselin JM, Hudak ML, Aschner JL, Shoemaker CT. High-frequency oscillatory ventilation versus conventional mechanical ventilation for very-low-birth-weight infants. *N Engl J Med*. 2002;347(9):643–652.
64. Wiswell TE, Graziani LJ, Kornhauser MS, et al. High-frequency jet ventilation in the early management of respiratory distress syndrome is associated with a greater risk for adverse outcomes. *Pediatrics*. 1996;98(6 Pt 1):1035–1043.
65. Rettwitz-Volk W, Veldman A, Roth B, et al. A prospective, randomized, multicenter trial of high-frequency oscillatory ventilation compared with conventional ventilation in preterm infants with respiratory distress syndrome receiving surfactant. *J Pediatr*. 1998;132(2):249–254.
66. Moriette G, Paris-Llado J, Walti H, et al. Prospective randomized multicenter comparison of high-frequency oscillatory ventilation and conventional ventilation in preterm infants of less than 30 weeks with respiratory distress syndrome. *Pediatrics*. 2001;107(2):363–372.
67. Johnson AH, Peacock JL, Greenough A, et al. High-frequency oscillatory ventilation for the prevention of chronic lung disease of prematurity. *N Engl J Med*. 2002;347(9):633–642.
68. Van Reempts P, Borstlap C, Laroche S, Van der Auwera JC. Early use of high frequency ventilation in the premature neonate. *Eur J Pediatr*. 2003;162(4):219–226.
69. Thome U, Kossel H, Lipowsky G, et al. Randomized comparison of high-frequency ventilation with high-rate intermittent positive pressure ventilation in preterm infants with respiratory failure. *J Pediatr*. 1999;135(1):39–46.
70. McCulloch PR, Forkert PG, Froese AB. Lung volume maintenance prevents lung injury during high frequency oscillatory ventilation in surfactant-deficient rabbits. *Am Rev Respir Dis*. 1988;137(5):1185–1192.
71. Gommers D, Hartog A, Schnabel R, De Jaegere A, Lachmann B. High-frequency oscillatory ventilation is not superior to conventional mechanical ventilation in surfactant-treated rabbits with lung injury. *Eur Respir Rev*. 1999;14(4):738–744.
72. Vazquez de Anda GF, Hartog A, Verbrugge SJ, Gommers D, Lachmann B. The open lung concept: pressure-controlled ventilation is as effective as high-frequency oscillatory ventilation in improving gas exchange and lung mechanics in surfactant-deficient animals. *Intensive Care Med*. 1999;25(9):990–996.
73. van Kaam AH, de Jaegere A, Haitsma JJ, Van Aalderen WM, Kok JH, Lachmann B. Positive pressure ventilation with the open lung concept optimizes gas exchange and reduces ventilator-induced lung injury in newborn piglets. *Pediatr Res*. 2003;53(2):245–253.

74. Jobe AH. Lung recruitment for ventilation: does it work, and is it safe? *J Pediatr*. 2009;154(5):635–636.

75. Cools F, Henderson-Smart DJ, Offringa M, Askie LM. Elective high frequency oscillatory ventilation versus conventional ventilation for acute pulmonary dysfunction in preterm infants. *Cochrane Database Syst Rev (Online)*. 2009;(3):CD000104.

76. Cools F, Askie LM, Offringa M, et al. Elective high-frequency oscillatory versus conventional ventilation in preterm infants: a systematic review and meta-analysis of individual patients' data. *Lancet*. 2010;375(9731):2082–2091.

77. Enomoto M, Keszler M, Sakuma M, et al. Effect of volume guarantee in preterm infants on high-frequency oscillatory ventilation: a pilot study. *Am J Perinatol*. 2017;34(1):26–30.

78. Iscan B, Duman N, Tuzun F, Kumral A, Ozkan H. Impact of volume guarantee on high-frequency oscillatory ventilation in preterm infants: a randomized crossover clinical trial. *Neonatology*. 2015;108(4):277–282.

79. Fabres J, Carlo WA, Phillips V, Howard G, Ambalavanan N. Both extremes of arterial carbon dioxide pressure and the magnitude of fluctuations in arterial carbon dioxide pressure are associated with severe intraventricular hemorrhage in preterm infants. *Pediatrics*. 2007;119(2):299–305.

80. Kaiser JR, Gauss CH, Pont MM, Williams DK. Hypercapnia during the first 3 days of life is associated with severe intraventricular hemorrhage in very low birth weight infants. *J Perinatol*. 2006;26(5):279–285.

81. Thome UH, Genzel-Boroviczeny O, Bohnhorst B, et al. Permissive hypercapnia in extremely low birthweight infants (PHELBI): a randomised controlled multicentre trial. *Lancet Respir Med*. 2015.

82. Kaiser JR, Gauss CH, Williams DK. Tracheal suctioning is associated with prolonged disturbances of cerebral hemodynamics in very low birth weight infants. *J Perinatol*. 2008;28(1):34–41.

83. Osorio W, Claure N, D'Ugard C, Athavale K, Bancalari E. Effects of pressure support during an acute reduction of synchronized intermittent mandatory ventilation in preterm infants. *J Perinatol*. 2005;25(6):412–416.

84. Ambalavanan N, Walsh M, Bobashev G, et al. Intercenter differences in bronchopulmonary dysplasia or death among very low birth weight infants. *Pediatrics*. 2011;127(1):e106–e116.

18

CHAPTER 19

Automation of Respiratory Support

Nelson Claure, Martin Keszler, and Eduardo Bancalari

- The settings during conventional ventilation and oxygen supplementation require frequent adjustments to adapt to the changing needs of the preterm infant.
- Because of the premature infant's respiratory instability and resource limitations, a balance between adequate respiratory support and the risk of adverse side effects is not always achieved.
- Automated modalities that adjust the respiratory support and oxygen supplementation to the infant's needs have been developed to address these limitations.
- Studies evaluating these modalities show promising short-term results, but further research is needed to determine whether these systems can improve longer-term respiratory, ophthalmic, and neurodevelopmental outcomes.

A high proportion of premature infants have respiratory failure and require mechanical respiratory support and supplemental oxygen. These therapies are associated with increased risk for lung and eye injury, particularly when they are used for prolonged periods. Excessive oxygen supplementation is also associated with greater risk for oxidative damage to the central nervous system and other organs.[1–5]

During neonatal intensive care, caregivers need to make frequent adjustments in respiratory support based on monitored parameters of ventilation and oxygenation to minimize the risk of adverse effects. Despite best efforts, the respiratory support often exceeds what is actually needed by the infant or at times may be insufficient. This is due to the intrinsic respiratory instability of the preterm infant, to the intermittent nature of monitoring, and to staff limitations that do not allow minute-to-minute adjustment of the respiratory support to meet the infant's needs.

To address these limitations, newer forms of neonatal respiratory support have been developed to automatically adapt respiratory support to the changing needs of the infant. The most promising of these approaches will be described in this chapter with emphasis on the available evidence and possible limitations.

Automation in Mechanical Ventilation

Despite the increasing use of noninvasive respiratory support, a considerable proportion of very preterm infants require intubation and mechanical ventilation after birth. As the initial respiratory failure improves, two divergent patterns are commonly observed. In some infants, the weaning process proceeds rapidly, but in others weaning is difficult and they continue mechanical respiratory support for long periods.

In addition to the severity of underlying lung disease, factors that prolong the need for respiratory support in preterm infants include immaturity of the respiratory control system, instability of lung volume, and unfavorable lung and chest wall mechanics. These conditions increase the respiratory instability, which combined with inconsistent weaning strategies and staff limitations, can lead to prolonged ventilation and increased risk for lung injury.

Standard modes of neonatal ventilation, such as intermittent mandatory ventilation (IMV), synchronized IMV (SIMV), and assist/control (A/C) ventilation, use inflation pressure as the primary control variable and are referred to as pressure-controlled (PC) modes. They provide a constant level of ventilatory support whereby the peak inflation pressure (PIP), ventilator cycling frequency, or both are constant. These modes require manual adjustments to adapt to the changing needs of the infants, but many times these are not frequent enough to maintain stable gas exchange. During the weaning process, the ventilator frequency and/or PIP are reduced and spontaneous inspiratory effort plays a greater role in maintaining ventilation. However, ventilation can be affected by an inconsistent respiratory drive and acute changes in lung mechanics. To overcome the limitations of intermittent manual adjustment of ventilator settings, automated modes have been proposed as means to continuously titrate respiratory support to the infant's changing needs.

Volume-Targeted Ventilation

Volume-targeted ventilation (VTV) includes modes of PC ventilation in which the peak inflation pressure or inflation time is automatically adjusted from one cycle to the next or within the cycle to maintain the tidal volume (V_T) close to a target level. Available modalities of VTV differ in whether V_T adjustment is based on the volume delivered to the patient during inspiration, the exhaled volume, or the volume delivered by the ventilator to the circuit rather than the patient.

In *volume guarantee (VG)* ventilation PIP is adjusted from one cycle to the next to maintain a target V_T. PIP of the subsequent cycle is adjusted based on the difference between the exhaled V_T of the previous cycle and the target V_T. VG targets the exhaled V_T to circumvent the overestimation of delivered V_T resulting from gas leaks around the endotracheal tube (ETT) during the inspiratory phase. PIP is automatically adjusted within a range set by the clinician. VG ventilation can be used in combination with A/C ventilation, PSV, SIMV, and IMV.

In *pressure-regulated–volume-control (PRVC)* ventilation an initial diagnostic cycle determines the respiratory system compliance and PIP is subsequently adjusted from cycle to cycle based on the difference between the inspiratory V_T and the target. The V_T is measured at the ventilator end of the patient circuit, resulting in overestimation of the V_T delivered to the patient. Use of the compliance compensation feature to estimate the infant's inspiratory V_T after compensation for the volume compressed in the circuit is available but may be unreliable in the presence of ETT leaks. The measured V_T during inspiration may be overestimated in the presence of leaks around the ETT. The newest version of PRVC now measures the V_T at the airway opening, which should provide more accurate estimation of delivered V_T. PRVC is exclusively an A/C mode.

In volume controlled (VC) ventilation the set volume is delivered into the ventilator circuit and the inspiratory phase ends when this volume is delivered. Pressure rises and reaches its peak just before exhalation. In newborn infants, the volume delivered to the circuit is much larger than V_T delivered to the infant because of compression of gas within the circuit and humidifier and possible loss of gas owing to ETT leak. VC can be used in combination with A/C, SIMV, or IMV.

The automatic adjustment of PIP in VTV maintains a more stable V_T, prevents excessive lung inflation, and leads to a more stable gas exchange in the face of changing lung mechanics and spontaneous respiratory effort. Fig. 19.1 shows typical adjustments in peak pressure to changes in spontaneous respiratory effort during VTV.

Studies in premature infants have shown reduced variability in V_T, fewer ventilator cycles delivering too large or small V_T, and less hypocapnia with VG compared with PC ventilation.[6–12]

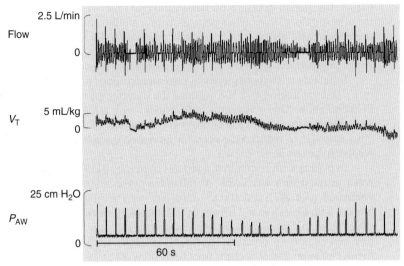

Fig. 19.1 Automatic adjustments in peak pressure in response to changes in spontaneous breathing effort during volume-targeted ventilation. Flow, tidal volume (V_T), and airway pressure (P_{AW}) tracings show downward adjustments in peak pressure as the infant's spontaneous inspiratory effort maintained V_T and upward adjustments in peak pressure when V_T decreased.

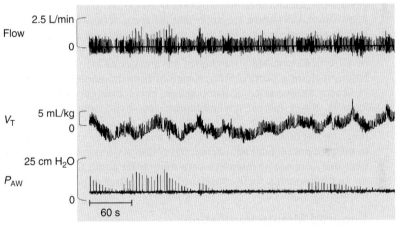

Fig. 19.2 Automatic adjustments in peak pressure during volume-targeted ventilation with a low target tidal volume (V_T). Tracings of flow, V_T, and airway pressure (P_{AW}) show a declining peak pressure as the infant maintained V_T above the target V_T. This resulted in periods when the infant was left receiving only positive end-expiratory pressure.

Another documented advantage of VTV is automatic weaning of PIP in real time, rather than intermittently in response to blood gas measurements. The effectiveness of this approach, however, appears to be dependent on the target V_T. Targeting a very low V_T resulted in rapid weaning of PIP, but this led to a compensatory rise in spontaneous breathing effort or resulted in higher transcutaneous partial pressure of carbon dioxide (PCO_2) levels in those infants unable to compensate consistently.[7]

Similarly, in a recent study a reduction in the target V_T from 5 to 4 mL/kg resulted in a greater than 50% increase in work of breathing.[13] Thus weaning should be done with caution because a target V_T that is too low could lead to a large reduction in PIP and result in periods when the infant receives minimal or no ventilatory support (Fig. 19.2). This and other studies underscore the importance of choosing an appropriate V_T for each patient and clinical situation. Patient size, postnatal age, the nature of the lung disease, and the choice of synchronized mode all affect the optimal V_T setting.[14–17] It is also important to appreciate that it is the patient's pH, not just the arterial partial pressure of carbon dioxide (Pa_{CO_2}), that is the primary regulator of respiratory drive. Thus patients with a significant base deficit will attempt to normalize their pH by achieving mild respiratory alkalosis. The low Pa_{CO_2} often prompts weaning of target V_T, which in turn results in automatic lowering of PIP and inadequate support when the patient generates a spontaneous V_T above the set value.

In infants with spontaneous hypoxemia episodes triggered by acute reductions in V_T and ventilation,[18,19] VG reduced the duration of the episodes compared with PC ventilation. This was particularly evident with a higher target V_T.[20,21] Although the automatic increase in PIP during VG did not prevent the occurrence of the hypoxemia episodes, it reduced the need for increased fraction of inspired oxygen F_{IO_2} to resolve hypoxemia.[21]

In infants with respiratory distress syndrome (RDS), use of VG during the first week resulted in lower levels of inflammatory cytokines in bronchoalveolar fluid compared with PC ventilation.[22] This has been attributed to reduced exposure to breaths with excessive V_T. However, inflammatory markers were shown to be higher when these infants underwent ventilated with VG at a low target V_T and low positive end-expiratory pressure (PEEP).[23] These findings indicate that avoidance of hypoventilation and atelectasis may be as relevant as avoiding overinflation.[24]

In randomized clinical trials in preterm infants with RDS, VTV resulted in faster weaning from mechanical ventilation compared conventional PC ventilation and a reduction in the composite of BPD or death.[22,25–30] These studies did not focus on the subpopulation of premature infants who at present are more likely to require mechanical ventilation after birth—that is, infants of less than 28 weeks' gestational age. Further investigation is necessary to confirm these findings in this population. Also, there are important differences between modalities of VTV that have been implemented and their relative advantages or limitations that have not been evaluated. Nonetheless, two meta-analyses that included a variety of modes of VTV demonstrated a number of advantages of VTV compared with PC ventilation, including decreased incidence of bronchopulmonary dysplasia, lower rate of severe intraventricular hemorrhage, lower incidence of periventricular leukomalacia, lower rate of pneumothorax, less hypocapnia, and shorter duration of mechanical ventilation.[30,31] Although these meta-analyses have some limitations, they suggest that automated, real-time adjustment of inflation pressure is superior to intermittent manual adjustment. As of this writing, all of the ventilators in common use in neonatal intensive care units offer some form of VTV, making VTV the first reasonably well-established and widely available modality of automated respiratory support.[32]

Targeted Minute Ventilation

Targeted minute ventilation (TMV) is a modality of respiratory support in which the cycling frequency of the ventilator is automatically adjusted to maintain minute ventilation at a target level. TMV is intended to reduce the respiratory support by providing fewer ventilator breaths when the infant is able to increase his or her contribution to minute ventilation. If minute ventilation exceeds the set target, the ventilator rate is automatically reduced to a lower limit or vice versa. In preterm infants recovering from RDS, TMV reduced the ventilator rate by 50% compared with SIMV[33] while total minute ventilation remained within the same range. Transient increases in ventilator rate were observed during TMV to prevent hypoventilation during periods of central apnea or reduced V_T. Typical adjustments of the ventilator rate during TMV are shown in Fig. 19.3.

TMV was combined with automatic adjustments to PIP to simultaneously maintain targets of minute ventilation and V_T, respectively. This modality was evaluated in an animal model that replicated the mechanisms leading to episodes of hypoxemia in preterm infants. Automatic increases in ventilator rate or PIP were effective in attenuating the severity of hypoxemia while the combined adjustments further improved ventilation stability and attenuated hypoxemia.[34] This strategy has yet to be evaluated in infants.

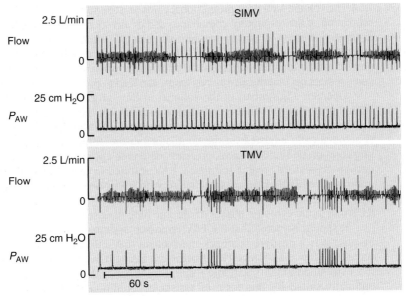

Fig. 19.3 Automatic adjustments in ventilator frequency during targeted minute ventilation *(TMV, bottom panel)* in contrast to the constant frequency during spontaneous intermittent mandatory ventilation *(SIMV, top panel)*. Tracings of flow and airway pressure *(P$_{AW}$)* show periods when the ventilator frequency is considerably reduced during TMV as the infant contribution to ventilation is consistent while transient increases in ventilator frequency maintain ventilation during periods of apnea.

Mandatory minute ventilation (MMV) is a modality in which the measured minute ventilation is compared with a set target level. Ventilator mandatory breaths stop when this level is exceeded by unassisted spontaneous breaths or by spontaneous breaths assisted with pressure support. When minute ventilation declines below the target, the ventilator delivers volume-targeted cycles at a constant rate to keep minute ventilation at the target. In near-term infants without lung disease, MMV reduced the ventilator rate compared with SIMV.[35] As of this writing, this mode has not been evaluated in premature infants with lung disease.

Adaptive mechanical backup ventilation is a modality in which the ventilator monitors spontaneous breathing and arterial oxygen saturation (Spo$_2$). In the occurrence of apnea or hypoxemia, the ventilator provides a backup rate until the episode is resolved. In preterm infants recovering from RDS, adaptive backup ventilation attenuated the frequency and duration of episodes of hypoxemia compared with conventional backup ventilation set to respond to apnea alone.[36] These findings suggest a role for hybrid ventilation modes to improve oxygenation stability.

The effects of different minute ventilation targets in premature infants have not been assessed. A target level below the infant's required total minute ventilation is likely to provide a background level of minimal respiratory support. On the other hand, a target level that is near or exceeds the infant's total minute ventilation could result in the ventilator taking over and inhibition of the infant's respiratory drive.

Proportional Assist Ventilation

The respiratory pump of the ventilated preterm infant must overcome increased resistive or elastic loads owing to the underlying lung disease to generate an adequate V_T. Proportional assist ventilation (PAV) is a modality whereby the ventilator pressure is automatically adjusted in proportion to the volume, flow, or both, generated by the respiratory pump. This enhances the infant's volume- or flow-generating ability and results in a reduction in the obstructive or restrictive loads that impede breathing. In PAV, the user determines the degree of mechanical unloading by setting the elastic (volume-proportional) and resistive (flow-proportional) gains in airway pressure.

The volume- and flow-proportional gains must be suited to each infant and require estimation of the respiratory compliance and/or airway resistance. Higher gains result in larger increases in airway pressure per unit of volume or flow generated by the infant. An excessively high elastic (volume) gain that exceeds the elastic recoil of the lungs can lead to a runaway increase in pressure, whereas a resistive (flow) gain that compensates beyond the airway resistance can lead to pressure oscillations.

Operator adjustments of the volume- or flow-proportional gains during PAV to maintain adequate ventilation parallel to some extent the adjustments in PIP during PSV or A/C ventilation to maintain an adequate V_T. During PAV the airway pressure is automatically adjusted by the ventilator but the clinician is responsible for setting appropriate limits for peak pressure, delivered volume, inspiratory time, and the backup mandatory breaths for apnea. PAV resulted in reduced breathing effort and improved ventilation and gas exchange with lower peak pressures compared with IMV, A/C ventilation, and SIMV in preterm infants during the weaning phase of RDS and in the evolving phases of chronic lung disease.[37–39]

It should be noted that the PAV approach assumes mature respiratory control, because it is a positive feedback mechanism that unloads the elastic and resistive forces to allow the subject with insufficient strength to generate the desired V_T. The inconsistent and highly variable respiratory drive of the preterm infant may not be optimally suited for this form of assistance. Additionally, because the system by necessity responds to inspiratory flow and volume, a large leak around the uncuffed ETT would be interpreted as a large inspiration and given correspondingly high level of inflation pressure, potentially leading to dangerously large V_T. Although PAV has been available for many years, it has not gained widespread acceptance, possibly because of its complexity and lack of documented advantage over other modalities.

Neurally Adjusted Ventilatory Assist

Neurally adjusted ventilatory assist (NAVA) is a modality where the ventilator pressure is automatically adjusted in proportion to the patient's respiratory effort as measured the electrical activity of the diaphragm (EA_{DIA}). The proportionality factor or NAVA gain determines the increase in pressure per microvolt of EA_{DIA}. Because the ventilator pressure increases or declines with the infant's inspiratory effort, NAVA is proposed as a way to enhance the inspiratory effort and optimize synchrony. Fig. 19.4 shows adjustments in ventilator pressure during NAVA. Like PAV, this is a positive feedback system, raising concern about amplifying the variability of the immature infant's respiratory effort.

NAVA has been shown to be effective in maintaining ventilation and gas exchange in premature infants comparably or better than modalities of conventional PC ventilation.[40–44] This has been attributed to the better synchrony between the infant's inspiration and the ventilator. However, no randomized trials with important clinical outcomes, such as bronchopulmonary dysplasia or intraventricular hemorrhage, have been conducted.

In NAVA, increasing the proportionality gain can produce an increase in V_T, a reduction in EA_{DIA}, or both. EA_{DIA} is monitored continuously and is used to assess the patient's inspiratory drive and adjust the NAVA gain as needed. However, data on the relation between the EA_{DIA} and inspiratory effort or volume generation and the variability between or within patients are scant for preterm infants. The EA_{DIA}, seen as an indicator of inspiratory effort, was reduced during NAVA compared with PC ventilation,[35,36] but it was higher compared with VTV.[37]

The reported findings on the use of NAVA are promising, but further research is needed to assess its physiologic and clinical effects in premature infants. In NAVA the level of support depends largely on the NAVA gain setting, but little is known about the effects of different NAVA gains or the methods to determine the most appropriate gain. Appropriate limits for PIP should be set to avoid excessive V_T resulting from the positive feedback when the infant becomes agitated, and apnea ventilation is necessary when respiratory effort is lacking. The extent to which EA_{DIA} can be compared between infants or within the same infant over time as an indicator

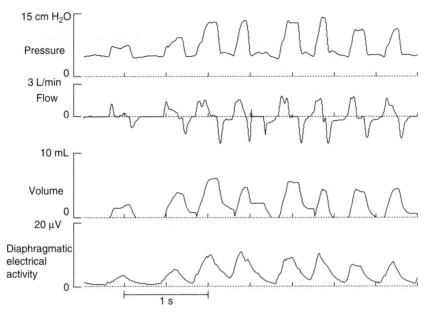

Fig. 19.4 Adjustments in ventilator pressure during neurally adjusted ventilatory assist. Tracings of pressure, flow, volume, and diaphragmatic electrical activity show changes in ventilator pressure in direct proportion to the magnitude of the diaphragmatic activity.

of inspiratory drive is unknown. Thus further research is needed to determine the interaction between NAVA and the extremely premature infant's immature respiratory control center. Use of noninvasive NAVA as a means of synchronizing noninvasive positive-pressure ventilation is gaining popularity because it is currently the only available method of synchronization of nasal ventilation available in the United States. Noninvasive NAVA is likely to be safer in immature infants, because excessive V_T is unlikely to be achieved with an open system.

Automated Adjustment of Supplemental Oxygen

Most premature infants with respiratory insufficiency require supplemental oxygen to maintain adequate oxygenation. However, the fraction of inspired oxygen (F_{IO_2}) can be excessive at times and induce hyperoxemia, which increases the risk for eye and lung injury and oxidative stress in other organs, including the central nervous system.[45–48] To avoid this problem, arterial oxygen saturation is continuously monitored by pulse oximetry (Spo_2) and F_{IO_2} is adjusted to keep Spo_2 within a prescribed range. However, multicenter data revealed that preterm infants receiving supplemental oxygen spent only 48% of the time with Spo_2 within the target range.[49–51] They spent 36% of the time with Spo_2 above (range 5%–90%) and 16% of the time below the target range (range 0%–47%). These data showed that maintenance of Spo_2 within the target range worsens over time and is slightly improved by tight Spo_2 alarms.[42] Maintenance of oxygenation within the intended range has been shown to be largely influenced by the nurse/patient ratio.[52]

Maintenance of Spo_2 within the target range becomes increasingly difficult over time due to frequent fluctuations in Spo_2. These fluctuations also increase the demand for staff effort, and frequently the adjustment in F_{IO_2} in response to episodes of hypoxemia is not optimal and infants are exposed to prolonged periods with Spo_2 above and below the target range.[53] In an attempt to attenuate the frequency of hypoxemia episodes, the clinical staff often tolerates Spo_2 levels above the target ranges, thus exposing infants to excessive oxygen, as illustrated in Fig. 19.5.

Systems for automatic adjustment of F_{IO_2} have been developed to improve the maintenance of Spo_2 within a target range and to reduce exposure to hyperoxemia and hypoxemia as well as supplemental oxygen in premature infants.[54–67] Fig. 19.6 shows representative automatic adjustments to F_{IO_2} in a preterm infant.

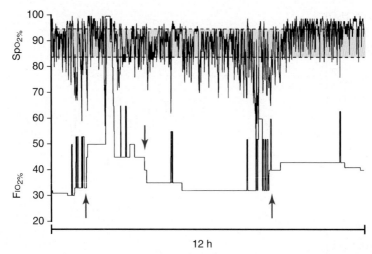

Fig. 19.5 Manual adjustments of F_{IO_2} during routine care. Recordings from a preterm infant with frequent fluctuations in Sp_{O_2} show typical adjustments in F_{IO_2} in response to episodes with Sp_{O_2} declining into hypoxemia *(below the bottom dotted line)* and changes in the baseline F_{IO_2} level *(red arrows)*. Increases in basal F_{IO_2} attenuated the severity of the hypoxemia spells but resulted in periods with Sp_{O_2} in hyperoxemia *(above the top dotted line)* and increased the exposure to higher F_{IO_2}. F_{IO_2}, Fraction of inspired oxygen; Sp_{O_2}, arterial oxygen saturation.

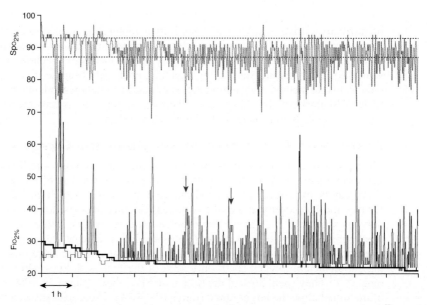

Fig. 19.6 Automatic adjustment of F_{IO_2} during a period of 12 hours in a premature infant. Recordings of Sp_{O_2} and F_{IO_2} show an initial reduction in the basal F_{IO_2} level *(thick line)* during the first 2 hours of automated control. Thereafter F_{IO_2} is automatically increased to keep Sp_{O_2} within the target range *(dotted lines)*. Only twice during the 12-hour period did the caregivers titrate F_{IO_2} by hand *(red arrows)*. F_{IO_2}, Fraction of inspired oxygen; Sp_{O_2}, arterial oxygen saturation.

Clinical studies showed that automatic F_{IO_2} control improved the maintenance of Sp_{O_2} within the target range compared with manual adjustments made by the infant's caregivers and maintained the range comparably or better than a fully dedicated research nurse (Table 19.1).[54–67] These studies documented consistent reductions in hyperoxemia with use of automatic control (Table 19.2). These findings confirm the tolerance of excessive Sp_{O_2} levels in premature infants during routine care. In these studies the exposure to supplemental oxygen was also reduced by automatic control.

Table 19.1 SpO_2 TARGETING DURING AUTOMATIC AND MANUAL FIO_2 CONTROL

Authors (Year)	SpO_2 Target Range (%)	Time Within Target Range (%)		Manual Changes in FIO_2/24 h		Manual Mode
		Auto	Manual	Auto	Manual	
Bhutani et al. (1992)	94–96	81	54	NA	48–72[a]	Routine
			69		288–720[a]	Dedicated
Morozoff and Evans (1992)	90–95	50	39	25[a]	194[a]	Routine
Sun et al. (1997)	Set value ± 3%	72	58	NA	NA	Routine
Claure et al. (2001)	88–96	75	66	0	696[a]	Dedicated
Urschitz et al. (2004)	87–96	91	82	7.2[a]	72[a]	Routine
			91		185[a]	Dedicated
Morozoff and Smyth (2009)	90–96	73	57	5[a]	89[a]	Routine
Claure et al. (2009)	88–95	58	42	42[a]	204[a]	Routine
Claure et al. (2011)	87–93[b]	47	39	10	112	Routine
Hallenberger et al. (2014)	All 4 centers:	72	61	52	77	Routine
	90–95	71	63			
	80–92	69	64			
	83–93	66	43			
	85–94	84	65			
Zapata et al. (2014)	85–93	58	34	0[a]	160[a]	Routine
Waitz et al. (2015)	88–96	76	69	NA	NA	Routine
Lal et al. (2015)	90–95	69	60	NA	NA	Routine
van Kaam et al. (2015)	89–93[b]	62	54	1	102	Routine
	91–95[b]	62	58	1	109	
Plottier et al. (2017)	91–95[b]	81	56	6[a]	55[a]	Routine

[a]Extrapolated to 24 h.
[b]Includes time with SpO_2 above target range while FIO_2 = 0.21.
FIO_2, Fraction of inspired oxygen; *NA*, not available; SpO_2, arterial oxygen saturation.

Table 19.2 TIME IN HYPEROXEMIA AND MEAN FIO_2 DURING AUTOMATIC AND MANUAL FIO_2 CONTROL

Authors (Year)	SpO_2 Range of Hyperoxemia	Time in Hyperoxemia (%)		Mean FIO_2		Manual Mode
		Auto	Manual	Auto	Manual	
Morozoff and Evans (1992)	>95%	23	39	NA	NA	Routine
Sun et al. (1997)	>98%	↓ or ~		NA	NA	Routine
Claure et al. (2001)	>96%	10	15	0.34	0.34	Dedicated
Urschitz et al. (2004)	>96%	1.3[a]	4.9[a]	NA	NA	Routine
			1.8[a]			Dedicated
Claure et al. (2009)	> 95%	9	31	0.29	0.34	Routine
	>97%	3	16			
Claure et al. (2011)	>93%[b]	21	37	0.32	0.37	Routine
	>98%[b]	0.7	5.6			
Hallenberger et al. (2014)	4 centers: >95% >92% >93% or >94%	16	16	NA	NA	Routine
Zapata et al. (2014)	>95%	27	55	0.37	0.44	Routine
Waitz et al. (2015)	>96%	6.6	10	0.32	0.30	Routine
Lal et al. (2015)	>95%	9.8	15	NA	NA	Routine
	>97%	0.3	4.8			
van Kaam et al. (2015)	TR 89%–93%:	21	25	0.31	0.30	Routine
	>93%[a]	0.2	0.7	0.35	0.33	
	>98%[b]	22	19			
	TR 91%–95%: >95%[b]	0.7	1.7			
	>98%[b]					
Plottier et al. (2017)	>95%[b]	5.1	25	0.27	0.27	Routine
	>98%[b]	0	0.5			

[a]Estimated.
[b]Excludes time with SpO_2 values while FIO_2 = 0.21.
FIO_2, Fraction of inspired oxygen; *NA*, not available; SpO_2, arterial oxygen saturation; *TR*, target range.

Table 19.3 TIME IN HYPOXEMIA AND FREQUENCY OF HYPOXEMIA EPISODES DURING AUTOMATIC AND MANUAL F_{IO_2} CONTROL

Authors (Year)	Spo₂ Range of Hypoxemia	Time in Hypoxemia (%) Auto	Time in Hypoxemia (%) Manual	Episodes of Hypoxemia (%, duration)	Episodes/24 h Auto	Episodes/24 h Manual	Manual Mode
Morozoff and Evans (1992)	<90%	27	22	NA			Routine
Claure et al. (2001)	<88%	17	19	<88%, >5 s	386	360[a]	Dedicated
	<75%	0	0.35	<85%, >5 s	257	257[a]	
				<75%, >5 s	31	31[a]	
Urschitz et al. (2004)	<87%	3.2[b]	6.7[b]	<87%, >5 s	223	305[a]	Routine
			3.9[b]			209[a]	Dedicated
Claure et al. (2009)	<88%	33	27	<88%, ≥10 s	552	360[a]	Routine
	<75%	4.6	6.6	<85%, >120 s	15	33[a]	
				<75%, >60 s	12	23[a]	
Claure et al. (2011)	<87%	32	23	<87%, ≥10 s	456	264	Routine
	<80%	9.8	9.5	<85%, >120 s	22	35	
	<75%	4.7	5.4	<75%, >60 s	3	10	
Hallenberger et al. (2014)	4 centers: <90% <80% <83% or <85%)	9	15	NA			Routine
Zapata et al. (2014)	<85%	14	11[b]	80%–85%	↑		Routine
				80%–85%, >30 s	↓		
				70%–75%	↓		
Waitz et al. (2015)	<88%	17	21	<88%, ≥10 s	552	360[a]	Routine
	<80%	3.1	4.3	<85%, >120 s	15	33[a]	
	<70%	0.7	1.0	<75%, >60 s	12	23[a]	
Lal et al. (2015)	<90%	21	25	NA			Routine
	<80%	4.5	4.4				
van Kaam et al. (2015)	TR 89%–93%: <89% <80% TR 91%–95%: <91% <80%	17 1.2 17 0.8	21 2.6 23 2.0	TR 89%–93%: <80%, >60 s TR 91%–95%: <80%, >60 s	4 4	15 13	Routine
Plottier et al. (2017)	<90%	14	19	<85%, >60 s	0	11[a]	Routine
	<80%	0	0.7	<80%, >60 s	0	3.1[a]	

[a]Extrapolated to 24 h.
[b]Estimated.
F_{IO_2}, Fraction of inspired oxygen; *NA*, not available; *Spo₂*, arterial oxygen saturation; *TR*, target range.

In some of these studies the reduction in hyperoxemia during automated F_{IO_2} control was accompanied by an increased frequency of brief fluctuations in Spo₂ below the target range compared with routine manual adjustment. As illustrated in Fig. 19.7, the prevalent maintenance of Spo₂ above the target range during routine care is in part aimed at preventing episodic hypoxemia. The extent to which these relatively mild episodes may raise the risks of adverse effects and offset the benefits of avoiding hyperoxemia is not known. On the other hand, automatic F_{IO_2} control consistently reduced the frequency of episodes of severe and/or prolonged hypoxemia (Table 19.3). These findings highlight the fact that automatic F_{IO_2} control cannot prevent the occurrence of hypoxemia episodes because these are largely triggered by changes in respiratory effort, airway obstruction, and agitation. However, a faster and more consistent automatic response can reduce the exposure to severe or prolonged hypoxemia.

An important goal of automatic F_{IO_2} control is reducing the concentration of oxygen in the inspired gas with the aim of reducing oxidative lung injury. In clinical studies F_{IO_2} has been consistently reduced by automatic control systems (see Table 19.2).

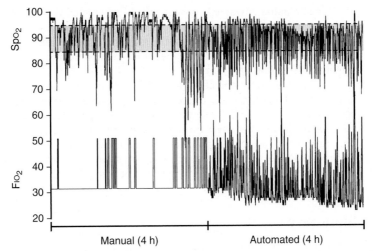

Fig. 19.7 Manual and automatic Fio$_2$ adjustments in an infant with frequent spontaneous episodes of hypoxemia. Recordings of Spo$_2$ and Fio$_2$ during routine care show frequent manual increases in Fio$_2$ in response to episodes of hypoxemia (Spo$_2$ declining *below the bottom dotted line*) while the basal Fio$_2$ was kept unchanged. The continuous high basal Fio$_2$ led to hyperoxemia (Spo$_2$ *above top dotted line*). During automated control, a gradual weaning of the basal Fio$_2$ avoided hyperoxemia, but it was accompanied by more frequent brief episodes of hypoxemia. *Fio$_2$,* Fraction of inspired oxygen; *Spo$_2$,* arterial oxygen saturation.

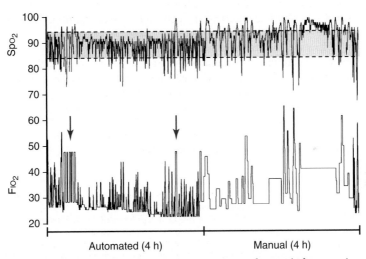

Fig. 19.8 Automated and manual Fio$_2$ adjustments in a preterm infant with frequent hypoxemia episodes. Recordings of Spo$_2$ and Fio$_2$ illustrate the workload involved in maintaining Spo$_2$ within a target range (indicated by the *dotted lines*) during routine care. In this example, few manual adjustments were needed during automated Fio$_2$ control *(red arrows),* which predominantly occurred during patient care procedures. *Fio$_2$,* Fraction of inspired oxygen; *Spo$_2$,* arterial oxygen saturation.

Automated Fio$_2$ control can also reduce workload. Clinical studies showed that Spo$_2$ targeting was improved even when there was a considerable effort on the part of the clinical staff or fully dedicated caregivers in manual Fio$_2$ titration (see Table 19.1). Fig. 19.6 illustrates the reduction in staff workload during automated control. The effort involved in manual Fio$_2$ titration can be very considerable when caring for infants with frequent episodes of hypoxemia. Studies have documented manual Fio$_2$ adjustments at intervals ranging from 7 to 120 minutes during routine care to every 2 minutes by a fully dedicated nurse. Fig. 19.8 illustrates how demanding the task is for the staff to maintain Spo$_2$ with manual FiO$_2$ adjustments. In infants with frequent episodes of hypoxemia, automatic control reduced the number of manual Fio$_2$ adjustments by 90%.

One potential unwanted consequence of automated F_{IO_2} control is that it could lead to a reduction in caregiver attentiveness. For this reason automatic systems should include monitoring features that alert the caregiver about changes in patient status—for example, a persistently higher F_{IO_2} to maintain Spo_2 within range or poor signal quality of the Spo_2 sensor.

A very important consideration in the use of automatic F_{IO_2} control systems in preterm infants is the selection of the target range of Spo_2. This is because the optimal range of Spo_2 for preterm infants has not been clearly defined. This is compounded by the fact that there is often considerable mismatch between the prescribed Spo_2 ranges and the actual Spo_2. Caution is recommended in selecting a target range for automatic F_{IO_2} control because some target ranges of Spo_2 may have significant physiologic effects that only become apparent when they are more effectively maintained by these systems.

Summary

Conventional modalities of ventilation that provide constant respiratory support require adjustment by a caregiver to adapt to the changing needs of the preterm infant. The automated modalities discussed in this chapter can potentially address these limitations. Studies evaluating these modalities show promising findings, but further evidence is needed in regards to the extent these modalities can impact the premature infant respiratory outcome.

Modalities of automated control are available for adult ventilation,[68,69] but implementation of these modalities is more challenging in newborns because of their small size, short respiratory time constants, use of uncuffed ETTs, and limited use of muscle relaxation and heavy sedation.

It is well established that maintenance of adequate oxygenation in the neonatal intensive care unit has limitations and that this may affect the outcome of the premature infant. Automatic F_{IO_2} control has been proposed as a tool to overcome these limitations. Short-term studies showed automatic F_{IO_2} control can achieve a better balance between maintaining Spo_2 targets and reducing exposure to the extreme ranges of Spo_2 and supplemental oxygen. Still, clinical trials are needed to determine the impact of extended use of this technology on ophthalmic, respiratory, and neurodevelopmental outcomes in preterm infants.

REFERENCES

1. Stoll BJ, Hansen NI, Bell EF, et al. Neonatal outcomes of extremely preterm infants from the NICHD Neonatal Research Network. *Pediatrics*. 2010;126:443–456.
2. Ehrenkranz RA, Walsh MC, Vohr BR, et al. Validation of the National Institutes of Health consensus definition of bronchopulmonary dysplasia. *Pediatrics*. 2005;116:1353–1360.
3. Walsh MC, Morris BH, Wrage LA, et al. National Institutes of Child Health and Human Development Neonatal Research Network. Extremely low birth weight neonates with protracted ventilation: mortality and 18-month neurodevelopmental outcomes. *J Pediatr*. 2005;146:798–804.
4. Lifschitz MH, Seilheimer DK, Wilson GS, et al. Neurodevelopmental status of low birth weight infants with bronchopulmonary dysplasia requiring prolonged oxygen supplementation. *J Perinatol*. 1987;7:127–132.
5. Schmidt B, Asztalos EV, Roberts RS, et al. Impact of bronchopulmonary dysplasia, brain injury, and severe retinopathy on the outcome of extremely low-birth-weight infants at 18 months: results from the trial of indomethacin prophylaxis in preterms. *JAMA*. 2003;289:1124–1129.
6. Abubakar KM, Keszler M. Patient-ventilator interactions in new modes of patient-triggered ventilation. *Pediatr Pulmonol*. 2001;32:71–75.
7. Herrera CM, Gerhardt T, Claure N, et al. Effects of volume-guaranteed synchronized intermittent mandatory ventilation in preterm infants recovering from respiratory failure. *Pediatrics*. 2002;110:529–533.
8. Keszler M, Abubakar K. Volume guarantee: stability of tidal volume and incidence of hypocarbia. *Pediatr Pulmonol*. 2004;38:240–245.
9. Cheema IU, Sinha AK, Kempley ST, Ahluwalia JS. Impact of volume guarantee ventilation on arterial carbon dioxide tension in newborn infants: A randomized controlled trial. *Early Hum Dev*. 2007;83:183–189.
10. Dawson C, Davies MW. Volume-targeted ventilation and arterial carbon dioxide in neonates. *J Paediatr Child Health*. 2005;41:518–521.
11. Cheema IU, Ahluwalia JS. Feasibility of tidal volume-guided ventilation in newborn infants: a randomized, crossover trial using the volume guarantee modality. *Pediatrics*. 2001;107:1323–1328.

12. Chowdhury O, Patel DS, Hannam S, et al. Randomised trial of volume-targeted ventilation versus pressure-limited ventilation in acute respiratory failure in prematurely born infants. *Neonatology.* 2013;104:290–294.

13. Patel DS, Rafferty GF, Lee S, Hannam S, Greenough A. Work of breathing and volume targeted ventilation in respiratory distress. *Arch Dis Child Fetal Neonatal Ed.* 2010;95:F443–F446.

14. Nassabeh-Montazami S, Abubakar K, Keszler M. The impact of instrumental dead-space in volume targeted ventilation of the extremely low birth weight infant. *Pediatr Pulmonol.* 2009;44:128–133.

15. Keszler M, Nassabeh-Montazami S, Abubakar K. Evolution of tidal volume requirement during the first three weeks of life in extremely low birth weight infants ventilated with volume-targeted ventilation. *Arch Dis Child Fetal Neonatal Ed.* 2009;94:F279–F282.

16. Sharma S, Abubakar KM, Keszler M. Tidal volume in infants with congenital diaphragmatic hernia supported with conventional mechanical ventilation. *Am J Perinatol.* 2015;32:577–582.

17. Sharma S, Clark S, Abubakar K, Keszler M. Tidal volume requirement in mechanically ventilated infants with meconium aspiration syndrome. *Am J Perinatol.* 2015;32:916–919.

18. Bolivar JM, Gerhardt T, Gonzalez A, et al. Mechanisms for episodes of hypoxemia in preterm infants undergoing mechanical ventilation. *J Pediatr.* 1995;127:767–773.

19. Dimaguila MA, DiFiore JA, Martin R, et al. Characteristics of hypoxemic episodes in very low birth weight infants on ventilatory support. *J Pediatr.* 1997;130:577–583.

20. Polimeni V, Claure N, D'Ugard C, et al. Effects of volume-targeted synchronized intermittent mandatory ventilation on spontaneous episodes of hypoxemia in preterm infants. *Biol Neonate.* 2006;89:50–55.

21. Jain D, Claure N, D'Ugard C, Bello J, Bancalari E. Volume guarantee ventilation: effect on preterm infants with frequent hypoxemia episodes. *Neonatology.* 2016;110:129–134.

22. Lista G, Colnaghi M, Castoldi F, et al. Impact of targeted-volume ventilation on lung inflammatory response in preterm infants with respiratory distress syndrome (RDS). *Pediatr Pulmonol.* 2004;37:510–514.

23. Lista G, Castoldi F, Fontana P, et al. Lung inflammation in preterm infants with respiratory distress syndrome: effects of ventilation with different tidal volumes. *Pediatr Pulmonol.* 2006;41(4):357–363.

24. Keszler M. Volume guarantee and ventilator-induced lung injury: Goldilocks' rules apply. *Commentary Pediatr Pulmonol.* 2006;41:364–366.

25. Piotrowski A, Sobala W, Kawczynski P. Patient-initiated, pressure-regulated, volume-controlled ventilation compared with intermittent mandatory ventilation in neonates: a prospective, randomised study. *Intensive Care Med.* 1997;23:975–981.

26. D'Angio CT, Chess PR, Kovacs SJ, et al. Pressure-regulated volume control ventilation vs synchronized intermittent mandatory ventilation for very low-birth-weight infants: a randomized controlled trial. *Arch Pediatr Adolesc Med.* 2005;159:868–875.

27. Sinha SK, Donn SM, Gavey J, et al. Randomised trial of volume controlled versus time cycled, pressure limited ventilation in preterm infants with respiratory distress syndrome. *Arch Dis Child Fetal Neonatal Ed.* 1997;77:F202–F205.

28. Singh J, Sinha SK, Donn SM, et al. Mechanical ventilation of very low birth weight infants: is volume or pressure a better target variable? *J Pediatr.* 2006;149:308–313.

29. Duman N, Tuzun F, Sutcuoglu S, Yesilirmak CD, Kumral A, Ozkan H. Impact of volume guarantee on synchronized ventilation in preterm infants: a randomized controlled trial. *Intensive Care Med.* 2012;38:1358–1364.

30. Wheeler KI, Klingenberg C, Morley CJ, Davis PG. Volume-targeted versus pressure-limited ventilation for preterm infants: a systematic review and meta-analysis. *Neonatology.* 2011;100:219–227.

31. Peng WS, Zhu HW, Shi H, et al. Volume-targeted ventilation is more suitable than pressure-limited ventilation for preterm infants: a systematic review and meta-analysis. *Arch Dis Child Fetal Neonatal Ed.* 2014;99:F158–F165.

32. Keszler M. Update on mechanical ventilatory strategies. *NeoReviews.* 2013;14:e237–e251. American Academy of Pediatrics online publication http://neoreviews.aappublications.org/content/14/5/e237.

33. Claure N, Gerhardt T, Hummler H, et al. Computer controlled minute ventilation in preterm infants undergoing mechanical ventilation. *J Pediatr.* 1997;131:910–913.

34. Claure N, Suguihara C, Peng J, et al. Targeted minute ventilation and tidal volume in an animal model of acute changes in lung mechanics and episodes of hypoxemia. *Neonatology.* 2009;95:132–140.

35. Guthrie SO, Lynn C, Lafleur BJ, et al. A crossover analysis of mandatory minute ventilation compared to synchronized intermittent mandatory ventilation in neonates. *J Perinatol.* 2005;25:643–646.

36. Herber-Jonat S, Rieger-Fackeldey E, Hummler H, Schulze A. Adaptive mechanical backup ventilation for preterm infants on respiratory assist modes—a pilot study. *Int Care Med.* 2006;32:302–308.

37. Musante G, Schulze A, Gerhardt T, et al. Proportional assist ventilation decreases thoracoabdominal asynchrony and chest wall distortion in preterm infants. *Pediatr Res.* 2001;49:175–180.

38. Schulze A, Rieger-Fackeldey E, Gerhardt T, et al. Randomized crossover comparison of proportional assist ventilation and patient triggered ventilation in extremely low birth weight infants with evolving chronic lung disease. *Neonatology.* 2007;92:1–7.

39. Schulze A, Gerhardt T, Musante G, et al. Proportional assist ventilation in low birth weight infants with acute respiratory disease: A comparison to assist/control and conventional mechanical ventilation. *J Pediatr.* 1999;135:339–344.

40. Beck J, Reilly M, Grasselli G, et al. Patient-ventilator interaction during neurally adjusted ventilatory assist in low birth weight infants. *Pediatr Res.* 2009;65:663–668.

41. Beck J, Reilly M, Grasselli G, et al. Patient-ventilator interaction during neurally adjusted ventilatory assist in low birth weight infants. *Pediatr Res.* 2009;65:663–668.

42. Stein H, Alosh H, Ethington P, White DB. Prospective crossover comparison between NAVA and pressure control ventilation in premature neonates less than 1500 grams. *J Perinatol.* 2013;33(6):452–456.

43. Lee J, Kim HS, Sohn JA, et al. Randomized crossover study of neurally adjusted ventilatory assist in preterm infants. *J Pediatr.* 2012;161(5):808–813.

44. Longhini F, Ferrero F, De Luca D, et al. Neurally adjusted ventilatory assist in preterm neonates with acute respiratory failure. *Neonatology.* 2014;107:60–67.

45. Flynn JT, Bancalari E, Snyder ES, et al. A cohort study of transcutaneous oxygen tension and the incidence and severity of retinopathy of prematurity. *N Engl J Med.* 1992;326:1050–1054.

46. Supplemental therapeutic oxygen for prethreshold retinopathy of prematurity (STOP-ROP), a randomized, controlled trial. I: primary outcomes. *Pediatrics.* 2000;105:295–310.

47. Askie LM, Henderson-Smart DJ, Irwig L, Simpson JM. Oxygen-saturation targets and outcomes in extremely preterm infants. *N Engl J Med.* 2003;349:959–967.

48. Collins MP, Lorenz JM, Jetton JR, Paneth N. Hypocapnia and other ventilation-related risk factors for cerebral palsy in low birth weight infants. *Pediatr Res.* 2001;50:712–719.

49. Hagadorn JI, Furey AM, Nghiem TH, et al. AVIOx Study Group. Achieved versus intended pulse oximeter saturation in infants born less than 28 weeks' gestation: the AVIOx study. *Pediatrics.* 2006;118:1574–1582.

50. Laptook AR, Salhab W, Allen J, et al. Pulse oximetry in very low birth weight infants: can oxygen saturation be maintained in the desired range? *J Perinatol.* 2006;26:337–341.

51. Lim K, Wheeler KI, Gale TJ, et al. Oxygen saturation targeting in preterm infants receiving continuous positive airway pressure. *J Pediatr.* 2014;164:730–736.

52. Sink DW, Hope SA, Hagadorn JI. Nurse:patient ratio and achievement of oxygen saturation goals in premature infants. *Arch Dis Child Fetal Neonatal Ed.* 2011;96:F93–F98.

53. van Zanten HA, Tan RN, Thio M, et al. The risk for hyperoxaemia after apnoea, bradycardia and hypoxaemia in preterm infants. *Arch Dis Child Fetal Neonatal Ed.* 2014;99:F269–F273.

54. Bhutani VK, Taube JC, Antunes MJ, Delivoria-Papadopoulos M. Adaptive control of the inspired oxygen delivery to the neonate. *Pediatr Pulmonol.* 1992;14:110–117.

55. Morozoff PE, Evans RW. Closed-loop control of SaO$_2$ in the neonate. *Biomed Instrum Technol.* 1992;26:117–123.

56. Sun Y, Kohane IS, Stark AR. Computer-assisted adjustment of inspired oxygen concentration improves control of oxygen saturation in newborn infants requiring mechanical ventilation. *J Pediatr.* 1997;131:754–756.

57. Claure N, Gerhardt T, Everett R, et al. Closed-loop controlled inspired oxygen concentration for mechanically ventilated very low birth weight infants with frequent episodes of hypoxemia. *Pediatrics.* 2001;107:1120–1124.

58. Urschitz MS, Horn W, Seyfang A, et al. Automatic control of the inspired oxygen fraction in preterm infants: a randomized crossover trial. *Am J Respir Crit Care Med.* 2004;170:1095–1100.

59. Claure N, D'Ugard C, Bancalari E. Automated adjustment of inspired oxygen in preterm infants with frequent fluctuations in oxygenation: a pilot clinical trial. *J Pediatr.* 2009;155:640–645.

60. Morozoff EP, Smyth JA. Evaluation of three automatic oxygen therapy control algorithms on ventilated low birth weight neonates. *Conf Proc IEEE Eng Med Biol Soc.* 2009;2009:3079–3082.

61. Claure N, Bancalari E, D'Ugard C, et al. Multicenter crossover study of automated adjustment of inspired oxygen in mechanically ventilated preterm infants. *Pediatrics.* 2011;127:e76–e83.

62. Hallenberger A, Poets CF, Horn W, Seyfang A, Urschitz MS, CLAC Study Group. Closed-loop automatic oxygen control (CLAC) in preterm infants: a randomized controlled trial. *Pediatrics.* 2014;133:e379–e385.

63. Zapata J, Gómez JJ, Araque Campo R, Matiz Rubio A, Sola A. A randomised controlled trial of an automated oxygen delivery algorithm for preterm neonates receiving supplemental oxygen without mechanical ventilation. *Acta Paediatr.* 2014;103(9):928–933.

64. Waitz M, Schmid MB, Fuchs H, Mendler MR, Dreyhaupt J, Hummler HD. Effects of automated adjustment of the inspired oxygen on fluctuations of arterial and regional cerebral tissue oxygenation in preterm infants with frequent desaturations. *J Pediatr.* 2015;166:240–244.

65. Lal M, Tin W, Sinha S. Automated control of inspired oxygen in ventilated preterm infants: crossover physiological study. *Acta Paediatr.* 2015;104:1084–1089.

66. van Kaam AH, Hummler HD, Wilinska M, et al. Automated versus manual oxygen control with different saturation targets and modes of respiratory support in preterm infants. *J Pediatr.* 2015;167:545–550.e1–e2.

67. Plottier GK, Wheeler KI, Ali SK, et al. Clinical evaluation of a novel adaptive algorithm for automated control of oxygen therapy in preterm infants on non-invasive respiratory support. *Arch Dis Child Fetal Neonatal Ed.* 2017;102:F37–F43.

68. Petter AH, Chiolero RL, Cassina T, et al. Automatic "respirator weaning" with adaptive support ventilation: the effect on duration of endotracheal intubation and patient management. *Anesth Analg.* 2003;97:1743–1750.

69. Lellouche F, Mancebo J, Jolliet P, et al. A multicenter randomized trial of computer-driven protocolized weaning from mechanical ventilation. *Am J Respir Crit Care Med.* 2006;174:894–900.

B

CHAPTER 20

Prenatal and Postnatal Steroids and Pulmonary Outcomes

Alan H. Jobe

- Antenatal steroids (ANS) are one of the oldest and most effective therapies in perinatal medicine.
- The randomized controlled trials (RCTs) are dated and do not necessarily apply for current clinical populations.
- There are minimal RCT data to support ANS use for deliveries before 28 weeks' gestational age.
- The risk/benefit ratio for gestation after 34 weeks is unclear.
- The dose and drug choice for ANS may not be optimal.
- Postnatal steroids (PNS) can effectively decrease bronchopulmonary dysplasia (BPD), but there are risks.
- The trend is to use lower doses and shorter periods of treatment.
- Four new trials of PNS begun shortly after birth are proof of principle that PNS decrease BPD.
- PNS should only be used for infants at high risk of severe BPD.

This chapter reviews knowledge gaps and new information about the two primary uses of corticosteroids in the perinatal period: antenatal (maternal) treatments (ANS) to decrease respiratory distress syndrome (RDS) and infant mortality, and postdelivery corticosteroid treatments (PNS) to prevent or treat bronchopulmonary dysplasia (BPD). Clinical and experimental information for both treatments is not optimal for current clinical practice as a result of the histories for the development and testing of corticosteroids for both antenatal and postnatal indications. Both therapies were used by clinicians in the early period of modern perinatal medicine without formal drug development and licensure. Thus optimal drug selection, dose, and patient selection remain poorly defined today. Much of the clinical information is quite old, and patient populations and clinical management have changed strikingly. Further, the therapies were evaluated and adopted before the era of modern molecular techniques were available, leaving large gaps in knowledge about the mechanisms of action and the potential risks of treatment. Corticosteroids are potent drugs with pleotropic effects on multiple organ systems that play essential roles in basal physiology, stress responses, and when used in higher doses, therapeutic effects. The major focus of the chapter is on the fetal and newborn lung, but cardiovascular and mortality outcomes cannot be separated from lung responses.

Antenatal Corticosteroids

Historical Overview

While evaluating the role of fetal exposures to corticosteroids on labor in sheep, Liggins reported in 1969 that fetal dexamethasone infusions caused preterm delivery of lambs that had unanticipatedly good lung aeration.[1] That result was consistent with other early reports that corticosteroids could mature developing organ systems in other animal models. His observation in sheep was quickly evaluated in a clinical trial reported in 1972 that randomly assigned 282 women to a maternal intramuscular treatment with the drug betamethasone (Celestone) that was used to suppress inflammation.[2] Celestone Soluspan is a mixture of two prodrug forms of the fluorinated corticosteroid betamethasone–betamethasone phosphate and a micronized suspension of betamethasone acetate. When injected intramuscularly, the betamethasone phosphate is rapidly dephosphorylated while the betamethasone acetate is slowly deacylated over many hours. Both compounds yield free betamethasone, which crosses the placenta to achieve a prolonged fetal exposure when given as a two-dose treatment of 12 mg at a 24-hour interval. This level of detail is important to understand today's approach for ANS dosing (see the following text).

The Liggins and Howie trial demonstrated decreased RDS and mortality in infants of an average gestational age of 35 weeks at delivery.[2] More than 20 trials were completed by 1993 that in aggregate demonstrated comparable effects without clear risks. However, ANS were not widely used in the United States until recommended by a National Institutes of Health Consensus Conference in 1994.[3] The majority of trials tested Celestone against placebo, but dexamethasone phosphate, a similar drug given as 4 doses of 6 mg every 12 hours, was used in some trials as summarized by the definitive meta-analysis of Roberts et al. in 2006 that was updated in 2017.[4] The primary outcomes of most of the trials were decreased RDS and mortality, although ANS also had benefits for decreased intraventricular hemorrhage and necrotizing enterocolitis. ANS became the standard of care for all women at risk of preterm delivery and ANS were recognized as a major advancement in perinatal medicine. There was minimal information developed for drug selection or dose in animal models or humans, and ANS remain unapproved by the U.S. Food and Drug Administration.

Mechanism of Action of ANS on Fetal Lungs

Multiple experimental studies with animals, human fetal lung explants, and isolated lung cells followed the initial Liggins observation in fetal sheep. Exposure to steroids induced the enzymes that contribute to surfactant synthesis and increased surfactant lipid and protein components in tissue and air spaces that became the explanation for the effects of ANS on fetal lungs.[5] However, in large animal models such as sheep and primates, improved lung function as assessed by increased gas volumes and improved lung mechanics occur within 15 to 24 hours, whereas surfactant amounts do not increase for 3 to 5 days.[6] ANS decrease lung mesenchyme tissue volume, and the barrier function of the air space epithelium improves rapidly after ANS in animal models, which contributed to improved lung function soon after ANS treatment.[7] At the molecular level, ANS upregulate and downregulate the expression of multiple genes, with the net effects of improved lung function after preterm delivery.[8] These multiple effects certainly cause improved lung function, but the ANS response is not simply an acceleration of normal lung development. Animal fetuses exposed to ANS have a transient decrease in saccular/alveolar septation and microvascular arborization that is similar to the phenotype of delayed lung development associated with BPD.[9] Alveolarization and microvascular development "catches up" in fetal sheep if they remain undelivered.[10] There is no information about how ANS-induced arrests in lung development associated with improved lung function might alter subsequent lung development after preterm delivery. Empirically very preterm infants exposed to ANS who do not have BPD seem to fare well, although their lung function is not equivalent to the lung function of term infants.[11] Further work using newer research techniques is needed to learn the effect of ANS on the fetal lung.

Dated Randomized Controlled Trials and Current Patient Populations

When ANS were initially used, RDS was a lethal disease for most infants and very preterm infants with or without RDS had very high mortality. The single ANS treatment trials versus placebo reported more than 25 years ago have RDS outcomes for just

Table 20.1 RCT DATA FOR ANTENATAL STEROIDS IN INFANTS BORN BEFORE 28 WEEKS

Result	Trials	Treated Patients	Controls	Relative Risk (95% CI)
Respiratory distress syndrome	4	48	54	0.79 (0.53–1.18)
Death	2	45	44	0.79 (0.56–1.12)
Intraventricular hemorrhage	1	34	28	3.4 (0.14–0.86)

CI, Confidence interval; *RCT,* randomized controlled trial.

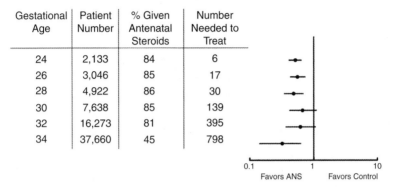

Gestational Age	Patient Number	% Given Antenatal Steroids	Number Needed to Treat
24	2,133	84	6
26	3,046	85	17
28	4,922	86	30
30	7,638	85	139
32	16,273	81	395
34	37,660	45	798

Fig. 20.1 Epidemiology of a large clinical experience for the effect of ANS on infant mortality (2009–2013). Across gestations from 24 to 34 weeks, ANS was associated with a similar decrease in infant death, but the number needed to treat increased greatly as gestational age increased. (Data from Travers CP, Clark RH, Spitzer AR, et al. Exposure to any antenatal corticosteroids and outcomes in preterm infants by gestational age: prospective cohort study. *BMJ.* 2017;356:j1039.)

102 randomized patients that delivered before 28 weeks' gestational age (Table 20.1). In contrast, today RDS at more than 28 weeks' gestation is generally easily managed with surfactant and current techniques for respiratory support. The recommendation at a 1994 Consensus Conference was to administer ANS for women at risk of preterm delivery between 24 and 34 weeks' gestational age, even though there were minimal data to support that recommendation.[3] We lack the randomized controlled trial (RCT) evidence that use of ANS benefits the pulmonary outcomes of the population of infants most targeted to receive ANS today.

Non-RCT information Regarding ANS and Outcomes

Other information is available to support ANS use at early gestational ages. Very immature animal models and in vitro explants of human fetal lungs have maturational responses to steroids, indicating that receptors and response pathways are present from early gestational ages.[12] Very large databases from neonatal networks are being extensively mined for outcomes of very low-birth-weight (VLBW) infants who were and were not exposed to ANS.[13,14] These analyses focus on mortality and outcomes such as intraventricular hemorrhage but not respiratory outcomes soon after birth, presumably because most infants at less than 28 weeks' gestation age receive some respiratory support and are imprecisely coded as having RDS.[15] A weakness of the studies is a lack of information about the severity of the early respiratory distress and any accurate categorization as to whether early deaths are caused by RDS.

Travers et al.[14] reported that ANS decreased mortality for all gestational ages from 24 to 34 weeks. The data are for the period from 2009 to 2013 for 61,571 infants, with about 84% of infants exposed to ANS, except at 34 weeks when the percent of exposure was 45% (Fig. 20.1). ANS exposure resulted in a remarkably consistent decreased mortality even at 34 weeks' gestation. A similar report from Carlo et al.[13] documented decreased mortality and intraventricular hemorrhage for more than 10,000 infants for the gestational age range from 22 to 25 weeks with 74% of the population exposed to ANS. No respiratory outcomes are reported other than

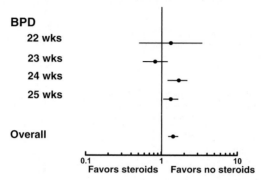

Antenatal Corticosteroid Effects on BPD
By Gestational Age
(1993–2009; 10,541 infants)

Fig. 20.2   Association of antenatal steroid use and the bronchopulmonary dysplasia (BPD) outcome. Across very early gestational ages, there was no decrease in BPD, and the overall effect was an increase in BPD. Data for 10,541 infants cared for in the Eunice Kennedy Shriver National Institute of Child Health and Human Development Neonatal Research Network from 1993 to 2009. (Data from Carlo WA, McDonald SA, Fanaroff AA, et al. Association of antenatal corticosteroids with mortality and neurodevelopmental outcomes among infants born at 22 to 25 weeks' gestation. JAMA. 2011;306:2348–2358.)

BPD, which is increased by use of ANS (Fig. 20.2). The association of increased BPD with ANS is quite uniform across the RCTs and epidemiology studies. The generally accepted explanation is that ANS improves survival in the most marginal infants who are at increased risk of developing BPD. However, the arrest of septation and microvascular development with ANS may contribute to this adverse lung outcome. The severity of BPD relative to ANS has not been analyzed and is worthy of evaluation.

The optimal interval from ANS treatment to delivery for maximal benefit based on the RCTs is 1 to 7 days.[4] A new analysis of a large European data set not randomized to ANS indicates that maximal benefit for decreasing death may be an exposure interval as short as 18 to 36 hours, with benefit after 3 hours.[16] Such rapid effects would be more consistent with acute steroid effects on cardiovascular function rather than for lung maturation.

A concern with the associations between ANS and the clinical outcomes is that the great majority of women are treated with ANS. The women not given ANS differ in ways that cannot be reliably adjusted for in the analyses. The women not exposed to ANS have different causes and severities of problems related to prematurity.[13] Many likely deliver before ANS can be given. The epidemiologic analyses may overestimate the benefits of ANS at early gestational ages. Another concern is treatment creep. The RCT data to support early gestational treatment with ANS are minimal, and RCTs for the use of ANS at "previable" gestational ages are nonexistent. Again, the epidemiology supports improved outcomes at gestations of 22 and 23 weeks, but that information likely reflects highly selected use of ANS in pregnancies being actively managed to achieve infant survival.[17]

Repeated ANS Treatments

The pregnancies of many women considered likely to deliver 1 to 7 days after ANS may continue for weeks or until term. A recent report noted that more than 50% of women given ANS did not deliver within 7 days.[18] The fact that the majority of women do not deliver in an optimal window for efficacy and many deliver at term is of substantial concern if this "off- target" treatment has adverse effects on the mother or infant. Multiple trials have evaluated Celestone for repeated ANS given at weekly intervals, at 2-week intervals, or when preterm delivery appeared to be imminent more than 7 days after the initial treatment. The benefits of steroids seem to be optimal at 1 to 7 days after ANS because some of the maturational effects seem to fade after 7 days, and repeated weekly treatments in animal models augment lung benefits.[19] The concerns with repeated treatments are cumulative injury to the fetal lung and neurodevelopment. A meta-analysis of 10 trials that randomized 4733 pregnancies demonstrated modest improvements in respiratory outcomes with no concerns for neurodevelopment.[20] However, several trials reported effects of repeated courses of ANS on birth weight and length, and one trial was stopped early for perceived adverse fetal growth effects.[21,22] There are fewer concerns about a single repeated dose of ANS, but the use of multiple weekly treatments likely is excessive. Further, a single dose of Celestone may be adequate for retreatment rather than the two-dose treatment.

ANS After 34 Weeks' Gestational Age

Although severe RDS is infrequent after 34 weeks' gestation and the treatment of RDS is generally successful, the odd ratios for RDS and transient tachypnea increase from normalized values of 1 at 38 to 40 weeks to 40 for RDS and 16 for transient tachypnea of the newborn at 34 weeks.[23] These late-gestation infants represent about 6% of the total delivery population and thus consume substantial resources. The definitive trial of ANS for women at risk of preterm delivery at 34^0 to 36^6 weeks' gestation randomly assigned 2831 women to the standard 2-dose Celestone treatment or placebo.[24] There was a modest benefit for the composite primary outcome of need for respiratory support, stillbirth, or death, which decreased from 14.4% to 11.6% ($P = .023$), with the difference being for respiratory problems. Fewer infants exposed to ANS than controls had severe respiratory morbidity or received surfactant treatment. However, 24% of ANS-exposed infants had transient hypoglycemia in contrast to 15% of controls. The Society for Maternal-Fetal Medicine statement recommends ANS selectively for late preterm birth,[25] but others have recommended caution because of the lack of follow-up and the relatively modest benefits.[26]

Another "late-gestation" use of ANS is before elective cesarean section at early term or term. Stutchfield et al.[27] randomly assigned 998 women to receive 2 doses of 12-mg betamethasone and found a decrease of about 50% for admittance of infants to a neonatal intensive care unit (NICU) and respiratory problems with the ANS. The benefit was for infants delivered before 39 weeks. A second trial randomly assigned 1280 women to receive 3 doses of 8-mg dexamethasone before elective cesarean section.[28] Administration of ANS was associated with a decrease in total NICU admissions from 3.9% to 1.6% ($P = .014$) and fewer NICU admissions for respiratory morbidity (number needed to treat = 43). From one perspective, the pathologic conditions prevented by ANS for elective cesarean sections are modest, but with cesarean deliveries exceeding 50% of all deliveries in some countries, the potential benefits are considerable. However, the therapy must be safe for used in the majority of women and fetuses, a high bar to confidently achieve.

Concerns Regarding Drug and Dose Choices for ANS

Liggins chose the 50/50 mixture of betamethasone phosphate plus betamethasone acetate for maternal intramuscular treatments to match the prolonged exposures with fetal infusions in sheep.[1,2] This dose and treatment interval were not validated by standard pharmacology. The other ANS treatment recommended by the World Health Organization (WHO) is 4 doses of 6-mg dexamethasone phosphate. There have been fewer clinical evaluations of this less expensive and widely available drug for ANS. Notably, there are no trials for repeated courses of treatment using dexamethasone.[20] Worldwide, different drug and dosing schedules are used without validation—for example, the United Kingdom uses betamethasone phosphate, an untested drug. Based on measurements of others indicating that drug doses are too high and our experience with betamethasone acetate, the slow-release component of Celestone,[29,30] it is likely that the perinatal community is using the wrong drugs at higher doses than necessary to achieve the pulmonary benefits of ANS. In fetal sheep models, 25% of the total betamethasone exposure given as one dose of betamethasone acetate is equivalent to the current clinical dose, and lower doses may be equally effective as a lung maturational agent.[29] Further, dexamethasone phosphate or betamethasone phosphate given as two doses is less effective for lung maturation in sheep models.[31] Concerns about risks of ANS should be minimized if lower dosing strategies can be developed.

Long-Term Outcomes After ANS

The 30-year outcomes of the original Liggins and Howie trial were reassuring,[32] but those infants were more mature than current populations. One concern is that the follow-up from the early trials focused on the infants who were delivered before term, with no follow-up of those who received off-target treatments and were delivered close to or at term. Braun et al.[33] observed that newborns delivered after 34 weeks after receiving ANS treatment weighed less than unexposed newborns. There are many other cohort or convenience comparisons of variables (e.g., responses to stress and aortic stiffness) that suggest adverse effects of ANS in later life.[34] Although these outcomes are consistent with results from animal models, a substantial concern is that the human populations have not been randomly assigned to ANS treatment. Because the great majority of women eligible for ANS are treated, a comparison population of unexposed children may not be representative. All observations are further confounded by prematurity. Global neurodevelopmental outcomes are reassuring even for infants exposed to repeated courses of ANS.[20]

Antenal Steroid Use in Low-Resource Environments

Most of the premature infants born worldwide are born in low-resource environments and have a very high mortality rate. The use of ANS is very spotty despite their use as a priority of the WHO and other groups attempting to improve maternal and infant outcomes. The recently completed Antenatal Corticosteroid Trial illustrated the difficulties and risks of using ANS in low-resource environments.[35] This trial randomly assigned almost 100,000 women in Pakistan, Africa, India, and Guatemala to the WHO-recommended ANS treatment of four doses of betamethasone after identification of risk of preterm delivery. Major problems were a lack of gestational age determination and identification of women at risk. Use of ANS did not improve outcomes for the smallest infants who had a perinatal mortality risk of more than 350 per 1000 births. More problematic was the increased mortality of off-target ANS-exposed infants who were large and mature, perhaps because of increased infection.[36] This experience is a caution that all exposed infants need to be followed for outcomes, not just those delivered prematurely. A safe treatment in one environment may be neither safe nor effective in a different environment.

Postnatal Steroids

Historical Review

There were brief reports of the use of systemic PNS before the first randomized trial by Avery et al. in 1985.[37] Only 8 pairs of infants were randomly assigned to a 42-day course of systemic dexamethasone with an initial dose of 0.5 mg/kg. The steroid-treated infants improved and ceased mechanical ventilation by 72 hours. This high-dose, long-tapering course was validated in a larger trial as superior to an 18-day course of dexamethasone in 1989 by Cummings et al.[38] The team of Doyle, Ehrenkranz, and Halliday have reported meta-analyses of PNS beginning in 2000, with updates continuing to the present.[39,40] These frequently updated reviews were critical to our understanding of a role for PNS in the care of very preterm infants at risk of developing BPD. Because of the frequent use of PNS and concerns about neuroinjury from PNS, the American Academy of Pediatrics and the Canadian Paediatric Association stated the following in 2002: "The routine use of systemic dexamethasone for the prevention or treatment of chronic lung disease in infants with very low birth weight is not recommended."[41] Although epidemiologic studies demonstrated a decrease in steroid use for infants born between 22 and 28 weeks' gestation from a high of 40% in 1996, steroids continue to be used in 10% to 15% of VLBW infants

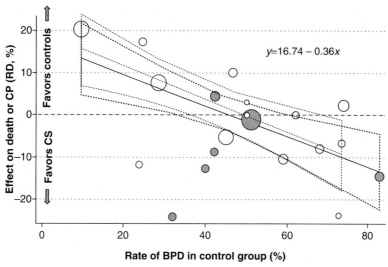

Fig. 20.3   Meta-regression analysis of 20 trials correlating the rate of bronchopulmonary dysplasia *(BPD)* in the control group with the effect of postnatal steroids on death or cerebral palsy *(CP)* expressed as the risk difference *(RD)* between control and steroid-treated infants. Each trial is represented by a *circle* and the size of the circle is proportional to the size of the trial. The higher the rate of BPD in the control group, the greater the likelihood of more benefit to be gained by prenatal steroids. Therefore at more than 50% BPD in the control population, the benefit of prenatal steroids exceeds the risk. (Figure from Doyle LW, Halliday HL, Ehrenkranz RA, et al. An update on the impact of postnatal systemic corticosteroids on mortality and cerebral palsy in preterm infants: effect modification by risk of bronchopulmonary dysplasia. *J Pediatr.* 2014;165:1258–1260.)

with respiratory failure.[42] A major contribution to the field was the meta-regression analysis in 2005 that was updated in 2014, demonstrating how the risk of BPD in a population modulated the risks of death and cerebral palsy (Fig. 20.3).[43] If the risks of adverse outcomes may be substantial, why do clinicians continue to use PNS? Shinwell et al.[44] demonstrated that in Israel as the use of PNS decreased, the incidence of BPD increased. The clear answer is that in trials and empirically PNS facilitates extubation of infants from ventilators. Ventilation of infants also is associated with poor outcomes. However, substantial numbers of infants receive PNS even though they are not receiving significant respiratory support.[45]

Pathophysiology of BPD: What Are We Treating With PNS?

Although an extensive discussion of BPD is beyond the scope of this chapter, BPD is recognized as the end result of lung injury and repair in VLBW infants.[46] Multiple antenatal variables contribute to postnatal injury mechanisms, such as oxygen exposure, mechanical stretch, and infection, to initiate and maintain chronic lung inflammation over weeks to months.[5] This injury/inflammation must be counteracted by repair mechanisms that support lung development for the infant to survive. PNS are potent synthetic steroids that are given systemically or as aerosols in pharmacologic doses primarily to decrease lung inflammation. However, steroids in developing animal models also interfere with air space septation and microvascular development.[9] Conceptually, PNS have been given from soon after birth to "prevent" BPD, after 7 days of age to "treat" and decrease the incidence of BPD, or more chronically after 36 weeks' gestational age for infants with BPD. The effects of PNS are certainly infant-age-at-treatment–specific and are much more complex than simply suppression of inflammation.

Meta-Analyses of Early and Late Treatments

Early treatments, defined by Doyle et al. as treatment at less than 8 days of age, have focused primarily on death and BPD as outcomes.[40] Although the use of PNS did not decrease death in 28 trials, their use did decrease BPD (relative risk [RR] 0.79, 95% confidence interval [CI] 0.71–0.88), but the complications of treatment were substantial and included hyperglycemia, hypertension, gastrointestinal perforation, and cerebral palsy. The simultaneous use of indomethacin and dexamethasone was associated with an increased risk of gastrointestinal perforation in several trials.[47] The consensus has been that early PNS are of minimal benefit and their use causes substantial adverse outcomes. However, new trials described in the following text may change that assessment.

PNS given after 7 days of age did not increase death in 19 trials, and benefits were earlier extubation (RR 0.64, 95% CI 0.56–0.74) and decreased BPD (RR 0.78, 95% CI 0.66–0.88).[39] Although hyperglycemia and hypertension were complications, gastrointestinal perforation and necrotizing enterocolitis were not. The neurodevelopmental outcomes were comparable between PNS-exposed and control infants except for abnormal neurologic examination results in four trials, which may not predict longer-term outcomes. The conclusion of the meta-analysis for late PNS is that the benefits exceed the risks for infants who cannot be weaned from the ventilator before 36 weeks. There is no systematic information about PNS use for infants who require very prolonged ventilation.

Drug, Dose, Route, and Duration of Therapy

Although the trials of PNS are numerous, resulting in meta-analyses that appear to be robust, the trials are quite heterogeneous with varied drug choice, dose, and duration of treatment. Most trials have used dexamethasone phosphate for intervals ranging from 10 to 42 days. Most of the neurodevelopmental outcome data are for infants treated with the high-dose, 42-day treatment beginning at 0.5 mg/kg per day. Many of the adverse outcomes—particularly hyperglycemia and hypertension—likely result from high-dose, long treatments. The adverse neurodevelopmental outcomes may also result from the high dose. A major problem for interpreting trial results is that control infants often were given open-label PNS. Thus for all outcomes, variable numbers of placebo-treated infants received PNS with poorly documented treatments. As with ANS, formal pharmacologic or pharmacodynamic studies have not been done for PNS.

The recent trend based on small trials has been to decrease the dose and duration of treatment.[48] The most influential lower-dose trial is the Dexamethasone: A Randomized Trial (DART) study, which randomly assigned infants to an initial dose of 0.15 mg/kg dexamethasone or placebo.[49] The steroid treatment then was decreased over a 10-day treatment. This international RCT was stopped early because of an inability to enroll patients after the therapy was not recommended by the American Academy of Pediatrics and the Canadian Paediatric Association—a most unfortunate outcome. The trial was planned for 814 patients and ended with just 35 patients in the treatment arm and 35 patients in the control arm. Nevertheless, the dexamethasone-treated infants had striking decreases in oxygen need and fewer PNS-treated infants experienced failed extubation. It is more than ironic that this failed trial has established the default standard of care for PNS use. Hyperglycemia and hypertension were not complications of this low-dose, short-duration PNS protocol. Even lower doses of dexamethasone for PNS may be equally effective but remain to be tested.

Hydrocortisone has been used more frequently in Europe for PNS than dexamethasone. There is less RCT information about hydrocortisone to treat BPD, and large trials are in progress. A new trial of early hydrocortisone is discussed in the following text.[50]

Aerosolized PNS are frequently used for infants with severe BPD using different steroids and delivery devices with a wide variance in use between neonatal services.[51] A meta-analysis evaluated 8 trials of inhaled PNS that included 232 infants. The aerosols were begun at more than 7 days of life and did not decrease death or BPD.[52] Of note, there also was no decrease in intubation failure or oxygen use, which are the short-term benefits of systemic PNS extubation. The aerosolized steroids may have decreased the use of systemic steroids.

How PNS Are Used

Based on my understanding of risks and benefits and the primary mechanism of action of PNS as potent antiinflammatory drugs, I suggest an initial course of

Table 20.2 SUMMARY OF RECENT EARLY STEROID TRIALS

Exposures and Outcomes	Fluticasone Inhaler (49)	Budesonide Aerosol (46)	Intravenous Hydrocortisone (46)	Budesonide + Surfactant (52)
Steroid exposure	Targeted to lung	Targeted to lung	Very low dose, but systemic	Targeted to lung
Duration of treatment	Until extubation	Off support or 32 weeks	10 days	With surfactant treatments
Death	Increased 2.5%	Increased 3.3%	Decreased 5%	Decreased 3%
Bronchopulmonary dysplasia	Decreased 10.8%	Decreased 10.2%	Decreased 4%	Decreased 21%

The numbers in parentheses are to reference.

20

PNS only for infants "stuck" on a ventilator and without overt infection. A target time to treatment is 2 to 3 weeks of age with a simple goal: cease ventilation and begin continuous positive airway pressure. I use the DART protocol of 0.15 mg/kg dexamethasone with the dose decreased and stopped by 10 days.[49] However, if the infant has not made progress toward extubation by 3 days, PNS is stopped. Once PNS has been started, then the obligation of the clinical team is to push for an optimized extubation trial. If the PNS fails to improve the infant's condition or the extubation attempt fails, then routine care continues for several more weeks until the infant's condition improves or the team, in desperation, starts another course of PNS. I do not use aerosolized steroids. An important perspective is that most of these chronically ventilated infants at 2 to 3 weeks of age will eventually stop ventilator use. They have more potential to heal their lungs than commonly appreciated.

Four New Trials of Early PNS

Surprisingly, although the meta-analysis results and the general consensus are that early use of PNS has a decidedly adverse risk/benefit ratio, innovative trials have recently been published that challenge not using PNS soon after birth to prevent BPD. Two trials used aerosolized steroids. Nakamura et al.[53] randomly assigned 211 infants at a mean gestational age of 26.1 weeks to a fluticasone metered inhaler given twice a day beginning on day 1 after birth and continued to extubation. There were no differences in death or death and oxygen use at discharge overall, but the combined outcome favored PNS for 24- to 26-week gestational age infants and infants exposed to chorioamnionitis (Table 20.2).

A second trial evaluated budesonide delivered by metered-dose inhaler.[54] The treatment was 2 doses/day from day 1 to 14 and 1 dose per day until 32 weeks or off oxygen and pressure support. This much larger trial randomly assigned 856 patients of 26 weeks mean gestational age. A nonsignificant 3.3% increase in deaths favored the placebo. The benefit was a significant 10.2% decrease in BPD with the steroid treatment. The authors were cautious about the benefits given the potential risk of increased death.

The use of hydrocortisone infusions at 1 mg/kg from day 1 for 7 days followed by 0.5 mg/kg to day 10 was evaluated by Baud et al.[50] in 521 randomly assigned infants of 26.4 weeks average gestational age. The benefits were earlier extubation and more survival without BPD; these benefits were larger for girls and for infants exposed to chorioamnionitis.

The most remarkable results were reported by Yeh et al.[55] for a strategy of mixing 0.25 mg/kg of micronized budesonide with surfactant for treatment of infants with RDS versus surfactant alone. They randomly assigned 265 infants of average gestational age of 26.7 weeks for the surfactant treatments at about 2 hours of age. Infants receiving surfactant plus budesonide had no difference in death but a remarkable decrease in BPD from 50% to 29%. Severe BPD also decreased significantly. One strength of this report is follow-up at 2 to 3 years in a subset of the infants that showed no adverse effects of the PNS on neurodevelopment.

For me these four trials are proof of principle that early PNS can decrease BPD. In the trials by Nakamura et al. and Bassler et al., the fetal exposure to chorioamnionitis resulted in larger and significant decreases in BPD.[53,54] I interpret this outcome as indicating that early PNS can effectively target the fetal lung inflammation associated with chorioamnionitis. Table 20.2 highlights some of the results from the trials. The aerosol and surfactant plus budesonide treatment strategies target the lungs and thus should have fewer complications. The 10-day hydrocortisone systemic therapy has the advantage of shorter exposures to PNS relative to the aerosols. The surfactant plus budesonide trial was the trial most targeted to the lung, had the shortest exposure, and resulted in the greatest decrease in BPD without increased mortality. The doses for the trials have not been evaluated for optimal effects, admittedly a difficult task in clinical neonatology. These trials challenge the notion that early PNS use is undesirable.

Summary and Future Directions

Corticosteroids are intimately entwined in the care of women at risk of preterm delivery and their preterm infants. Endogenous steroids are essential for fetal and newborn survival. ANS decrease infant death and multiple complications of prematurity, although the standard treatments are likely using the wrong dosing strategies. Caution is warranted for the use of ANS in low-resource environments unless gestation is known and at least basic care is available for the mother and infant. PNS are used because they work, and lower dosing strategies need to be evaluated. An often-overlooked reality is that the majority of very preterm infants are exposed as fetuses to ANS. Other "steroid use opportunities" beyond treatments to prevent or treat BPD with PNS are hydrocortisone to support blood pressure and dexamethasone for airway edema or elective extubation.[56] Thus infants may be exposed to steroids for a number of reasons, and the sickest and most immature infants will have the most reasons. For the future, we need to judiciously use steroids at the lowest doses and for the shortest durations possible. Specific organ targeting such as the addition of budesonide to surfactant is particularly attractive to minimize risk. A perspective on steroids in perinatal medicine is provided by the (modified) apocryphal statement by Galen: "All who receive steroids recover in a short time, except those whom steroids do not help, who all die. It is obvious, therefore, that steroids fail only in incurable cases."

REFERENCES

1. Liggins GC. Premature delivery of foetal lambs infused with glucocorticoids. *J Endocrinol.* 1969;45(4):515–523.
2. Liggins GC, Howie RN. A controlled trial of antepartum glucocorticoid treatment for prevention of the respiratory distress syndrome in premature infants. *Pediatrics.* 1972;50(4):515–525.
3. Effect of corticosteroids for fetal maturation on perinatal outcomes. NIH consensus development panel on the effect of corticosteroids for fetal maturation on perinatal outcomes. *JAMA.* 1995;273(5):413–418.
4. Roberts D, Brown J, Medley N, Dalziel SR. Antenatal corticosteroids for accelerating fetal lung maturation for women at risk of preterm birth. *Cochrane Database Syst Rev.* 2017;3:CD004454.
5. Jobe AH. Animal models, learning lessons to prevent and treat neonatal chronic lung disease. *Front Med (Lausanne).* 2015;2:49.
6. Ikegami M, Polk D, Jobe A. Minimum interval from fetal betamethasone treatment to postnatal lung responses in preterm lambs. *Am J Obstet Gynecol.* 1996;174(5):1408–1413.
7. Willet KE, Jobe AH, Ikegami M, Kovar J, Sly PD. Lung morphometry after repetitive antenatal glucocorticoid treatment in preterm sheep. *Am J Respir Crit Care Med.* 2001;163(6):1437–1443.
8. Pew BK, Harris RA, Sbrana E, et al. Structural and transcriptomic response to antenatal corticosteroids in an Erk3-null mouse model of respiratory distress. *Am J Obstet Gynecol.* 2016;215(3):384. e381–384.e389.
9. Massaro D, Massaro GD. Dexamethasone accelerates postnatal alveolar wall thinning and alters wall composition. *Am J Physiol.* 1986;251(2 Pt 2):R218–R224.
10. Jobe AH, Polk DH, Ervin MG, Padbury JF, Rebello CM, Ikegami M. Preterm betamethasone treatment of fetal sheep: outcome after term delivery. *J Soc Gynecol Investig.* 1996;3(5):250–258.
11. Fawke J, Lum S, Kirkby J, et al. Lung function and respiratory symptoms at 11 years in children born extremely preterm: the EPICure study. *Am J Respir Crit Care Med.* 2010;182(2):237–245.
12. Gonzales LW, Ballard PL, Ertsey R, Williams MC. Glucocorticoids and thyroid hormones stimulate biochemical and morphological differentiation of human fetal lung in organ culture. *J Clin Endocrinol Metab.* 1986;62(4):678–691.
13. Carlo WA, McDonald SA, Fanaroff AA, et al. Association of antenatal corticosteroids with mortality and neurodevelopmental outcomes among infants born at 22 to 25 weeks' gestation. *JAMA.* 2011;306(21):2348–2358.

14. Travers CP, Clark RH, Spitzer AR, Das A, Garite TJ, Carlo WA. Exposure to any antenatal corticosteroids and outcomes in preterm infants by gestational age: prospective cohort study. *BMJ.* 2017;356:j1039.

15. Bancalari EH, Jobe AH. The respiratory course of extremely preterm infants: a dilemma for diagnosis and terminology. *J Pediatr.* 2012;161(4):585–588.

16. Norman M, Piedvache A, Borch K, et al. Association of short antenatal corticosteroid administration-to-birth intervals with survival and morbidity among very preterm infants: results from the EPICE cohort. *JAMA Pediatr;* 2017.

17. Mori R, Kusuda S, Fujimura M, Neonatal Research Network Japan. Antenatal corticosteroids promote survival of extremely preterm infants born at 22 to 23 weeks of gestation. *J Pediatr.* 2011;159(1):110–114.e111.

18. Makhija NK, Tronnes AA, Dunlap BS, Schulkin J, Lannon SM. Antenatal corticosteroid timing: accuracy after the introduction of a rescue course protocol. *Am J Obstet Gynecol.* 2016;214(1):120.e121–e126.

19. Ikegami M, Jobe AH, Newnham J, Polk DH, Willet KE, Sly P. Repetitive prenatal glucocorticoids improve lung function and decrease growth in preterm lambs. *Am J Respir Crit Care Med.* 1997;156(1):178–184.

20. Crowther CA, McKinlay CJ, Middleton P, Harding JE. Repeat doses of prenatal corticosteroids for women at risk of preterm birth for improving neonatal health outcomes. *Cochrane Database Syst Rev.* 2015;(7):CD003935.

21. Murphy KE, Willan AR, Hannah ME, et al. Effect of antenatal corticosteroids on fetal growth and gestational age at birth. *Obstet Gynecol.* 2012;119(5):917–923.

22. Wapner RJ, Sorokin Y, Thom EA, et al. Single versus weekly courses of antenatal corticosteroids: evaluation of safety and efficacy. *Am J Obstet Gynecol.* 2006;195(3):633–642.

23. Consortium on Safe L Hibbard JU, Wilkins I, et al. Respiratory morbidity in late preterm births. *JAMA.* 2010;304(4):419–425.

24. Gyamfi-Bannerman C, Thom EA. Antenatal betamethasone for women at risk for late preterm delivery. *N Engl J Med.* 2016;375(5):486–487.

25. Society for Maternal-Fetal Medicine Publications Committee. Implementation of the use of antenatal corticosteroids in the late preterm birth period in women at risk for preterm delivery. *Am J Obstet Gynecol.* 2016;215(2):B13–B15.

26. Kamath-Rayne BD, Rozance PJ, Goldenberg RL, Jobe AH. Antenatal corticosteroids beyond 34 weeks gestation: What do we do now? *Am J Obstet Gynecol.* 2016;215(4):423–430.

27. Stutchfield P, Whitaker R, Russell I. Antenatal Steroids for Term Elective Caesarean Section Research Team. Antenatal betamethasone and incidence of neonatal respiratory distress after elective caesarean section: pragmatic randomised trial. *BMJ.* 2005;331(7518):662.

28. Nada AM, Shafeek MM, El Maraghy MA, Nageeb AH, Salah El Din AS, Awad MH. Antenatal corticosteroid administration before elective caesarean section at term to prevent neonatal respiratory morbidity: a randomized controlled trial. *Eur J Obstet Gynecol Reprod Biol.* 2016;199:88–91.

29. Jobe AH, Nitsos I, Pillow JJ, Polglase GR, Kallapur SG, Newnham JP. Betamethasone dose and formulation for induced lung maturation in fetal sheep. *Am J Obstet Gynecol.* 2009;201(6):611.e611–e617.

30. Samtani MN, Lohle M, Grant A, Nathanielsz PW, Jusko WJ. Betamethasone pharmacokinetics after two prodrug formulations in sheep: implications for antenatal corticosteroid use. *Drug Metab Dispos.* 2005;33(8):1124–1130.

31. Schmidt AF, Kemp MW, Kannan PS, et al. Antenatal dexamethasone vs. betamethasone dosing for lung maturation in fetal sheep. *Pediatr Res.* 2017;81(3):496–503.

32. Dalziel SR, Walker NK, Parag V, et al. Cardiovascular risk factors after antenatal exposure to betamethasone: 30-year follow-up of a randomised controlled trial. *Lancet.* 2005;365(9474):1856–1862.

33. Braun T, Sloboda DM, Tutschek B, et al. Fetal and neonatal outcomes after term and preterm delivery following betamethasone administration. *Int J Gynaecol Obstet.* 2015;130(1):64–69.

34. Kelly BA, Lewandowski AJ, Worton SA, et al. Antenatal glucocorticoid exposure and long-term alterations in aortic function and glucose metabolism. *Pediatrics.* 2012;129(5):e1282–e1290.

35. Althabe F, Belizan JM, McClure EM, et al. A population-based, multifaceted strategy to implement antenatal corticosteroid treatment versus standard care for the reduction of neonatal mortality due to preterm birth in low-income and middle-income countries: the ACT cluster-randomised trial. *Lancet.* 2015;385(9968):629–639.

36. Althabe F, Thorsten V, Klein K, et al. The Antenatal Corticosteroids Trial (ACT)'s explanations for neonatal mortality—a secondary analysis. *Reprod Health.* 2016;13(1):62.

37. Avery GB, Fletcher AB, Kaplan M, Brudno DS. Controlled trial of dexamethasone in respirator-dependent infants with bronchopulmonary dysplasia. *Pediatrics.* 1985;75(1):106–111.

38. Cummings JJ, D'Eugenio DB, Gross SJ. A controlled trial of dexamethasone in preterm infants at high risk for bronchopulmonary dysplasia. *N Engl J Med.* 1989;320(23):1505–1510.

39. Doyle LW, Ehrenkranz RA, Halliday HL. Late (>7 days) postnatal corticosteroids for chronic lung disease in preterm infants. *Cochrane Database Syst Rev.* 2014;(5):CD001145.

40. Doyle LW, Ehrenkranz RA, Halliday HL. Early (<8 days) postnatal corticosteroids for preventing chronic lung disease in preterm infants. *Cochrane Database Syst Rev.* 2014;(5):CD001146.

41. Committee on Fetus and Newborn. Postnatal corticosteroids to treat or prevent chronic lung disease in preterm infants. *Pediatrics.* 2002;109(2):330–338.

42. Stoll BJ, Hansen NI, Bell EF, et al. Trends in care practices, morbidity, and mortality of extremely preterm neonates, 1993–2012. *JAMA.* 2015;314(10):1039–1051.

20

43. Doyle LW, Halliday HL, Ehrenkranz RA, Davis PG, Sinclair JC. An update on the impact of postnatal systemic corticosteroids on mortality and cerebral palsy in preterm infants: effect modification by risk of bronchopulmonary dysplasia. *J Pediatr.* 2014;165(6):1258–1260.

44. Shinwell ES, Lerner-Geva L, Lusky A, Reichman B. Less postnatal steroids, more bronchopulmonary dysplasia: a population-based study in very low birthweight infants. *Arch Dis Child Fetal Neonatal Ed.* 2007;92(1):F30–F33.

45. Virkud YV, Hornik CP, Benjamin DK, et al. Respiratory support for very low birth weight infants receiving dexamethasone. *J Pediatr.* 2017;183:26–30.e23.

46. McEvoy CT, Jain L, Schmidt B, Abman S, Bancalari E, Aschner JL. Bronchopulmonary dysplasia: NHLBI workshop on the primary prevention of chronic lung diseases. *Ann Am Thorac Soc.* 2014;11(suppl 3):S146–S153.

47. Stark AR, Carlo WA, Tyson JE, et al. Adverse effects of early dexamethasone treatment in extremely-low-birth-weight infants. National institute of child health and human development neonatal research network. *N Engl J Med.* 2001;344(2):95–101.

48. Durand M, Mendoza ME, Tantivit P, Kugelman A, McEvoy C. A randomized trial of moderately early low-dose dexamethasone therapy in very low birth weight infants: dynamic pulmonary mechanics, oxygenation, and ventilation. *Pediatrics.* 2002;109(2):262–268.

49. Doyle LW, Davis PG, Morley CJ, McPhee A, Carlin JB, Investigators DS. Low-dose dexamethasone facilitates extubation among chronically ventilator-dependent infants: a multicenter, international, randomized, controlled trial. *Pediatrics.* 2006;117(1):75–83.

50. Baud O, Maury L, Lebail F, et al. Effect of early low-dose hydrocortisone on survival without bronchopulmonary dysplasia in extremely preterm infants (PREMILOC): a double-blind, placebo-controlled, multicentre, randomised trial. *Lancet.* 2016;387(10030):1827–1836.

51. Slaughter JL, Stenger MR, Reagan PB, Jadcherla SR. Utilization of inhaled corticosteroids for infants with bronchopulmonary dysplasia. *PLoS One.* 2014;9(9):e106838.

52. Onland W, Offringa M, van Kaam A. Late (>/= 7 days) inhalation corticosteroids to reduce broncho-pulmonary dysplasia in preterm infants. *Cochrane Database Syst Rev.* 2012;(4):CD002311.

53. Nakamura T, Yonemoto N, Nakayama M, et al. Early inhaled steroid use in extremely low birthweight infants: a randomised controlled trial. *Arch Dis Child Fetal Neonatal Ed.* 2016.

54. Bassler D, Plavka R, Shinwell ES, et al. Early inhaled budesonide for the prevention of bronchopul-monary dysplasia. *N Engl J Med.* 2015;373(16):1497–1506.

55. Yeh TF, Chen CM, Wu SY, et al. Intratracheal administration of budesonide/surfactant to prevent bronchopulmonary dysplasia. *Am J Respir Crit Care Med.* 2016;193(1):86–95.

56. Finer NN, Powers RJ, Ou CH, et al. Prospective evaluation of postnatal steroid administration: a 1-year experience from the California perinatal quality care collaborative. *Pediatrics.* 2006;117(3):704–713.

B

CHAPTER 21

Cell-Based Therapy for Neonatal Lung Diseases

Karen C. Young, Bernard Thébaud, and Won Soon Park

- The postnatal lung contains populations of stem cells with the capacity to reconstitute the lung following injury.
- Prematurity and its antecedent factors may alter lung stem cell programming leading to dysfunctional repair.
- Preterm infants in whom bronchopulmonary dysplasia develops exhibit decreased and/or dysfunctional stem cells.
- Preclinical studies provide robust evidence that stem cells reduce lung injury and improve survival in experimental models of bronchopulmonary dysplasia via paracrine-mediated mechanisms.
- Mesenchymal stem cells are an attractive population for lung repair as they are immunoprivileged, easily isolated, and have pleiotropic therapeutic effects.
- Early clinical evidence demonstrates the safety and feasibility of mesenchymal stem cell therapy for bronchopulmonary dysplasia. However, barriers for implementation, including optimal dosing, patient, timing, and culture techniques, need to be overcome for successful translation.

The lungs are remarkably complex organs with more than 40 different cell types uniquely organized to facilitate gas transport and exchange. This intrinsic complexity along with low cell turnover has led to challenges in understanding lung stem cell biology.[1,2] Despite this, real progress has been made in the past decade and recent reports indicate that following injury, the damaged lung epithelium has the capacity to repair itself by a population of resident lung stem cells, with possibly minor contribution of bone marrow (BM)-derived stem cells. More data are also accumulating on the complex niches within which stem cells reside and the molecular mechanisms that regulate stem cell self-renewal and differentiation, and their impact on disease pathogenesis.[3,4] Evidence is also mounting that environmental perturbations alter stem cell function and fate, leading to dysfunctional repair and remodeling.

Aberrant stem cell reprogramming in preterm infants and their antecedent diseases now support the notion that early alterations in stem cell function contribute to bronchopulmonary dysplasia (BPD) pathogenesis. New exciting preclinical data provide evidence that stem cell–based therapies reduce lung injury in BPD models. Among the cells being tested, mesenchymal stem cells have shown tremendous promise owing to their ability to replenish the endogenous stem niche, their immunomodulatory properties, and their availability. Clinical trials in several countries using mesenchymal stem cell–based therapies are now underway in preterm infants. This chapter discusses recent advances in lung stem cell biology, our current understanding of the impact of BPD on endogenous stem cells, and the application as well as challenges of implementing stem cell–based therapies for BPD.

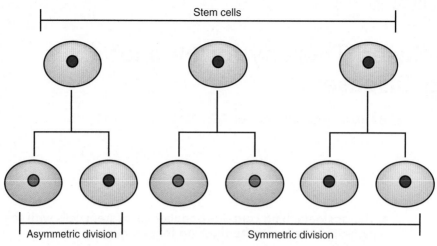

Fig. 21.1 Stem cell division. Stem cells may divide asymmetrically or symmetrically. During symmetric division, the stem cells divide and produce two daughter stem cells or two differentiated daughter progeny. Alternatively, during asymmetric division, the stem cell produces one differentiated daughter progeny and one stem cell.

Stem Cells

In the early 1900s the Russian histologist Alexander Maximow discovered that all blood cells have a common ancestral origin.[5] Since then our knowledge of stem cell biology has grown exponentially, and stem cells are now known to be essential for organogenesis and tissue homeostasis. By definition, stem cells must have the ability to both replenish themselves through self-renewal and to differentiate into mature progeny.[6–8] They may divide symmetrically or asymmetrically, giving rise to a stem cell and a more committed progenitor cell (Fig. 21.1).[9,10] They may also be classified as totipotent, pluripotent, or multipotent (Fig. 21.2).[10] Totipotent stem cells are capable of differentiating into all adult and embryonic tissues, including extraembryonic tissues such as trophectoderm.[11,12] In mammals, only the zygote and the first cleavage blastomeres are totipotent.[12] Pluripotent stem cells are capable of differentiating into derivatives of all three germ layers (ectoderm, mesoderm, and endoderm) and are typically derived from embryos at different embryonic stages of development.[13] Multipotent stem cells are able to differentiate into multiple cell types of one lineage.[14] The most prominent example remains hematopoietic stem cells, which are capable of differentiating into all cell types of the hematopoietic system.[15] Stem cells may also be categorized as embryonic or adult stem cells. Embryonic stem cells are derived from blastocysts in the developing embryo and are pluripotent.[16] Adult stem cells are found in tissues in specialized microenvironments.[17,18] These cells are typically multipotent and following an asymmetric cell division, they produce a population of transit-amplifying progenitor cells.[19] They may act as intermediates between dedicated stem cells and mature differentiated cells. Within tissues, there may also be facultative stem cells or progenitors, which are normally quiescent differentiated cells, but following injury, they may self-renew and give rise to other differentiated progeny.[2,20]

Endogenous Lung Stem Cells

The postnatal lung contains stem cells capable of reconstituting the lung following injury[21] (Table 21.1) and these are predominantly facultative stem cells. These endogenous lung stem cells are limited in their differentiation potential, have potency restricted to lung cell lineages and topographically, are localized to specific anatomic regions and tissue micro-environments.[22] Despite attempts to identify a dedicated lung stem cell, there is no clear evidence of such a cell. Instead, it is more likely that there are several niches of multipotent cells with the

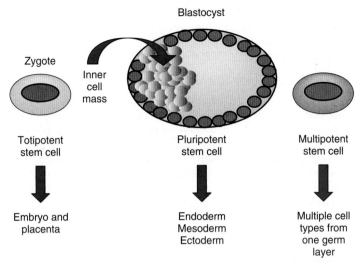

Fig. 21.2   Stem cell potency. Totipotent stem cells (zygote or first cleavage blastomeres) can give rise to all cells in the embryo and placenta. Pluripotent stem cells (e.g., embryonic stem cells) can give rise to the entire embryo and all cell lineages (endoderm, mesoderm, and ectoderm). Multipotent stem cells typically give rise to cells in one cell lineage.

Table 21.1   SUMMARY OF LUNG EPITHELIAL PROGENITOR CELL POPULATIONS

Cell Type	Marker Genes	Location	Differentiation Potential	Role in BPD	References
Basal cells	Trp63, Krt5, Krt14, NGFR, Pdpn	Trachea	Self, ciliated, club	Unknown	23–26
Club cells	Scgb1a1, Cyp2f2	Bronchiole	Self, ciliated	Unknown, killed by naphthalene	28,29
Variant club cells	Scgb1a1, Cyp2f2^{low}	Near neuroepithelial bodies	Self, ciliated, club	Unknown but survive naphthalene injury	31,32
BASCs	SP-C, Scgb1a1		Self, club, ciliated, AEC2	Unchanged in rodent hyperoxia-models of BPD but gives rise to AEC2 cells following bleomycin injury and increases after intratracheal MSC therapy in rodent hyperoxia BPD models	46–50
Integrin α6β4 alveolar progenitors	Itgα6, Itgβ4	Conducting airways, BADJ, alveolar wall	Self, club, ciliated, AEC2, AEC1	Unknown but may contribute to alveolar repair following bleomycin-induced lung injury	44,45
Distal airway stem cells	Trp63, Krt5, Krt14, NGFR, Pdpn	Distal airways	Self, club, ciliated, AEC2, AEC1	Unknown but migrate and give rise to alveolar cells following severe influenza	40–42
AEC2	SP-C	Alveoli	Self, AEC1	Proliferates in response to hyperoxia and gives rise to AEC1 cells	33–36,37,121

AECA, Alveolar type 1 epithelial cells; *AEC2,* alveolar type 2 epithelial cells; *BADJ,* bronchoalveolar duct junction; *BASC,* bronchoalveolar stem cell; *BPD,* bronchopulmonary dysplasia, *MSC,* mesenchymal stem cells; *NGFR,* nerve growth factor receptor; *SP-C,* surfactant protein C.

potential to reenter the cell cycle during injury. It is also conceivable that prematurity and its associated exposures dysregulate signaling pathways that modulate stem cell programming, leading to perturbation of these endogenous niches and dysfunctional repair.

Airway Candidate Stem Cells

Within the proximal gas-conducting system (the trachea and main bronchi) is a distinct population of undifferentiated basal cells expressing cytokeratins 5 and 14, transcription factor 63, and nerve growth factor that functions as bronchiolar stem cells.[23–26] These basal cells self-renew and give rise to ciliated and club cells (formerly known as Clara cells)[27] under steady-state conditions and following sulfur dioxide inhalation injury. Within the distal airways, lineage tracing experiments show that club cells self-renew and differentiate into ciliated cells.[28,29] Evidence also points to different club cell populations with variable proliferative capacity and lineage potential.[30,31] One club cell subpopulation is resistant to the toxin, naphthalene, which poisons the cytochrome P450 enzyme.[31] These cells have been termed "variant club cells" and are located around the neuroendocrine bodies and at the bronchoalveolar duct junction. Variant club cells are quiescent in the steady state; however following naphthalene-induced injury they proliferate quite rapidly.[32] The role of these cells in BPD is unknown.

Alveolar Candidate Stem Cells

Within the alveoli, substantial in vivo and in vitro evidence suggest that alveolar type 2 epithelial cells (AEC2) are the progenitors of alveolar type 1 epithelial cells (AEC1).[33–36] AEC2 cells play a crucial role in replenishing the AEC1 population under both steady-state and injury conditions, and lineage tracing experiments reveal that AEC2 cells not only self-renew but also give rise to AEC1 progeny.[37] In three-dimensional (3D) culture, AEC2 cells form alveolospheres containing cells that express both AEC2 and AEC1 cell markers.[37] Emerging data also show different subpopulations of AEC2 cells with variable regenerative potential. In whole lung and primary cultures of adult rat AEC2 cells, there is a hyperoxia-resistant subpopulation of telomerase-positive AEC2 that expands in response to injury.[38] AEC2 cells expressing high surface levels of telomerase but low epithelial (E)-cadherin are more proliferative and less likely to undergo hyperoxic damage compared with AEC2 cells that express high levels of E-cadherin.[39]

More recently, rare populations of undifferentiated basally located distal airway stem cells expressing cytokeratin 5, transcription factor 63, and cytokeratin 14 have also been identified as potential alveolar progenitors.[40–42] These cells originate from SOX2+ airway progenitors[43] and are inactive under steady-state conditions, but they proliferate and migrate into the alveoli following severe influenza-induced lung injury, differentiating into both airway and alveolar lineages.[40–42] Additional populations of multipotent epithelial stem cells that express the laminin receptor $\alpha6\beta4$ have also been described.[44,45] These cells are localized within the epithelium of the conducting airways and alveoli and have the capacity to give rise to AEC2 cells, suggesting the possibility that these multipotent distal airway stem cells may contribute to alveolar repair.

Other candidate alveolar progenitors include rare populations of epithelial cells located at the bronchoalveolar duct junction, so-called bronchoalveolar stem cells (BASCs).[46] These cells express both surfactant protein C (SP-C) as well as secretoglobin (Scgb1a1), are resistant to naphthalene, and proliferate rapidly after naphthalene- and bleomycin-induced lung injury[47] Although BASCs are unchanged in hyperoxia-induced lung injury[48] and their role in lung development is unclear, BASCs are able to give rise to AEC2 cells following bleomycin-induced lung injury, albeit to a minor degree.[49,50] In specialized culture media, BASCs give rise to cells that express pro-SP-C, aquaporin 5, as well as Scgb1a1, suggesting that these cells could give rise to cells in the conducting as well as gas exchange portion of the lung. However, more research is needed to elucidate the regenerative capacity of these alveolar progenitor cells in BPD, their interactions with cells in the lung vasculature and mesenchymal compartment, and the molecular mechanisms that drive these alveolar progenitors toward quiescence or activation.

Lung Mesenchymal Stem Cells

Originally characterized in 1968 by Friedenstein and colleagues, mesenchymal stem cells (MSCs) were first described as a population of BM stromal cells that were adherent, fibroblastic in appearance, and clonogenic.[51] Because there are no specific cell markers for MSCs, the International Society for Cellular Therapy established minimal criteria for defining MSCs: (1) adherence to plastic under standard tissue culture conditions; (2) expression of cell surface markers, CD105, CD90, and CD73, and no expression for HLA-DR, CD79α, CD45, CD34, CD14, CD19, and CD11b; and (3) the capacity to differentiate into osteoblasts, chondroblasts, and adipocytes under appropriate in vitro conditions.[52]

Although these criteria were mainly used to describe BM-derived MSC, emerging data now suggest that most organs have endogenous MSC populations, albeit with varying functionality, differentiation potential, and phenotype, depending on micro-environmental cues.[53,54] MSCs have been isolated from fetal and adult lungs based on their adherence to plastic,[55] expression of adenosine-binding cassette G (ABCG2),[56] Hoechst 33342 dye efflux,[57] and their osteogenic, chondrogenic, and adipogenic differentiation potential.[56,58] Compared with BM-MSCs, lung-derived MSCs seem to be constitutively more prone to epithelial differentiation[59] and have a distinct pattern of *Hox* gene expression implicated in lung development.[60] Although lung and BM-MSCs reduce elastase injury to the same extent,[61] lung MSCs express more intercellular adhesion molecule 1 (ICAM-1), platelet-derived growth factor receptor alpha (PDGFRα), and integrin α2 than BM-MSCs,[61] conferring potential differences in MSC adherence, migration, and invasion. Moreover, lung MSCs are now believed to be a part of a diverse population of mesenchymal progenitors[62] directly involved in regulating the growth and function of epithelial progenitor cells.[63]

The role of lung MSCs in BPD is still being clarified. Lung MSCs are decreased in the lungs of newborn rodents exposed to hyperoxia,[64] yet increased MSCs in the tracheal aspirate of preterm infants predicts an increased risk for BPD by more than 25-fold.[65] Moreover, MSCs isolated from the lungs of preterm infants differentiate into myofibroblasts under the influence of the pro-fibrotic factor, transforming growth factor beta.[66] Similarly, MSCs isolated from human lung allografts undergo pro-fibrotic differentiation in response to cytokines associated with bronchiolitis obliterans,[67] but a significant decrease in lung MSCs is evident in the lungs of rodents with bleomycin-induced pulmonary fibrosis and replacement of lung MSCs attenuates fibrosis.[68] One potential explanation for these apparent contradictory findings is the presence of different subpopulations of lung MSCs with variable epithelial-supportive capacity and myofibroblastic differentiation potential.[69] Conceivably, depletion of lung MSCs may interfere with the endogenous regenerative response; conversely, lung microenvironmental cues may influence MSC behavior and function, potentially driving them toward a more dysfunctional fibrotic phenotype.

Lung Endothelial Progenitors

Endothelial progenitors (EPCs) were first described by Asahara et al. in 1997.[70] This group described a population of peripheral blood mononuclear cells that could differentiate into endothelial cells. These cells expressed the hematopoietic stem marker, CD34, as well as the endothelial cell marker, vascular endothelial growth factor receptor 2 (VEGFR2), and were shown to contribute to physiologic and pathologic neovascularization.[70] Since then various different markers have been used to identify this population, and although still marred with controversy, current data suggest that there is a hierarchy of EPCs based on their proliferative potential.[71] One subset appears early in culture, displays endothelial markers, but does not form vessels in vivo.[72] These cells exert mainly paracrine effects on endothelial cells. Another subset, termed endothelial colony-forming cells (ECFCs),[71] gives rise to colonies 7 to 21 days after plating, has robust proliferative potential, and forms vessels when transplanted in vivo.[71] These cells can not only be isolated from umbilical cord and aorta vessel walls,[73] but recent evidence also points to similar cells within the pulmonary microvasculature.[74] This is intriguing given the importance of angiogenesis in lung development and repair. Indeed, prior studies have linked circulating EPC quantity with adult lung disease outcomes. Patients with end-stage chronic lung disease have reduced circulating EPCs[75] and patients with idiopathic pulmonary fibrosis showed a marked EPC depletion, particularly when pulmonary hypertension is evident.[76] Interestingly, ECFCs isolated from neonatal rats with hyperoxia-induced BPD-like lung injury proliferate less and form fewer capillary-like networks, suggesting that functional deficiency in ECFCs may contribute to BPD pathogenesis.[77] This is further supported by evidence of decreased and dysfunctional cord ECFCs in preterm infants in whom BPD subsequently develops.[78,79]

Cell Therapies for Bronchopulmonary Dysplasia

Evidence from Preclinical Studies

The recent insights into stem cell biology have unraveled the therapeutic potential of stem cells. Specifically, MSCs have attracted much attention because of their ease of isolation, culture, and expansion; allogeneic use; and pleiotropic therapeutic effects. The latter is of particular interest for a multifactorial disease such as BPD, in which multiple pathophysiologic mechanisms contribute to impaired alveolar and lung vascular development.

Early proof-of-concept studies in neonatal rodents exposed to hyperoxia showed that rodent BM-MSCs administered intravenously (IV) or intratracheally (IT) prevent the arrest in lung vascular and alveolar growth in this model (Fig. 21.3).[64,80] An interesting source of MSCs, especially when treating neonatal diseases, is represented by perinatal tissue. The placenta and umbilical cord are usually discarded after birth, yet they contain a large number of various cells, including MSCs, with therapeutic potential and can be harvested without harm to the mother or the newborn. After the above-mentioned proof-of-concept studies, MSCs derived from the umbilical cord (UC) Wharton jelly and from the umbilical cord blood (UCB) have been studied extensively in experimental BPD models. Similar to the therapeutic

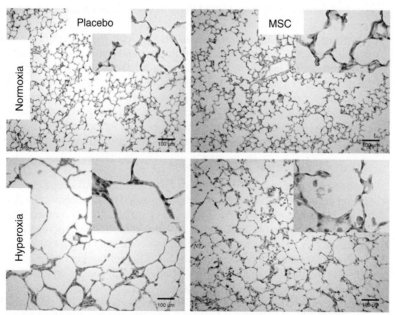

Fig. 21.3 Mesenchymal stem cells (MSCs) improve hyperoxia-induced alveolar simplification. The lung sections demonstrate improved alveolar structure following administration of MSCs to neonatal rats with hyperoxia-induced lung injury.

benefit reported for BM-MSCs, UC- and UCB-derived MSCs demonstrated comparable effects in hyperoxia-induced neonatal lung injury in rodents[81–85]: improved alveolar and lung vascular structure and even restoration of alveolar growth after established lung injury, attenuation of lung fibrosis, reduced lung inflammation, and improved exercise capacity. The therapeutic benefit persisted into adulthood with no evidence of tumor formation or adverse effects on lung architecture.[81,85] Since then numerous investigators have attempted to optimize the use of MSCs by exploring the best timing, dose, and route of administration as outlined further in the following text. A consistent finding, however, was the low rate of lung engraftment of MSCs. Increasing evidence suggests that MSCs act via a paracrine mechanism to protect the developing lung from injury.[86] Table 21.2 provides a summary of the preclinical evidence.

Mechanisms of Repair

Similar observation of low organ engraftment of transplanted MSCs had already been observed in the heart and the central nervous system. The working hypothesis became that MSCs release bioactive molecules that modulate organ repair. Proof-of-concept experiments in vitro showed that cell-free conditioned media derived from MSCs prevent hyperoxia-induced alveolar epithelial cell apoptosis, accelerate alveolar epithelial cell wound healing, and preserve endothelial cord formation on Matrigel Matrix (Corning, Oneonta, New York) during hyperoxia.[64]

This paracrine effect was then confirmed in vivo. The efficacy of intraperitoneal administration of MSCs in protecting the neonatal rodent lung already suggested some paracrine activity of these cells.[82,87] Direct in vivo evidence was provided by studies in which a single IV injection of cell-free MSC-derived conditioned media improved lung function, alveolar injury, and pulmonary hypertension.[80,88] A single IT injection of BM-MSCs or BM-MSC-free conditioned media protected from oxygen-induced alveolar and vascular injury with a persistent benefit up to 3 months.[89] Likewise, cell-free conditioned media derived from human UCB-MSCs injected daily intraperitoneally prevented and reversed arrested alveolar growth and lung function in hyperoxia-exposed rats with persistent safety and therapeutic benefit up to 6 months.[81]

Thus rather than replacing injured cells and differentiating into lung cells, MSCs release factors that protect resident lung cells from injury or modulate the function of inflammatory cells. For example, BM-MSCs and BM-MSC-derived conditioned media increase the number of BASCs in neonatal mice exposed to hyperoxia.[90] In addition, MSCs can modulate the phenotype of macrophages from a M1 (proinflammatory) to an M2 (healer) phenotype in various disease conditions,[91,92] but this has not yet been investigated in neonates. Also, the interactions between MSCs and other immune cells remain unexplored in neonates.

The identification of soluble factors in the conditioned media may allow the discovery of novel repair mechanisms and therapeutic interventions.[93] Likewise, the variety of factors released by MSCs explains their pleiotropic effects and further underscores the rationale for MSC therapy for BPD. MSCs produce factors known to promote lung growth and repair such as keratinocyte growth factors,[94] vascular endothelial growth factor,[95,96] or adiponectin.[97] Novel molecules secreted by MSCs have already been identified and have shown therapeutic benefit in various disease models, such as stanniocalcin-1[98] (a potent antioxidant) or tumor necrosis factor α (TNF-α)–stimulated gene/protein 6 (TSG-6)[99] (a potent antiinflammatory protein). These discoveries open interesting therapeutic avenues into manufacturing superior therapeutic cells. For example, preconditioning of BM-MSCs ex vivo in hyperoxia for 24 hours enhanced the release of stanniocalcin-1 in the conditioned media and boosted the therapeutic benefit of preconditioned MSCs on lung architecture in hyperoxic neonatal rodents compared with non-preconditioned media.[100]

The recognition of the paracrine effect of MSCs has also renewed the excitement regarding extracellular vesicles, which are crucial for cell-to-cell communication. In particular, MSCs, like many other cells, release membrane-derived nanosized

Table 21.2   MESENCHYMAL STEM CELLS FOR BRONCHOPULMONARY DYSPLASIA: SUMMARY OF PRECLINICAL EVIDENCE

Cell Population	Cell Dose	Timing of Administration	Model	Route of Delivery	Effects of Therapy	Suggested Mechanisms of Repair	References
Mouse BM MSCs or CM	5×10^4	Postnatal day (P)4	Neonatal rats in hyperoxia P1–P14	Intravenous (IV)	CM have more pronounced improvement in alveolar and vascular structure than MSCs	Paracrine-mediated	122
Rat BM MSCs	1×10^5	P4 (prevention) P14 (treatment)	Neonatal rats in hyperoxia P1–P14, studied on P21 (prevention) or P45 (treatment)	Intratracheal (IT)	Early but not late MSC administration preserves lung architecture and survival. Both early and late administration improve exercise capacity	Paracrine-mediated	123
Human UCB MSCs	5×10^3 5×10^4 5×10^5	P5	Neonatal rats in hyperoxia Birth–P14	IT	Higher-dose MSCs have more pronounced effects on alveolar structure	Modulation of host inflammatory and antioxidant responses	83
Male rat BM MSCs or CM	2×10^6	P9	Neonatal rats in hyperoxia P2–P16; evaluated at P16, P30, and P100	IT	MSC and CM similarly improve lung architecture at P16 and P30; however, MSCs have more pronounced effects than CM at P100	Reduced inflammation	89
Male and female rat BM MSCs	1×10^6	P7	Neonatal rats in hyperoxia P2–P21	IT	Improved alveolar structure, increased vascular density, reduced pulmonary hypertension (PH) and remodeling	Female MSCs have greater antiinflammatory and pro-angiogenic effects than male MSCs	104
Human UCB MSCs	5×10^5 (IT) 2×10^6 (IV)	P5	Neonatal rats in hyperoxia Birth–P14	IT or IV	IT administration improves body weight and is better than IV in improving alveolar structure	IT administration has greater MSC retention and is better than IV in reducing inflammation and apoptosis	118
Human UCT MSCs	0.1×10^6 0.5×10^6 1×10^6	P5	Newborn SCID mice in hyperoxia Birth–P7; evaluated 8 weeks after MSC transplantation	Intranasally or IP	High-dose IP MSCs restore lung compliance, elastance, and pressure-volume loops. Intranasal or low-dose MSCs have no significant effects	Paracrine-mediated	124
Human UCB MSCs	5×10^5	P3 (early) P10 (late) P3 + P10	Neonatal rats in hyperoxia 90% for 2 weeks and 60% for 1 week	IT	More pronounced improvement in alveolar structure, oxidative stress, inflammation with early compared with late MSCs	Paracrine-mediated	84
Human cord PCs or UCB MSCs	3×10^5 (early) 6×10^5 (late)	P4 (early) P14 (late)	Neonatal rats in hyperoxia P4–P14; evaluated at P22 (prevention) or P35 (regeneration)	IT	Both early and late MSCs and PCs improved alveolar structure and lung function. No tumors evident at 6 months	Paracrine-mediated	116

BM, Bone marrow; *CM*, conditioned medium; *IP*, intraperitoneal; *MSC*, mesenchymal stem cell; *PC*, perivascular cell; *SCID*, severe combined immunodeficiency syndrome; *UCB*, umbilical cord blood; *UCT*, umbilical cord tissue.

exosomes, acting as cargoes that contain not only the combination of bioactive molecules but also microRNA (miRNA).[101] miRNAs are small noncoding RNA molecules involved in transcriptional regulation of gene expression, and this may explain the long-term effect of single injections of MSC-derived conditioned media. miRNA may represent interesting therapeutic targets in the prevention of BPD through activation or silencing of specific genes with beneficial or deleterious effects on lung development.[102] In adult lung injury models, MSC-derived exosomes attenuate lung macrophage influx, decrease proinflammatory cytokine levels in the bronchoalveolar lavage, and prevent pulmonary vascular remodeling and hypoxic-induced pulmonary hypertension in mice.[103] The therapeutic benefit of exosomes is currently being investigated in neonatal lung injury models.

The impact of gender in MSC efficacy is also being explored. Female BM-MSCs secrete more pro-angiogenic and antiinflammatory factors than male BM-MSCs.[104] In neonatal rats with hyperoxia-induced lung injury, female BM-MSCs are superior to male BM-MSCs in reducing lung inflammation, improving pulmonary hypertension, and attenuating vascular remodeling.[104] These beneficial effects are particularly more pronounced in male recipients, suggesting that female cells[104] may be a potent BM-MSC population for BPD complicated by severe pulmonary hypertension.

From Bench to Bedside: Evidence from a Phase I Clinical Trial

The above-mentioned preclinical evidence supporting the role of MSC transplantation as a potential therapy for BPD without short- and long-term toxicity or tumorigenicity[81,82,84,85,105] provided the foundation for the first clinical trial in preterm newborns.[106] This study was an open-label, single-center clinical trial that assessed the safety and feasibility of a single IT transplantation of allogenic human UCB-derived MSCs for BPD. MSCs were transplanted into 9 very preterm infants at high risk for developing BPD (mean gestational age 25.3 ± 0.9 weeks, range 24–26 weeks; mean birth weight 793 ± 127 g, range 630–1030 g) at a mean age of 10.4 ± 2.6 days (range 7–14 days) after birth. All of the infants were receiving ventilator support, the settings of which could not be decreased owing to significant respiratory distress within 24 hours before enrollment. The first three patients received a low dose of MSCs (1×10^7 cells/kg in 2 mL/kg of saline solution), while the remaining six patients received a high dose (2×10^7 cells/kg in 4 mL/kg of saline solution). The MSCs were administered IT into the left and right lungs in two fractions via a feeding tube, the same method used to administer surfactant. The treatment was well tolerated without any serious adverse effects or dose-limiting toxicity up to 84 days following transplantation. The incidence of serious adverse effects did not significantly differ in the low- and high-dose groups. The levels of interleukin 6 (IL-6), IL-8, matrix metalloproteinase-9, TNF-α, and transforming growth factor beta 1 in the tracheal aspirates collected on day 7 were significantly reduced compared with baseline and day 3 posttransplantation levels. Furthermore, compared with a historical control group matched for gestational age, birth weight, and respiratory severity score, BPD severity was significantly lower in transplant recipients. Overall, these findings suggest that IT allogenic human UCB-derived MSC transplantation in very preterm infants at high risk for developing BPD is safe and feasible.

Long-term follow-up studies extending up to 2 years (clinical trial No. NCT01632475) and 5 years of age (clinical trial No. NCT02023788) are currently underway to assess the long-term safety of MSC treatment in the subjects of these phase I trials. Furthermore, a phase II double-blind, randomized, multicenter, controlled clinical trial investigating the efficacy and safety of low-dose MSC transplantation compared with a control group for the treatment of BPD is also in progress (clinical trial No. NCT0182957). Another study following these phase II clinical trial patients to 5 years of age has also begun with the goal of gathering further long-term safety and efficacy data (clinical trial No. NCT01897987). Favorable results from these current clinical trials are greatly anticipated and are expected to pave the way for future clinical translation of stem cell therapies for BPD.

Barriers to Implementation

Clinical introduction of cell-based therapies could be a paradigm shift in neonatal medicine and in the treatment of BPD. However, barriers to clinical implementation, including optimization of the cells delivered to the right patients via the right route, at the right time, and right dose need to be overcome for the success of future clinical translation.[106–113]

Optimal Cells

Determining the optimal cells for transplantation is the most critical issue for successful clinical translation. MSCs have been extensively investigated, and their therapeutic efficacy has consistently been proven in BPD animal models.[64,82,114–116] Because donor cells do not engraft,[117] allogenic transplantation of MSCs is considered safe. Moreover, considering the time-consuming and costly isolation and expansion processes involved in the generation of autologous MSCs, allogenic therapy might have a logistic advantage for its ability to be used off the shelf in a clinical setting. MSCs are broadly distributed in the body; UCB-derived MSCs exhibited better efficacy in attenuating hyperoxic lung injuries and greater paracrine potency compared with fat-derived MSCs in newborn rats.[115] Production of a high-quality, standardized, clinical-grade product using good manufacturing practice (GMP) criteria is another important factor in the success of MSCs in a clinical setting.[111]

Based on present evidence, both the Korean Ministry of Food and Drug Safety and the United States Food and Drug Administration approved the use of allogenic human UCB-derived MSCs manufactured with strict GMP compliance for use in phase I/II BPD clinical trials conducted in Korea[106] and the United States (clinical trial No. NCT02381366). Standardization of the isolation, expansion, and production of these cells in GMP facilities would be necessary for the introduction of other cell types, such as endothelial progenitor cells and amnion epithelial cells, as well as cell-derived products such as exosomes, showing promising effects in BPD models.

Right Patient

Despite its potential benefits, cautious risk/benefit evaluations must be made before using MSC transplantation in the most vulnerable preterm infants. Therefore identification of the preterm infants at highest risk for BPD is a very important step in the application of these potentially beneficial rescue/preventive strategies. Because early gestational age and prolonged respiratory support must be cited as the most important predictors of BPD development among extremely preterm infants,[113] infants of 24 to 2 weeks' gestation requiring continuous ventilator support were enrolled in a phase I clinical trial conducted by Chang et al.[106] However, the clinical courses of these infants may vary widely and not all progress to development of BPD. Additional clinical predictors and/or biomarkers[112] will be necessary to further stratify these infants and determine who will ultimately progress to BPD, thus avoiding unnecessary treatment exposure.

Right Time

Even though the therapeutic efficacy of MSC transplantation in the prevention and rescue of experimental BPD has already been shown, the optimal timing of administration is a key issue that remains to be clarified. Pierro et al.[116] reported that although the long-term benefits of the rescue approach have not been investigated, MSCs or their conditioning media were not only effective for prevention at P4, their use at P14 as a rescue approach both prevented and rescued hyperoxic alveolar growth arrest. Chang and colleagues compared the therapeutic efficacy of early versus late MSC administration at P3 or P10 as well as at both of these time points.[84] Their study found significant attenuation of hyperoxic lung injuries only with early but not with late MSC transplantation, and combined early and late transplantation did not have a synergistic effect. In a study by van Haaften et al.,[64] MSC transplantation at P4 for prevention significantly attenuated neonatal hyperoxic lung injuries, whereas transplantation at P14 for regeneration showed no effect. Taken together, the therapeutic time window for MSC transplantation in the treatment of BPD appears to be narrow. Thus in a clinical setting, early identification of the highest-risk preterm infants and administration of MSCs within the first few days of life seem preferable to later administration in infants with established BPD.

Right Route

Several routes, including local IT instillation,[64,82] systemic IV injection[80,118] and intraperitoneal administration,[82] have been tested to determine the optimal route of MSC transplantation. As injured lung tissue produces chemotactic factors, systemically transplanted MSCs migrate[119] and localize to the injured lung.[120] The most convenient and minimally invasive systemic IV approach might be more therapeutically advantageous compared with a local IT approach, especially in very unstable preterm infants with BPD. Most preterm infants at high risk of BPD are intubated and receive ventilator support, and since MSCs can be instilled in the same way as surfactant, IT MSC transplantation during the first days of life might not be so invasive in the extremely preterm infants.[106] Furthermore, despite a fourfold lower dose and more frequent donor cell engraftment, better paracrine potency and attenuation of hyperoxic lung injuries were observed with local IT MSC transplantation than with systemic administration.[82,118] Based on superior therapeutic efficacy observed with local IT compared with systemic IV or intraperitoneal transplantation as demonstrated in these preclinical data, MSCs were delivered IT in the first phase I clinical trial.[106]

Right Dose

Because previous studies[82,118] have shown that the MSC therapeutic dose could be reduced more than fourfold by choosing a local IT route over systemic IV or intraperitoneal administration, the route of MSC administration might be a major determinant of optimal dosing. Chang et al.[105] compared the therapeutic efficacy of three different doses of human UCB-derived MSCs (5×10^3, 5×10^4, and 5×10^5 cells per animal, reflecting 0.5 to 50×10^6 cells per kg body weight) given IT to hyperoxic newborn rat pups at P5. The best therapeutic effects were seen in the mid- and high-dose treatment groups. Based on this evidence, a single IT administration of 1×10^7 cells/kg (low-dose, 3 infants) and 2×10^7 cells (high-dose, 6 infants) were used in the phase I clinical trial; no dose-limiting toxicity or serious adverse events were observed with either dose.[106] In light of these findings, further preclinical and clinical studies examining the optimal MSC dose of clinical benefit to human preterm neonates with BPD are anticipated.

Conclusion

In recent years, various translational studies have broadened the knowledge and understanding of stem cell therapy in neonatal lung injury, and clinical trials are harnessing the therapeutic potential of stem cell therapies for BPD. The exciting progress in both preclinical and clinical research has brought human stem cell BPD therapy one step closer to clinical translation. However, a better understanding of the potential protective mechanism of stem cells in BPD and the resolution of several issues, such as manufacturing processes, clinical indication, timing, dose, and modes of action, are required to permit safe clinical translation of stem cell therapy for this disorder. It will be essential to proceed sequentially rather than in haste with relentless efforts to overcome all obstacles in making stem cell therapy the next treatment breakthrough for BPD.

REFERENCES

1. Bowden DH. Cell turnover in the lung. *Am Rev Respir Dis.* 1983;128:S46–S48.
2. Rawlins EL, Okubo T, Que J, et al. Epithelial stem/progenitor cells in lung postnatal growth, maintenance, and repair. *Cold Spring Harb Symp Quant Biol.* 2008;73:291–295.
3. Whitsett J. A lungful of transcription factors. *Nat Gen.* 1998;20:7.
4. Maeda Y, Dave V, Whitsett JA. Transcriptional control of lung morphogenesis. *Physiol Rev.* 2007;87:219–244.

5. Konstantinov IE. In search of Alexander A. Maximow: the man behind the unitarian theory of hematopoiesis. *Perspect Biol Med.* 2000;43:269–276.
6. Goss AM, Morrisey EE. Wnt signaling and specification of the respiratory endoderm. *Cell Cycle.* 9:10–11.
7. Weissman IL. Stem cells: units of development, units of regeneration, and units in evolution. *Cell.* 2000;100:157–168.
8. Morrison SJ, Shah NM, Anderson DJ. Regulatory mechanisms in stem cell biology. *Cell.* 1997;88:287–298.
9. Till JE, McCulloch EA, Siminovitch L. A stochastic model of stem cell proliferation, based on the growth of spleen colony–forming cells. *Proc Natl Acad Sci U S A.* 1964;51:29–36.
10. Smith A. A glossary for stem-cell biology. *Nature.* 2006;441:1060–1060.
11. Kelly SJ. Studies of the developmental potential of 4- and 8-cell stage mouse blastomeres. *J Exp Zool.* 1977;200:365–376.
12. Modlinski JA. The fate of inner cell mass and trophectoderm nuclei transplanted to fertilized mouse eggs. *Nature.* 1981;292:342–343.
13. Donovan PJ, Gearhart J. The end of the beginning for pluripotent stem cells. *Nature.* 2001;414:92–97.
14. Rawlins EL, Okubo T, Xue Y. The role of Scgb1a1+ Clara cells in the long-term maintenance and repair of lung airway, but not alveolar, epithelium. *Cell Stem Cell.* 2009;4:525–534.
15. Wu AM, Siminovitch L, Till JE, McCulloch EA. Evidence for a relationship between mouse hemopoietic stem cells and cells forming colonies in culture. *Proc Natl Acad Sci U S A.* 1968;59:1209–1215.
16. Thomson JA, et al. Embryonic stem cell lines derived from human blastocysts. *Science.* 1998;282:1145–1147.
17. Moore KA, Lemischka IR. Stem cells and their niches. *Science.* 2006;311:1880–1885.
18. Li L, Xie T. Stem cell niche: structure and function. *Annu Rev Cell Dev Biol.* 2005;21:605–631.
19. Potten CS, Loeffler M. Stem cells: attributes, cycles, spirals, pitfalls and uncertainties. Lessons for and from the crypt. *Development.* 1990;110:1001–1020.
20. Rawlins EL, Hogan BL. Epithelial stem cells of the lung: privileged few or opportunities for many? *Development.* 2006;133:2455–2465.
21. Hogan Brigid LM, et al. Repair and regeneration of the respiratory system: complexity, plasticity, and mechanisms of lung stem cell function. *Cell Stem Cell.* 2014;15:123–138.
22. Watt FM, Hogan, Brigid LM. Out of Eden: stem cells and their niches. *Science.* 2000;287:1427–1430.
23. Rock JR, Onaitis MW, Rawlins EL. Basal cells as stem cells of the mouse trachea and human airway epithelium. *Proc Natl Acad Sci U S A.* 2009;106:12771–12775.
24. Hong KU, Reynolds SD, Watkins S, Fuchs E, Stripp BR. Basal cells are a multipotent progenitor capable of renewing the bronchial epithelium. *Am J Pathol.* 2004;164:577–588.
25. Hong KU, Reynolds SD, Watkins S, Fuchs E, Stripp BR. In vivo differentiation potential of tracheal basal cells: evidence for multipotent and unipotent subpopulations. *Am J Physiol Lung Cell Mol Physiol.* 2004;286:L643–L649.
26. Schoch KG, et al. A subset of mouse tracheal epithelial basal cells generates large colonies in vitro. *Am J Physiol Lung Cell Mol Physiol.* 2004;286:L631–L642.
27. Borthwick DW, Shahbazian M, Todd Krantz Q, Dorin JR, Randell SH. Evidence for stem-cell niches in the tracheal epithelium. *Am J Respir Cell Mol Biol.* 2001;24:662–670.
28. Rawlins EL, et al. The role of Scgb1a1+ Clara cells in the long-term maintenance and repair of lung airway, but not alveolar, epithelium. *Cell Stem Cell.* 2009;4:525–534.
29. Evans MJ, Cabral-Anderson LJ, Freeman G. Role of the Clara cell in renewal of the bronchiolar epithelium. *Lab Invest.* 1978;38:648–653.
30. Giangreco A, Reynolds SD, Stripp BR. Terminal bronchioles harbor a unique airway stem cell population that localizes to the bronchoalveolar duct junction. *Am J Pathol.* 2002;161:173–182.
31. Hong KU, Reynolds SD, Giangreco A, Hurley CM, Stripp BR. Clara cell secretory protein-expressing cells of the airway neuroepithelial body microenvironment include a label-retaining subset and are critical for epithelial renewal after progenitor cell depletion. *Am J Respir Cell Mol Biol.* 2001;24:671–681.
32. Reynolds SD, Giangreco A, Power JH. Neuroepithelial bodies of pulmonary airways serve as a reservoir of progenitor cells capable of epithelial regeneration. *Am J Pathol.* 2000;156:269.
33. Adamson IY, Bowden DH. The type 2 cell as progenitor of alveolar epithelial regeneration. A cytodynamic study in mice after exposure to oxygen. *Lab Invest.* 1974;30:35–42.
34. Tryka AF, Witschi H, Gosslee DG, McArthur AH, Clapp NK. Patterns of cell proliferation during recovery from oxygen injury. Species differences. *Am Rev Respir Dis.* 1986;133:1055–1059.
35. Adamson IY, Bowden DH. The type 2 cell as progenitor of alveolar epithelial regeneration. A cytodynamic study in mice after exposure to oxygen. *Lab Invest.* 1974;30:35.
36. Adamson IY, Bowden DH. Derivation of type 1 epithelium from type 2 cells in the developing rat lung. *Lab Invest.* 1975;32:736.
37. Barkauskas CE, et al. Type 2 alveolar cells are stem cells in adult lung. *J Clin Invest.* 2013;123:3025–3036.
38. Driscoll B, Buckley S, Bui KC, Anderson KD, Warburton D. Telomerase in alveolar epithelial development and repair. *Am J Physiol Lung Cell Mol Physiol.* 2000;279:L1191–L1198.
39. Reddy R, et al. Isolation of a putative progenitor subpopulation of alveolar epithelial type 2 cells. *Am J Physiol Lung Cell Mol Physiol.* 2004;286:L658–L667.
40. Vaughan AE, et al. Lineage-negative progenitors mobilize to regenerate lung epithelium after major injury. *Nature.* 2015;517:621–625.

41. Zuo W, et al. p63+Krt5+ distal airway stem cells are essential for lung regeneration. *Nature*. 2015;517:616–620.
42. Kumar Pooja A, et al. Distal airway stem cells yield alveoli in vitro and during lung regeneration following H1N1 Influenza Infection. *Cell*. 2011;147:525–538.
43. Ray S, et al. Rare SOX2(+) airway progenitor cells generate KRT5(+) cells that repopulate damaged alveolar parenchyma following influenza virus infection. *Stem Cell Reports*. 2016;7:817–825.
44. McQualter JL, Yuen K, Williams B, Bertoncello I. Evidence of an epithelial stem/progenitor cell hierarchy in the adult mouse lung. *Proc Natl Acad Sci U S A*. 2010;107:1414–1419.
45. Chapman HA, et al. Integrin α6β4 identifies an adult distal lung epithelial population with regenerative potential in mice. *J Clin Invest*. 2011;121:2855–2862.
46. Kim CF, Jackson EL, Woolfenden AE. Identification of bronchioalveolar stem cells in normal lung and lung cancer. *Cell*. 2005;121:823–835.
47. Kim CFB, et al. Identification of bronchioalveolar stem cells in normal lung and lung cancer. *Cell*. 2005;121:823–835.
48. Rawlins EL, et al. The role of Scgb1a1(+) Clara cells in the long-term maintenance and repair of lung airway, but not alveolar, epithelium. *Cell Stem Cell*. 2009;4:525–534.
49. Rock JR, et al. Multiple stromal populations contribute to pulmonary fibrosis without evidence for epithelial to mesenchymal transition. *Proc Natl Acad Sci U S A*. 2011;108:E1475–E1483.
50. Zheng D, et al. Regeneration of alveolar type I and II cells from Scgb1a1-expressing cells following severe pulmonary damage induced by bleomycin and influenza. *PLoS One*. 2012;7:e48451.
51. Friedenstein AJ, Petrakova KV, Kurolesova AI, Frolova GP. Heterotopic of bone marrow. analysis of precursor cells for osteogenic and hematopoietic tissues. *Transplantation*. 1968;6:230–247.
52. Dominici M, et al. Minimal criteria for defining multipotent mesenchymal stromal cells. The international society for cellular therapy position statement. *Cytotherapy*. 2006;8:315–317.
53. Lama VN, et al. Evidence for tissue-resident mesenchymal stem cells in human adult lung from studies of transplanted allografts. *J Clin Invest*. 2007;117:989–996.
54. Young HE, et al. Mesenchymal stem cells reside within the connective tissues of many organs. *Dev Dynam*. 1995;202:137–144.
55. Hennrick KT, et al. Lung cells from neonates show a mesenchymal stem cell phenotype. *Am J Respir Crit Care Med*. 2007;175:1158–1164.
56. Jun D, et al. The pathology of bleomycin induced fibrosis is associated with loss of resident lung mesenchymal stem cells which regulate effector T-cell proliferation. *Stem Cells (Dayton, Ohio)*. 2011;29:725–735.
57. Summer R, Fitzsimmons K, Dwyer D, Murphy J, Fine A. Isolation of an adult mouse lung mesenchymal progenitor cell population. *Am J Respir Cell Mol Biol*. 2007;37:152–159.
58. Majka SM, et al. Identification of novel resident pulmonary stem cells: form and function of the lung side population. *Stem Cells*. 2005;23:1073–1081.
59. Ricciardi M, et al. Comparison of epithelial differentiation and immune regulatory properties of mesenchymal stromal cells derived from human lung and bone marrow. *PLoS one*. 2012;7:e35639.
60. Bozyk PD, et al. Mesenchymal stromal cells from neonatal tracheal aspirates demonstrate a pattern of lung-specific gene expression. *Stem Cells Dev*. 2011;20:1995–2007.
61. Hoffman AM, et al. Lung-derived mesenchymal stromal cell post-transplantation survival, persistence, paracrine expression, and repair of elastase-injured lung. *Stem Cells Dev*. 2011;20:1779–1792.
62. Kumar ME, et al. Defining a mesenchymal progenitor niche at single cell resolution. *Science (New York, N.Y.)*. 2014;346:1258810.
63. Hegab AE, Arai D, Gao J, et al. Mimicking the niche of lung epithelial stem cells and characterization of several effectors of their in vitro behavior. *Stem Cell Res*. 2015;15:109–121.
64. van Haaften T, et al. Airway delivery of mesenchymal stem cells prevents arrested alveolar growth in neonatal lung injury in rats. *Am J Respir Crit Care Med*. 2009;180:1131–1142.
65. Popova AP, et al. Isolation of tracheal aspirate mesenchymal stromal cells predicts bronchopulmonary dysplasia. *Pediatrics*. 2010;126:e1127–e1133.
66. Popova AP, et al. Autocrine production of TGF-β1 promotes myofibroblastic differentiation of neonatal lung mesenchymal stem cells. *Am J Physiol Lung Cell Mol Physiol*. 2010;298:L735–L743.
67. Walker N, et al. Resident tissue-specific mesenchymal progenitor cells contribute to fibrogenesis in human lung allografts. *Am J Pathol*. 2011;178:2461–2469.
68. Jun D, et al. The pathology of bleomycin-induced fibrosis is associated with loss of resident lung mesenchymal stem cells that regulate effector T-cell proliferation. *Stem Cells*. 2011;29:725–735.
69. McQualter JL, et al. TGF-β signaling in stromal cells acts upstream of FGF-10 to regulate epithelial stem cell growth in the adult lung. *Stem Cell Res*. 2013;11:1222–1233.
70. Asahara T, et al. Isolation of putative progenitor endothelial cells for angiogenesis. *Science*. 1997;275:964–966.
71. Ingram DA, et al. Identification of a novel hierarchy of endothelial progenitor cells using human peripheral and umbilical cord blood. *Blood*. 2004;104:2752–2760.
72. Yoder MC, et al. Redefining endothelial progenitor cells via clonal analysis and hematopoietic stem/progenitor cell principals. *Blood*. 2007;109:1801.
73. Ingram DA, et al. Vessel wall–derived endothelial cells rapidly proliferate because they contain a complete hierarchy of endothelial progenitor cells. *Blood*. 2005;105:2783.
74. Alvarez DF, et al. Lung microvascular endothelium is enriched with progenitor cells that exhibit vasculogenic capacity. *Am J Physiol Lung Cell Mol Physiol*. 2008;294:L419.
75. Fadini GP, et al. Circulating progenitor cells are reduced in patients with severe lung disease. *Stem Cells*. 2006;24:1806–1813.

21

76. Fadini GP, Schiavon M, Rea F, Avogaro A, Agostini C. Depletion of endothelial progenitor cells may link pulmonary fibrosis and pulmonary hypertension. *Am J Respir Crit Care Med.* 2007;176:724–725.

77. Alphonse RS, et al. Existence, functional impairment, and lung repair potential of endothelial colony-forming cells in oxygen-induced arrested alveolar growth. *Circulation.* 2014;129:2144–2157.

78. Baker CD, et al. Cord blood angiogenic progenitor cells are decreased in bronchopulmonary dysplasia. *Eur Respir J.* 2012;40:1516.

79. Borghesi A, et al. Circulating endothelial progenitor cells in preterm infants with bronchopulmonary dysplasia. *Am J Respir Crit Care Med.* 2009;180:540–546.

80. Aslam M, et al. Bone marrow stromal cells attenuate lung injury in a murine model of neonatal chronic lung disease. *Am J Respir Crit Care Med.* 2009;180:1122–1130.

81. Pierro M, et al. Short-term, long-term and paracrine effect of human umbilical cord-derived stem cells in lung injury prevention and repair in experimental bronchopulmonary dysplasia. *Thorax.* 2012.

82. Chang YS, et al. Human umbilical cord blood-derived mesenchymal stem cells attenuate hyperoxia-induced lung injury in neonatal rats. *Cell Transplant.* 2009;18:869–886.

83. Chang YS, et al. Intratracheal transplantation of human umbilical cord blood derived mesenchymal stem cells dose-dependently attenuates hyperoxia-induced lung injury in neonatal rats. *Cell Transplant.* 2011;20:1843–1854.

84. Chang YS, et al. Timing of umbilical cord blood derived mesenchymal stem cells transplantation determines therapeutic efficacy in the neonatal hyperoxic lung injury. *PLoS One.* 2013;8:e52419.

85. Ahn SY, et al. Long-term (postnatal day 70) outcome and safety of intratracheal transplantation of human umbilical cord blood-derived mesenchymal stem cells in neonatal hyperoxic lung injury. *Yonsei Med J.* 2013;54:416–424.

86. Fung ME, Thebaud B. Stem cell-based therapy for neonatal lung disease: it is in the juice. *Pediatr Res.* 2014;75:2–7.

87. Zhang X, et al. Role of bone marrow-derived mesenchymal stem cells in the prevention of hyperoxia-induced lung injury in newborn mice. *Cell Biol Int.* 2012;36:589–594.

88. Hansmann G, et al. Mesenchymal stem cell-mediated reversal of bronchopulmonary dysplasia and associated pulmonary hypertension. *Pulm Circ.* 2012;2:170–181.

89. Sutsko RP, et al. Long-term reparative effects of mesenchymal stem cell therapy following neonatal hyperoxia-induced lung injury. *Pediatr Res.* 2013;73:46–53.

90. Tropea KA, et al. Bronchioalveolar stem cells increase after mesenchymal stromal cell treatment in a mouse model of bronchopulmonary dysplasia. *Am J Physiol Lung Cell Mol Physiol.* 2012;302:L829–L837.

91. Ionescu L, et al. Stem cell conditioned medium improves acute lung injury in mice: in vivo evidence for stem cell paracrine action. *Am J Physiol Lung Cell Mol Physiol.* 2012;303:L967–L977.

92. Nemeth K, et al. Bone marrow stromal cells attenuate sepsis via prostaglandin E(2)-dependent reprogramming of host macrophages to increase their interleukin-10 production. *Nat Med.* 2009;15:42–49.

93. Caplan AI, Correa D. The MSC: an injury drugstore. *Cell Stem Cell.* 2011;9:11–15.

94. Lee JW, Fang X, Gupta N, Serikov V, Matthay MA. Allogeneic human mesenchymal stem cells for treatment of *E. coli* endotoxin-induced acute lung injury in the ex vivo perfused human lung. *Proc Natl Acad Sci U S A.* 2009;106:16357–16362.

95. Chang YS, et al. Critical role of vascular endothelial growth factor secreted by mesenchymal stem cells in hyperoxic lung injury. *Am J Respir Cell Mol Biol.* 2014;51:391–399.

96. Thebaud B, et al. Vascular endothelial growth factor gene therapy increases survival, promotes lung angiogenesis, and prevents alveolar damage in hyperoxia-induced lung injury: evidence that angiogenesis participates in alveolarization. *Circulation.* 2005;112:2477–2486.

97. Ionescu LI, et al. Airway delivery of soluble factors from plastic-adherent bone marrow cells prevents murine asthma. *Am J Respir Cell Mol Biol.* 2012;46:207–216.

98. Block GJ, et al. Multipotent stromal cells are activated to reduce apoptosis in part by upregulation and secretion of stanniocalcin-1. *Stem Cells.* 2009;27:670–681.

99. Lee RH, et al. Intravenous hMSCs improve myocardial infarction in mice because cells embolized in lung are activated to secrete the anti-inflammatory protein TSG-6. *Cell Stem Cell.* 2009;5:54–63.

100. Waszak P, et al. Preconditioning enhances the paracrine effect of mesenchymal stem cells in preventing oxygen-induced neonatal lung injury in rats. *Stem Cells Dev.* 2012;21:2789–2797.

101. Chaput N, Thery C. Exosomes: immune properties and potential clinical implementations. *Semin Immunopathol.* 2011;33:419–440.

102. Olave N, et al. Regulation of alveolar septation by microRNA-489. *Am J Physiol Lung Cell Mol Physiol.* 2016;310:L476–L487.

103. Lee C, et al. Exosomes mediate the cytoprotective action of mesenchymal stromal cells on hypoxia-induced pulmonary hypertension. *Circulation.* 2012;126:2601–2611.

104. Sammour I, et al. The Effect of gender on mesenchymal stem cell (MSC) efficacy in neonatal hyperoxia-induced lung injury. *PLoS One.* 2016;11:e0164269.

105. Chang YS, et al. Intratracheal transplantation of human umbilical cord blood-derived mesenchymal stem cells dose-dependently attenuates hyperoxia-induced lung injury in neonatal rats. *Cell Transplant.* 2011;20:1843–1854.

106. Chang YS, et al. Mesenchymal stem cells for bronchopulmonary dysplasia: phase 1 dose-escalation clinical trial. *J Pediatr.* 2014;164:966–972.e966.

107. Ahn SY, Chang YS, Park WS. Stem cell therapy for bronchopulmonary dysplasia: bench to bedside translation. *J Korean Med Sci.* 2015;30:509–513.
108. Strueby L, Thebaud B. Mesenchymal stromal cell-based therapies for chronic lung disease of prematurity. *Am J Perinatol.* 2016;33:1043–1049.
109. Mitsialis SA, Kourembanas S. Stem cell-based therapies for the newborn lung and brain: possibilities and challenges. *Semin Perinatol.* 2016;40:138–151.
110. Mobius MA, Thebaud B. Cell therapy for bronchopulmonary dysplasia: promises and perils. *Paediatr Respir Rev.* 2016.
111. Mendicino M, Bailey AM, Wonnacott K, Puri RK, Bauer SR. MSC-based product characterization for clinical trials: an FDA perspective. *Cell Stem Cell.* 2014;14:141–145.
112. D'Angio CT, et al. Blood cytokine profiles associated with distinct patterns of bronchopulmonary dysplasia among extremely low birth weight infants. *J Pediatr.* 2016;174:45–51.e45.
113. Laughon MM, et al. Prediction of bronchopulmonary dysplasia by postnatal age in extremely premature infants. *Am J Respir Crit Care Med.* 2011;183:1715–1722.
114. Abman SH, Matthay MA. Mesenchymal stem cells for the prevention of bronchopulmonary dysplasia: delivering the secretome. *Am J Respir Crit Care Med.* 2009;180:1039–1041.
115. Ahn SY, et al. Cell type-dependent variation in paracrine potency determines therapeutic efficacy against neonatal hyperoxic lung injury. *Cytotherapy.* 2015;17:1025–1035.
116. Pierro M, et al. Short-term, long-term and paracrine effect of human umbilical cord-derived stem cells in lung injury prevention and repair in experimental bronchopulmonary dysplasia. *Thorax.* 2013;68:475–484.
117. Waszak P, et al. Preconditioning enhances the paracrine effect of mesenchymal stem cells in preventing oxygen-induced neonatal lung injury in rats. *Stem Cells Dev.* 2012;21:2789–2797.
118. Sung DK, et al. Optimal route for human umbilical cord blood-derived mesenchymal stem cell transplantation to protect against neonatal hyperoxic lung injury: gene expression profiles and histopathology. *PLoS One.* 2015;10:e0135574.
119. Rojas M, et al. Bone marrow-derived mesenchymal stem cells in repair of the injured lung. *Am J Respir Cell Mol Biol.* 2005;33:145–152.
120. Ortiz LA, et al. Mesenchymal stem cell engraftment in lung is enhanced in response to bleomycin exposure and ameliorates its fibrotic effects. *Proc Natl Acad Sci U S A.* 2003;100:8407–8411.
121. Desai TJ, Brownfield DG, Krasnow MA. Alveolar progenitor and stem cells in lung development, renewal and cancer. *Nature.* 2014;507:190–194.
122. Aslam M, et al. Bone marrow stromal cells attenuate lung injury in a murine model of neonatal chronic lung disease. *Am J Respir Crit Care Med.* 2009;180:1122–1130.
123. van Haaften T, et al. Airway delivery of mesenchymal stem cells prevents arrested alveolar growth in neonatal lung injury in rats. *Am J Respir Crit Care Med.* 2009;180:1131–1142.
124. Liu L, et al. Intranasal versus intraperitoneal delivery of human umbilical cord tissue–derived cultured mesenchymal stromal cells in a murine model of neonatal lung injury. *Am J Pathol.* 2014;184:3344–3358.

21

CHAPTER 22

A Physiology-Based Approach to the Respiratory Care of Children With Severe Bronchopulmonary Dysplasia

Leif D. Nelin, Steven H. Abman, and Howard B. Panitch

- The incidence of bronchopulmonary dysplasia (BPD) remains high, but the nature of the disease has evolved from the traditional form marked by extensive fibroproliferative changes to one of alveolar simplification and less scarring.
- There is a wide spectrum of severity of BPD; thus better definition of specific phenotypes is needed.
- BPD is associated with multiple co-morbidities, including poor growth, metabolic bone disease, aerodigestive disorders, pulmonary hypertension and neurodevelopmental impairment.
- The complex needs of these infants are quite different from those of the typical preterm infant are best served by a multidisciplinary team approach focused on BPD care.
- Many current therapies for BPD lack a solid evidence base; more research is urgently needed.

Bronchopulmonary dysplasia (BPD), the chronic lung disease of infancy that follows preterm birth, was first characterized by Northway and colleagues 50 years ago.[1] In that era, prematurity-associated lung disease contributed to high mortality (60%) in relatively late-gestation preterm infants by today's standards (32–34 weeks' gestation). Currently survival for these late preterm infants is nearly 100%, with a 94% survival of preterm infants born even at 28 weeks.[2] This remarkable success of modern care has increased survival of even the most extremely low gestational age newborns at the limits of viability (currently 22–23 weeks' gestation), which likely accounts for the persistent rate of BPD at 43% of preterm infants born before 29 weeks' gestation.[2] As a result, BPD remains the most common morbidity of preterm birth, occurring in an estimated 10,000 to 15,000 infants per year in the United States alone.[3] This has important health care implications as infants with BPD require prolonged neonatal intensive care unit (NICU) hospitalizations; are frequently readmitted during the first 2 years for respiratory infections, asthma, and related problems; and often have persistent lung function abnormalities and exercise intolerance as adolescents and young adults.

Although the overall incidence of BPD has not declined over the past decade, the nature of the disease and number of infants with severe BPD (sBPD) have changed with current clinical practice. Infants with chronic lung disease after premature birth have a different clinical course and pathology from that traditionally observed in infants dying with BPD during the pre-surfactant era.[3–6] The classic progressive stages of disease, including prominent fibroproliferative changes, that first characterized BPD are often absent now, and the disease has changed to being predominantly defined as a disruption of distal lung growth, referred to as "the new BPD."[7] The new BPD often develops in preterm newborns who may have required minimal or even no ventilator support and relatively low inspired oxygen concentrations during the

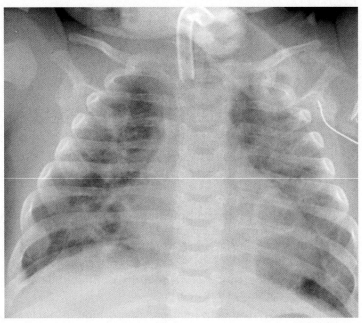

Fig. 22.1 Chest radiograph showing advanced findings of severe, ventilator-dependent bronchopulmonary dysplasia.

early postnatal days.[6,7] At autopsy, the lung histology of infants who die with the new BPD displays more uniform and milder injury, but impaired alveolar and vascular growth remain prominent. The new BPD is likely the result of disrupted antenatal and postnatal lung growth, which along with abnormalities of central and small airways, causes persistent abnormalities of lung architecture and function. Long-term pulmonary outcomes are incompletely understood, but recent work suggests a persistent high rate of abnormal lung function through late childhood continues in the post-surfactant era.[8]

Although improved care has generally led to milder respiratory courses, infants with BPD can still develop severe lung disease, as reflected by chronic respiratory failure with high mortality and related morbidities (Fig. 22.1). Ongoing clinical care and research has largely focused on issues regarding the prevention of BPD in preterm infants; however, strategies to improve care and outcomes of preterm infants in whom particularly severe disease develops remain a major challenge. The management of infants with sBPD has received less attention regarding clinical studies and interventions compared with preventive strategies, yet these infants constitute a critical population who remain at high risk for extensive morbidities and late mortality.

Therefore, the goal of this chapter is to characterize the epidemiology, pulmonary, and cardiovascular pathophysiology of sBPD, especially in ventilator-dependent infants, and to discuss therapeutic strategies for their management as based on the underlying physiology.

Definitions and Scope of Severe BPD

BPD is typically defined by the presence of chronic respiratory signs, a persistent requirement for supplemental oxygen, and an abnormal chest radiograph at 1 month of age or at 36 weeks postmenstrual age (PMA) in patients born before 32 weeks' gestation. This definition lacks specificity and fails to account for important clinical distinctions related to the extremes of prematurity and wide variability in criteria for the use of prolonged oxygen therapy. The need for supplemental oxygen at 1 month in infants born at 24 or 25 weeks' gestation may represent lung or respiratory control immaturity and not reflect the results of "lung injury," and chronic respiratory disease may or may not develop in such infants. A National Institutes of Health

(NIH)-sponsored conference in 2000 led to the current widely used definition of BPD that categorizes the severity of BPD according to the level of respiratory support required at 36 weeks PMA.[4] An advantage of this classification is that BPD is defined as a spectrum of disease with early markers that may be predictive of long-term pulmonary morbidity. Past studies suggest that this grading of BPD severity is associated with the degree of abnormal lung function during infancy[9]; however, recent studies suggest that antenatal factors are key determinants for late respiratory disease independent of the diagnosis of BPD.[10]

Another approach to determine the severity of BPD is to assess chest radiographs, but for many infants with chronic supplemental oxygen dependency, the chest radiograph demonstrates only small volumes with hazy lung fields. Various scoring systems have been developed and may predict chronic oxygen dependency and troublesome respiratory symptoms at follow-up.[11,12] Further work is clearly needed to identify early physiologic, structural, and genetic or biochemical markers of BPD, which are predictive of critical long-term endpoints, such as the presence of late respiratory disease evidenced by prolonged mechanical ventilation and oxygen therapy, recurrent hospitalizations, reactive airways disease, respiratory medications, and/or exercise intolerance during childhood.

The current NIH classification system defines "severe" BPD as the need for supplemental oxygen above a fraction of inspired oxygen (F_{IO_2}) of 0.30 with or without positive-pressure ventilation and/or continuous positive airway pressure (CPAP) at 36 weeks PMA in patients born before 32 weeks' gestation.[4] Currently data on the proportion of infants who meet these criteria are relatively limited. In addition, early respiratory deaths after the first week of life but before 36 weeks PMA may represent the most severe form of BPD, yet are not included in databases because they fail to reach the standard endpoint.

In addition, some of the most severely affected infants are those who require sustained mechanical ventilation. Although they are included in the severe classification of BPD according to NIH definitions, the proportion of infants with the most severe disease requiring high levels of respiratory support is uncertain and optimal approaches to their care are incompletely understood. This is an important issue as mortality increases with the duration of mechanical ventilation.[13] Thus a subgroup of infants with sBPD exists that can be defined by a sustained need for mechanical ventilator support at 36 weeks PMA, which has recently been labeled as "type 2 sBPD" to differentiate infants with especially severe lung disease.[3]

The limited incidence data for sBPD suggest that 16% to 30% of extremely low-birth-weight infants have sBPD. The original validation study of the NIH consensus definition of BPD found that 16% of infants born before 32 weeks and weighing less than 1000 g had sBPD (Table 22.1).[4] Two reports using birth cohorts from Scandinavia found that the incidence of sBPD was 20% to 25% in preterm infants born at or before 28 weeks.[14,15] In 2013 the Children's Hospitals Neonatal Consortium (CHNC) reported a 16% incidence of sBPD in patients born before 32 weeks, of whom the 91% who survived to discharge, 66% were discharged using supplemental oxygen, 4% required mechanical ventilation, and 5% received tracheostomy.[16] The BPD Collaborative, a network of sites with multidisciplinary care programs for sBPD, recently reported a point prevalence of sBPD of 37%, ranging from 11% to 58% across centers.[17] This same group reported that 41% of the patients born before 32 weeks' gestation with sBPD had a persistent need for ventilator support at 36 weeks PMA, or type 2 sBPD. More recently the National Heart, Lung, and Blood Institute Prematurity and Respiratory Outcomes Program (PROP), involving a cohort of 724 infants born before 29 weeks' gestational age from 6 academic U.S. centers, reported an incidence of sBPD of 30.6%; 37% of those followed through the first year had persistent respiratory disease.[18]

Few studies have examined the proportion of infants with type 2 sBPD who continue with high levels of respiratory support at and after 36 weeks PMA. In patients born before 27 weeks' gestation admitted to a level IV NICU caring exclusively for outborn infants, 22% required mechanical ventilation at 36 weeks PMA and 16% had a tracheostomy.[19] The variables associated with the need for prolonged mechanical ventilation have not been extensively examined, but in this cohort patients who

Table 22.1   VENTILATOR STRATEGIES IN BRONCHOPULMONARY DYSPLASIA

Early (prevention)	Strategies to prevent acute lung injury:
	1. Low tidal volumes (4–6 mL/kg)
	2. Short inspiratory times
	3. Increased PEEP as needed for lung recruitment without overdistention (as reflected by high peak airway pressures)
	4. Achieve lower F_{IO_2}
	Goals for gas exchange:
	1. Adjust F_{IO_2} to target lower oxygen saturations (88%–92%)
	2. Permissive hypercapnia
Late (established BPD)	Strategies for effective gas exchange:
	1. Marked regional heterogeneity:
	• Larger tidal volumes (10–12 mL/kg)
	• Longer inspiratory time ($\geq$0.6 s)
	2. Airways obstruction:
	• Slower rates allow better emptying, especially with larger tidal volumes
	• Complex roles for PEEP with dynamic airway collapse
	3. Interactive effects of vent strategies:
	• Changes in rate, tidal volume, inspiratory and expiratory times, pressure support are highly interdependent
	• Overdistention can increase agitation and paradoxically worsen ventilation
	4. Permissive hypercapnia to facilitate weaning

BPD, Bronchopulmonary dysplasia; *F_{IO_2},* fraction of inspired oxygen; *PEEP,* positive end-expiratory pressure.

required ventilation at 36 weeks were of lower birth weight and were more likely to need dopamine or insulin and to have had a fungal infection, but there was no difference in gestational age, Apgar scores at 1 and 5 minutes, age at NICU admission, indomethacin prophylaxis and/or treatment, need for patent ductus arteriosus ligation, intraventricular hemorrhage, severe intraventricular hemorrhage, or necrotizing enterocolitis between patients treated with intermittent positive-pressure ventilation at 36 weeks and those not requiring intermittent positive-pressure ventilation at 36 weeks. Thus the smaller and sicker extremely premature infants are at the highest risk for developing type 2 sBPD.

Using an estimated incidence of sBPD of 16% for infants born before 32 weeks suggests that sBPD develops in approximately 13,000 patients annually in the United States alone.[3] Epidemiologic data are limited, but estimates suggest that roughly 8000 children in the United States receive mechanical ventilation at home.[20] Based on 2011 data from the state of Pennsylvania's Ventilator Assisted Children's Home Program, 36% of ventilator-dependent children were diagnosed with chronic lung disease; 77% of these specifically had a diagnosis of sBPD.[20] From these data it can be extrapolated that approximately 2000 infants and children with sBPD are dependent on mechanical ventilation at home in the United States.

sBPD is directly linked with worse long-term outcomes, such as need for rehospitalization, need for pulmonary medications, poor neurodevelopmental outcomes, need for home ventilation, and others. In one study the incidence of cerebral palsy was 11% and 27% in those with mild and severe BPD, respectively.[9] A report of patients cared for in the Comprehensive Center for BPD at Nationwide Children's Hospital showed that 12% of patients with moderate BPD had cognitive scores on the Bayley Scales of Infant Development at 18 to 24 months below 70, whereas 15% of patients with severe BPD had cognitive scores below 70.[21]

Pathogenesis of Severe BPD

Preterm infants are especially susceptible to lung injury from mechanical ventilation, oxidative stress, and inflammation because of the extreme structural and biochemical immaturity of the preterm lung. As Northway et al. first observed, BPD has multifactorial etiologies, including hyperoxia, ventilator-induced lung injury, inflammation, and infection.[1] Animal studies suggest that lung injury caused by each of these adverse stimuli is at least partly mediated through increased oxidative stress that further augments inflammation, promotes lung injury, and impairs growth factor signaling pathways.[22,23] Antenatal factors, such as maternal smoking, chorioamnionitis, preeclampsia, and intrauterine growth restriction, are clear contributing factors to the risk for BPD and perhaps its severity.[10,18,24–29] A recent longitudinal study of 587 preterm infants born before 34 weeks found that maternal smoking increased the risk for BPD twofold and was associated with prolonged mechanical ventilation and respiratory support during the NICU stay.[10] In this study, preexisting maternal hypertension was associated with a twofold increase in odds for BPD. Further studies are needed to determine how different etiologic mechanisms alter the risk for BPD as well as its severity.

Among at-risk infants, the duration and approach to mechanical ventilation, including the use of high inspired oxygen, high peak inspiratory pressures, lower positive end-expiratory pressures, and higher ventilation rate, are also associated with BPD, relationships that could be causal or simply reflect the underlying severity of acute respiratory disease.[30] Mechanical ventilation can induce lung injury through volutrauma, in which phasic stretch or overdistention of the lung can induce lung inflammation, permeability edema, and subsequent structural changes that mimic human BPD, even in the absence of high levels of supplemental oxygen.[31,32] Aggressive mechanical ventilation with hypocarbia has been associated with the development of BPD, as reports have shown an inverse relationship between low partial pressure of carbon dioxide ($Paco_2$) levels and BPD development.[33] High tidal volumes should be avoided both during mechanical ventilation in the early stages of respiratory distress syndrome (RDS) in the NICU and during resuscitation in the delivery room.[34] Although small tidal volumes may reduce the risk for ventilator-induced lung injury in preterm infants, failure to recruit and maintain adequate functional residual capacity (FRC) even with low tidal volumes is injurious in experimental models.[35] Despite some data suggesting that alternate strategies such as nasal continuous positive airway pressure (nCPAP) and other noninvasive ventilation modes may reduce the risk for BPD, there remains striking center-to-center variability and meta-analysis has not shown uniform benefits.[36]

The association of volutrauma with the development of BPD has led to the use of strategies such as permissive hypercapnia to minimize lung injury.[37] Various ventilator devices and strategies have been assessed regarding their ability to reduce BPD. Meta-analysis of randomized trials has demonstrated that patient-triggered ventilation does not reduce the incidence of BPD but, if started in the recovery phase of RDS, it significantly shortens weaning from mechanical ventilation. The results of randomized trials of high-frequency oscillatory ventilation (HFOV) or high-frequency jet ventilation have been inconsistent.[38,39] Two large studies that incorporated prenatal steroid and surfactant replacement therapy yielded different results. In one, which restricted entry to very low-birth-weight infants with moderate to severe hypoxemic respiratory failure following surfactant administration, there was a significant benefit from HFOV of higher survival without BPD and shorter duration of ventilation.[40] No substantial benefit or adverse effects of HFOV were found in the other study, however, which randomly assigned premature infants (<29 weeks) within 1 hour of birth regardless of the degree of lung disease.[41] An explanation for those conflicting results may be that in the current era that includes the use of modified conventional ventilation strategies, pulmonary benefit from HFOV may be demonstrable only in infants with moderate to severe disease. Clearly, the strategies applied for either conventional or HFOV are more important than the device itself. HFOV is frequently used as "rescue" therapy in premature newborns with severe respiratory failure despite treatment with exogenous surfactant and conventional ventilation. Whether such an approach reduces the risk to develop BPD or improves long-term outcomes requires additional investigation.

An optimal ventilation mode has not yet emerged to prevent BPD, but it is clear from physiologic studies that tidal volumes and inspired oxygen concentrations should be reduced as low as possible to avoid hypocarbia, volutrauma, and oxygen toxicity, while applying strategies to optimize lung recruitment. Two meta-analyses suggest that volume-targeted ventilation reduces the duration of mechanical ventilation and significantly reduces the incidence of BPD.[42,43] An alternative approach to reduce the risk of developing BPD has been to avoid intubation and mechanical ventilation by using early nCPAP. For example the Surfactant, Positive Pressure, and Oxygenation Randomized Trial (SUPPORT) found that patients who received early CPAP without intubation and surfactant therapy had decreased need for intubation or postnatal corticosteroids for BPD, required fewer days of mechanical ventilation, and were more likely to be alive and free from the need for mechanical ventilation by 7 days of age.[44] Many centers now minimize their use of mechanical ventilation, preferring nCPAP with or without administration of exogenous surfactant, and report low incidences of BPD in high-risk infants. Because the risk for BPD is associated with the need for mechanical ventilation and centers that use less mechanical ventilation have a lower incidence of BPD, avoiding or minimizing mechanical ventilation during the early course of extreme prematurity may prevent BPD or lessen its severity. As discussed later, however, ventilator strategies during the early stages of respiratory distress are strikingly different from approaches needed to optimize gas exchange and treat chronic respiratory failure in the setting of established BPD.

Pathophysiology of Severe BPD

Respiratory Function

Multiple abnormalities of lung structure and function contribute to late respiratory disease in BPD. Chronic respiratory signs in children with moderate and severe BPD include tachypnea with shallow breathing, retractions, and paradoxical breathing pattern; coarse rhonchi, rales, and wheezes are typically heard on auscultation. The increased respiratory rate and shallow breathing increase dead-space ventilation. Nonuniform damage to the airways and distal lungs results in variable time constants for different areas of the lungs, and inspired gas may be distributed to relatively poorly perfused lung, thereby worsening ventilation-perfusion matching. Decreased lung compliance appears to correlate strongly with morphologic and radiographic changes in the lung. Dynamic lung compliance is markedly reduced in infants with established BPD, even in those who no longer require oxygen therapy.[45] The reduction in dynamic compliance is due to small airway narrowing, interstitial fibrosis, edema, and atelectasis.

Newer mechanical ventilation strategies have resulted in less central airway damage in infants with the new BPD, but significant tracheomalacia and abnormalities of conducting airway structure persist in the current era. Increases in airway smooth muscle have been found within the first month of life in infants with BPD,[46,47] and epithelial cell height was found to be greater than in controls.[47] The combination of smooth muscle hypertrophy and thickened airway walls, together with fewer alveolar wall attachments supporting small airway patency, predispose BPD infants to increased airway resistance, which can be demonstrated even during the first week after birth in preterm neonates at risk for BPD.[48] Although there is not complete agreement among various studies, most have demonstrated that pulmonary or respiratory system resistance is elevated within the first 2 weeks in those ventilator-dependent infants in whom BPD subsequently develops compared with those in whom BPD does not develop.[48–52] This abnormality in lung mechanics persists: older infants with BPD have been found to have an increased total respiratory and expiratory resistance with severe flow limitation, especially at low lung volumes.[51]

The presence of tracheobronchomalacia may also result in airflow limitation. It is important for the clinician to recognize this entity, because the airflow limitation is worsened by bronchodilator therapy.[53] The presence of tracheobronchomalacia in BPD infants has been associated with longer courses of mechanical ventilation, longer NICU stays, and more complicated NICU courses.[54] In the early stages the functional lung volume is often reduced as the result of atelectasis, but during the later stages of BPD there is gas trapping with hyperinflation.[49,50,55] The use of pulmonary function testing to follow the progression of BPD and the response to therapeutic interventions has increased but is still not commonly applied in the clinical setting owing to the technical challenges, expense, and need for sedation.

Although the new BPD has been characterized as an arrest of distal lung and vascular growth, most of these observations were based on lung histology and evidence was lacking that provided direct physiologic data to support this finding. Balinotti and colleagues have demonstrated reduced lung surface area in infants with BPD by using novel methods of assessing diffusion capacity.[56] Thus established BPD is primarily characterized by reduced surface area and heterogeneous lung units, in which regional variations in airway resistance and tissue compliance lead to highly variable time constants throughout the lung.[57] As a result, mechanical ventilation of infants with sBPD requires strikingly different ventilator strategies from those commonly used early in infants with RDS to prevent BPD. Strategies for severe BPD generally favor longer inspiratory times, larger tidal volumes, higher positive end-expiratory pressure (PEEP), and lower rates to allow more effective gas exchange and respiratory function.

Lung Mechanics in Severe BPD

Diverse methods have been used to assess lung mechanics in infants with established BPD during tidal breathing. These include measurements of dynamic resistance and compliance of the lung with the use of esophageal pressure catheters; single- and multiple-breath occlusion for measuring respiratory system resistance and compliance; plethysmography measurement of airway resistance; interrupter and forced oscillation methods for measuring respiratory system resistance; and weighted spirometry. Airway obstruction has also been determined from respiratory inductive plethysmography measurements of phase-angle differences in chest wall and abdominal dimensions. These approaches have been reviewed in detail.[58,59] Normalized measures of both static and dynamic lung compliance are reduced in established BPD. This may be due to fibrosis, atelectasis, changes in parenchyma and airway properties, or diminished coupling between lung parenchyma and airways owing to edema.[60]

Past studies have reported increased airway resistance in infants with established BPD.[49,50,61,62] Specific compliance and conductance generally improve over the first 2 to 3 years of life. However, concerns persist regarding limitations of infant pulmonary function testing, especially for routine clinical use. Measures of compliance and resistance can be variable as these values are generally determined over a limited tidal volume range and are dependent on the lung volume at which these measurements are made; thus hyperinflation will be associated with lower lung or respiratory system compliance. Additionally, in BPD patients with airway obstruction, measurements of dynamic compliance are markedly affected by respiratory rate (e.g., "frequency dependence") because of the heterogeneity of time constants of regional lung units. This heterogeneity is reflected in the substantial curvilinearity of the passive expiratory flow-volume curve obtained by the single-breath occlusion method in infants with BPD. Jarriel et al. have pointed out that respiratory system mechanics in these patients are much better characterized by a "two-compartment" rather than a linear "one-compartment" model (see below).[57] The abnormalities in compliance and especially resistance in BPD infants significantly alter how the lung fills and empties; the respiratory system time constant of 24 BPD infants mechanically ventilated for 38 ± 4 days increased from 0.14 ± 0.01 seconds at 10 to 20 days of life to 0.33 ± 0.02 seconds at 6 months, 0.48 ± 0.03 seconds at 1 year, and 0.50 ± 0.03 seconds at 2 years ($p < .0001$).[49]

Lung Volumes in Severe BPD

FRC has been measured in infants with BPD by body plethysmography and with nitrogen washout and gas dilution methods.[58] In contrast to plethysmography, washout and gas dilution methods measure only gas that communicates with the conducting airways during tidal breathing. These measurements may underestimate the actual lung volume at FRC because they do not measure volumes of gas trapped behind closed airways and can underestimate volumes in severely obstructed poorly ventilated areas.[63-66] Measurements before 1 year of age using gas dilution and washout methods have consistently reported reduced FRC in infants with both old and new BPD.[49,61,64,65] In contrast, plethysmography studies have demonstrated normal or elevated FRC values.[67,68] Reductions in gas dilution and nitrogen washout measurements of FRC probably reflect the amount of noncommunicating trapped gas not measured in infants with obstructive disease rather than being indicative of a true restrictive defect. Reduction in the difference between the two methods is probably indicative of improvements in airway function, less gas trapping, and better gas exchange.[55] Thus functional abnormalities in infants with severe BPD are primarily obstructive rather than restrictive, but precise measurements are especially complicated in severe disease because of heterogeneity of airway and lung parenchymal abnormalities.

Recently the use of the raised volume rapid thoracic compression method for performing spirometry in sedated infants has provided an alternative approach to measure fractional lung volumes, including total lung capacity (TLC) and residual volume (RV).[69] Robin et al. have reported the results of fractional lung volume measurements in 28 patients with new BPD.[68] Mean RV and RV/TLC ratio were found to be significantly elevated in infants with BPD compared with normal control infants while mean TLC was in the normal range. In contrast, FRC as measured by plethysmography was found to be only marginally elevated compared to the normal control infants. In addition, TLC continued to increase over the second year of life in infants with BPD, yet the severity of air trapping, as reflected by the RV/TLC ratio, remained unchanged.[69] Thus infants with the new BPD have obstructive airway disease with gas trapping that persists over time and is strikingly abnormal in severe BPD.

Forced Flows in Severe BPD

Measurements of forced flows have been made in infants with BPD using the rapid thoracic compression (RTC) method to produce partial flow-volume curves over the tidal range and the forced deflation and raised volume rapid thoracic compression techniques to produce forced expiratory flows over the full vital capacity range. The use of these tests in infants with BPD has been reviewed and guidelines for the two RTC methods have been published.[70,71] The RTC technique to produce partial expiratory flow volume curves was applied to infants with BPD, demonstrating that average maximal flows measured at FRC ($V'max_{FRC}$) were reduced by approximately 50% when compared to normal infants.[67] A reduction in $V'max_{FRC}$ in infants with BPD has been a consistent finding in subsequent studies, and longitudinal measurements over the first 2 years of life demonstrated very modest increases in absolute flows in individual infants with BPD who often do not keep pace with the expected rate of increase with growth.[45] On average, the rate of increase for infants with BPD was substantially below that measured in normal infants over the same interval. Thus at follow-up, measurements of $V'max_{FRC}$ in the infants with BPD had fallen even farther below those measured in normal infants. Reduction in forced flow can also reflect severity of the underlying disease: toddlers with BPD still dependent on supplemental oxygen use after 2 years of age had significantly lower volume-corrected forced flows ($V'max_{FRC/FRC}$) than those BPD toddlers who were weaned from supplemental oxygen.

Lung Imaging in Severe BPD

The chest radiographic characteristics of infants with BPD have changed substantially since the original description by Northway et al.[1] Although the chest radiograph of BPD as classically described is still seen in infants with severe disease, radiographic changes in smaller, less mature infants with new BPD are much more variable and are often characterized by irregularly distributed areas of fine infiltrates and mild hyperlucency. Chest radiographs often underestimate and correlate poorly with the extent of the pathologic changes in infants with established BPD.[72,73] High-resolution computed tomography (HRCT) is a more sensitive technique for detecting structural abnormalities in the lungs of patients with established BPD than plain chest radiography (Fig. 22.2).[74,75] Correlations between abnormalities seen on HRCT and measures of lung function and clinical severity suggest that HRCT may be useful in clinical management and as an outcome measure in this population. CT imaging is helpful for identifying unsuspected abnormalities in the lungs of individual patients with BPD, but its ultimate utility as a tool for clinical management and as an outcome measure for research investigations is not yet clear. Radiation exposure from CT imaging is substantially greater than that received from standard chest radiographs.[76] Through the development of novel scanning algorithms,

Age 6 months   Age 14 months   Age 23 months

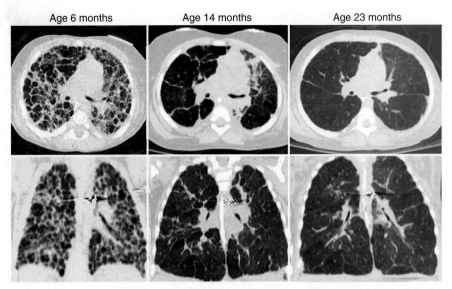

Fig. 22.2   High-resolution computed tomography (HRCT) scans done at 25 cm H_2O during a breath-hold in the same patient with severe bronchopulmonary dysplasia at three different ages. The *top row* shows transverse sections and the *bottom row* shows coronal sections from the same area. These scans demonstrate that despite ongoing mechanical ventilator support with lung growth and repair the findings on HRCT improve over time, although the scan at 23 months of age remains abnormal.

however, the radiation exposure from CT imaging has been greatly reduced,[77–79] such that in cystic fibrosis diagnostic HRCT can be done at a radiation dose similar to that of a chest radiograph, and similar algorithm development is ongoing for patients with BPD.

The Cardiovascular System in Severe BPD

Acute lung injury impairs growth, structure, and function of the developing pulmonary circulation after premature birth.[80,81] Endothelial cells are particularly susceptible to oxidant injury owing to hyperoxia or inflammation. The media of small pulmonary arteries may also undergo striking changes, including smooth muscle cell proliferation, precocious maturation of immature pericytes into mature smooth muscle cells, and incorporation of fibroblasts into the vessel wall and surrounding adventitia.[82] Structural changes in the lung vasculature contribute to high pulmonary vascular resistance (PVR) caused by narrowing of the vessel diameter and decreased vascular compliance. Decreased angiogenesis may limit vascular surface area, causing further elevations of PVR, especially in response to high cardiac output with exercise or stress. The pulmonary circulation in BPD patients is further characterized by abnormal vasoreactivity, which also increases PVR.[81] Abnormal pulmonary vasoreactivity is evidenced by a marked vasoconstrictor response to acute hypoxia.[81,82] Cardiac catheterization studies have shown that even mild hypoxia causes marked elevations in pulmonary artery pressure, even in infants with modest basal levels of pulmonary hypertension (PH). Maintaining oxygen saturation levels above 92% to 94% effectively lowers the pulmonary artery pressure.[81] Strategies to lower pulmonary artery pressure or to minimize lung injury to the pulmonary vasculature may limit the subsequent development of PH in BPD.

Early injury to the lung circulation leads to the rapid development of PH, which contributes significantly to the morbidity and mortality of severe BPD. Even in early reports of BPD, PH, and cor pulmonale were recognized as being associated with high mortality.[83,84] Persistent echocardiographic evidence of PH beyond the first few months has been associated with up to 40% mortality in infants with BPD.[85] High mortality rates have also been reported in infants with BPD and severe PH, especially in those who require prolonged ventilator support.[81,85] In addition to the adverse effects of PH on the clinical course of infants with BPD, the lung circulation is further characterized by persistence of abnormal or "dysmorphic" growth of the pulmonary circulation, including a relative paucity of small pulmonary arteries with an altered pattern of distribution within the interstitium of the distal lung.[86-88] In infants with severe BPD, decreased vascular growth occurs in conjunction with marked reductions in alveoli, suggesting that the new BPD is primarily characterized by growth arrest of the developing lung. This reduction of alveolar-capillary surface area impairs gas exchange—thereby increasing the need for prolonged supplemental oxygen and ventilator therapy, causing marked hypoxemia with acute respiratory infections and late exercise intolerance—and further increases the risk for developing severe PH. Experimental studies have further shown that early injury to the developing lung can impair angiogenesis,[89-91] which further contributes to decreased alveolarization and simplification of distal lung air space (the "vascular hypothesis"[87]). Thus abnormalities of the lung circulation in BPD are not only related to the presence or absence of PH, but more broadly, pulmonary vascular disease after premature birth as manifested by decreased vascular growth and structure also contributes to the pathogenesis and abnormal cardiopulmonary physiology of BPD.

A recently emerging cause of PH in patients with BPD is pulmonary vein stenosis (PVS).[92-94] Mahgoub et al.[93] described 39 former preterm infants with a median gestational age of 28 weeks and a median birth weight of 1100 g with PVS; 74% of these infants had BPD. In their cohort, freedom from death or restenosis was 73% at 1 year and 55% at 2 years. Another retrospective review of 213 patients with sBPD found that 5% had PVS with a survival to discharge of 50% compared with 86% survival of sBPD patients with PH without PVS.[92]

In addition to pulmonary vascular disease and right ventricular hypertrophy, other cardiovascular abnormalities associated with BPD include left ventricular hypertrophy, systemic hypertension, and the development of prominent systemic-to-pulmonary collateral vessels.[95,96] Infants with sBPD can develop left ventricular hypertrophy in the absence of right ventricular hypertrophy. Systemic hypertension in BPD may be mild, transient, or striking and usually responds to medication. Left ventricular diastolic dysfunction can contribute to lung edema, diuretic dependency, and PH in some infants with BPD.[97] In addition, atrial septal defects commonly complicate the course of infants with BPD and have variable contributions to underlying disease severity. Prominent bronchial or other systemic-to-pulmonary collateral vessels were noted in early morphometric studies of infants with BPD and can be readily identified in many infants during cardiac catheterization. Although these collateral vessels are generally small, large collaterals may contribute to significant shunting of blood flow to the lung, resulting in edema and the need for higher levels of supplemental oxygen. Collateral vessels have been associated with high mortality in some patients with both sBPD and PH. Some infants have improved after embolization of large collateral vessels, as reflected by a reduced need for supplemental oxygen, ventilator support, or diuretics. The contribution of collateral vessels to the pathophysiology of BPD, however, is poorly understood.

Evaluation and Treatment of Severe BPD

A general evaluation and treatment for infants with significant BPD is described in the following text (see Table 22.1). An important consideration in the treatment of sBPD is that recovery from this disease will be relatively slow—months to years rather than days to weeks. Therefore patience is required when caring for these patients with complicated conditions. In other words, management of infants with severe BPD requires a chronic care model, which is strikingly different in philosophy and treatment goals from the approach used in the acute care model that is generally followed in the NICU. This approach includes strategies for weaning from mechanical ventilation, assessing the need for chronic ventilator support, the role of tracheostomy, and related issues.

Supplemental oxygen remains a mainstay of therapy for infants with BPD, yet the most appropriate target for oxygen saturation levels remains controversial. Growing concern regarding the adverse effects of even moderate levels of oxygen therapy has led many neonatologists to accept oxygen saturations below 85% to 90% early after the birth of preterm newborns. However, it should also be kept in mind that patients with established sBPD are usually beyond 36 weeks PGA, past the time when retinopathy of prematurity is a major concern. Prolonged monitoring of oxygenation while infants are awake, asleep, and during feedings to ensure the avoidance of hypoxemia is necessary while adjusting oxygen therapy. In those infants with established sBPD, we recommend targeting oxygen saturation above 94% to provide more consistent treatment of underlying PH, to minimize lability and cyanotic episodes, and to enhance growth.

In most NICUs, nCPAP and/or high-flow nasal cannula (HFNC) are used to maintain adequate oxygenation and ventilation while avoiding the need for prolonged ventilation or reintubation for ventilator support. Whereas several studies have examined the role of early nCPAP in lieu of endotracheal intubation during the first week after birth, there are no studies regarding benefits of the prolonged use of nCPAP in established BPD with chronic respiratory failure. Although nCPAP may provide adequate support, in some infants with BPD, signs of severe respiratory distress persist despite nCPAP or HFNC therapy, including marked dyspnea, head-bobbing, retractions, tachypnea, intermittent cyanosis and carbon dioxide retention. These infants may benefit from reintubation and considerations of tracheostomy for chronic ventilator support if subsequent attempts at weaning are not successful. The timing and patient selection for tracheostomy and commitment to more prolonged ventilator support varies widely between centers.[98] Tracheostomy and chronic ventilator support may provide a stable airway to allow for more effective ventilation and less respiratory distress, and to enhance cardiopulmonary function as reflected by lower oxygen requirements and less PH. Greater respiratory stability often improves tolerance of respiratory treatments, physical therapies, and handling by staff and family members, thereby improving maternal-infant interactions and neurodevelopmental outcomes. Successful management of chronic ventilator–dependent children requires well-organized, multidisciplinary teams to address the complexity of issues.[3,21]

Mechanical Ventilation

In contrast to a low–tidal volume and high-PEEP approach to acute RDS for minimizing acute lung injury, most clinicians favor a strategy of larger tidal volumes delivered at slower rates with longer inspiratory and expiratory times in sBPD (Box 22.1). This strategy is directly related to the striking differences in lung physiology that characterize infants with established BPD from newborns with acute respiratory failure. Striking heterogeneity of lung disease, characterized by marked regional variability in time constants, provides the physiologic rationale for this strategy in

---

Box 22.1   GENERAL TREATMENT STRATEGIES FOR SEVERE BRONCHOPULMONARY DYSPLASIA

- Family-centered chronic care model
- Focus on neurodevelopment:
    - Optimize pulmonary status/respiratory support
    - Long-term ventilator settings
    - Consider need for tracheostomy if long-term mechanical ventilation is necessary
    - Optimize oxygenation, targeting SpO_2 at 92%–95%
    - Use short courses of diuretics to treat episodes of pulmonary edema
    - Treat airway reactivity with inhaled bronchodilators and/or inhaled steroids
    - Reserve systemic steroids for acute deteriorations
- Pulmonary hypertension:
    - Avoid hypoxemia
    - Use inhaled nitric oxide for short-term therapy
    - Treatment will need to be long-term; sildenafil most studied
    - If response to sildenafil alone is poor, consider adding bosentan and/or prostacyclin
    - Determine need for cardiac catheterization (see text)
- Nutritional status:
    - Optimize nutrition: fluid restriction with high–caloric density feeds
- Gastroesophageal reflux:
    - Medical management
    - Consider surgical management if severe or unresponsive to medical management

SpO₂, Oxygen saturation measured by pulse oximetry.

established BPD for improving the distribution of ventilation, minimizing physiologic dead space and gas trapping, and improving gas exchange. This represents a distinct change in strategy from the higher rates and lower tidal volumes commonly used early in the course of respiratory distress in the premature infant. However, no objective studies have been published to substantiate this approach. The overall goal of this ventilator strategy is to provide support while preventing complications and optimizing lung growth and recovery for patients with the most severe form of BPD—that is, those patients who continue to require intermittent positive-pressure ventilation) many weeks into their initial hospitalization.

Ventilation with larger tidal volumes and increased inspiratory times often improves the distribution of ventilation while minimizing dead-space ventilation (Fig. 22.3). This strategy can reduce chronic retractions and respiratory distress and

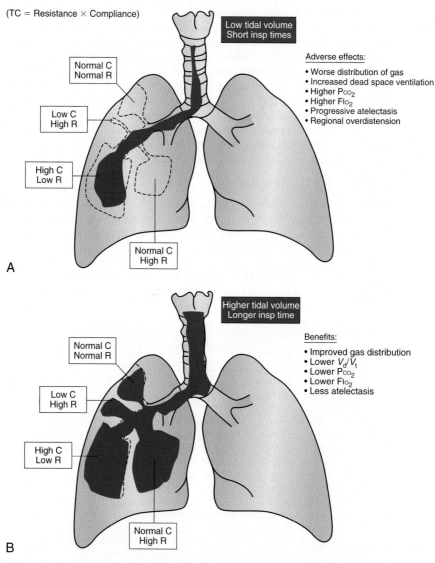

HETEROGENEITY OF LUNG DISEASE IN ESTABLISHED BPD: ROLE OF VARIABLE TIME CONSTANTS

(TC = Resistance × Compliance)

Low tidal volume Short insp times

Normal C
Normal R

Low C
High R

High C
Low R

Normal C
High R

Adverse effects:
- Worse distribution of gas
- Increased dead space ventilation
- Higher P_{CO_2}
- Higher F_{IO_2}
- Progressive atelectasis
- Regional overdistension

A

Higher tidal volume Longer insp time

Normal C
Normal R

Low C
High R

High C
Low R

Normal C
High R

Benefits:
- Improved gas distribution
- Lower V_d/V_t
- Lower P_{CO_2}
- Lower F_{IO_2}
- Less atelectasis

B

Fig. 22.3 Theoretical effects of mechanical ventilator strategies for severe bronchopulmonary dysplasia *(BPD)*. As illustrated in A, small tidal volume breaths often increase dead-space ventilation, leading to atelectasis, hypercapnia, and high oxygen requirements in the setting of heterogeneous lung disease in severe BPD. Increased tidal volumes and inspiratory times may enhance distribution of gas, leading to lower oxygen requirements, improved ventilation, and less atelectasis (B). *C,* Compliance; *FIO₂,* fraction of inspired oxygen; *PCO₂,* partial pressure of carbon dioxide; *R,* resistance; *TC,* time constant; *Vd/Vt,* dead-space ventilation/total ventilation.

may decrease recurrent cyanotic spells in some patients. However, hyperinflation is typically present in severe, ventilator-dependent BPD. As a result, the patient is breathing on a relatively flat portion of the pressure-volume loop, such that generating large pressures results in only small changes in tidal volumes. Furthermore, lung hyperinflation will increase PVR owing to compression of the alveolar vessels. Thus hyperinflation of the lung worsens not only lung mechanics, but also ventilation-perfusion matching and pulmonary hemodynamics. To effectively reduce hyperinflation in sBPD, strategies must also allow for adequate time for exhalation to allow the lungs to empty with relatively lower ventilator rates and increased expiratory times. Therefore slower rates are needed to accommodate increases in tidal volume and inspiratory time, thus allowing adequate expiratory time and avoiding gas trapping, inadvertent PEEP, and dynamic hyperinflation (Fig. 22.4). Requirements for PEEP are highly variable among ventilator-dependent BPD infants but are generally higher than in the acute phase of RDS. Infants with sBPD often have evidence of tracheomalacia or bronchomalacia, for which increased PEEP will decrease central airway closure (Fig. 22.5).[99–102] However, high PEEP can complicate gas trapping and will not be tolerated without sufficient expiratory times and low ventilator rates. In some infants with BPD, the combination of marked alteration in lung mechanics and increase in respiratory drive results in dynamic hyperinflation and intrinsic PEEP even with a large tidal volume–low mandatory rate strategy. When identified, increasing the set PEEP to at least 80% of the intrinsic PEEP can improve the infant's ability to trigger the ventilator, thereby enhancing patient-ventilator synchrony and reducing the infant's respiratory work.

As discussed earlier, patients with type 2 sBPD are likely to have either a prolonged need for mechanical ventilation or marginal respiratory status on less invasive forms of support such as HFNC or CPAP, thus necessitating a tracheostomy. Indeed, the BPD Collaborative reported a point prevalence of tracheostomy in sBPD of 12%,[17] and the CHNC reported that 13.5% of patients with sBPD underwent

Dynamic hyperinflation in severe BPD

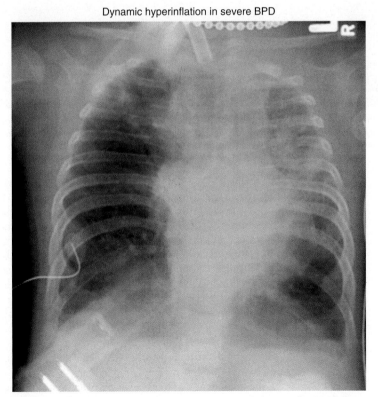

Fig. 22.4 Chest radiograph demonstrating marked gas trapping and dynamic hyperinflation in severe bronchopulmonary dysplasia (BPD).

BRONCHOGRAM/PEEP STUDY

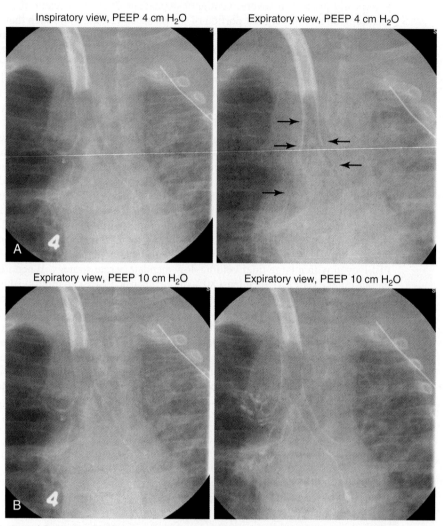

Fig. 22.5 Bronchogram studies for assessing effects of positive end-expiratory pressure *(PEEP)* on central airways caliber. As shown on A, low PEEP support is associated with small airway diameter on expiration and expiratory airway closure (marked by *arrows*). Higher PEEP appears to reduce airway closure.

tracheostomy placement.[98] There are no data or evidence of efficacy regarding the optimal timing of tracheostomy in infants with sBPD. Furthermore, the majority of NICU providers equate tracheostomy with a poor outcome.[98] Interestingly, in adult ICU care, early tracheostomy, defined as performed at 10 days or earlier, is associated with lower mortality and increased likelihood of discharge from the ICU at 28 days compared with late tracheostomy.[103] Similar conclusions have been reached in pediatric ICU care.[104] Furthermore, in a review of the Neonatal Research Network database involving 304 infants who underwent tracheostomy among a group of 8683 preterm neonates followed to 18 to 22 months corrected age, the risk of death or neurodevelopmental impairment was less in those who underwent tracheostomy placement before versus after 120 days.[105] This leads us to wonder if "earlier" tracheostomy would improve survival, neurodevelopmental outcome, and/or time to discharge from the hospital for patients with sBPD in the NICU, as suggested by retrospective studies from one center.[106,107]

In one study, the median age at tracheostomy placement in patients with sBPD was 46 weeks postmenstrual age (interquartile range 43–52 weeks).[98] As the majority of patients with sBPD are born before 28 weeks, these findings suggest that patients may be ventilated with an endotracheal tube for extended time periods, perhaps as long as 6 or 7 months, or require repeated reintubations in the NICU. These relatively long times will likely have adverse effects on neurodevelopment given that sedation is frequently used for intubated patients, developmental and oral skills are difficult to advance with an endotracheal tube in place, and restraints often have to be applied to prevent the infant from unplanned self-extubations.[108] Furthermore, patients with less than optimal support while being treated with HFNC or CPAP often have difficulty interacting with their environment and therefore developing normally. A recent report on mortality in pediatric tracheostomy patients found that BPD was an independent predictor of mortality.[109] Lee et al.,[110] however, reported that in infants with tracheostomies, survivors had a lower postnatal age and PGA at the time of tracheostomy than did nonsurvivors.

Tracheostomy placement is obviously a difficult and complicated decision, and it should be viewed as a means for delivering sustained respiratory support to relieve respiratory distress and provide the respiratory stability necessary to optimize neurodevelopmental outcomes in the subset of sBPD patients requiring continued mechanical ventilation. The optimal timing of tracheostomy placement remains to be determined; however, we suggest that if a patient born before 28 weeks remains on continuous mechanical ventilatory support through 40 weeks, discussions about tracheostomy should begin with the parents realizing that it will likely take several weeks to reach a definitive decision on tracheostomy. However, as recently noted, an often-overlooked issue in such studies or in clinical practice is that the placement of a tracheostomy alone is not sufficient for the overall optimization of care through interdisciplinary teams and critical approaches to ventilator and overall management (see later text).[3,106]

The contribution of gastroesophageal reflux (GER) in sBPD remains controversial. Patients with sBPD should be evaluated for GER with radiologic studies (barium swallow studies, upper gastrointestinal series), pH or impedance probes, and/or swallow studies. Because GER with chronic aspiration may contribute to ongoing lung injury, we recommend considering gastrostomy with fundoplication in this fragile group of infants owing to the high morbidity and mortality related to sBPD. Many would also recommend gastrostomy and fundoplication in the setting of sBPD that is failing to improve if clinical suspicion remains high in the face of negative studies. Jadcherla et al. recently reported that GER may cause symptoms in BPD even without the refluxate reaching the pharynx, and that the likelihood of symptoms was related to the clearance time of the acid refluxate.[111] These findings suggest that medical treatment of GER may improve symptoms in patients with BPD.

Drug Therapies

Multiple pharmacologic therapies have been used in the management of BPD, including diuretics, bronchodilators, and steroids. In most cases, despite observations suggesting acute improvement with many of these interventions, data are limited regarding long-term safety and efficacy of many drugs used in infants with BPD.

Diuretics can improve lung compliance and airway resistance by reducing pulmonary edema. Two Cochrane reviews assessed the effects of loop diuretics (furosemide) and those acting on the distal renal tubule (thiazides and spironolactone) for preventing or treating BPD in preterm infants.[112,113] A small study suggested that furosemide (1 mg/kg every 12 hours intravenously or 2 mg/kg every 12 hours orally) can increase weaning from the ventilator when compared with placebo.[114] Aerosolized furosemide can acutely improve lung mechanics, but data are lacking regarding its chronic use.[115] Furosemide has beneficial effects that are independent of its diuretic properties; it induces prostaglandin formation from renal and vascular endothelium that results directly in vasodilation, promoting a shift of fluid from alveoli to the venous compartment.[116] Thiazides and spironolactone can improve lung function, but this has not been a consistent finding.[117,118] The use of alternate-day furosemide may sustain improvements in lung function while minimizing risks for electrolyte imbalance and nephrocalcinosis.[119] Although diuretics generally cause short-term improvements of lung compliance, there is little evidence of sustained reduction in ventilator support, length of hospital stay, or other long-term outcomes. The need for chronic diuretic use may reflect a contribution of left ventricular diastolic dysfunction to recurrent pulmonary edema.[97]

Infants with BPD have airway smooth muscle hypertrophy and often have signs of bronchial hyperreactivity that acutely improves with bronchodilator therapy, but response rates are variable.[120–122] Data showing long-term benefit of bronchodilators, including β-agonists and anticholinergic agents, for the prevention or treatment of BPD are lacking.[122] In addition to their roles in apnea, aminophylline and caffeine can reduce airway resistance in infants with BPD and may have an additive effect with diuretics. Methylxanthines can improve weaning of infants from mechanical ventilation,[123] but jitteriness, seizures, and GER are known side effects.

Corticosteroid therapy, primarily directed at reducing lung inflammation, is one of the most controversial areas of BPD care.[124,125] The use of systemic corticosteroids to prevent BPD early in the course of care of preterm infants is currently discouraged by the American Academy of Pediatrics because of adverse effects on neurodevelopment.[126] In established BPD, corticosteroids are generally used to reduce lung inflammation. The side effects of poor head growth and neurocognitive outcomes with early and prolonged high-dose strategies are unacceptable risks for preterm infants at risk for BPD. However, steroid bursts (e.g., prednisone 1–2 mg/kg per day for 3–5 days) may be helpful in the management of infants with sBPD with acute deteriorations of lung function. Although commonly used in infants with asthma, inhaled steroids have not consistently shown improvement in lung function in BPD.[127] However, two small studies have shown that inhaled steroids can improve the rate of successful extubation and reduce the need for systemic steroids.[128,129] Fluticasone propionate is a more potent steroid, but when given by inhalation was associated with only one positive effect, a lower chest radiograph score, while also associated with the negative effect of a higher systolic blood pressure.[130] Intriguingly, older children and adolescents with BPD and a history of recurrent wheezing do not demonstrate elevated markers of eosinophilic inflammation[131] or experience bronchospasm in response to mast cell stimulation,[132] making the role of inhaled corticosteroid therapy in these patients less certain.

Treatment of Pulmonary Hypertension

Recommendations for the evaluation and care of PH-associated BPD have recently been published.[133] The initial clinical strategy for the management of PH in infants with BPD begins with treating the underlying lung disease, including an extensive evaluation for chronic reflux and aspiration, structural airway abnormalities (such as tonsillar and adenoidal hypertrophy, vocal cord paralysis, subglottic stenosis, tracheomalacia, and other lesions); assessments of bronchial reactivity; improving lung edema and airway function; or any other intervening factors. Periods of acute hypoxemia, whether intermittent or prolonged, can often contribute to late PH in BPD. A sleep study may be necessary to determine the presence of noteworthy episodes of hypoxemia and whether hypoxemia has predominantly obstructive, central, or mixed causes. Additional studies that may be required include flexible bronchoscopy for the diagnosis of anatomic and dynamic airway lesions (such as tracheomalacia) that can contribute to hypoxemia and poor clinical responses to oxygen therapy. Upper gastrointestinal series, pH or impedance probe, and swallow studies may be indicated to evaluate for GER and aspiration that can contribute to ongoing lung injury. For patients with BPD and severe PH who are unable to maintain near-normal ventilation or require high levels of F_{IO_2} despite conservative treatment, strong consideration should be given to chronic mechanical ventilatory support in an attempt to halt progression of PH (Box 22.2).

Despite the growing use of pulmonary vasodilator therapy for the treatment of PH in BPD, data demonstrating efficacy are extremely limited, and the use of these agents should only follow thorough diagnostic evaluations and aggressive management of the underlying lung disease. We strongly encourage cardiac catheterization before initiation of chronic pulmonary vasodilator therapy. Current therapies used for PH therapy in infants with BPD generally include inhaled nitric oxide (iNO), sildenafil, endothelin-receptor antagonists (ETRAs), and calcium channel blockers (CCBs).

Box 22.2   PULMONARY HYPERTENSION IN SEVERE BRONCHOPULMONARY DYSPLASIA

- Screening echocardiography:
  - Septal flattening, tricuspid regurgitant jet velocity, cor pulmonale
- If no pulmonary hypertension, perform echocardiography every 1–2 months until significant improvement in respiratory status
- If pulmonary hypertension/cor pulmonale present:
  - Optimize respiratory support, avoid hypoxemia
  - Start inhaled nitric oxide at 20 ppm
- Switch to sildenafil:
  - Start at 0.5 mg/kg q8h and advance as needed to 2 mg/kg q6h if no systemic hypotension
  - Wean patient from inhaled nitric oxide
- If unable to wean patient from inhaled nitric oxide:
  - Continue inhaled nitric oxide and sildenafil or consider endothelin receptor antagonist or prostacyclin analog
- Cardiac catheterization:
  - Evaluate pulmonary hemodynamics, left heart function, presence of pulmonary vein stenosis, aortopulmonary collaterals, and response to acute vasodilator challenge

22

Note that if PVS is an important contributor to PH in the patient with sBPD, these vasodilators will either have little effect or could worsen the patient's clinical status, underscoring the importance of cardiac catheterization before initiation of vasodilator therapy. CCBs (such as nifedipine) benefit some patients with PH, and short-term effects of CCBs in infants with BPD have been reported.[134] In comparison with a study of acute iNO reactivity in infants with BPD, the acute response to CCBs was poor and systemic hypotension developed in some infants.[135]

In general, we use sildenafil or bosentan (an ETRA) for chronic therapy of PH in infants with BPD. Sildenafil, a highly selective type 5 phosphodiesterase inhibitor, augments cyclic guanosine monophosphate content in vascular smooth muscle, and has been shown to benefit adults with PH as monotherapy and in combination with standard treatment regimens.[136] In a study of 25 infants with chronic lung disease and PH (18 with BPD), prolonged sildenafil therapy as part of an aggressive program to treat PH was associated with improvement in PH by echocardiogram in most (88%) patients without significant rates of adverse events.[137] Although the time to improvement was variable, many patients were able to be weaned from mechanical ventilator support and other PH therapies, especially iNO, during the course of sildenafil treatment without worsening of PH. The recommended starting dose for sildenafil is 0.5 mg/kg per dose every 8 hours. If there is no evidence of systemic hypotension, this dose can be gradually increased over 2 weeks to achieve the desired pulmonary hemodynamic effect or a maximum of 2 mg/kg per dose every 6 to 8 hours. Other agents, such as ETRAs and prostacyclin analogs, are sometimes used in infants who are unable to respond to other approaches, but data on their dosage, safety, and efficacy in this population are largely lacking.

Interdisciplinary Care

Severe BPD is associated with poor nutrition and neurodevelopmental outcomes and increased family stress. Therefore optimal care of infants with established BPD should include a multidisciplinary team, consisting of neonatologists, pulmonologists, respiratory therapists, nutritionists, occupational therapists, speech therapists, physical therapists, social workers, and others.[3] It is imperative to involve the family in the interdisciplinary care of the patient with established BPD early in the hospitalization to improve the family's comfort with the disease process. This family-centered care will hasten discharge home, decrease the need for rehospitalization, and improve family dynamics. Regular team meetings should occur throughout the NICU course, not simply at the time of discharge.

Nutritional care is critical not only to maintain growth for the patient but also to foster lung healing and repair. We recommend displaying a growth chart at the bedside of patients hospitalized with established BPD to facilitate the daily assessment of nutritional needs. The goal should be 15 to 20 g/kg per day for infants younger than 37 weeks PGA and 20 to 30 g/day for infants 37 weeks PGA or older. These patients are often fluid restricted; however, they usually require 120 to 150 kcal/kg per day to achieve adequate growth and lung repair, such that high caloric density feedings are required. Whenever possible, the mother's own breast milk should be used in these patients, even if it needs to be heavily fortified.

In patients with established BPD, neurodevelopmental assessments and care are of marked benefit toward optimizing care.[3,21] Consultation and application of behavioral interventions are often important factors in many aspects of the care plan, including the decision regarding the need for placement of a tracheostomy for chronic mechanical ventilation. Patients with sBPD treated with long-term nasal CPAP or those who have persistent distress and recurrent cyanotic episodes with less invasive respiratory support will not be able to interact well with the environment or work on motor skills. Intensive neurodevelopmental care for patients with established BPD should include developmental therapies 3 to 5 times a week while they are hospitalized. These developmental treatments should focus on creating an age-appropriate sensory and social environment. A formal neurodevelopmental assessment should be carried out at approximately 40 weeks PMA; therapies are directed at improving areas of developmental delay. Behavioral aspects of nursing care and routine handling can minimize the frequency or severity of recurrent cyanotic episodes and irritability with agitation. Noxious stimuli should be minimized in these patients (e.g., arterial or heel sticks), and opioids and sedatives should be used with caution.

Long-Term Outcomes

There are limited data examining the long-term respiratory outcomes of patients with sBPD. A study of 86 survivors of extreme preterm birth (<1000 g or gestational age ≤28 weeks) at 10 or 18 years of age found significantly higher HRCT scores as well as more opacities and hypoattenuated areas in subjects with a history of moderate or severe BPD than in those with a history of no or mild BPD.[138] Similarly, Wong et al.[139] described abnormal HRCT scans with emphysematous changes in 19 subjects aged 17 to 33 years who were born with birth weights less than 1500 g between 1980 and 1987 with the diagnosis of moderate-to-severe BPD; the abnormal CT scans were correlated with abnormalities in pulmonary function. Thus there is evidence that sBPD is associated with lifelong changes in pulmonary structure and function.[140] However, more studies are needed to accurately determine the long-term course of premature neonates with sBPD and their relative contribution to the growing adult population with chronic obstructive pulmonary disease.

REFERENCES

1. Northway WH Jr, Rosan RC, Porter DY. Pulmonary disease following respirator therapy of hyaline-membrane disease. Bronchopulmonary dysplasia. *New Eng J Med.* 1967;276:357–368.
2. Stoll BJ, Hansen NI, Bell EF, et al. Trends in care practices, morbidity, and mortality of extremely preterm neonates, 1993–2012. *JAMA.* 2015;314:1039–1051.
3. Abman SH, Collaco JM, Shepherd EG, Keszler M, Cuevas-Guaman M, et al. Bronchopulmonary dysplasia C. Interdisciplinary care of children with severe bronchopulmonary dysplasia. *J Pediatr.* 2017;181:12 e11–28 e11.
4. Jobe AH, Bancalari E. Bronchopulmonary dysplasia. *Am J Respir Crit Care Med.* 2001;163:1723–1729.
5. Rojas MA, Gonzalez A, Bancalari E, Claure N, Poole C, Silva-Neto G. Changing trends in the epidemiology and pathogenesis of neonatal chronic lung disease. *J Pediatr.* 1995;126:605–610.
6. Charafeddine L, D'Angio CT, Phelps DL. Atypical chronic lung disease patterns in neonates. *Pediatrics.* 1999;103:759–765.
7. Jobe AH. The new bronchopulmonary dysplasia. *Curr Opin Pediatr.* 2011;23:167–172.
8. Doyle LW, Carse E, Adams AM, Ranganathan S, Opie G, Cheong JLY. Ventilation in extremely preterm infants and respiratory function at 8 years. *New Eng J Med.* 2017;377:329–337.
9. Ehrenkranz RA, Walsh MC, Vohr BR, et al. Validation of the National Institutes of Health consensus definition of bronchopulmonary dysplasia. *Pediatrics.* 2005;116:1353–1360.

22

10. Morrow LA, Wagner BD, Ingram DA, et al. Antenatal determinants of bronchopulmonary dysplasia and late respiratory disease in preterm infants. *Am J Respir Crit Care Med.* 2017;196:364–374.

11. Laughon MM, Langer JC, Bose CL, et al. Prediction of bronchopulmonary dysplasia by postnatal age in extremely premature infants. *Am J Respir Crit Care Med.* 2011;183:1715–1722.

12. Isayama T, Lee SK, Yang J, et al. Revisiting the definition of bronchopulmonary dysplasia: effect of changing panoply of respiratory support for preterm neonates. *JAMA Pediatr.* 2017;171:271–279.

13. Walsh MC, Morris BH, Wrage LA, et al. Extremely low birthweight neonates with protracted ventilation:mortality and 18-month neurodevelopmental outcomes. *J Pediatr.* 2005;146:798–804.

14. EXPRESS Group. Incidence of and risk factors for neonatal morbidity after active perinatal care: extremely preterm infants study in Sweden (EXPRESS). *Acta Paediatr.* 2010;99:978–992.

15. Farstad T, Bratlid D, Medbo S, Markestad T. Bronchopulmonary dysplasia—prevalence, severity and predictive factors in a national cohort of extremely premature infants. *Acta Paediatr.* 2011;100:53–58.

16. Padula MA, Grover TR, Brozanski B, et al. Therapeutic interventions and short-term outcomes for infants with severe bronchopulmonary dysplasia born at <32 weeks' gestation. *J Perinatol.* 2013;33:877–881.

17. Guaman MC, Gien J, Baker CD, Zhang H, Austin ED, Collaco JM. Point prevalence, clinical characteristics, and treatment variation for infants with severe bronchopulmonary dysplasia. *Am J Perinatol.* 2015;32:960–967.

18. Keller RL, Feng R, DeMauro SB, et al. Bronchopulmonary dysplasia and perinatal characteristics predict 1-year respiratory outcomes in newborns born at extremely low gestational age: a prospective cohort study. *J Pediatr.* 2017;187:89–97.e83.

19. Yossef L, Shepherd, EG, Lynch S, Reber KM, Nelin LD. Factors associated with long-term mechanical ventilation in extremely preterm infants. *J Neonatal Perinatal Med.*, in press

20. Boroughs D, Dougherty JA. Decreasing accidental mortality of ventilator-dependent children at home:a call to action. *Home Healthc Nurse.* 2012;30:103–111;quiz 112–103.

21. Shepherd EG, Knupp AM, Welty SE, Susey KM, Gardner WP, Gest AL. An interdisciplinary bronchopulmonary dysplasia program is associated with improved neurodevelopmental outcomes and fewer rehospitalizations. *J Perinatol.* 2012;32:33–38.

22. Delaney C, Wright RH, Tang JR, et al. Lack of EC-SOD worsens alveolar and vascular development in a neonatal mouse model of bleomycin-induced bronchopulmonary dysplasia and pulmonary hypertension. *Pediatr Res.* 2015;78:634–640.

23. Salaets T, Richter J, Brady P, et al. Transcriptome analysis of the preterm rabbit lung after seven days of hyperoxic exposure. *PLoS One.* 2015;10:e0136569.

24. Reiss I, Landmann E, Heckmann M, Misselwitz B, Gortner L. Increased risk of bronchopulmonary dysplasia and increased mortality in very preterm infants being small for gestational age. *Arch Gynecol Obstetr.* 2003;269:40–44.

25. Van Marter LJ, Leviton A, Kuban KC, Pagano M, Allred EN. Maternal glucocorticoid therapy and reduced risk of bronchopulmonary dysplasia. *Pediatrics.* 1990;86:331–336.

26. Zeitlin J, El Ayoubi M, Jarreau PH, et al. Impact of fetal growth restriction on mortality and morbidity in a very preterm birth cohort. *J Pediatr.* 2010;157:733–739.e731.

27. Bose C, Van Marter LJ, Laughon M, et al. Fetal growth restriction and chronic lung disease among infants born before the 28th week of gestation. *Pediatrics.* 2009;124:e450–e458.

28. Lee HJ, Kim EK, Kim HS, Choi CW, Kim BI, Choi JH. Chorioamnionitis, respiratory distress syndrome and bronchopulmonary dysplasia in extremely low birth weight infants. *J Perinatol.* 2011;31:166–170.

29. Hansen AR, Barnes CM, Folkman J, McElrath TF. Maternal preeclampsia predicts the development of bronchopulmonary dysplasia. *J Pediatr.* 2010;156:532–536.

30. Keszler M. Mechanical ventilation strategies. *Semin Fetal Neonatal Med.* 2017;22:267–274.

31. Deptula N, Royse E, Kemp MW, et al. Brief mechanical ventilation causes differential epithelial repair along the airways of fetal, preterm lambs. *Am J Physiol Lung Cell Mol Physiol.* 2016;311:L412–L420.

32. Hillman NH, Polglase GR, Pillow JJ, Saito M, Kallapur SG, Jobe AH. Inflammation and lung maturation from stretch injury in preterm fetal sheep. *Am J Physiol Lung Cell Mol Physiol.* 2011;300:L232–L241.

33. Garland JS, Buck RK, Allred EN, Leviton A. Hypocarbia before surfactant therapy appears to increase bronchopulmonary dysplasia risk in infants with respiratory distress syndrome. *Arch Pediatr Adolesc Med.* 1995;149:617–622.

34. Keszler M, Sant'Anna G. Mechanical ventilation and bronchopulmonary dysplasia. *Clin Perinatol.* 2015;42:781–796.

35. Tingay DG, Lavizzari A, Zonneveld CE, et al. An individualized approach to sustained inflation duration at birth improves outcomes in newborn preterm lambs. *Am J Physiol Lung Cell Mol Physiol.* 2015;309:L1138–L1149.

36. Isayama T, Iwami H, McDonald S, Beyene J. Association of noninvasive ventilation strategies with mortality and bronchopulmonary dysplasia among preterm infants: a systematic review and meta-analysis. *JAMA.* 2016;316:611–624.

37. Ryu J, Haddad G, Carlo WA. Clinical effectiveness and safety of permissive hypercapnia. *Clin Perinatol.* 2012;39:603–612.

38. Cools F, Offringa M, Askie LM. Elective high frequency oscillatory ventilation versus conventional ventilation for acute pulmonary dysfunction in preterm infants. *Cochrane Database Syst Rev.* 2015:CD000104.

39. Rojas-Reyes MX, Orrego-Rojas PA. Rescue high-frequency jet ventilation versus conventional ventilation for severe pulmonary dysfunction in preterm infants. *Cochrane Database Syst Rev.* 2015: CD000437.

40. Courtney SE, Durand DJ, Asselin JM, Hudak ML, Aschner JL, Shoemaker CT. High-frequency oscillatory ventilation versus conventional mechanical ventilation for very-low-birth-weight infants. *New Eng J Med.* 2002;347:643–652.

41. Johnson AH, Peacock JL, Greenough A, et al. High-frequency oscillatory ventilation for the prevention of chronic lung disease of prematurity. *New Eng J Med.* 2002;347:633–642.

42. Peng W, Zhu H, Shi H, Liu E. Volume-targeted ventilation is more suitable than pressure-limited ventilation for preterm infants: a systematic review and meta-analysis. *Arch Dis Child Fetal Neonatal Ed.* 2014;99:F158–F165.

43. Wheeler K, Klingenberg C, McCallion N, Morley CJ, Davis PG. Volume-targeted versus pressure-limited ventilation in the neonate. *Cochrane Database Syst Rev.* 2010:CD003666.

44. Finer NN, Carlo WA, Walsh MC, et al. Early CPAP versus surfactant in extremely preterm infants. *N Engl J Med.* 2010;362:1970–1979.

45. Thunqvist P, Gustafsson P, Norman M, Wickman M, Hallberg J. Lung function at 6 and 18 months after preterm birth in relation to severity of bronchopulmonary dysplasia. *Pediatr Pulmonol.* 2015;50:978–986.

46. Sward-Comunelli SL, Mabry SM, Truog WE, Thibeault DW. Airway muscle in preterm infants:changes during development. *J Pediatr.* 1997;130:570–576.

47. Tiddens HA, Hofhuis W, Casotti V, Hop WC, Hulsmann AR, de Jongste JC. Airway dimensions in bronchopulmonary dysplasia: implications for airflow obstruction. *Pediatr Pulmonol.* 2008;43:1206–1213.

48. Goldman SL, Gerhardt T, Sonni R, et al. Early prediction of chronic lung disease by pulmonary function testing. *J Pediatr.* 1983;102:613–617.

49. Baraldi E, Filippone M, Trevisanuto D, Zanardo V, Zacchello F. Pulmonary function until two years of life in infants with bronchopulmonary dysplasia. *Am J Respir Crit Care Med.* 1997;155:149–155.

50. Gerhardt T, Hehre D, Feller R, Reifenberg L, Bancalari E. Serial determination of pulmonary function in infants with chronic lung disease. *J Pediatr.* 1987;110:448–456.

51. Lui K, Lloyd J, Ang E, Rynn M, Gupta JM. Early changes in respiratory compliance and resistance during the development of bronchopulmonary dysplasia in the era of surfactant therapy. *Pediatr Pulmonol.* 2000;30:282–290.

52. Van Lierde S, Smith J, Devlieger H, Eggermont E. Pulmonary mechanics during respiratory distress syndrome in the prediction of outcome and differentiation of mild and severe bronchopulmonary dysplasia. *Pediatr Pulmonol.* 1994;17:218–224.

53. Panitch HB, Keklikian EN, Motley RA, Wolfson MR, Schidlow DV. Effect of altering smooth muscle tone on maximal expiratory flows in patients with tracheomalacia. *Pediatri Pulmonol.* 1990;9:170–176.

54. Hysinger EB, Friedman NL, Padula MA, et al. Tracheobronchomalacia is associated with increased morbidity in bronchopulmonary dysplasia. *Ann Am Thor Soc.* 2017.

55. Wauer RR, Maurer T, Nowotny T, Schmalisch G. Assessment of functional residual capacity using nitrogen washout and plethysmographic techniques in infants with and without bronchopulmonary dysplasia. *Intensive Care Med.* 1998;24:469–475.

56. Balinotti JE, Tiller CJ, Llapur CJ, et al. Growth of the lung parenchyma early in life. *Am J Respir Crit Care Med.* 2009;179:134–137.

57. Jarriel WS, Richardson P, Knapp RD, Hansen TN. A nonlinear regression analysis of nonlinear, passive-deflation flow-volume plots. *Pediatr Pulmonol.* 1993;15:175–182.

58. Gappa M, Pillow JJ, Allen J, Mayer O, Stocks J. Lung function tests in neonates and infants with chronic lung disease: lung and chest-wall mechanics. *Pediatr Pulmonol.* 2006;41:291–317.

59. Tepper RS, Pagtakhan RD, Taussig LM. Noninvasive determination of total respiratory system compliance in infants by the weighted-spirometer method. *Am Rev Respir Dis.* 1984;130:461–466.

60. Adams EW, Harrison MC, Counsell SJ, et al. Increased lung water and tissue damage in bronchopulmonary dysplasia. *J Pediatr.* 2004;145:503–507.

61. Moriette G, Gaudebout C, Clement A, et al. Pulmonary function at 1 year of age in survivors of neonatal respiratory distress: a multivariate analysis of factors associated with sequelae. *Pediatr Pulmonol.* 1987;3:242–250.

62. Farstad T, Brockmeier F, Bratlid D. Cardiopulmonary function in premature infants with bronchopulmonary dysplasia—a 2-year follow up. *Eur J Pediatr.* 1995;154:853–858.

63. Mead J. Contribution of compliance of airways to frequency-dependent behavior of lungs. *J Appl Physiol.* 1969;26:670–673.

64. Hulskamp G, Pillow JJ, Dinger J, Stocks J. Lung function tests in neonates and infants with chronic lung disease of infancy: functional residual capacity. *Pediatr Pulmonol.* 2006;41:1–22.

65. Stocks J, Godfrey S, Beardsmore C, Bar-Yishay E, Castile R. Plethysmographic measurements of lung volume and airway resistance. ERS/ATS Task Force on Standards for Infant Respiratory Function Testing. European Respiratory Society/American Thoracic Society. *Eur Respir J.* 2001; 17:302–312.

66. Morris MG, Gustafsson P, Tepper R, Gappa M, Stocks J. The bias flow nitrogen washout technique for measuring the functional residual capacity in infants. ERS/ATS Task Force on Standards for Infant Respiratory Function Testing. *Eur Respir J.* 2001;17:529–536.

67. Hofhuis W, Huysman MW, van der Wiel EC, et al. Worsening of V'maxFRC in infants with chronic lung disease in the first year of life: a more favorable outcome after high-frequency oscillation ventilation. *Am J Respir Crit Care Med.* 2002;166:1539–1543.

68. Robin B, Kim YJ, Huth J, et al. Pulmonary function in bronchopulmonary dysplasia. *Pediatr Pulmonol.* 2004;37:236–242.

69. Filbrun AG, Popova AP, Linn MJ, McIntosh NA, Hershenson MB. Longitudinal measures of lung function in infants with bronchopulmonary dysplasia. *Pediatr Pulmonol.* 2011;46:369–375.

70. Lum S, Hulskamp G, Merkus P, Baraldi E, Hofhuis W, Stocks J. Lung function tests in neonates and infants with chronic lung disease: forced expiratory maneuvers. *Pediatr Pulmonol.* 2006;41:199–214.

71. Sly PD, Tepper R, Henschen M, Gappa M, Stocks J. Tidal forced expirations. ERS/ATS Task Force on Standards for Infant Respiratory Function Testing. European Respiratory Society/American Thoracic Society. *Eur Respir J.* 2000;16:741–748.

72. Oppermann HC, Wille L, Bleyl U, Obladen M. Bronchopulmonary dysplasia in premature infants. A radiological and pathological correlation. *Pediatr Radiol.* 1977;5:137–141.

73. Edwards DK, Colby TV, Northway WH Jr. Radiographic-pathologic correlation in bronchopulmonary dysplasia. *J Pediatr.* 1979;95:834–836.

74. Mahut B, De Blic J, Emond S, et al. Chest computed tomography findings in bronchopulmonary dysplasia and correlation with lung function. *Arch Dis Child Fetal Neonatal Ed.* 2007;92:F459–F464.

75. Kubota J, Ohki Y, Inoue T, et al. Ultrafast CT scoring system for assessing bronchopulmonary dysplasia:reproducibility and clinical correlation. *Radiat Med.* 1998;16:167–174.

76. Raman P, Raman R, Newman B, Venkatraman R, Raman B, Robinson TE. Development and validation of automated 2D–3D bronchial airway matching to track changes in regional bronchial morphology using serial low-dose chest CT scans in children with chronic lung disease. *J Digit Imaging.* 2010;23:744–754.

77. de Jong PA, Long FR, Nakano Y. Computed tomography dose and variability of airway dimension measurements: how low can we go? *Pediatr Radiol.* 2006;36:1043–1047.

78. Long FR. High-resolution computed tomography of the lung in children with cystic fibrosis: technical factors. *Proc Am Thorac Soc.* 2007;4:306–309.

79. de Gonzalez AB, Kim KP, Samet JM. Radiation-induced cancer risk from annual computed tomography for patients with cystic fibrosis. *Am J Respir Crit Care Med.* 2007;176:970–973.

80. Abman SH. Pulmonary hypertension in chronic lung disease of infancy. Pathogenesis, pathophysiology, and treatment. In: Bland RD, Coalson JJ, eds. *Chronic Lung Disease of Infancy.* New York: Marcel Dekker; 2000:619–668.

81. Parker TA, Abman SH. The pulmonary circulation in bronchopulmonary dysplasia. *Semin Neonatol.* 2003;8:51–61.

82. Tomashefski Jr JF, Oppermann HC, Vawter GF, Reid LM. Bronchopulmonary dysplasia: a morphometric study with emphasis on the pulmonary vasculature. *Pediatr Pathol.* 1984;2:469–487.

83. Halliday HL, Dumpit FM, Brady JP. Effects of inspired oxygen on echocardiographic assessment of pulmonary vascular resistance and myocardial contractility in bronchopulmonary dysplasia. *Pediatr.* 1980;65:536–540.

84. Gorenflo M, Vogel M, Obladen M. Pulmonary vascular changes in bronchopulmonary dysplasia: a clinicopathologic correlation in short- and long-term survivors. *Pediatr Pathol.* 1991;11:851–866.

85. Khemani E, McElhinney DB, Rhein L, et al. Pulmonary artery hypertension in formerly premature infants with bronchopulmonary dysplasia: clinical features and outcomes in the surfactant era. *Pediatrics.* 2007;120:1260–1269.

86. Bhatt AJ, Pryhuber GS, Huyck H, Watkins RH, Metlay LA, Maniscalco WM. Disrupted pulmonary vasculature and decreased vascular endothelial growth factor, Flt-1, and TIE-2 in human infants dying with bronchopulmonary dysplasia. *Am J Respir Crit Care Med.* 2001;164:1971–1980.

87. Abman SH. Bronchopulmonary dysplasia: "a vascular hypothesis." *Am J Respir Crit Care Med.* 2001;164:1755–1756.

88. De Paepe ME, Mao Q, Powell J, et al. Growth of pulmonary microvasculature in ventilated preterm infants. *Am J Respir Crit Care Med.* 2006;173:204–211.

89. Jakkula M, Le Cras TD, Gebb S, et al. Inhibition of angiogenesis decreases alveolarization in the developing rat lung. *Am J Physiol Lung Cell Mol Physiol.* 2000;279:L600–L607.

90. Menon RT, Shrestha AK, Shivanna B. Hyperoxia exposure disrupts adrenomedullin signaling in newborn mice: implications for lung development in premature infants. *Biochem Biophys Res Commun.* 2017;487:666–671.

91. Perveen S, Patel H, Arif A, Younis S, Codipilly CN, Ahmed M. Role of EC-SOD overexpression in preserving pulmonary angiogenesis inhibited by oxidative stress. *PLoS One.* 2012;7:e51945.

92. Swier NL, Richards B, Cua CL, et al. Pulmonary vein stenosis in neonates with severe bronchopulmonary dysplasia. *Am J Perinatol.* 2016;33:671–677.

93. Mahgoub L, Kaddoura T, Kameny AR, et al. Pulmonary vein stenosis of ex-premature infants with pulmonary hypertension and bronchopulmonary dysplasia, epidemiology, and survival from a multicenter cohort. *Pediatr Pulmonol.* 2017;52:1063–1070.

94. Drossner DM, Kim DW, Maher KO, Mahle WT. Pulmonary vein stenosis: prematurity and associated conditions. *Pediatrics.* 2008;122:e656–e661.

95. Abman SH, Warady BA, Lum GM, Koops BL. Systemic hypertension in infants with bronchopulmonary dysplasia. *J Pediatr.* 1984;104:928–931.

96. Anderson AH, Warady BA, Daily DK, Johnson JA, Thomas MK. Systemic hypertension in infants with severe bronchopulmonary dysplasia: associated clinical factors. *Am J Perinatol.* 1993;10:190–193.

97. Mourani PM, Ivy DD, Rosenberg AA, Fagan TE, Abman SH. Left ventricular diastolic dysfunction in bronchopulmonary dysplasia. *J Pediatr.* 2008;152:291–293.

98. Murthy K, Porta NFM, Lagatta JM, et al. Inter-center variation in death or tracheostomy placement in infants with severe bronchopulmonary dysplasia. *J Perinatol.* 2017;37:723–727.

99. Davis S, Jones M, Kisling J, Angelicchio C, Tepper RS. Effect of continuous positive airway pressure on forced expiratory flows in infants with tracheomalacia. *Am J Respir Crit Care Med.* 1998;158:148–152.

100. Doull IJ, Mok Q, Tasker RC. Tracheobronchomalacia in preterm infants with chronic lung disease. *Arch Dis Child Fetal Neonatal Ed.* 1997;76:F203–F205.

101. McCoy KS, Bagwell CE, Wagner M, Sallent J, O'Keefe M, Kosch PC. Spirometric and endoscopic evaluation of airway collapse in infants with bronchopulmonary dysplasia. *Pediatr Pulmonol.* 1992;14:23–27.

102. Panitch HB, Allen JL, Alpert BE, Schidlow DV. Effects of CPAP on lung mechanics in infants with acquired tracheobronchomalacia. *Am J Respir Crit Care Med.* 1994;150:1341–1346.

103. Andriolo BN, Andriolo RB, Saconato H, Atallah AN, Valente O. Early versus late tracheostomy for critically ill patients. *Cochrane Database Syst Rev.* 2015;1:CD007271.

104. Holloway AJ, Spaeder MC, Basu S. Association of timing of tracheostomy on clinical outcomes in PICU patients. *Pediatr Crit Care Med.* 2015;16:e52–e58.

105. DeMauro SB, D'Agostino JA, Bann C, et al. Developmental outcomes of very preterm infants with tracheostomies. *J Pediatr.* 2014;164:1303–1310.e1302.

106. Gien J, Kinsella J, Thrasher J, Grenolds A, Abman SH, Baker CD. Retrospective analysis of an interdisciplinary ventilator care program intervention on survival of infants with ventilator-dependent bronchopulmonary dysplasia. *Am J Perinatol.* 2017;34:155–163.

107. Baker CD, Martin S, Thrasher J, et al. Standardized discharge process decreases length of stay for ventilator-dependent children. *Pediatrics.* 2016;137.

108. DeMauro SB, Wei JL, Lin RJ. Perspectives on neonatal and infant tracheostomy. *Semin Fetal Neonatal Med.* 2016;21:285–291.

109. Funamura JL, Yuen S, Kawai K, et al. Characterizing mortality in pediatric tracheostomy patients. *Laryngoscope.* 2017;127:1701–1706.

110. Lee JH, Smith PB, Quek MB, Laughon MM, Clark RH, Hornik CP. Risk factors and in-hospital outcomes following tracheostomy in infants. *J Pediatr.* 2016;173:39–44.e31.

111. Jadcherla SR, Gupta A, Fernandez S, et al. Spatiotemporal characteristics of acid refluxate and relationship to symptoms in premature and term infants with chronic lung disease. *Am J Gastroenterol.* 2008;103:720–728.

112. Brion LP, Primhak RA, Ambrosio-Perez I. Diuretics acting on the distal renal tubule for preterm infants with (or developing) chronic lung disease. *Cochrane Database Syst Rev.* 2002:CD001817.

113. Brion LP, Primhak RA. Intravenous or enteral loop diuretics for preterm infants with (or developing) chronic lung disease. *Cochrane Database Syst Rev.* 2002:CD001453.

114. McCann EM, Lewis K, Deming DD, Donovan MJ, Brady JP. Controlled trial of furosemide therapy in infants with chronic lung disease. *J Pediatr.* 1985;106:957–962.

115. Brion LP, Primhak RA, Yong W. Aerosolized diuretics for preterm infants with (or developing) chronic lung disease. *Cochrane Database Syst Rev.* 2006:CD001694.

116. Cotton R, Suarez S, Reese J. Unexpected extra-renal effects of loop diuretics in the preterm neonate. *Acta Paediatr.* 2012;101:835–845.

117. Kao LC, Warburton D, Cheng MH, Cedeno C, Platzker AC, Keens TG. Effect of oral diuretics on pulmonary mechanics in infants with chronic bronchopulmonary dysplasia: results of a double-blind crossover sequential trial. *Pediatrics.* 1984;74:37–44.

118. Engelhardt B, Blalock WA, DonLevy S, Rush M, Hazinski TA. Effect of spironolactone-hydrochlorothiazide on lung function in infants with chronic bronchopulmonary dysplasia. *J Pediatr.* 1989;114:619–624.

119. Rush MG, Engelhardt B, Parker RA, Hazinski TA. Double-blind, placebo-controlled trial of alternate-day furosemide therapy in infants with chronic bronchopulmonary dysplasia. *J Pediatr.* 1990;117:112–118.

120. Sosulski R, Abbasi S, Bhutani VK, Fox WW. Physiologic effects of terbutaline on pulmonary function of infants with bronchopulmonary dysplasia. *Pediatr Pulmonol.* 1986;2:269–273.

121. Wilkie RA, Bryan MH. Effect of bronchodilators on airway resistance in ventilator-dependent neonates with chronic lung disease. *J Pediatr.* 1987;111:278–282.

122. Clouse BJ, Jadcherla SR, Slaughter JL. Systematic review of inhaled bronchodilator and corticosteroid therapies in infants with bronchopulmonary dysplasia: implications and future directions. *PLoS One.* 2016;11:e0148188.

123. Henderson-Smart DJ, Davis PG. Prophylactic methylxanthines for extubation in preterm infants. *Cochrane Database Syst Rev.* 2003:CD000139.

124. Doyle LW, Ehrenkranz RA, Halliday HL. Early (<8 days) postnatal corticosteroids for preventing chronic lung disease in preterm infants. *Cochrane Database Syst Rev.* 2014:CD001146.

125. Doyle LW, Ehrenkranz RA, Halliday HL. Late (>7 days) postnatal corticosteroids for chronic lung disease in preterm infants. *Cochrane Database Syst Rev.* 2014:CD001145.

126. Watterberg KL. Policy statement—postnatal corticosteroids to prevent or treat bronchopulmonary dysplasia. *Pediatrics.* 2010;126:800–808.

127. Shah SS, Ohlsson A, Halliday HL, Shah VS. Inhaled versus systemic corticosteroids for the treatment of chronic lung disease in ventilated very low birth weight preterm infants. *Cochrane Database Syst Rev.* 2012:CD002057.

128. Cole CH, Colton T, Shah BL, et al. Early inhaled glucocorticoid therapy to prevent bronchopulmonary dysplasia. *N Engl J Med.* 1999;340:1005–1010.

129. Jonsson B, Eriksson M, Soder O, Broberger U, Lagercrantz H. Budesonide delivered by dosimetric jet nebulization to preterm very low birthweight infants at high risk for development of chronic lung disease. *Acta Paediatr.* 2000;89:1449–1455.

130. Dugas MA, Nguyen D, Frenette L, et al. Fluticasone inhalation in moderate cases of bronchopulmonary dysplasia. *Pediatrics.* 2005;115:e566–e572.

131. Halvorsen T, Skadberg BT, Eide GE, Roksund O, Aksnes L, Oymar K. Characteristics of asthma and airway hyper-responsiveness after premature birth. *Pediatr Allergy Immunol.* 2005;16:487–494.

132. Kim DK, Choi SH, Yu J, Yoo Y, Kim B, Koh YY. Bronchial responsiveness to methacholine and adenosine 5′-monophosphate in preschool children with bronchopulmonary dysplasia. *Pediatric pulmonology.* 2006;41:538–543.

133. Krishnan U, Feinstein JA, Adatia I, et al. Evaluation and management of pulmonary hypertension in children with bronchopulmonary dysplasia. *J Pediatr.* 2017;188:24–34.e21.

134. Johnson CE, Beekman RH, Kostyshak DA, Nguyen T, Oh DM, Amidon GL. Pharmacokinetics and pharmacodynamics of nifedipine in children with bronchopulmonary dysplasia and pulmonary hypertension. *Pediatr Res.* 1991;29:500–503.

135. Mourani PM, Ivy DD, Gao D, Abman SH. Pulmonary vascular effects of inhaled nitric oxide and oxygen tension in bronchopulmonary dysplasia. *Am J Respir Crit Care Med.* 2004;170:1006–1013.

136. Galie N, Ghofrani HA, Torbicki A, et al. Sildenafil citrate therapy for pulmonary arterial hypertension. *N Engl J Med.* 2005;353:2148–2157.

137. Mourani PM, Sontag MK, Ivy DD, Abman SH. Effects of long-term sildenafil treatment for pulmonary hypertension in infants with chronic lung disease. *J Pediatr.* 2009;154:379–384, 384 e371–e372.

138. Aukland SM, Rosendahl K, Owens CM, Fosse KR, Eide GE, Halvorsen T. Neonatal bronchopulmonary dysplasia predicts abnormal pulmonary HRCT scans in long-term survivors of extreme preterm birth. *Thorax.* 2009;64:405–410.

139. Wong PM, Lees AN, Louw J, et al. Emphysema in young adult survivors of moderate-to-severe bronchopulmonary dysplasia. *Eur Respir J.* 2008;32:321–328.

140. Islam JY, Keller RL, Aschner JL, Hartert TV, Moore PE. Understanding the short- and long-term respiratory outcomes of prematurity and bronchopulmonary dysplasia. *Am J Respir Crit Care Med.* 2015;192:134–156.

22

Index

A

ABCA3. *see* Adenosine triphosphate-binding
    cassette transporter 3
Acidosis, effect of, 296–297
Acinetobacter species
    in lung microbiome, 98
    ventilator-assisted pneumonia and, 153
Actinobacteria, in lung microbiome, 98–99, 99f
Adaptive mechanical backup ventilation, 325
Adenosine triphosphate-binding cassette
    transporter 3 (ABCA3), 13
Adolescence, pulmonary function in, 165–166,
    165t
Adult stem cells, 348
Adulthood, early, pulmonary function in,
    165–166, 165t
AEC1. *see* Alveolar type 1 epithelial cells
AEC2. *see* Alveolar type 2 epithelial cells
Aerosolization, 223, 223t
Aerosolized steroids
    postnatal, 342
    prenatal, 343
Air leaks, infant-ventilator asynchrony and, 271
Airway
    candidate stem cells, in cell-based therapy, 350
    devices, 176–177
    epithelial lineages, development of, 13
    laryngeal mask, 182–183, 182t
        delivery of surfactant by, 224
Alcohol abuse, maternal, lung development
    and, 57
Alveogenesis
    elastin deposition in, 11–12, 12f
    myofibroblast differentiation in, 11–13, 12f
    regulatory mechanisms of, 11–13, 11f–12f
Alveolar candidate stem cells, in cell-based
    therapy, 350–351
Alveolar capillary dysplasia, 78
Alveolar macrophage, 50
Alveolar septation, 11–12
Alveolar stage, of lung development, 10, 11f
Alveolar type 1 epithelial cells (AEC1), 350
Alveolar type 2 epithelial cells (AEC2), 349t
Alveolocapillary barrier, 3
Angiogenesis, 13–14
    in severe bronchopulmonary dysplasia, 371
Angiopoietins (Ang), 15
Antenatal corticosteroids, 335–339
    in current population, 336–337

Antenatal corticosteroids *(Continued)*
    historical overview of, 335–336
    mechanism of action, on fetal lungs, 336
    non-randomized controlled trial for,
        337–338, 337f–338f
    PDA and, 132
        BPD risk, 135
    randomized controlled trials for, 336–337, 337t
Antenatal ductal closure, pulmonary
    vasculature and, 75
Antenatal inflammation/infection, 39–55
    fetal exposure to, 41–44, 41f, 43f–44f, 43t
        early gestational responses, 47
        experimental results, 44–45, 45f–46f
        immune response and modulation, 50–52,
            51f
    overview, 39
Antenatal steroids
    after 34 weeks' gestational period, 339–340
    as BPD risk factor, 122
    drug and dose choices for, 339–340
    long-term outcomes after, 340
    in low-resource environments, 340
    repeated, 338–339
Antibiotics
    for *Ureaplasma* infection, 108
    for ventilator-associated pneumonia,
        152–154, 153b
Antigen, ureaplasmal MB, 103
Antimicrobials, for ventilator-associated
    pneumonia, 154
Apnea, 177, 178f
    in early postnatal life, underreporting of,
        241–242
    neonatal, clinical challenges in defining,
        241–242
    neonatal sepsis and, 241
Apnea of prematurity, 198, 239–250
    blood transfusions for, 246
    caffeine for, 244–245, 245b
    carbon dioxide therapy for, 246
    controversies in therapy of, 244–247
    defined, 241
    discharge practice for, 247
    doxapram for, 246–247
    intermittent hypoxemia and bradycardia
        associated with
        longer-term outcomes and, 243
        neonatal outcomes and, 242–243, 242f

Note: Page numbers followed by "f" refer to illustrations; page numbers followed by "t" refer to
tables; page numbers followed by "b" refer to boxes.

Apnea of prematurity *(Continued)*
   kangaroo care for, 246
   mechanistic insights into morbidity and,
      243–244
   mechanosensory stimulation for, 246
   noninvasive ventilation for, 245
   oxygen administration for, 245
Arabella NCPAP Infant Flow System, 200
Arachidonic acid-prostacyclin pathway, 72
Arterial oxygenation, BPD and
   prognosis, 126
   targets, impact of, 121
Asphyxia, 299
   defined, 176
   hypotension in, 189
   in postnatal pulmonary vascular
      development, 78
Aspiration, meconium, airway management in,
   179–180
Assist/control (A/C) ventilation, 274, 275f,
   311, 322
Assisted ventilation modes, choice of, 312
Asthma, after preterm birth, 162–163
Atelectasis, BPD and, 116
Atelectrauma, 307–308
Atrial septal defects, in severe
   bronchopulmonary dysplasia, 372
Automation, of respiratory support, 321–334
   automated adjustment of supplemental
      oxygen, 327–332, 328f, 329t–330t, 331f
   mechanical ventilation, 321–327
   neurally adjusted ventilatory assist, 326–327,
      327f
   proportional assist ventilation, 325–326
   targeted minute ventilation, 324–325, 325f
   volume-controlled ventilation, 323f
Autotriggering, 278
Avoid Mechanical Ventilation trial, 225
Azithromycin, for *Ureaplasma* infection, 108

B

Bacterial overgrowth, ventilator-assisted
   pneumonia and, 150, 151f
Bacteroidetes, in lung microbiome, 98–99, 99f
Bags
   polyethylene, for warming, 176–179
   for positive-pressure ventilation, 180
Barotrauma, 307–308
Basal cells, 349t
BASCs. *see* Bronchoalveolar stem cells
Betamethasone, 335–336
   lung maturation and, 35, 53, 54f
Betamethasone acetate, 335–336
Betamethasone phosphate, 335–336, 339–340
Betamethasone phosphate plus betamethasone
   acetate, 339–340
Biomarkers, bronchopulmonary dysplasia and,
   87
Biotrauma, 307–308
Birth, cardiorespiratory interactions at,
   290–292, 290t
Birth weight, ventilator-associated pneumonia,
   149
Blood transfusions, for apnea of prematurity, 246
BMP. *see* Bone morphogenetic protein
Bone marrow (BM) mesenchymal stem cells,
   for bronchopulmonary dysplasia, 354t
Bone morphogenetic protein (BMP), in
   branching morphogenesis, 8
BPD. *see* Bronchopulmonary dysplasia

Bradycardia, apnea of prematurity and, 241
   intermittent hypoxemia and, association
      between
      longer-term outcomes and, 243
      neonatal outcomes and, 242–243, 242f
Brain injury
   during early transition and potential clinical
      implication, 300–301
   hypoxemia and, 257
Branching morphogenesis, 7–8
   BMP in, 8
   epithelial-mesenchymal interactions in, 7
   FGF10-FGFR2b in, 7–8
   Shh in, 8
   Sprouty in, 8
   TGF-β, 8–9
   Wnt in, 9
Breast milk, ventilator-associated pneumonia
   and, 156
Breathing
   periodic, 240
   sleep-disordered, 243
Bronchial vascular system, 13
Bronchoalveolar stem cells (BASCs), 349t
Bronchopulmonary dysplasia (BPD), 4, 87–96,
   88f, 307
   antenatal corticosteroids and, 34–35, 37f
   cell-based therapy for, 352–353
      barriers to implementation of, 356
      evidence from phase I clinical trial, 355
      evidence from preclinical studies,
         352–353, 352f, 354t
      mechanisms of repair, 353–357
      optimal cells for, 356–357
   chorioamnionitis and, 42, 43t, 53t
   clinical and research implications,
      115–130
   clinical presentation of, 115–116
   CTGF in, 15–16, 19
   definition of, 115
      National Institutes of Health Workshop,
         119t
   development of, 16–18, 17f
   diagnosis of, 116–127
   disease process, 88–89
   economics and, 93
   genomics of, 89–90
   IL-1β in, 18
   infant demographics of, 122
   innate immunity, 16–18
   long-term outcomes in, 163–168
   lung microbiome and, 98–99, 100f
   metabolomics of, 91–92
   microbiomics and, 92–93
   new, 164
   outcomes of, 121
   pathogenesis of, 16f, 52
   populations at risk for, 124–125
   postdelivery corticosteroid treatments for,
      335
   prediction for, 121–122
   predictive models of, 124
   prevention of, *Ureaplasma* eradication in,
      107–108
   prognosis for long-term impairment,
      125–127
   proteomics of, 91
   pulmonary oxygen toxicity and, 261
   risk factors for
      before birth, 122
      postnatal, 122–123

Bronchopulmonary dysplasia (BPD)
  (Continued)
  severe
    cardiovascular system in, 371–372
    definitions and scope of, 364–366
    evaluation and treatment of, 366t,
        372–380
    forced flows in, 370
    long-term outcomes of, 380
    lung imaging in, 370–371, 371f
    lung mechanics in, 369
    lung volumes in, 369–370
    pathogenesis of, 366–368
    pathophysiology of, 368–372
    physiology-based approach for, 363–386
    respiratory function in, 368–369
    ventilator strategies in, 366t
    ventilator-dependent, 364f
  signaling in, 18–19
  supplemental oxygen criteria for, 117–121,
      118f, 120f
  transcriptomics of, 90–91
  Ureaplasma infection in, 105–107
  VEGF in, 20
Bubble CPAP, 200
Budesonide, 343

C
Caffeine
  for apnea of prematurity, 244–245, 245b
  in central respiratory control, 240
Canalicular stage, of lung development, 10
Capnography, during cardiac compressions,
    187
Carbapenem-resistant *Acinetobacter* species,
    ventilator-assisted pneumonia and, 153
Carbon dioxide (CO_2)
  for apnea of prematurity, 246
  during early transition and potential clinical
      implication, 300–301
  responsiveness to, respiratory neural output
      and, 240
Cardiac catheterization, for pulmonary
    hypertension, in bronchopulmonary
    dysplasia, 379b
Cardiac output, impact of lung disease and
    ventilator support on components of, 293t
Cardiorespiratory events, impaired executive
    function and, 242
Cardiorespiratory interactions, at birth,
    290–292, 290t
Cardiorespiratory system, 289
Cardiovascular interaction, physiology of,
    292–297
  afterload, 294–295
  contractility, 294
  preload, 293–294, 294f
Cardiovascular system
  effect, on respiratory system, 297–299
  in severe bronchopulmonary dysplasia,
      371–372
Catheter, intratracheal, surfactant
    administration via, 204
Catheterization, tracheal, surfactant
    administration via, 224–230, 224t
  avoidance of bradycardia in, 232
  bradycardia in, 232
  clinical trials of, 225–229, 226t–227t
    Avoid Mechanical Ventilation Trial in, 225
    NINSAPP Trial in, 229

Catheterization, tracheal, surfactant
    administration via *(Continued)*
    summation of, 229–230
    Take Care Study, 225–228
  depth of catheter insertion for, 225
  effectiveness of, 228f, 230
  future research directions for, 233–235
  hypoxia in, 232
  laboratory studies of, 230–231
  observational and cohort studies of, 225
  premedication for, 231
  procedural complications of, 232
  recommendations for, 232–233
  repeated, 232
  scientific and practical considerations for,
      230–232
  surfactant reflux in, 232
Celestone, 335–336, 339–340
Cell-based therapy, for neonatal lung disease,
    347–362
  airway candidate stem cells in, 350
  alveolar candidate stem cells in, 350–351
  for bronchopulmonary dysplasia, 352–353
    barriers to implementation of, 356
    evidence from phase I clinical trial, 355
    evidence from preclinical studies,
        352–353, 352f, 354t
    mechanisms of repair, 353–357
    optimal cells for, 356–357
  endogenous lung stem cells in, 348–352,
      349t
    lung endothelial progenitors in, 351–352
    lung mesenchymal stem cells in, 351
    stem cells in, 348, 348f–349f
Central chemosensitivity, 240–241
Central respiratory control, 239–240
Cerebral blood flow, during early transition and
    potential clinical implication, 300–301
Chemosensitivity, central and peripheral,
    240–241
Chest compressions, 185–187
  blood pressure during, 188, 188f
  capnography during, 187
  compression-to-ventilation ratio in, 186–187
  compression-ventilation coordination in, 187
  $ETCO_2$ capnography during, 187
  technique of, 185–186, 186f
  two-thumb technique for, 185–186, 186f
Chest radiograph, of severe bronchopulmonary
    dysplasia (BPD), 364f, 365, 370–371
Chorioamnion, 39–40
Chorioamnionitis, 241
  antenatal corticosteroids and, 53–55,
      53t, 54f
  as BPD risk factor, 122
  bronchopulmonary dysplasia and, 42
  clinical, 39, 40f
  diagnosis of, 39–41, 40f
  experimental chronic, 49, 50f
  funisitis and, 39
  histologic, 39, 40f
  in preterm infants, 52
  severe bronchopulmonary dysplasia (BPD)
      and, 366–367
  Ureaplasma infection in, 103–104
Cigarette smoking. *see* Smoking
Circuit flow, excessive/insufficient, 278–279
Clinical chorioamnionitis, 39, 40f
Club cells, 349t
Cochrane systematic review, 265

Colistin, aerosolized, for ventilator-associated pneumonia, 154
Collateral vessels, severe bronchopulmonary dysplasia and, 372
Color, in initial assessment, 177
Conditioned medium (CM), for bronchopulmonary dysplasia, 354t
Congenital diaphragmatic hernia, 76–78, 77f, 299
Congenital heart disease, 299–300
Connective tissue growth factor (CTGF), in bronchopulmonary dysplasia, 19
Continuous distending pressure, for respiratory distress syndrome, 201–202, 202f
Continuous oxygen, BPD and, 117, 118f
Continuous positive airway pressure (CPAP), 222, 233f, 309–310
    bubble, 200
    effects of, 295–296
    nasal, for apnea of prematurity, 245
    nasal HFT *vs.*, 211, 211f
    in resuscitation, 182
    role of, in preterm infants, 198
    for surfactant, 203–213
        era, 202
        INSURE technique and, 211
        with nasal, 203
    weaning, 205–206
Conventional mechanical ventilation, patient-ventilator interaction during, 270, 270f
Coronary perfusion pressure, in resuscitation, 187–188
Corrected age, BPD and, 121
Corticosteroids
    antenatal, 34–38, 35t, 36f–38f, 37t–38t, 335–339
        chorioamnionitis and, 53–55, 53t, 54f
        in current population, 336–337
        historical overview of, 335–336
        mechanism of action, on fetal lungs, 336
        non-randomized controlled trial for, 337–338, 337f–338f
        randomized controlled trials for, 336–337, 337t
    for severe bronchopulmonary dysplasia, 378
CPAP. *see* Continuous positive airway pressure
CTGF. *see* Connective tissue growth factor
Cumulative oxygen supplementation, combined with oxygen requirement, at 36 weeks postmenstrual age, 118f, 119–121, 120f
Cyanobacteria, in lung microbiome, 98–99, 99f
Cytokines
    chorioamnionitis and, 241
    intermittent hypoxemia and, 244
    in *Ureaplasma* infection, 103–104, 106

D

DART study. *see* Dexamethasone: A Randomized Trial (DART) study
Death, oxygen saturation and, 264–265, 264t
Delivery room
    respiratory and cardiovascular support in, 171–196
    stabilization, 309–310
Dexamethasone: A Randomized Trial (DART) study, 342
Dexamethasone phosphate
    antenatal, 336, 339–340
    postnatal, 342
Diaphragmatic hernia, congenital, 299

Distal airway stem cells, 349t
Diuretics, for severe bronchopulmonary dysplasia, 377–378
Dose, for mesenchymal stem cell transplantation, 357
Down syndrome, pulmonary vascular development and, 74
Doxapram, for apnea of prematurity, 246–247
Drying and stimulation, in resuscitation, 179–180
Ductal-dependent cyanotic heart disease, 299–300
Dysbiosis, defined, 97–98
Dysplasia
    alveolar capillary, 78
    bronchopulmonary, 4, 87–96, 88f, 307
        antenatal corticosteroids and, 34–35, 37f
        cell-based therapy for, 352–353
        chorioamnionitis and, 42, 43t, 53t
        clinical and research implications, 115–130
        clinical presentation of, 115–116
        CTGF in, 15–16, 19
        definition of, 115, 119t
        development of, 16–18, 17f
        diagnosis of, 116–127
        disease process, 88–89
        economics and, 93
        genomics of, 89–90
        IL-1β in, 18
        infant demographics of, 122
        innate immunity, 16–18
        long-term outcomes in, 163–168
        lung microbiome and, 98–99, 100f
        metabolomics of, 91–92
        microbiomics and, 92–93
        new, 164
        outcomes of, 121
        pathogenesis of, 16f, 52
        populations at risk for, 124–125
        postdelivery corticosteroid treatments for, 335
        postnatal risk factors for, 122–123
        prediction for, 121–122
        predictive models of, 124
        prevention of, *Ureaplasma* eradication in, 107–108
        prognosis for long-term impairment, 125–127
        proteomics of, 91
        pulmonary oxygen toxicity and, 261
        risk factors before birth, 122
        severe. *see* Severe bronchopulmonary dysplasia
        signaling in, 18–19
        supplemental oxygen criteria for, 117–121, 118f, 120f
        transcriptomics of, 90–91
        Ureaplasma infection in, 105–107
        VEGF in, 20

E

EADia. *see* Electrical activity of diaphragm
ECFCs. *see* Endothelial colony-forming cells
Echocardiography, for pulmonary hypertension, in bronchopulmonary dysplasia, 379b
Economics, bronchopulmonary dysplasia and, 93
Ectrauma, 307–308
Elastic fiber density, in *Ureaplasma* infection, 105

Elastin, in alveogenesis, 11–12
Electrical activity of diaphragm (EADia), 273
    in neurally adjusted ventilatory assist, 326
Embryonic stage, of lung development, 5
Embryonic stem cells, 348
EME Infant Flow Nasal CPAP device, 200
End-inspiratory asynchrony, 275–277,
    276f–277f
Endogenous lung stem cells, in cell-based
    therapy, 348–352, 349t
Endogenous serotonin (5-HT), in pulmonary
    vasculature, 71
Endoglin, 20
Endothelial colony-forming cells (ECFCs),
    351–352
Endothelial injury, PDA and, 134–135
Endothelial progenitor cells (EPCs), 70,
    351–352
    in cell-based therapy, 351–352
Endothelin (ET-1), pulmonary vascular
    development and, 73–74
Endothelium-derived vasodilator, 68f
Endotoxin, intraamniotic
    betamethasone and, 53
    lung maturation and, 44, 45f–46f
Endotracheal intubation. see also Mechanical
    ventilation
    after failed nasal CPAP, 204–205
    noninvasive respiratory support vs., 198
    routine, vs. nasal CPAP, 202–203
    for surfactant administration, nasal CPAP
    vs., 203
Endotracheal tube (ETT), 182–183, 182t, 307
    surfactant administration without, 222–224,
    223t
    ventilator-assisted pneumonia and,
    150, 151f
Enterobacter spp., ventilator-assisted
    pneumonia and, 149–150
EPCs. see Endothelial progenitor cells
Ephrins, in vascular development, 15
Epinephrine, in resuscitation, 188
Epithelial-endothelial interaction, in alveolar
    development, 14–15
Epithelial-mesenchymal interaction, in
    branching morphogenesis, 7, 7f
Erythromycin, for Ureaplasma infection,
    107–108
ETCO2, during cardiac compressions, 187
ETT. see Endotracheal tube
Excessive circuit flow, 278–279
Exercise tolerance, pulmonary function and,
    167
Exogenous surfactant therapy, PDA and,
    132
Expiratory asynchrony, 270–271, 271f
Extremely low birth weight (ELBW) infants
    lung microbiome and, 98–99, 100f
    severe bronchopulmonary dysplasia (BPD)
    in, 365
Extremely preterm infants, optimal
    oxygenation in, 261–268
    guidelines for practice in, 266
    observational studies of, 262–263
    oxygen saturation targeting trials, meta-
    analyses of, 264–265, 264t
    randomized controlled trials for, 263–264
    achieved oxygen saturation in, 265–266,
    265f
    subgroup analyses of, 265
    SUPPORT trial for, 263

F
Face mask, 181
Fetal alcohol syndrome, lung development
    and, 57
Fetal growth restriction, as BPD risk factor,
    122
Fetal inflammatory response syndrome,
    chorioamnionitis and, 43t
Fetal lung, transition from fetal to neonatal
    life, 3
Fetal pulmonary circulation
    development of, 65
    physiology of, 65–67, 66f
    pulmonary vascular development, 65–86
    abnormal, 72–74, 73f
    disruption of, 74–76
    function, mediators of early, 70–71
    mediators of, 67–70, 69f
    postnatal, 71–72
    stages of, 65, 66f
    transitional, 71–72
Fibroblast growth factor 10, 6
    in branching morphogenesis, 7–8
Fisher & Paykel system, 210
Flk-1, 14–15
Flow cycling, 274, 277f
Flow-inflating bags, for positive-pressure
    ventilation, 176–177, 180
Flow-proportional gains, in proportional assist
    ventilation (PAV), 326
Flow sensors, in synchronized mechanical
    ventilation, 273
Flow starvation, 278–279
Flow triggering, in synchronized mechanical
    ventilation, 273
Flt-1, 14–15
Fluticasone propionate, for severe
    bronchopulmonary dysplasia, 378
Forced flows, in severe bronchopulmonary
    dysplasia, 370
Forkhead box (Fox) family, in pulmonary
    vascular development, 70
Fraction of inspired oxygen (FIO2)
    adjustment of, 327, 328f, 329t–330t, 331f
    in oxygen therapy, 255, 256f
Full term infants, lung microbiome and, 98–99,
    100f
Funisitis, 39
Furosemide, for severe bronchopulmonary
    dysplasia, 377–378
Fusobacteria, in lung microbiome, 98–99,
    99f–100f

G
GABA. see Gamma-aminobutyric acid
Gamma-aminobutyric acid (GABA), in central
    respiratory control, 240
Gas exchange, in infant-ventilator asynchrony,
    271
Gasping, 177, 178f
Gastric bacteria, ventilator-assisted pneumonia
    and, 150–152
Genital mycoplasmas, lung injury and,
    102–108
Genomics, of bronchopulmonary dysplasia,
    89–90
Glutamate, in central respiratory control, 240
Glutathione sulfonamide (GSA), ventilator-
    assisted pneumonia and, 157
Glycine, in central respiratory control, 240

"Golden minute," 180
G-protein-coupled receptor, 13
Graseby pressure capsule, 273
GSA. *see* Glutathione sulfonamide

H

Hand hygiene, ventilator-associated pneumonia
    and, 154
Head's paradoxical reflex, activation of, 270,
    270f
Heart disease, congenital, 299–300
Heart rate
    in initial assessment, 177
    in positive-pressure ventilation, 180
Heat loss prevention, 177–179
Hematopoietic stem cells, 348
Hepatocyte growth factor, in alveolar
    development, 14–15
Hering-Breuer vagal inhibitory reflex,
    activation of, 270, 270f
HFNC. *see* High-flow nasal cannula
HFNV. *see* High-frequency nasal ventilation
HFOV. *see* High-frequency oscillatory
    ventilation
HFV. *see* High-frequency ventilation
HIFs. *see* Hypoxia-inducible factors
High-flow nasal cannula (HFNC), for severe
    bronchopulmonary dysplasia, 373
High-frequency nasal ventilation (HFNV),
    noninvasive, 207
    clinical reports on, 208, 208t
    device-specific comments regarding, 209
    gas exchange during, 207–208
    laryngeal effects of, 208
    in NICU, 208–209
High-frequency oscillatory ventilation
    (HFOV), in severe bronchopulmonary
    dysplasia, 367
High-frequency ventilation (HFV),
    314–315
High-resolution computed tomography
    (HRCT), for severe bronchopulmonary
    dysplasia (BPD), 370–371, 371f
Histologic chorioamnionitis, 39, 40f
Hox5 genes, in lung patterning, 9–10
HRCT. *see* High-resolution computed
    tomography
Human cord perivascular cells, for
    bronchopulmonary dysplasia, 354t
Hydrocortisone, 342
    infusions, 343
Hypercapnia, permissive, effect of, 296–297
Hyperoxia
    in postnatal pulmonary vascular
        development, 79–80
    severe bronchopulmonary dysplasia (BPD)
        and, 366–367
Hypertension, pulmonary, 65–66, 298, 299f,
    302f
    echocardiography for, in severe
        bronchopulmonary dysplasia, 379b
    in severe bronchopulmonary dysplasia, 371
    treatment of, 378–379, 379b
Hyperthermia, 177–179
Hypoplasia, pulmonary, in preterm infants, 75
Hypotension, management of, 189
Hypothermia, prevention of, 177–179
Hypoventilation, in mechanical ventilation,
    252f
Hypovolemia, in resuscitation, 189

Hypoxemia
    apnea of prematurity and, 241
        longer-term outcomes, bradycardia and,
            association between, 243
        neonatal outcomes, bradycardia and,
            association between, 242–243, 242f
    episodes, spontaneous, volume guarantee
        ventilation for, 324
    in mechanical ventilation, 251
        after extubation, 253, 254f
        behavioral disturbances and, 252, 256
        FIO$_2$ and, 255, 256f
        mechanisms of, 252f
        supplemental oxygen in, 255–256, 256f
        ventilation strategies for, 254, 255f
Hypoxia, in postnatal pulmonary vascular
    development, 79
Hypoxia-inducible factors (HIFs), 67–68, 69f

I

Ibuprofen, for PDA, 137
Immune response
    and modulation, from fetal exposures to
        inflammation, 50–52, 51f
    to *Ureaplasma* infection, 107
Indomethacin, prophylactic, for PDA, 136–137
Infant Flow Driver, 200
Infants
    BPD and, 116
    selection of, for surfactant delivery via
        tracheal catheterization, 230f, 232–233,
        234b
Infant-ventilator asynchrony, 270–272, 271f
Infant-ventilator maladaptation, 275–280
Infection, severe bronchopulmonary dysplasia
    (BPD) and, 366–367
Infertility, *Ureaplasma* infection and, 103
Inflammation
    mechanisms of, respiratory control and, 241
    severe bronchopulmonary dysplasia (BPD)
        and, 366–367
Inflation pressure, 322
In-line suctioning devices, ventilator-associated
    pneumonia and, 155–156
Innate immune tolerance, 51–52
Innate immunity
    Ureaplasma infection susceptibility, 107
    ventilator-assisted pneumonia and, 150
Inspiratory asynchrony, 270–271, 271f
Insufficient circuit flow, 278–279
INSURE technique, 222
Integrin α6β4 alveolar progenitors, 349t
Interdisciplinary care, in severe
    bronchopulmonary dysplasia, 379–380
Intermittent hypoxia (IH)
    growth in preterm infants and, 243
    inflammatory pathways and, 241
    in preterm infants, 242, 242f
Intermittent mandatory ventilation
    (IMV), 322
    infant-ventilator asynchrony during, 270
    nasal, 284
    synchronized, 272f, 273–274, 274f
Internal flow sensors, in synchronized
    mechanical ventilation, 273
International Liaison Committee on
    Resuscitation (ILCOR) guidelines,
    309–310
Intratracheal catheter, surfactant administration
    via, 204

Intrauterine growth restriction
  bronchopulmonary dysplasia and, 55–57, 56f
  severe bronchopulmonary dysplasia (BPD)
    and, 366–367
Intraventricular hemorrhage (IVH)
  chorioamnionitis and, 53t
  infant-ventilator asynchrony and, 271
IVH. *see* Intraventricular hemorrhage

K

Kangaroo care, for apnea of prematurity, 246
Klebsiella spp., ventilator-assisted pneumonia
  and, 149–150

L

Labor, preterm, *Ureaplasma* infection and,
  103–104
Lactobacillus, 92–93
  in lung microbiome, 98–99
Laryngeal mask airway, 182–183, 182t
  delivery of surfactant by, 224
Left ventricular (LV) afterload, effects of
  intrathoracic pressure on, 292f
Left ventricular (LV) hypertrophy, in severe
  bronchopulmonary dysplasia, 372
Left-to-right shunting, PDA and, 132–133
Liggins and Howie trial, 336
Linezolid, for ventilator-associated pneumonia,
  152–153
Long inspiratory time, 275–277,
  276f–277f
Long-term pulmonary outcomes, 161–170
  controversies in, 161
  for late preterm infants, 162–163
  pulmonary function in
    in adolescence or early adulthood,
      165–166, 165t
    in childhood, 163–164, 164t
    with increasing age, 166–167
  research requirements for, 168
  for very preterm infants, 163–168
    cigarette smoking and, 167–168
    exercise tolerance, 167
    exogenous surfactant and, 167
    rehospitalization rates, 163
Low-resource environments, antenatal steroids
  in, 340
Lung bud initiation, molecular regulation of,
  5–6
Lung development, 1–64
  adverse events, 32–33, 33f
  alveolar septation in, 11–12
  branching morphogenesis in, 7–8
  disruption of, 15–20
  epithelial-endothelial interaction in, 14–15
  fluctuations in oxygenation and, 257
  inflammatory responses, 46–47, 47t
  lung bud initiation in, 5–6
  lung maturation and, 33–34
  microRNA in, 21
  overview, 31–32, 32f
  phases of, 4f
  postnatal, 3
  stages of, 4–10, 5f
    alveolar, 10, 11f
    canalicular stage, 10
    embryonic, 5
    pseudoglandular, 6–7
    saccular, 10
  tracheoesophageal separation in, 5–6, 5f

Lung disease
  environmental factors and, 56–57
  impact of, 293t
Lung injury
  severe bronchopulmonary dysplasia (BPD)
    and, 366–367
  ventilation strategies for, 307–320
Lung maturation, 33–34
  environmental factors and, 56–57
  inflammation-mediated, 48–49, 48f
Lungs
  fetal, transition from fetal to neonatal life,
    3. *see also* Transition from fetal to
    neonatal life
  function, BPD and, 126
  imaging, in severe bronchopulmonary
    dysplasia, 370–371, 371f
  mechanics, in severe bronchopulmonary
    dysplasia, 369
  volume
    loss of, in mechanical ventilation, 252,
      253f
    in severe bronchopulmonary dysplasia,
      369–370

M

Mainstream (proximal) flow sensors, in
  synchronized mechanical ventilation, 273
Mandatory minute ventilation (MMV), 325
MAP. *see* Mean airway pressure
Masks, face, 181
Maternal hyperoxygenation test, 67
Maternal smoking, severe bronchopulmonary
  dysplasia (BPD) and, 366–367
Mean airway pressure (MAP), effects of,
  295–296
Mechanical ventilation, 269, 291, 295
  adverse effects of, 198
  automation in, 321–327
  as BPD risk factor, 122–123
  bronchopulmonary dysplasia (BPD) due to,
    367
  conventional, 270, 270f
  duration of, pneumonia and, 149
  evidence-based approach to, 315–316
  historical perspective on, 198–199
  hypoventilation in, 251–252, 252f
  hypoxemia in, 251. *see also* Hypoxemia
  lung volume loss in, 252, 253f
  noninvasive respiratory support and, 310
  oxygen saturation in, 252f
  oxygenation instability after, 253, 254f
  for severe bronchopulmonary dysplasia and,
    373–377, 373b, 374f–376f
  SpO_2 in, 253
  strategies, 310
  synchronized, 272–280, 272f, 311–312
    assist/control ventilation in, 274, 275f
    autotriggering in, 278
    delayed triggering, 277
    end-inspiratory asynchrony in, 275–277,
      276f–277f
    excessive or insufficient circuit flow in,
      278–279
    excessive peak inflation pressure in, 279,
      279f
    excessive positive end-expiratory pressure
      in, 279–280, 280f
    flow sensors in, 273
    Graseby pressure capsule in, 273

Mechanical ventilation *(Continued)*
  infant-ventilator maladaptation in, 275–280
  long inspiratory time in, 275–277
  methods of, 273
  modalities of, 273–275
  pressure-support ventilation in, 274–275
  synchronized intermittent mandatory ventilation, 273–274, 274f
  trigger failure in, 278
  Ureaplasma infection and, 107
  ventilator-associated lung injury and, 307–310
  volume-targeted, hypoxemia and, 254
Mechanosensory stimulation, for apnea of prematurity, 246
Meconium staining, airway management in, 179–180
Mesenchymal stem cell (MSC)
  in cell-based therapy, 351
  transplantation
    for bronchopulmonary dysplasia, 354t
    dose, 357
    in hyperoxia-induced alveolar simplification, 352f
    for preterm infants, 356
    route, 357
    timing of administration of, 356–357
Metabolomics, of bronchopulmonary dysplasia, 87, 91–92
Methicillin-resistant *S. aureus* (MRSA), as cause of ventilator-associated pneumonia, 152–153
Microbiome
  lung, newborn, 98, 99f–100f
  in lung injury, 97–114
Microbiomics, bronchopulmonary dysplasia and, 92–93
Microbiota, defined, 97–98
MMV. *see* Mandatory minute ventilation
Morbidity, mechanistic insights into, intermittent hypoxemia and, 243–244
Motor delays, intermittent hypoxia and, 257
Mouse bone marrow (BM) mesenchymal stem cells, for bronchopulmonary dysplasia, 354t
MRSA. *see* Methicillin-resistant *S. aureus*
Multipotent stem cells, 348
Mycoplasma species, chorioamnionitis and, 39–40
Mycoplasmas, genital, lung injury and, 102–108
Myofibroblast, in alveologenesis, 11–12

N
Nasal cannulas, for nasal CPAP, 201
Nasal continuous positive airway pressure (NCPAP), 199–203. *see also* Noninvasive ventilation
  BPD and, 123
  complications of, 205
  devices for, 199–201, 199f–200f
    trauma from, 204
  failure of, 204–205
  for postextubation support, 204
    with nasal IPPV, 206, 206f
  prophylactic surfactant and, 203
  for respiratory distress syndrome, 201–202, 202f
    brief early intubation for surfactant *vs.*, 203–213

Nasal continuous positive airway pressure (NCPAP) *(Continued)*
    continuous distending pressure and, 201–202, 202f
    surfactant administration and, 204
    in surfactant era, 202
  routine intubation *vs.*, 202–203
  for severe bronchopulmonary dysplasia, 367–368, 373
  supporting pressure in, 201
  weaning from, 205–206
Nasal high-flow therapy (NHFT), for preterm infants, 209–210, 209f
  as an alternative treatment, 213
  CPAP *vs.*, 211, 211f
  evidence from randomized trial for, 210–213
    delivery room, stabilization in, 210
    for extubation failure prevention, 211–213, 212f
    as primary respiratory support, 211
  function of, 210
  mechanism of action of, 210
  NIPPV *vs.*, 211
  potential concerns with use of, 212–213
  safety of, 212
Nasal high-frequency oscillatory ventilation (HVOF), 310
Nasal intermittent positive-pressure ventilation (NIPPV), 206–207, 310. *see also* Noninvasive ventilation
  in apnea of prematurity, 206–207
  with nasal CPAP, 206
  NHFT *vs.*, 211
  postextubation, 206, 206f
  in respiratory distress syndrome, 206–207
NAVA. *see* Neurally adjusted ventilatory assist
NCPAP. *see* Nasal continuous positive airway pressure
Necrotizing enterocolitis, oxygen saturation and, 264t
Neonatal intensive care units (NICUs)
  HFNV use in, 208–209
  oxygen saturation in, 262
Neonatal lung disease, cell-based therapy for, 347–362
  airway candidate stem cells in, 350
  alveolar candidate stem cells in, 350–351
  for bronchopulmonary dysplasia, 352–353
    barriers to implementation of, 356
    evidence from phase I clinical trial, 355
    evidence from preclinical studies, 352–353, 352f, 354t
    mechanisms of repair, 353–357
    optimal cells for, 356–357
  endogenous lung stem cells in, 348–352, 349t
  lung endothelial progenitors in, 351–352
  lung mesenchymal stem cells in, 351
  stem cells in, 348, 348f–349f
Neonatal lung injury, *Ureaplasma* spp. and, 104–105, 105b
Neonatal-onset multisystem inflammatory diseases (NOMIDs), 18
Neonatal Oxygen Prospective Meta-analysis (NeOProM) Collaboration, 263
Neonatal Resuscitation Program (NRP), 309–310
Neurally adjusted ventilatory assist (NAVA), 326–327, 327f
  patient-ventilator interaction during, 281–283, 282f–283f
Neuromodulators, in central respiratory control, 240

Neurotransmitters, in central respiratory control, 240
Newborn life, transition to, 173–175, 174f–175f
Newborn mortality, chorioamnionitis and, 53t
NF-κB. *see* Nuclear factor kappa B
NHFT. *see* Nasal high-flow therapy
NICHD-NRN Benchmarking Trial, 124
NICUs. *see* Neonatal intensive care units
NIPPV. *see* Nasal intermittent positive-pressure ventilation
Nitric oxide
    in alveolar development, 14–15
    in *Ureaplasma* infection, 106
NIV. *see* Noninvasive ventilation
Nkx2.1, 5–6
NOMID. *see* Neonatal-onset multisystem inflammatory diseases
Nonintubated Surfactant Application (NINSAPP) trial, for tracheal catheterization, 229
Noninvasive respiratory support, 310
Noninvasive ventilation (NIV)
    for apnea of prematurity, 245
    patient-ventilator interaction during, 283–284, 284f–285f
    of preterm infants, 197–220
        for apnea of prematurity, 198
        brief history of, 198–199
        future directions in, 213
        high-frequency nasal ventilation in. *see* High-frequency nasal ventilation
        intubation *vs.*, 198
        nasal CPAP in. *see* Nasal continuous positive airway pressure (NCPAP)
        nasal high-flow therapy in. *see* Nasal high-flow therapy
        nasal IPPV in. *see* Nasal intermittent positive-pressure ventilation (NIPPV)
    for respiratory failure, 197–198
Nonsteroidal antiinflammatory drugs (NSAIDs), pulmonary vascular development and, 76
NRP. *see* Neonatal Resuscitation Program
NSAIDs. *see* Nonsteroidal antiinflammatory drugs
Nuclear factor kappa B (NF-κB), 70
    in *Ureaplasma* infection, 106

O

Oligohydramnios, in preterm infants, 75
Open lung strategy, importance of, 313–314
Optimal cells, for bronchopulmonary dysplasia, 356–357
Oral secretions, removal of, ventilator-assisted pneumonia and, 156
Oxidative stress
    inflammatory pathways and, 241
    severe bronchopulmonary dysplasia (BPD) and, 366–367
Oxygen, 79
    at 36 weeks postmenstrual corrected age, 117–119
    administration of, for apnea of prematurity, 245
        positioning for, 245
    blended, 184
    supplemental, for severe bronchopulmonary dysplasia, 372–373
    use, as BPD risk factor, 122–123

Oxygen hood, nasal CPAP for postextubation support *vs.*, 204
Oxygen saturation (SpO$_2$)
    maintenance of, 327
    in mechanical ventilation, 252f, 253
    in neonatal intensive care units, 262
    in oxygen therapy, 183, 184t
    in randomized controlled trials, 265–266, 265f
    retinopathy of prematurity and, 262
    SUPPORT trial in, 263
    targeting trials in, meta-analyses of, 264–265, 264t
Oxygen therapy, FIO$_2$ in, 255, 256f
Oxygen toxicity, 183
    pulmonary, in bronchopulmonary dysplasia, 261
Oxygenation
    blended oxygen in, 184
    instability
        consequences of, 257
        environmental disturbance reduction for, 256
        management of, 254–256
        in premature infants, 251–260
        in spontaneously breathing infants, after mechanical ventilation, 253, 254f
        supplemental oxygen for, 255–256, 256f
        in ventilated infants, 251–253
        ventilation strategies for, 254, 255f
    optimal, in extremely preterm infants, 261–268
        guidelines for practice in, 266
        observational studies of, 262–263
        oxygen saturation targeting trials, meta-analyses of, 264–265, 264t
        randomized controlled trials in, 263–264
        subgroup analyses of, 265
        SUPPORT trial in, 263
    pulse oximetry in, 183
    in resuscitation, 183–184, 184t
    targeting, observational studies of, 262–263

P

Paracetamol, for PDA, 137
Patent ductus arteriosus (PDA), 290, 298
    acute effects and long-term consequences, 131–146
    as BPD risk factor, 122–123
    bronchopulmonary dysplasia and, 135–136, 136f
    closure of
        spontaneous, 137
        surgical, 138–139
    incidence of, 132
    management of, and respiratory outcome, 136–139, 138f
    in preterm infants, 132
        critically ill, 139
    pulmonary consequences of, 133–135
        acute, 133–134
        long-term, 134–135
    respiratory management for infants, 139–140
    systemic consequences of, 132–133, 133f
    treatment of
        caffeine, 139
        corticosteroids, 132
        gestational age, 140
        indomethacin, 136–137
        surfactant, 132

Patient positioning, ventilator-assisted pneumonia and, 150
Patient-ventilator interaction, 269–288
  during conventional mechanical ventilation, 270, 270f
  infant-ventilator asynchrony and, 270–272, 271f
  during neurally adjusted ventilatory assist, 281–283, 282f–283f
  during noninvasive ventilation, 283–284, 284f–285f
  during synchronized mechanical ventilation, 272–280, 272f
    assist/control ventilation in, 274, 275f
    autotriggering in, 278
    delayed triggering, 277
    end-inspiratory asynchrony in, 275–277, 276f–277f
    excessive or insufficient circuit flow in, 278–279
    excessive peak inflation pressure in, 279, 279f
    excessive positive end-expiratory pressure in, 279–280, 280f
    flow sensors in, 273
    Graseby pressure capsule in, 273
    infant-ventilator maladaptation in, 275–280
    long inspiratory time in, 275–277
    methods of, 273
    modalities of, 273–275
    pressure-support ventilation in, 274–275
    synchronized intermittent mandatory ventilation, 273–274, 274f
    trigger failure in, 278
  during volume targeted ventilation, 280–281, 281f
PAV. *see* Proportional assist ventilation
PBF. *see* Pulmonary blood flow
PDA. *see* Patent ductus arteriosus
PDGF. *see* Platelet-derived growth factor
Peak inflation pressure (PIP), 322
  excessive, 279, 279f
PEEP. *see* Positive end-expiratory pressure
Periodic breathing, 240
Peripheral chemosensitivity, 240–241
Periventricular/intraventricular hemorrhage (P/IVH), 300–301
Permissive hypercapnia
  effect of, 296–297
  mild, mechanical ventilation and, 315
Persistent pulmonary hypertension of the newborn (PPHN), 290–291
Pharyngeal instillation, 223, 223t
PIP. *see* Peak inflation pressure
P/IVH. *see* Periventricular/intraventricular hemorrhage
Placental insufficiency, pulmonary vasculature and, 75
Platelet-derived growth factor (PDGF), in alveolar septation, 11–12
Pluripotent stem cells, 348
PMA. *see* Postmenstrual age
Pneumonia, ventilator-associated, 147–160
  birth weight and, 149
  definition of, 148, 149b
  epidemiology of, 148–149
  future research directions for, 157
  outcomes in, 156–157
  pathogenesis of, 149–152, 150b, 151f
  prevention of, 154–156, 155b

Pneumonia, ventilator-associated *(Continued)*
  risk factors for, 149
  treatment of, 152–157, 153b
  ventilation duration and, 149
Pneumothorax, from nasal CPAP, 205
Polyethylene wrap, for warming, 177–179
Positive end-expiratory pressure (PEEP), 173–175, 174f, 309–310
  effects of, 295–296
  excessive, 279–280, 280f
  oxygenation instability and, 254
Positive-pressure respiratory support, BPD and, 125
Postmenstrual age (PMA), severe bronchopulmonary dysplasia (BPD) in, 364–365
Postnatal steroids, 340–344
  for bronchopulmonary dysplasia, 341
  drug, dose, route, and duration of therapy with, 342
  historical review, 340–341, 341f
  meta-analyses of early and late treatments of, 341–342
  pulmonary outcomes of, 335–346
  use of, 342–343
PPHN. *see* Persistent pulmonary hypertension of the newborn
Pre-Bötzinger complex, 239–240
Predictive models, of BPD, 124
Preeclampsia, severe bronchopulmonary dysplasia (BPD) and, 366–367
Premature birth, PDA and, 133
Premature infants
  apnea in, 239–250
    blood transfusions for, 246
    caffeine for, 244–245, 245b
    carbon dioxide therapy for, 246
    controversies in therapy of, 244–247
    defined, 241
    discharge practice for, 247
    doxapram for, 246–247
    kangaroo care for, 246
    longer-term outcomes for, intermittent hypoxemia and bradycardia associated with, 243
    mechanistic insights into morbidity and, 243–244
    mechanosensory stimulation for, 246
    neonatal outcomes for, intermittent hypoxemia and bradycardia associated with, 242–243, 242f
    noninvasive ventilation for, 245
    oxygen administration for, 245
  BPD and, 126
  respiratory control in, 239–250
Prematurity, ventilator-associated pneumonia, 149
Prenatal steroids
  new trials of, 343–344, 343t
  pulmonary outcomes of, 335–346
Pressure-controlled (PC) modes, in neonatal ventilation, 322
Pressure-regulated-volume-control (PRVC) ventilation, 322
Pressure-support ventilation (PSV), 274–275, 311–312
Preterm baboons, PDA and, 135
Preterm birth
  in postnatal pulmonary vascular development, 78–79
  Ureaplasma infection in, 103–104

Preterm infants
  chorioamnionitis in, 52
  long-term pulmonary outcomes, 161–170
    controversies in, 161
    for late preterm infants, 162–163
    research requirements for, 168
    for very preterm infants, 163–168
  oligohydramnios/pulmonary hypoplasia in,
    75
  pulmonary function in, long-term pulmonary
    outcomes
    in adolescence or early adulthood,
      165–166, 165t
    in childhood, 163–164, 164t
    with increasing age, 166–167
  Ureaplasma spp. and, 104, 105b
  for very preterm infants, long-term
    pulmonary outcomes
    cigarette smoking and, 167–168
    exercise tolerance, 167
    exogenous surfactant and, 167
    rehospitalization rates, 163
Proportional assist ventilation (PAV),
  automation of, 325–326
Proteobacteria, 92–93
  in lung microbiome, 98, 99f–100f
Proteomics, of bronchopulmonary dysplasia,
  87, 91
Pseudoglandular stage, in lung development,
  6–7
Pseudomonas aeruginosa, ventilator-assisted
  pneumonia and, 149–150
PSV. *see* Pressure-support ventilation
Pulmonary artery pressure, in severe
  bronchopulmonary dysplasia, 371
Pulmonary blood flow (PBF), 173
  increased, PDA and, 134–135
Pulmonary-cardiovascular interaction,
  289–306
  after transition and potential clinical
    implications, 301
  cardiorespiratory interactions at birth,
    290–292
  cardiovascular system on respiratory system,
    effect of, 297–299
  congenital heart disease and, 299–300
  physiology of, 292–297
    afterload, 293t, 294–295
    contractility, 293t, 294
    preload, 293–294, 293t, 294f
  respiratory system on cardiovascular system,
    effect of, 295
  during transition and potential clinical
    implications, 300–301
Pulmonary circulation, fetal
  development of, 65
  physiology of, 65–67, 66f
  pulmonary vascular development, 65–86
    abnormal, 72–74, 73f
    disruption of, 74–76
    function, mediators of early, 70–71
    mediators of, 67–70, 69f
    postnatal, 71–72
    stages of, 65, 66f
  transitional, 71–72
Pulmonary function, in very preterm infants
  in adolescence or early adulthood, 165–166,
    165t
  in childhood, 163–164, 164t
  with increasing age, 166–167
Pulmonary hemorrhage, PDA and, 134

Pulmonary hypertension, 65–66, 298, 299f,
  302f
  echocardiography for, in severe
    bronchopulmonary dysplasia, 379b
  in severe bronchopulmonary dysplasia, 371
  treatment of, 378–379, 379b
Pulmonary hypoplasia, in preterm infants, 75
Pulmonary outcomes, long-term, of preterm
  infants, 161–170
  controversies in, 161
  for late preterm infants, 162–163
  pulmonary function in
    in adolescence or early adulthood,
      165–166, 165t
    in childhood, 163–164, 164t
    with increasing age, 166–167
  research requirements for, 168
  for very preterm infants, 163–168
    cigarette smoking and, 167–168
    exercise tolerance, 167
    exogenous surfactant and, 167
    rehospitalization rates, 163
Pulmonary oxygen toxicity, in
  bronchopulmonary dysplasia, 261
Pulmonary vascular development, in neonatal
  circulation, 65–86
  abnormal, 72–74, 73f
  disruption of, 74–76
    alveolar capillary dysplasia, 78
    antenatal ductal closure, 75
    congenital diaphragmatic hernia, 76–78,
      77f
    genetic, 74
    maternal drug exposure, 76
    oligohydramnios/ pulmonary hypoplasia,
      75
    placental insufficiency, 75
  function, mediators of early, 70–71
  mediators of, 67–70, 69f
    endothelial progenitor cells (EPCs), 70
    nuclear factor kappa B (NF-κB) as, 70
    VEGF as, 69
  postnatal, 71–72
    disruption of, 78–80
  stages of, 65, 66f
Pulmonary vasoreactivity, in severe
  bronchopulmonary dysplasia, 371
Pulmonary vein stenosis
  in postnatal pulmonary vascular
    development, 79
  severe bronchopulmonary dysplasia and, 372
Pulmonary veins, in fetus, 67, 68f
Pulmonary venous return, 290
Pulse oximetry, 183
  in resuscitation, 176–177
Pulse pressure variation, 292

R

Radiant warmers, 177–179
Rapid thoracic compression (RTC), in severe
  bronchopulmonary dysplasia, 370
Rat bone marrow (BM) mesenchymal stem
  cells, for bronchopulmonary dysplasia,
  354t
RDS. *see* Respiratory distress syndrome
Reflexes, respiratory, conventional mechanical
  ventilation and, 270
Respiratory assessment
  initial, 177, 180
  in positive-pressure ventilation, 180

Respiratory control
  central, 239–240
  neonatal, biologic challenges in
      characterizing, 239–241
    central and peripheral chemosensitivity
        and, 240–241
    central respiratory control and, 239–240
    contribution from inflammatory
        mechanisms and, 241
    in premature infants, 239–250
Respiratory distress syndrome (RDS),
      197–198, 222
  chorioamnionitis and, 43t, 53t
  lung maturation, 33–34
  nasal IPPV for, 206–207
  nasal NCPAP for, 201–202, 202f. see also
      Nasal continuous positive airway
      pressure (NCPAP)
  brief early intubation for surfactant vs.,
      203–213
  continuous distending pressure and,
      201–202, 202f
  surfactant administration and, 204
  in surfactant era, 202
  treatment of, surfactant in, 202
  volume guarantee ventilation in, 324
Respiratory function, severe bronchopulmonary
      dysplasia and, 368–369
Respiratory health problems, after preterm
      birth, 163
Respiratory interaction, physiology of,
      292–297
  afterload, 293t, 294–295
  contractility, 293t, 294
  preload, 293–294, 293t, 294f
Respiratory pause, apnea of prematurity and, 241
Respiratory reflexes, conventional mechanical
      ventilation and, 270
Respiratory support
  automation of, 321–334
    automated adjustment of supplemental
        oxygen, 327–332, 328f, 329t–330t,
        331f
    mechanical ventilation, 321–327
    neurally adjusted ventilatory assist,
        326–327, 327f
    proportional assist ventilation, 325–326
    targeted minute ventilation,
        324–325, 325f
    volume-controlled ventilation, 323f
  continuous distending pressure in, 201–202,
      202f
Respiratory syncytial virus infection, after late
      preterm birth, 162
Respiratory system, effect, on cardiovascular
      system, 295
Resuscitation
  anticipating need for, 176
  chest compressions in, 185–187
  coronary perfusion pressure in, 187–188
  CPAP in, 182
  epinephrine in, 188
  equipment for, 176–177
  "golden minute" in, 180
  initial assessment in, 177
  intubation in, 182–183, 182t
  medications for, 187–189
  positive-pressure ventilation in, 180–182
    assessment during, 180
    equipment for, 176–177
    inflation pressure in, 181

Resuscitation (Continued)
    inflation time in, 181
    ventilation rate in, 181
  preparation for, 176–177
  routine care vs., 177–179
  special situations in, 189–190
  steps in, 177–180, 178f
    clear airway, 179–180
    dry and stimulate, 179–180
    maintain normal temperature, 177–179
    position, 179
    provide warmth, 177–179
  volume infusion in, 189
Retinoic acid, in lung bud initiation, 6
Retinopathy of prematurity (ROP)
  oxygen saturation and, 262, 264t
  oxygenation and, 257
ROP. see Retinopathy of prematurity
Rosiglitazone, for BPD, 19

S
Saccular stage, of lung development, 10
sBPD. see Severe bronchopulmonary dysplasia
Self-inflating bags, for positive-pressure
      ventilation, 176–177, 180
Septation, 11–12
Serotonin, in central respiratory control, 240
Severe bronchopulmonary dysplasia (sBPD)
  cardiovascular system in, 371–372
  chest radiograph showing, 364f
  definitions and scope of, 364–366
  evaluation and treatment of, 366t, 372–380
    drug therapies in, 377–378
    interdisciplinary care in, 379–380
    mechanical ventilation in, 373–377, 373b,
        374f–376f
    pulmonary hypertension in, 378–379,
        379b
  forced flows in, 370
  long-term outcomes of, 380
  lung imaging in, 370–371, 371f
  lung mechanics in, 369
  lung volumes in, 369–370
  pathogenesis of, 366–368
  pathophysiology of, 368–372
  physiology-based approach, 363–386
  respiratory function in, 368–369
  ventilator strategies in, 366t
Signaling
  in bronchopulmonary dysplasia, 18–19
  in lung development, in branching
      morphogenesis, 7–8
  in neonatal injury, 18–19
Sildenafil, for pulmonary hypertension, in
      bronchopulmonary dysplasia, 379b
SIMV. see Synchronized intermittent
      mandatory ventilation
Sleep-disordered breathing, 243
Small for gestational age, bronchopulmonary
      dysplasia and, 55–57, 56f
Smoking
  maternal, lung maturation and, 56–57
  pulmonary function and, 167–168
Sonic hedgehog (Shh), 6
Spironolactone, for severe bronchopulmonary
      dysplasia, 377–378
SpO$_2$. see Oxygen saturation
Spontaneous breathing, in surfactant
      distribution, 234
Spontaneous PDA closure, 137

Sprouty, in branching morphogenesis, 8
SSRIs, in pulmonary vascular development, 76
Staphylococcus aureus, ventilator-assisted
    pneumonia and, 149–150
Staphylococcus epidermidis, 157
Staphylococcus spp. (Firmicutes), in lung
    microbiome, 98, 99f–100f
Stem cells
    in cell-based therapy, 348, 348f–349f
    reprogramming, in preterm infants, 347
Stenosis, pulmonary vein, in postnatal
    pulmonary vascular development, 79
Steroids
    antenatal
        after 34 weeks' gestational period,
            339–340
        drug and dose choices for, 339–340
        long-term outcomes after, 340
        in low-resource environments, 340
        repeated, 338–339
    postnatal, 340–344
        for bronchopulmonary dysplasia, 341
        drug, dose, route, and duration of therapy
            with, 342
        historical review, 340–341, 341f
        meta-analyses of early and late treatments
            of, 341–342
        use of, 342–343
    prenatal, new trials of early, 343–344, 343t
    for severe bronchopulmonary
        dysplasia, 378
Stimulation, in resuscitation, 179–180
Suctioning, 179
    in meconium staining, 179–180
    routine, 179–180
Supplemental oxygen
    automated adjustment of, 327–332, 328f,
        329t–330t, 331f
    BPD and
        diagnosis based on, 117–121
        indications for, 117
        as risk factor, 123
SUPPORT. *see* Surfactant, Positive Pressure,
    and Oxygenation Randomized Trial
Surfactant, 300
    administration of, by intratracheal catheter,
        204
    antenatal corticosteroids and, 34–35
    CPAP in, 203–213
        era, 202
        INSURE technique and, 211
        with nasal, 203
    effects of, 167
Surfactant, Positive Pressure, and Oxygenation
    Randomized Trial (SUPPORT), 123
    in oxygen saturation, 263
    in severe bronchopulmonary dysplasia
        (BPD), 367–368
Surfactant delivery, newer strategies for,
    221–238
    aerosolization, 223
    to infants treated by CPAP, 222
    by laryngeal mask airway, 224
    pharyngeal instillation, 223
    techniques for, without endotracheal tube,
        222–224, 223t
    via brief tracheal catheterization, 224–230,
        224t
        avoidance of bradycardia in, 232
        bradycardia in, 232
        clinical trials of, 225–229, 226t–227t

Surfactant delivery, newer strategies for
    (Continued)
        depth of catheter insertion for, 225
        effectiveness of, 228f, 230
        future research directions for, 233–235
        hypoxia in, 232
        laboratory studies of, 230–231
        observational and cohort studies of, 225
        premedication for, 231
        procedural complications of, 232
        recommendations for, 232–233
        repeated, 232
        scientific and practical considerations for,
            230–232
        surfactant reflux in, 232
    via thin catheter, 224
Surfactant system, 13
Synchronized intermittent mandatory
    ventilation (SIMV), 272f, 273–274, 274f,
        311, 322
Synchronized mechanical ventilation, patient-
    ventilator interaction during, 272–280, 272f
Synchronized ventilation, modes of, 311–312
    assist/control, 311
    assisted ventilation modes, 312
    high-frequency ventilation, 314–315
    open lung strategy, 313–314
    pressure-support ventilation, 311–312
    synchronized intermittent mandatory
        ventilation, 311
    volume-targeted ventilation, 312–313, 313t
Systemic hypertension, in severe
    bronchopulmonary dysplasia, 372
Systemic-to-pulmonary collateral vessels, in
    severe bronchopulmonary dysplasia, 372
Systemic-to-pulmonary communication, after
    birth, PDA and, 134

T
Targeted minute ventilation (TMV), automation
    of, 324–325, 325f
Thiazides, for severe bronchopulmonary
    dysplasia, 377–378
Thyroid transcription factor 1, in
    tracheoesophageal separation, 5–6
Tidal volume (V_T)
    effect of, 296
    severe bronchopulmonary dysplasia (BPD)
        and, 367
    in volume-controlled ventilation, 322
    in volume-targeted ventilation, 322
Tie1, 15
Tie2, 15
TLRs. *see* Toll-like receptors
TMV. *see* Targeted minute ventilation
Toll-like receptors (TLRs)
    endotoxins and, 46
    in *Ureaplasma* infection, 107
Totipotent stem cells, 348
Tracheal aspirates, ventilator-assisted
    pneumonia and, 149–150
Tracheal catheterization, surfactant
    administration via, 224–230, 224t
    avoidance of bradycardia in, 232
    bradycardia in, 232
    clinical trials of, 225–229, 226t–227t
        Avoid Mechanical Ventilation Trial in, 225
        NINSAPP Trial in, 229
        summation of, 229–230
        Take Care Study, 225–228

Tracheal catheterization, surfactant
    administration via *(Continued)*
  depth of catheter insertion for, 225
  effectiveness of, 228f, 230
  future research directions for, 233–235
  hypoxia in, 232
  laboratory studies of, 230–231
  observational and cohort studies of, 225
  premedication for, 231
  procedural complications of, 232
  recommendations for, 232–233
  repeated, 232
  scientific and practical considerations for,
      230–232
  surfactant reflux in, 232
Tracheobronchomalacia, in severe
    bronchopulmonary dysplasia, 368
Tracheoesophageal separation, molecular
    regulation of, 5–6
Transcription factor, in lung development, 5–6
Transcriptomics, of bronchopulmonary
    dysplasia, 87, 90–91
Transforming growth factor beta (TGF-β)
  in branching morphogenesis, 8–9
  in bronchopulmonary dysplasia, 17f, 18–19
  PDA and, 135
Transition from fetal to neonatal life, fetal
    lung, 3
Tricuspid regurgitation (TR), for estimating
    pressure gradient, 301
Tumor necrosis factor-α, in *Ureaplasma*
    infection, 103–104
Two-thumb technique, 185–186, 186f

U

Umbilical cord blood (UCB) mesenchymal
    stem cells, for bronchopulmonary
    dysplasia, 354t
Umbilical cord milking, 291
Umbilical cord tissue (UCT) mesenchymal
    stem cells, for bronchopulmonary
    dysplasia, 354t
Ureaplasma species, 102–108
  BPD and, 105–107
    eradication, 107–108
  chorioamnionitis and, 39–40
  infection, susceptibility to, 107
  intraamniotic, lung maturation and, 46, 47t
  intrauterine inflammation and, 103–104
  in lung microbiome, 98, 99f
  neonatal lung injury and, 104–105, 105b
  preterm birth and, 103–104
  ventilator-assisted pneumonia and, 156–157
Ureaplasmal MB antigen, 103

V

VALI. *see* Ventilator-associated lung injury
Vancomycin, for ventilator-associated
    pneumonia, 152–153
Variable-flow nasal CPAP device, 200
Variant club cells, 349t
Vascular development. *see also* Lung
    development; Pulmonary vascular
    development
  angiopoietins in, 15
  regulation, 13–15
  Tie in, 15
  vascular morphogenesis, 13–14
  VEGF-mediated epithelial-endothelial
      interaction in, 14–15

Vascular endothelial growth factor (VEGF), 69
  in epithelial-endothelial interaction, 14–15
  PDA and, 135
  in *Ureaplasma* infection, 106
  in vascular development, 15
Vascular endothelial growth factor receptor 2
    (VEGFR2), 351–352
Vascular morphogenesis, of lung, 13–14
Vascular system
  bronchial, 13
  pulmonary, 13
Vasculogenesis, 13–14
VEGF. *see* Vascular endothelial growth factor
VEGFR2. *see* Vascular endothelial growth
    factor receptor 2
Venous return, cardiorespiratory interactions
    and, 290
Ventilation, synchronized, modes of, 311–312
  assist/control, 311
  assisted ventilation modes, 312
  high-frequency ventilation, 314–315
  importance of open lung strategy, 313–314
  pressure-support ventilation, 311–312
  synchronized intermittent mandatory
      ventilation, 311
  volume-targeted ventilation, 312–313, 313t
Ventilator-associated lung injury (VALI),
    307–310
  delivery room stabilization for, 309–310
  mechanism of injury in, 307, 308f
  reduction, 309
Ventilator-associated pneumonia, 147–160
  birth weight and, 149
  definition of, 148, 149b
  epidemiology of, 148–149
  future research directions for, 157
  outcomes in, 156–157
  pathogenesis of, 149–152, 150b, 151f
  prevention of, 154–156, 155b
  risk factors for, 149
  treatment of, 152–157, 153b
  ventilation duration and, 149
Ventilator cycling frequency, 322
Ventilator-induced lung injury, severe
    bronchopulmonary dysplasia (BPD) and,
    366–367
Verrucomicrobia, in lung microbiome, 98–99,
    99f
Very low-birth-weight (VLBW) infants,
    antenatal steroids in, 337
Volume-controlled ventilation, automation of,
    323f
Volume guarantee (VG) ventilation, 313, 322
Volume infusion, in resuscitation, 189
Volume-proportional gains, in proportional
    assist ventilation (PAV), 326
Volume-targeted ventilation (VTV), 312–313,
    313t, 322–324
  hypoxemia and, 254
  patient-ventilator interaction during,
      280–281, 281f
Volutrauma, 307–308
  severe bronchopulmonary dysplasia (BPD)
      and, 367
VTV. *see* Volume-targeted ventilation

W

Weaning, from nasal CPAP, 205
Weight, birth, ventilator-associated pneumonia,
    149
Wnt, in branching morphogenesis, 9